Rhinoplasty and Septoplasty

Dedication

To Hye Jeong Jeon, MD
Best friend and wife, whose loving support made this book possible

To Jae Kyeong and Ho Kyeong
My loving sons

Rhinoplasty and Septoplasty

Yong Ju Jang

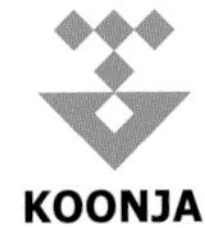

KOONJA

Contributors

Editor and Main Author **Jang, Yong Ju, MD, PhD**

Professor
Department of Otolaryngology
Asan Medical Center
University of Ulsan College of Medicine
Seoul, Korea

Contributors

Hyun, Sang Min, MD
Shimmian Rhinoplasty Clinic
Seoul, Korea

Jung, Yong Gi, MD, PhD
Assistant Professor
Department of Otorhinolaryngology-Head and Neck Surgery
Samsung Changwon Hospital
Sungkyunkwan University School of Medicine
Changwon, Korea

Kim, In-Sang, MD, PhD
Dr. Be Aesthetic Clinic
Seoul, Korea

Kim, Ji Heui, MD, PhD
Instructor
Department of Otolaryngology
Asan Medical Center
University of Ulsan College of Medicine
Seoul, Korea

Kim, Ji Sun, MD, PhD
Assistant Professor
Department of Otolaryngology-Head and Neck Surgery
Eulji University College of Medicine
Seoul, Korea

Kim, Jun Mo, MD, PhD
Artline Aesthetic Clinic
Clinical Professor
Department of Otolaryngology
Asan Medical Center
University of Ulsan College of Medicine
Seoul, Korea

Kim, Jung-Soo, MD, PhD
Professor
Department of Otorhinolaryngology-Head and Neck Surgery
Kyungpook National University School of Medicine
Daegu, Korea

Ku, Seung-Woo, MD, PhD
Associate Professor
Department of Anesthesiology and Pain Medicine
Asan Medical Center
University of Ulsan College of Medicine
Seoul, Korea

Kwon, Jae Hwan, MD, PhD
Associate Professor
Department of Otolaryngology-Head and Neck Surgery
Kosin University College of Medicine
Busan, Korea

Lee, Sung Bu, MD
Department of Otolaryngology
Yuseong Sun General hospital
Daejeon, Korea

Loh, Ian, MD
ENT consultant
Singapore Changi General Hospital
Singapore

Song, Hyung Min, MD, PhD
VIP International Plastic Surgery Center
Seoul, Korea

Moon, Hyoung Jin, MD, PhD
Navi Plastic Surgery Clinic
Clinical Professor
Yonsei University College of Medicine
Seoul, Korea

Min, Jin-Young, MD, PhD
Research Associate
Northwestern University Feinberg School of Medicine
Chicago, USA

Yeo, Nam-Kyung, MD, PhD
Assistant Professor
Department of Otolaryngology
Gangneung Asan Hospital
University of Ulsan College of Medicine
Gangneung, Korea

Yi, Jong Sook, MD
Assistant Professor
CHA Bundang Medical Center
CHA University
Bundang, Korea

Yu, Myeong Sang, MD, PhD
Assistant Professor
Department of Otorhinolaryngology-Head and Neck Surgery
School of Medicine, Konkuk University
Chungju, Korea

Preface

It has already been seven years since I published "Practical Septorhinoplasty" in 2007. Since letting the book into my readers' hands, I have had a lasting sense of dissatisfaction regarding its completeness. I also felt a strong sense of duty to pass on to my readers some conceptual changes and new surgical techniques I developed over the years. In that process, I was compelled to write a new book, and just at that moment Koonja Publishing Inc. proposed publishing a revised edition of "Practical Septorhinoplasty", at which I mustered up the courage to publish the book with a new title and major content revision.

I was supposed to wrap up planning and editing around early 2013, but due to various lectures and conferences abroad and personal research projects, editing was slower than anticipated. Thankfully I was able to finalize the manuscript by the spring of 2014 and get this burden off my chest.

This new book, titled "Rhinoplasty and Septoplasty" is a combination of my personal surgical philosophy and techniques. Readers will be able to clearly experience the world of rhinoseptoplasty through this book. Areas in which I lacked sufficient expertise were reinforced through several marvelous chapters submitted by many of my greatest colleagues.

One thing I learned after becoming immersed in the field of rhinoplasty is that it is rarely beneficial to have strong dogmas or biases towards certain methods. It is essential that surgeons approach various surgical methods with an open mind and humbly accept the subtle and unpredictable changes that inevitably follow a rhinoseptoplasty procedure. For the past two dozen years I've spent as a rhinoplasty surgeon, I've felt like a student of rhinoseptoplasty and it seems I will continue to be one. That is because the field of rhinoseptoplasty has never allowed me to loosen my academic rigor and passion and has kept arrogance at bay.

I hope this somewhat confessional book "Rhinoplasty and Septoplasty" can be a meaningful guide and companion for my readers who have set on the exciting yet arduous path of rhinoplasty.

I am deeply indebted to the authors who helped create this book. I am confident their contributions will bear fruit in the changes and realizations the readers will go through. I also express my sincere gratitude to Dr. Eduard M. Alfanta, who immensely helped in the English editing of this book. Finally, my thanks go out to my patients, who through their relationships with me shared both joy and frustration. Every patient has been my greatest mentor.

February, 2014, Yong Ju Jang
Seoul, Korea

Table of Contents

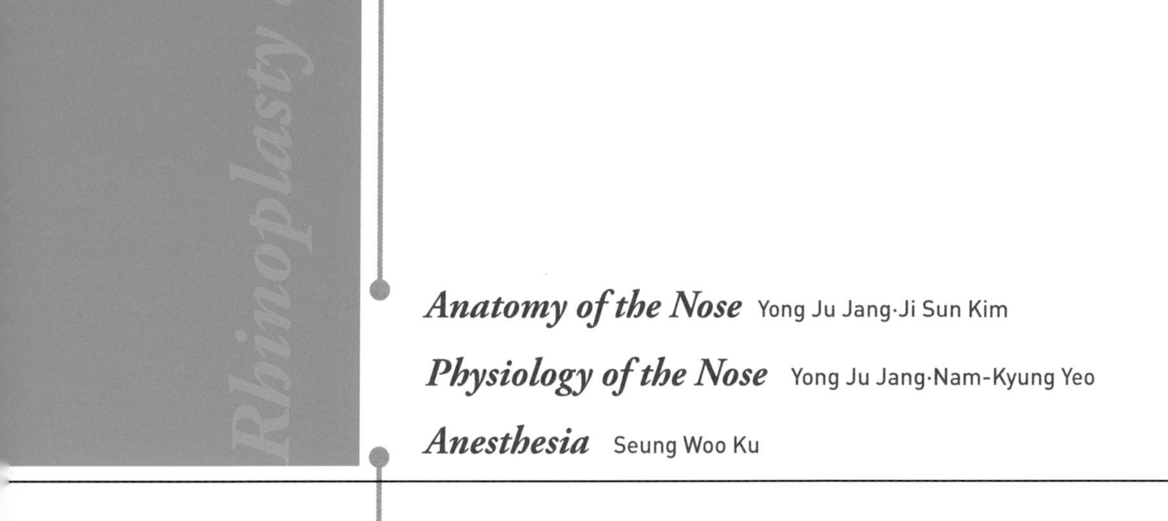

Section 01

Basics

Anatomy of the Nose

Yong Ju Jang · Ji Sun Kim

A prerequisite for successful rhinoplasty is a thorough understanding of the internal and external anatomy of the nose. This chapter is devoted to the description of all the internal and external anatomical features that make up the nose. In describing the anatomy of the nose with regard to direction, the part of the nose facing towards the head will be described as cephalic; the part facing downwards and away from the head as caudal. Also, in the case of frontal observation of the nose, the part nearer to the observer is defined as anterior while the opposite is defined as posterior *(Figure 1)*.

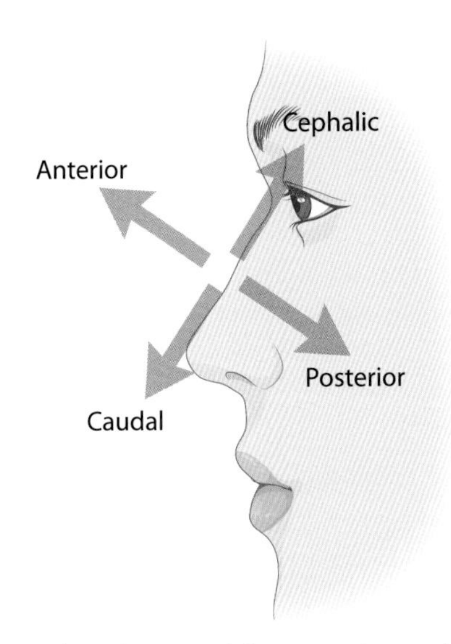

Figure 1 Definition of directions in nasal anatomy.

The nose is a prominently contoured pyramidal structure situated centrally on the face. It is composed of skin, mucosa, bone, cartilage, and intervening supporting tissue, including fat, muscle, and connective tissue *(Figure 2)*. The measurements of the Korean nose showed that young Koreans had a nasal length to nasal tip projection to dorsal height ratio of 2:0.97:0.61. The average nasolabial and nasofrontal angles were 78.5° and 126°, respectively, in young male Koreans; and 82.7° and 133.6°, respectively, in young female Koreans. When compared to the Caucasian nose, the average nasolabial and nasofrontal angles were 96.8° and 129°, respectively, in Caucasian males and 101.8° and 135.3°, respectively, in Caucasian females *(Figure 2)*.

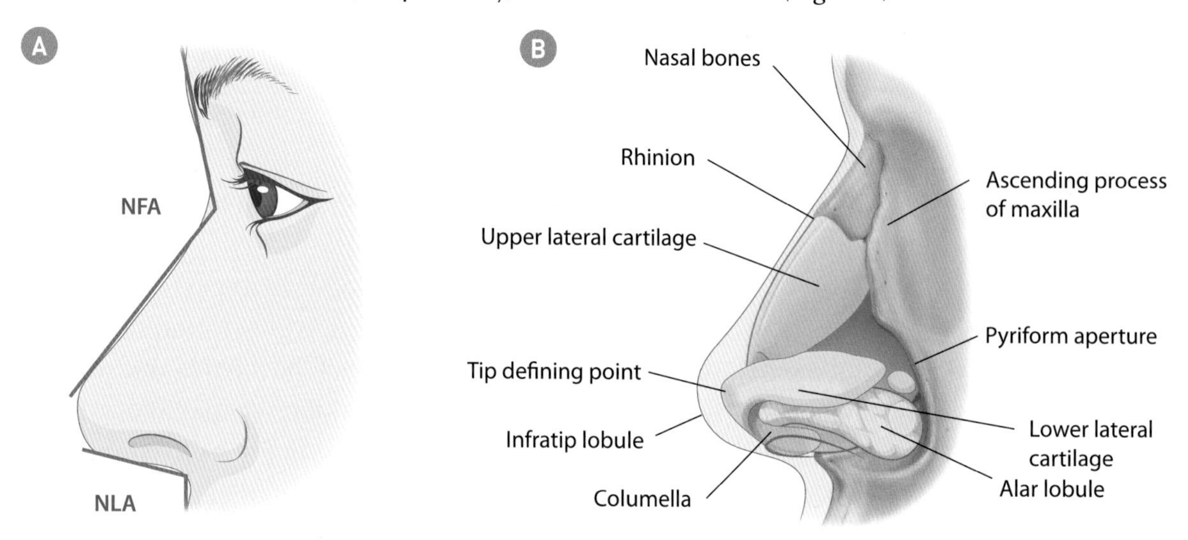

Figure 2 Surface anatomy of the nose from the lateral view. NFA-nasofrontal angle, NLA-nasolabial angle (A). Nasal framework (B).

I. Skin Soft Tissue Envelope

The skin soft tissue envelope of the nose consists of the following layers; skin, superficial fatty layer, fibromuscular layer, deep fatty layer, and the periosteum or perichondrium *(Figure 3)*.

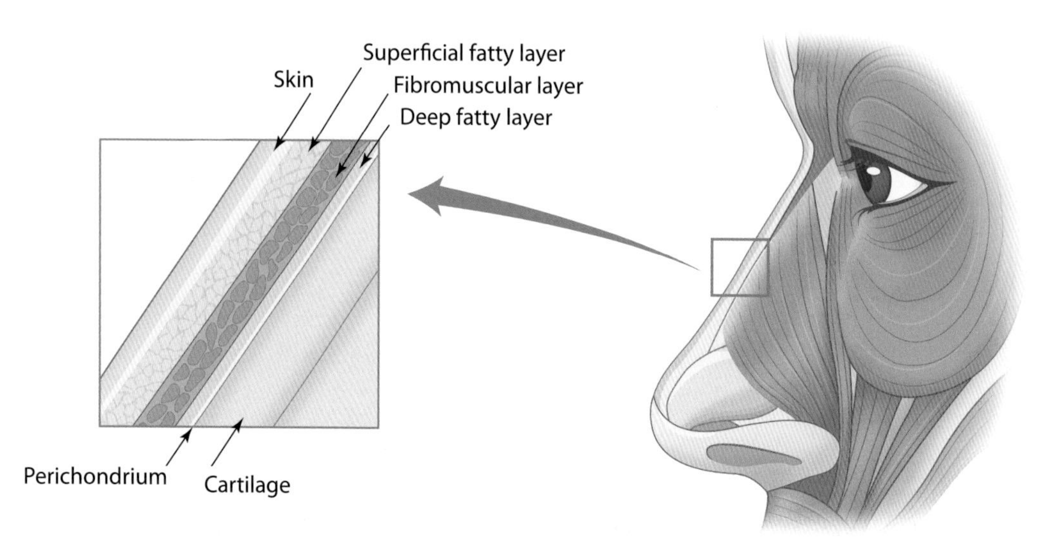

Figure 3 Cross section of nasal skin soft tissue envelope.

Included among these layers is the fibromuscular layer as well the superficial musculoaponeurotic system (SMAS) which divides the fatty layer into the superficial and deep layers. This layer is continuous to the SMAS that envelops the face and is attached to the facial muscles, frontal belly of the occipitofrontalis and platysma. Because major arteries or nerves, which are distributed around the nose, pass through the SMAS or the fatty layer, the most appropriate plane for making a dissection for rhinoplasty would be between the deep fatty layer and perichondrium below the SMAS. The advantage of this dissection plane is that the elevation of the flap is relatively easy, the risk of injuring the arteries or nerves is low, and the surgical field is excellent. Dissecting at this plane also allows for the prevention of deformities that can be caused by the contraction of tissue after surgery.

The skin of the nose is one of the important elements that must be evaluated prior to rhinoplasty. In particular, the thickness of the skin has an important aesthetic significance. There is a great variation in skin thickness among individuals. Some patients have thick skin while others have thin skin. In patients with thick skin, there is a strong tendency towards the post-surgical formation of edema and scarring as compared to patients with thin skin. In patients with thin skin, subtle unevenness of cartilage grafts or the bony dorsum can be easily seen through the skin. The skin of the nose is thick at the nasion, becomes thinner around the rhinion and then thick again at the supratip area. A study of nasal skin thickness in Caucasians reported that the mean skin thickness was thick at the nasion (1.3 mm), thins over the rhinion (0.6 mm), thickens over the nasal tip (1.2 mm), and thins again over the columella (0.8 mm). The skin thickness of the patients who underwent rhinoplasty at Asan Medical Center were examined using CT scan. Our study found the mean nasal skin thicknesses of 3.3 mm at the nasion, 2.4 mm at the rhinion, 2.9 mm at the nasal tip, and 2.3 mm at the columella *(Figure 4, Table 1)*. The mean nasal skin thickness was thicker in males than females at the nasion, rhinion, and nasal tip with statistical significance *(Table 1)*.

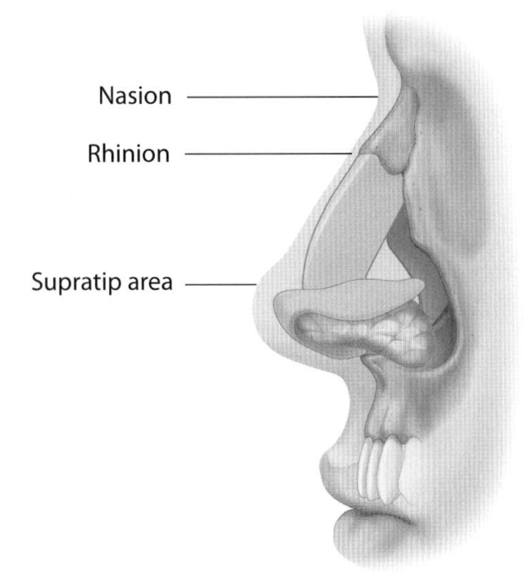

Figure 4 The skin of the nose is thick at the nasion, becomes thinner around the rhinion, and then thick again at the supratip area.

Table 1 Nasal skin thickness at the different regions

Skin thickness (mm)	Nasion	Rhinion	Nasal tip	Columella
Male	3.7	2.6	3.0	2.3
Female	2.2	1.7	2.7	2.1

There was a weak positive correlation between nasion skin thickness and age (the skin thickens with increasing age). No correlations were found between age and skin thickness at the rhinion, nasal tip, or columella. To analyze the effect of skin thickness on tip surgery outcome, tip surgery postoperative outcomes were classified as excellent, good, or poor and the mean skin thicknesses of these 3 outcome groups were determined. Surgical outcomes were excellent in 45 (58.4%) patients, good in 17 (25.5%) patients, and poor in 15 (19.5%) patients. The nasal tip and columella skin thicknesses were thinnest in the excellent group (nasal tip = 2.8 mm, columella = 2.2 mm), intermediate in the good group (nasal tip = 3.1 mm, columella = 2.4 mm), and thickest in the poor group (nasal tip = 3.4 mm, columella = 2.6 mm) *(Table 2)*. These findings indicate that thicker skin at the nasal tip and columella were associated with poor surgical outcomes.

Table 2 Nasal skin thickness and tip surgery outcome

	Excellent (n=45)	Good (n=17)	Poor (n=15)	*P*-value
Skin thickness (mm)				
Nasion	3.2	3.5	3.4	0.700
Rhinion	2.3	2.5	2.6	0.430
Nasal tip	2.8	3.1	3.4	< .001
Columella	2.2	2.4	2.6	0.010

In addition to skin thickness, the degree of adhesion between the skin and underlying skeletal structure has an influence on the surgical process. In the skin-soft tissue envelope of the nose, the part that covers the bony nasal pyramid is loosely attached while the skin attached to the alar cartilage and the tip is more firmly attached. The elasticity of the skin, likewise, is an important factor in determining the success of rhinoplasty. For young patients, the shrinkage and remodeling of the skin and subcutaneous tissue is complete within just a few weeks after rhinoplasty. However, among older patients, there are instances wherein the lost elasticity of the skin does not return even after many months following rhinoplasty. In some instances of extreme loss of elasticity, the excessive skin may have to be excised if the nose is to be shaped satisfactorily.

II. Muscles

The zygomatic and the temporal branch of the facial nerve (CN VII) innervates the muscles located at the nose. The elevator muscles include the procerus, levator labii superioris alaeque nasi, and anomalous nasi *(Figure 5)*. These muscles rotate the nasal tip in a cephalic direction and dilate the nostrils. The procerus muscle has a dual origin. The medial fibers originate from the aponeurosis of the transverse nasalis and the periosteum of the nasal bones. The lateral fibers originate from perichondrium of the upper lateral cartilages and the musculature of the upper lip. The procerus inserts into the glabellar skin. The levator labii superioris alaeque nasi originates from the medial part of the orbicularis oculi and frontal process of the maxilla and inserts into the melolabial fold, ala nasi, and skin and muscle of the upper lip. The depressor muscles of the nose include the alar nasalis and the depressor septi nasi. These muscles lengthen the nose and dilate the nostrils. The depressor septi nasi originates from the maxillary periosteum above the central and lateral incisors and inserts into the membranous septum and the footplates of the medial crura. The compressor muscles include the transverse portion of the nasalis and the compressor narium minor. These muscles rotate the nasal tip in a caudal direction and narrow the nostrils. The zygomaticus muscle has the effect of pulling the orbicularis oris, and indirectly help the movement of the nose.

Of the various muscles of the nose, the muscles that are clinically the most significant are the levator labii alaeque nasi and depressor septi nasi. The levator labii alaeque nasi has the function of opening the external nasal valve. Impaired alar flaring by facial paralysis may cause nasal obstruction. The depressor septi nasi muscle may accentuate drooping of the nasal tip and

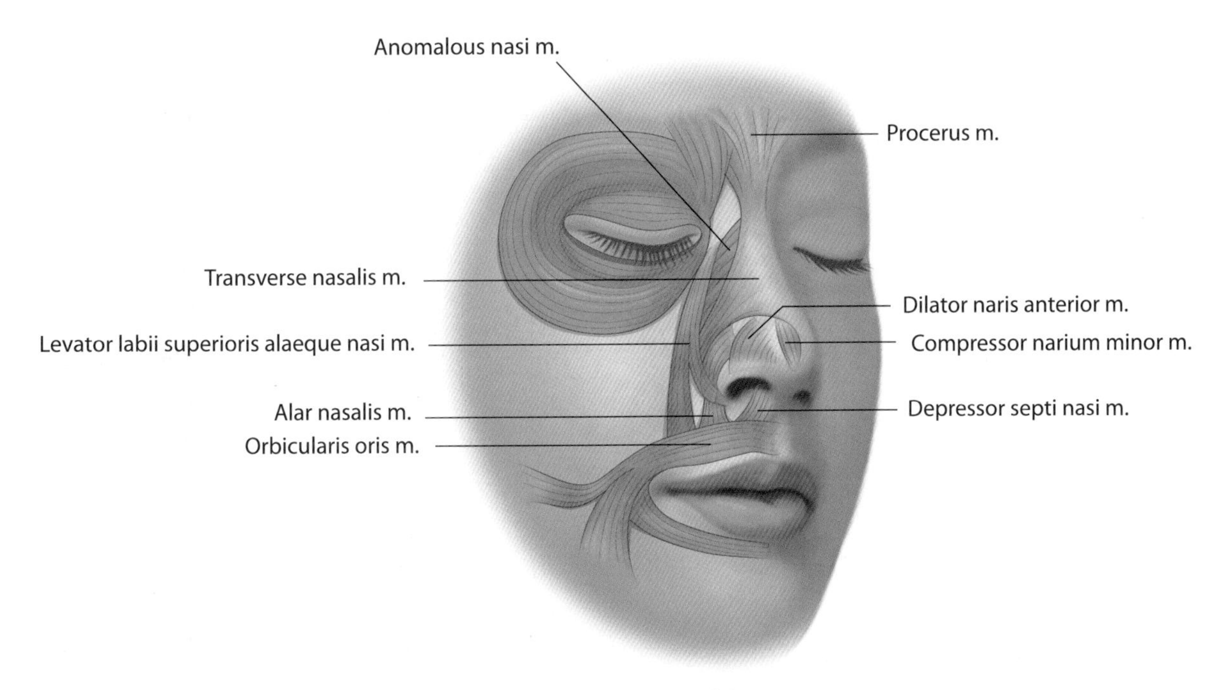

Figure 5 Major muscles of the nose.

shortening of the upper lip on animation. The preoperative examination of rhinoplasty patients should easily identify those patients who demonstrate a drooping nasal tip and shortened upper lip on animation, particularly when smiling. When this phenomenon is severe, it is called "rhino-gingivolabial syndrome of the smile", which consists of the following characteristics: (1) drooping of the nasal tip, (2) elevation and shortening of the upper lip, and (3) increased exposure of the maxillary gingiva. This is caused by hypertrophy of the depressor septi nasi with an anomalous insertion reaching the nasal tip; and hypertrophy of the nasalis whose posterior fibers intermingle with the orbicularis oris. Treatment is the transection of the depressor septi nasi. In severe cases, partial resection of the orbicularis oris muscle is known to be helpful. During rhinoplasty, if the depressor septi nasi is left unsevered in patients with a short columella, a postoperative polly beak deformity can occur. This muscle is also associated with the hypermobile tip, which denotes excessive mobility of the tip secondary to lip motion.

III. Blood Vessels

1. Arterial Supply to the External Nose

The arterial supply to the nose is quite abundant and is supplied by the ophthalmic artery, a branch of the internal carotid artery, as well as by the facial artery, a branch of the external carotid artery *(Figure 6)*. The ophthalmic artery supplies the external branch of the anterior ethmoidal artery as well as the dorsal nasal artery and is largely distributed around the cephalic area of the

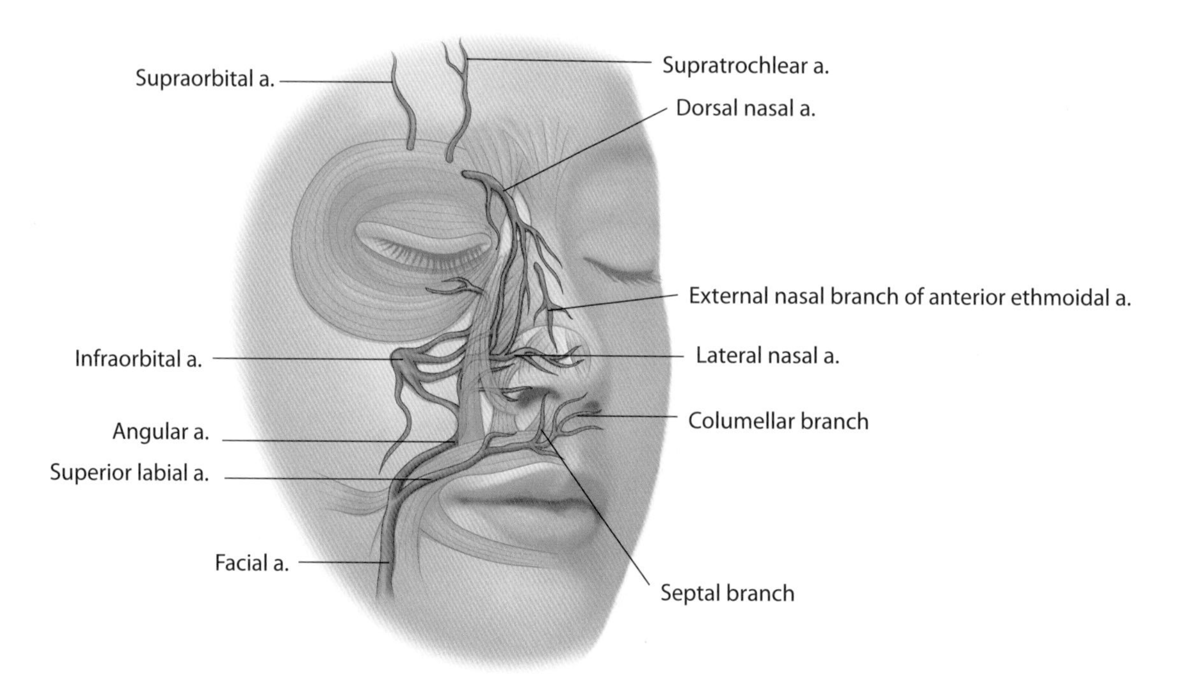

Figure 6 Arterial supply of the external nose.

nose. The caudal part is mainly supplied by the angular artery and the superior labial artery, both of which are the branches of the facial artery. The superior labial artery and angular artery supplies the columellar and the lateral nasal artery, respectively. The columellar artery often bleeds in the transcolumellar incision with an external rhinoplasty approach. The intraoperative cauterization of the columellar artery rarely leads to necrosis of nasal tip skin because of the abundant collaterals. Caution is advised in alar base resection, if the alar base incision extends more than 2 mm above the alar groove, and the lateral nasal artery is at risk.

2. Arterial Supply to the Internal Nose

There are several arteries supplying the internal nose *(Figure 7)*. Among them is the anterior and posterior ethmoidal arteries, which are branches of the ophthalmic artery originating from the internal carotid artery. Arteries that originate from the external carotid system are the sphenopalatine and greater palatine arteries, branches of the internal maxillary artery; as well as the anterior septal artery, a branch of the superior labial artery that derives from the facial artery.

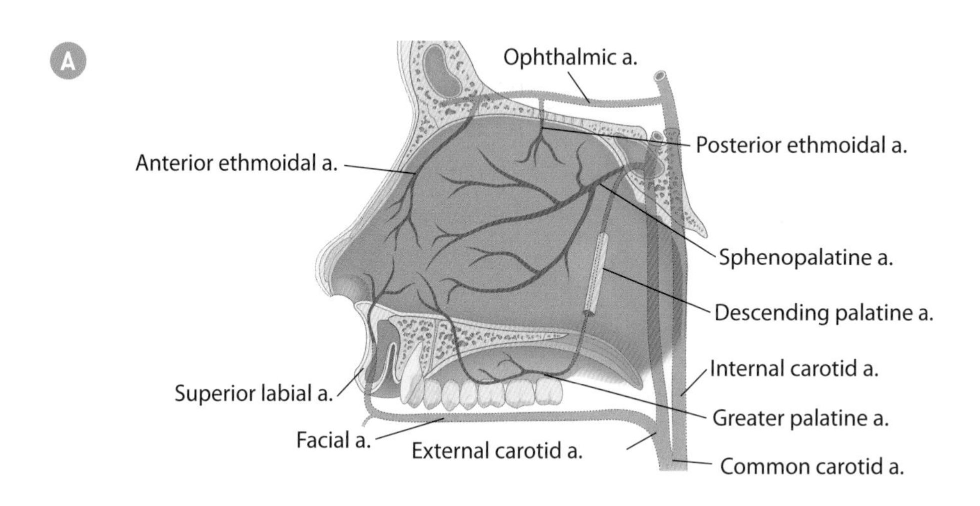

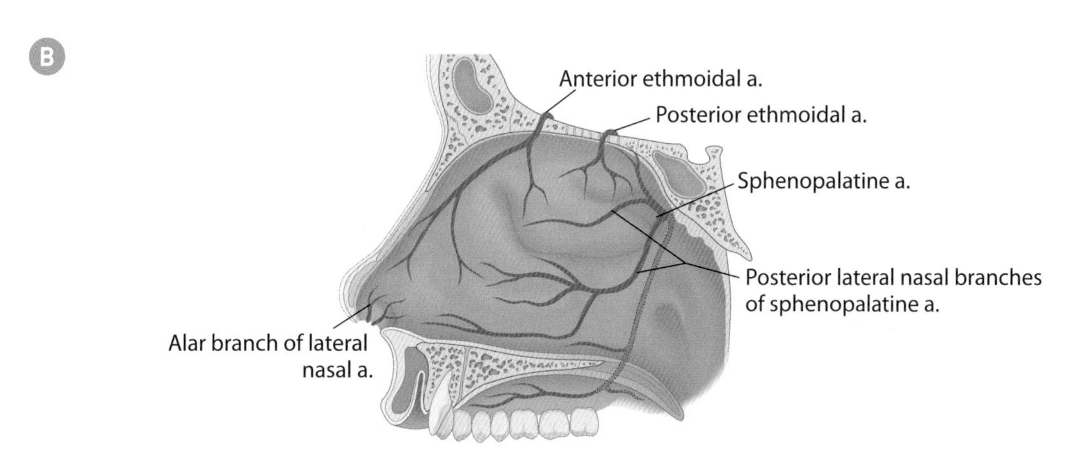

Figure 7 Arterial supply of the interior of the nose. Septum (A) and lateral nasal wall (B).

The anterior and posterior ethmoidal arteries that derive from the internal carotid artery system supply blood to the entire lateral nasal wall. The sphenopalatine and the greater palatine arteries of the external carotid system are branches of the internal maxillary artery. The sphenopalatine artery enters the nose through the sphenopalatine foramen. The internal lateral nasal area gets its blood supply from the posterior lateral nasal branch of sphenopalatine artery; while the posterior part of the nasal septum gets its blood supply from the posterior septal branch. Bleeding from the sphenopalatine artery is the most common cause for severe posterior epistaxis. Another branch of the internal maxillary artery is the greater palatine artery, also known as the descending palatine artery, which passes through the nasopalatine foramen. The greater palatine and the superior labial arteries anastomose in the Kisselbach's plexus area which is located at the caudal part of the septum. The sphenopalatine and the anterior ethmoidal arteries also branch out to the Kisselbach's plexus and approximately 90% of nosebleeds occur in this area. The septal cartilage is dependent on the lining of the mucoperichondrium for its blood supply. Therefore during septoplasty, bilateral elevation of the septal mucoperichondrium may increase the risk of infection or cartilage necrosis.

IV. Nerves

The trigeminal nerve (CN V) branches are the sensory nerves for the exterior of the nose. The ophthalmic division (V1) is responsible for the ophthalmic nerve dermatome (dorsum and most of the tip). The maxillary division (V2) innervates the lateral nasal region. The ophthalmic division (V1) starts from the trigeminal ganglion to reach the nose and is known as the ophthalmic nerve. An offshoot of this nerve, the nasocilliary nerve, continues as the anterior ethmoidal nerve within the orbit. This, in turn, divides into the lateral and the septal branches. The lateral branch acts as the sensory nerve for the turbinate sidewall and the mucosa of the meatus. The terminal branch of the lateral anterior ethmoidal nerve passes between the upper lateral cartilage and nasal bone to reach the skin of the lower external nasal area, including the tip. This is called the external nasal branch of the anterior ethmoidal nerve. The septal branch of the anterior ethmoidal nerve acts as the sensory nerve to the septal mucosa. The supplementary branches of V1, which is responsible for the dorsum of the nose, derive from the supraorbital and supratrochlear nerves to act as the sensory nerve of the inner wall of the eyeball, the lateral nasal wall, all the way to the nasofrontal angle. The infraorbital nerve (V2) acts as the sensory nerve for the alar rim and external nose. Therefore, the important sensory nerves for the nose are the external nasal branch of anterior ethmoidal nerve and the infraorbital nerve. In order to perform local anesthesia to this area, it is important to be able to adequately block these nerves *(Figures 8, 9)*. The sphenopalatine ganglion branch act as the sensory nerve for the rest of the internal nasal area. The sphenopalatine ganglion is located behind the middle turbinate close to the pterygopalatine fossa and sphenopalatine foramen. The nerve from the sphenopalatine ganglion is divided into two groups. One group is the lateral posterior-superior nasal nerve, which is distributed to the superior, middle, and inferior turbinates and the

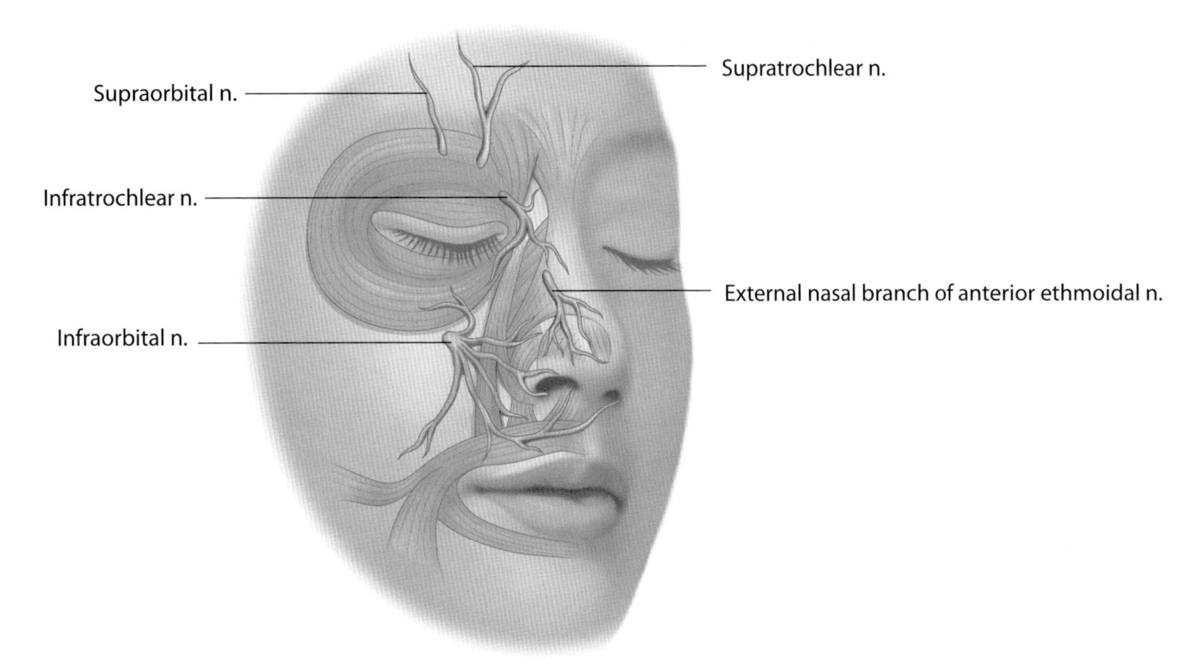

Figure 8 Sensory innervations of the external nose.

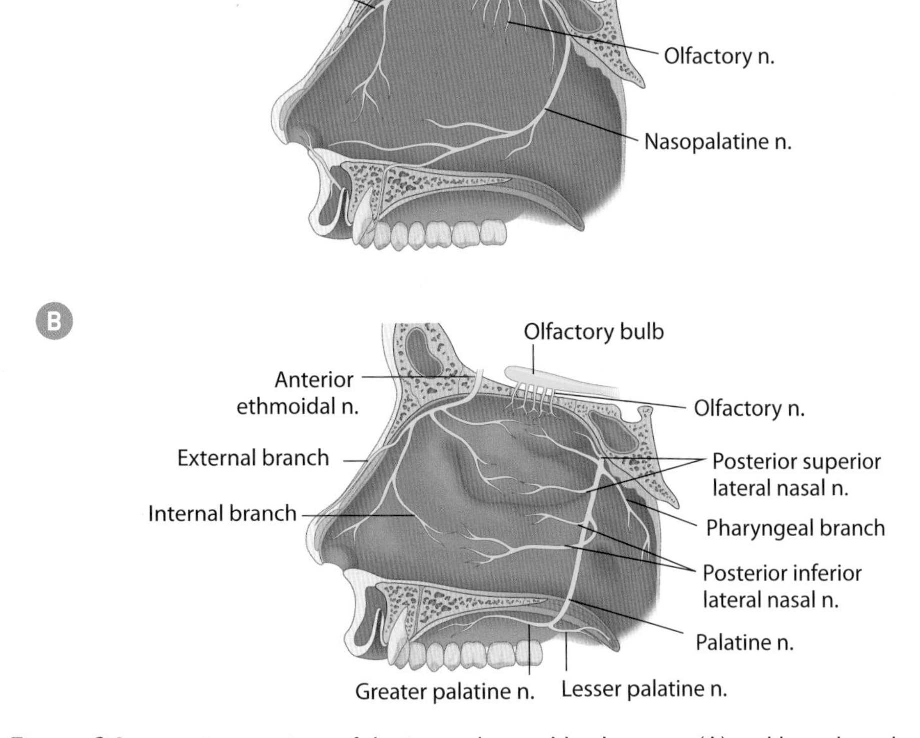

Figure 9 Sensory innervations of the internal nose. Nasal septum (A) and lateral nasal wall (B).

superior, and middle meatus. The other group is the nasal branch innervating the septum. The nasal branch of the greater palatine nerve begins as a branch of the sphenopalatine ganglion, goes down through the greater palatine canal and reaches to the soft tissues of the hard palate. The two nasal branches of the greater palatine nerve pass through canaliculi to reach to the nose. These nerves are responsible for the sensation of the inferior meatus and inferior turbinate within the nasal cavity.

V. Cartilages and Bones

The bony pyramid of the nose comprises the nasal bone and the frontal process of maxilla. The cartilaginous portion is made up of the quadrangular, upper lateral, and lower lateral cartilages *(Figure 10)*.

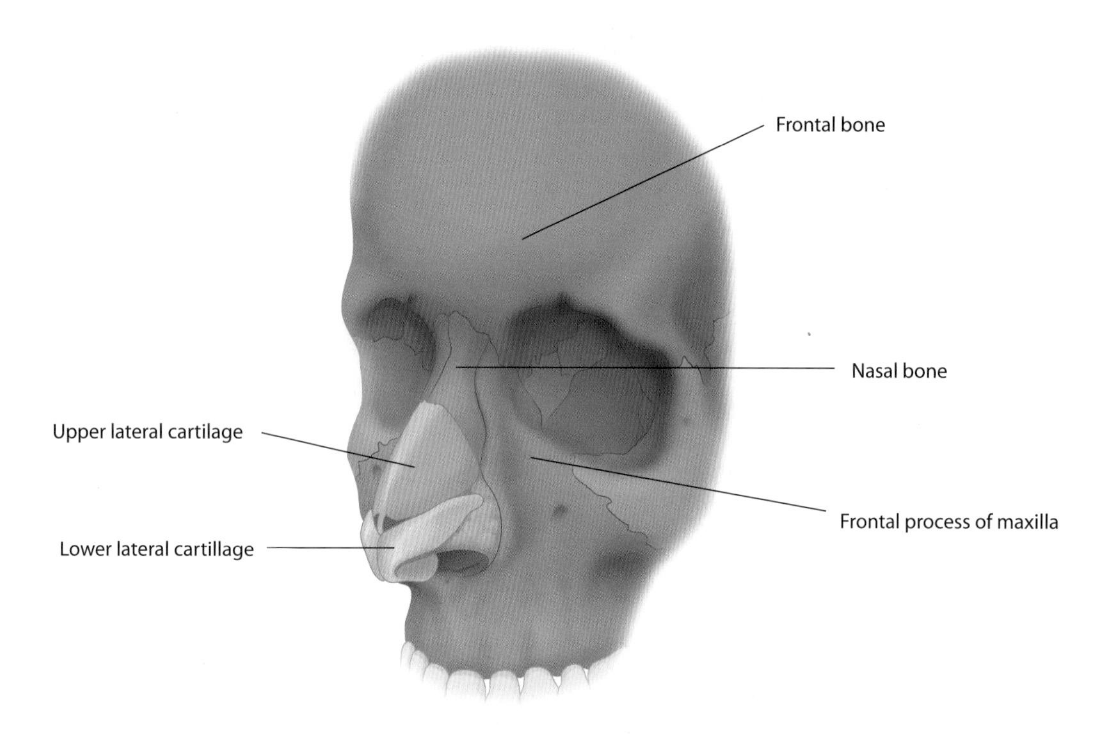

Figure 10 Bones and cartilages of the nose.

1. Nasal Bone

The bony vault of the nose is made up of a pair of oblong shaped nasal bones and the frontal process of the maxilla. The bony vault is normally of a pyramidal shape and become thicker towards the cephalic direction. The size, symmetry, and shape of the nasal bone varies greatly from person to person. Of the overall bony pyramid, only 1/3 of it is made up of the paired nasal bones, the rest is composed of the frontal process of the maxilla, nasal processes of the frontal bone, and the perpendicular plate of the ethmoid. The cephalic border of the thick nasal bone has a jagged appearance and is connected to the nasal part of the frontal bone. The caudal border of the nasal bone is connected to the upper lateral cartilages. The border of the external lateral area of the nasal bone is connected to the frontal process of the maxilla. The medial border, which is thicker at the cephalic than the caudal part, is connected to the opposite nasal bone. As the nasal bone is thicker at the cephalic than at the caudal part, nasal bone fractures frequently occur at the transitional zone between the thick and thin areas. The periosteum covers the nasal bones and is firmly attached to them. Dissecting without damaging the periosteum during surgery involves making an incision with a blade at the periosteum just above the caudal edge of the nasal bone and then elevating it using a periosteal elevator. The area where the nasal bones and the nasal process of the frontal bone meet is the area of the radix and is the narrowest region of the nose. In order to get an aesthetically acceptable result from rhinoplasty, this region must retain a certain level of width and height. Because the thickness of the nasal bone of this region is expected to impede the smooth progress of the osteotome during osteotomy, cutting the frontal bone by osteotomy is virtually impossible.

2. Frontal Process of the Maxilla

The frontal process of the maxilla stretches upwards from the body of the maxilla, forming the pyriform aperture, to meet the lower border of the lateral nasal wall. The pyriform aperture is a pear-shaped opening with the apex pointing cephalad. The inferior caudal margin on the facial midline establishes the border of the anterior nasal spine. The posterolateral border of the frontal process of the maxilla along the groove that forms with the lacrimal bone constitutes the groove that includes the lacrimal duct. Therefore, in performing lateral osteotomy, care must be taken not to invade this groove in order to avoid damaging the lacrimal apparatus.

3. Vomer

The vomer is a thin and flat bone, almost triangular in shape that forms the posteroinferior part of the septum. It is the main component which should be corrected in septoplasty because a deviation of the vomer often exists in patients with septal deviation. It doesn't matter that the vomer is removed rather aggressively because it has less effect on the whole support of nose than the perpendicular plate of ethmoid and anterior nasal spine *(Figure 11).*

4. Ethmoid Bone

The ethmoid bone is composed of three major parts: the perpendicular plate, crista galli, and the cribriform plate. On either side of the crista galli are the ethmoid sinuses. The superior and middle turbinates are also components of the ethmoid bone. This area should be corrected importantly in septoplasty. Especially, in patients with a high septal deviation, the perpendicular plate of ethmoid must be carefully removed to correct the deviation because it is almost the main component of the deviation *(Figure 11)*.

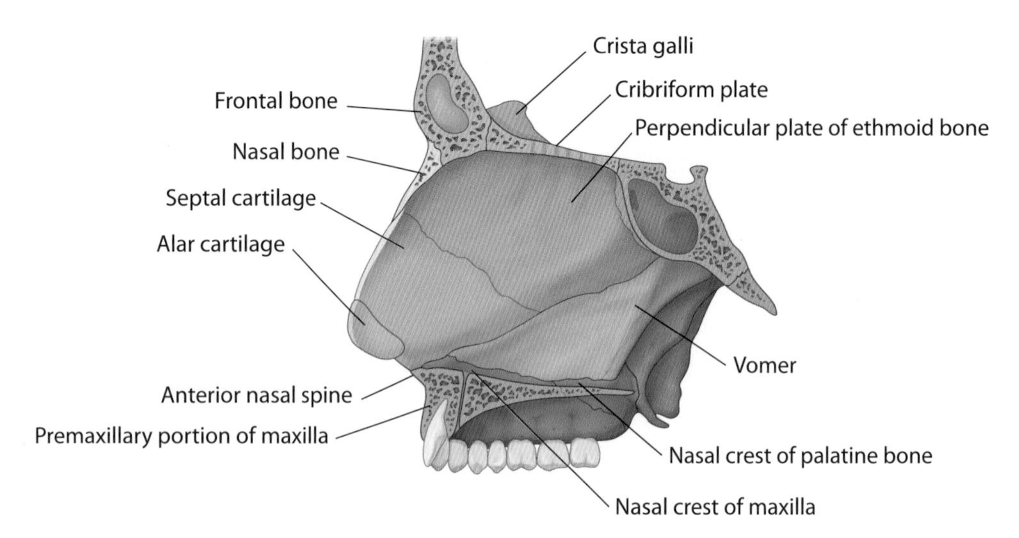

Figure 11 Structure of the nasal septum.

5. Septal Cartilage (Quadrangular Cartilage)

The nasal septum is a median structure that divides the nasal cavity into two chambers. The membranous septum, which is closest to the caudal area, is spread out in a wedge shape between the columella and the caudal border of the septal cartilage. The flexibility of the tissue and the mobility of the membranous septum allow the columella to be easily drawn away from the nasal septum and the nasal septum to be easily glided to the side, front, or back. The septal cartilage, greatly responsible for creating nasal obstruction, plays an important role in supporting the nasal dorsum and the tip, like a pillar in a building. The septal cartilage comprises the caudal half of the nasal septum. However, in some patients, the septal cartilage is very small and the septum is composed mainly of bone. In a study with authors' external rhinoplasty patients, intraoperative measurement of the harvested septal cartilage with preservation of 10 mm wide L-strut was performed. The mean caudal length of the harvested septal cartilage was 15.1 mm, the mean dorsal length was 18.2 mm, and the mean area was 520.9 mm^2. It was suspected that the size of the external nose has correlation with the size of septal cartilage, however, upon studying, we observed a lack of correlation between the size of the external nose and the quantity and size of harvestable septal cartilage. In rhinoplasty, there are big differences in the ease of surgery between patients with thick septal cartilage and patients with thin septal cartilage. Thin cartilage is difficult to use as multiple grafts. This is often found in female patients with poorly developed noses. The mucoperichondrium of the septal cartilage especially at the posterior part is tightly adherent to the vomer and the periosteum of the premaxilla.

The mobility of the nasal septum and the flexibility of the upper lateral cartilages play an important role in absorbing shocks applied to the nose. The dorsal border of the cartilaginous nasal septum becomes wider as it moves towards the nasal bone and forms the supraseptal groove by dividing into an almost Y-shape. This supraseptal groove becomes wider at the junction with the nasal bone and gradually disappears towards the septal angle *(Figure 12)*.

6. Upper Lateral Cartilage

The cartilaginous vault is made up of the upper lateral cartilages and the septal cartilage. The area where the upper lateral cartilages is strongly bound to the nasal bone is called the keystone area, and this region is made up of the upper lateral cartilages, nasal bone, septum, and the perpendicular plate of the ethmoid bone. As the keystone area plays an important role of supporting the nasal dorsum, care must be taken during the dorsal hump reduction or medial osteotomy so as not to damage this area. The upper lateral cartilage is Y-shaped at the junction with the nasal bone and transforms into an I-shape as it moves downward. The upper lateral cartilages extend underneath the nasal bone by about 6-8 mm at the keystone area. The upper lateral cartilages are closely connected to the septum and are fused together. If this fusion is traced caudally, the upper lateral cartilages are separated from the septum by a 10-15° angle. This area is the most elastic region between the upper lateral cartilages and the septum, giving the nasal valve its elasticity *(Figure 12)*.

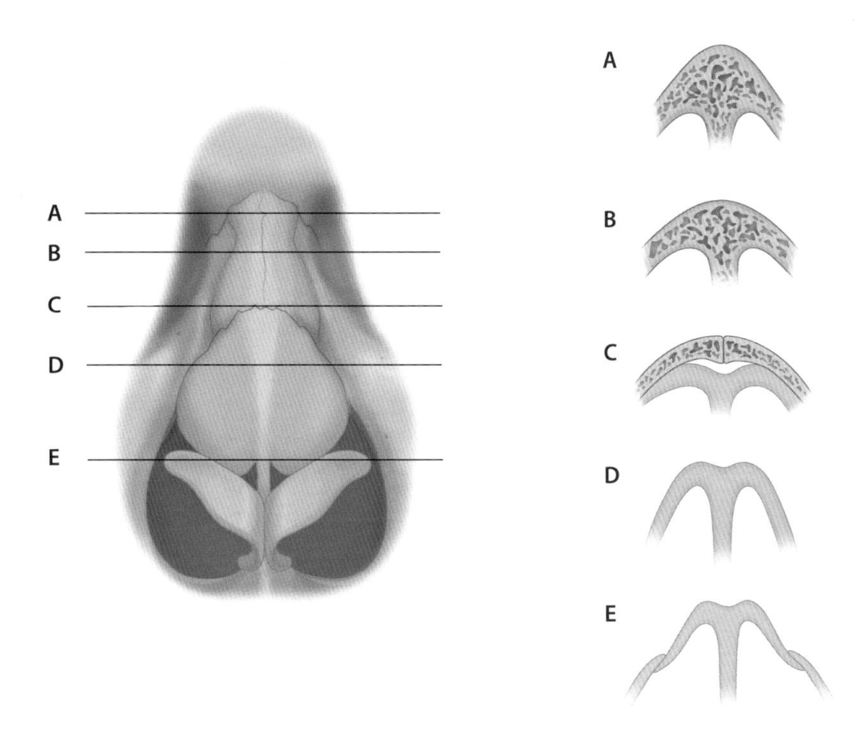

Figure 12 Cross section of different areas of the nasal dorsum. There is overlap of cartilage and bone in the rhinion (C).

7. Lower Lateral Cartilage (Alar Cartilage)

The alar cartilages or lower lateral cartilages are the structures that form the basic framework of the nasal tip. This cartilage is divided into the medial crus, middle crus, and the lateral crus *(Figure 13)*. The medial crus is the primary component of the columella and provides tip support. The medial crus can be subdivided into the footplate segment and the columellar segment. Seen from below, the columellar junction is found between the paired vertically oriented medial crura and the divergent angular middle crua. The overall length of columellar segment has a significant correlation with the visual length of the nostril. The middle crus begins at the columellar lobular junction and ends at the lateral crus. It can be subdivided into a lobular segment and a domal segment. The middle crura are bound together by the interdomal ligament, and lack of intervening soft tissue may give the tip a bifid appearance. On lateral view, the cephalic border of the domal segment of the middle crus is responsible for the prominence of the tip defining point. Thus, the shape, length, and angulation of the middle crura determine the configuration of the infratip lobule and the position of the tip-defining points. The lateral crus acts like a framework that

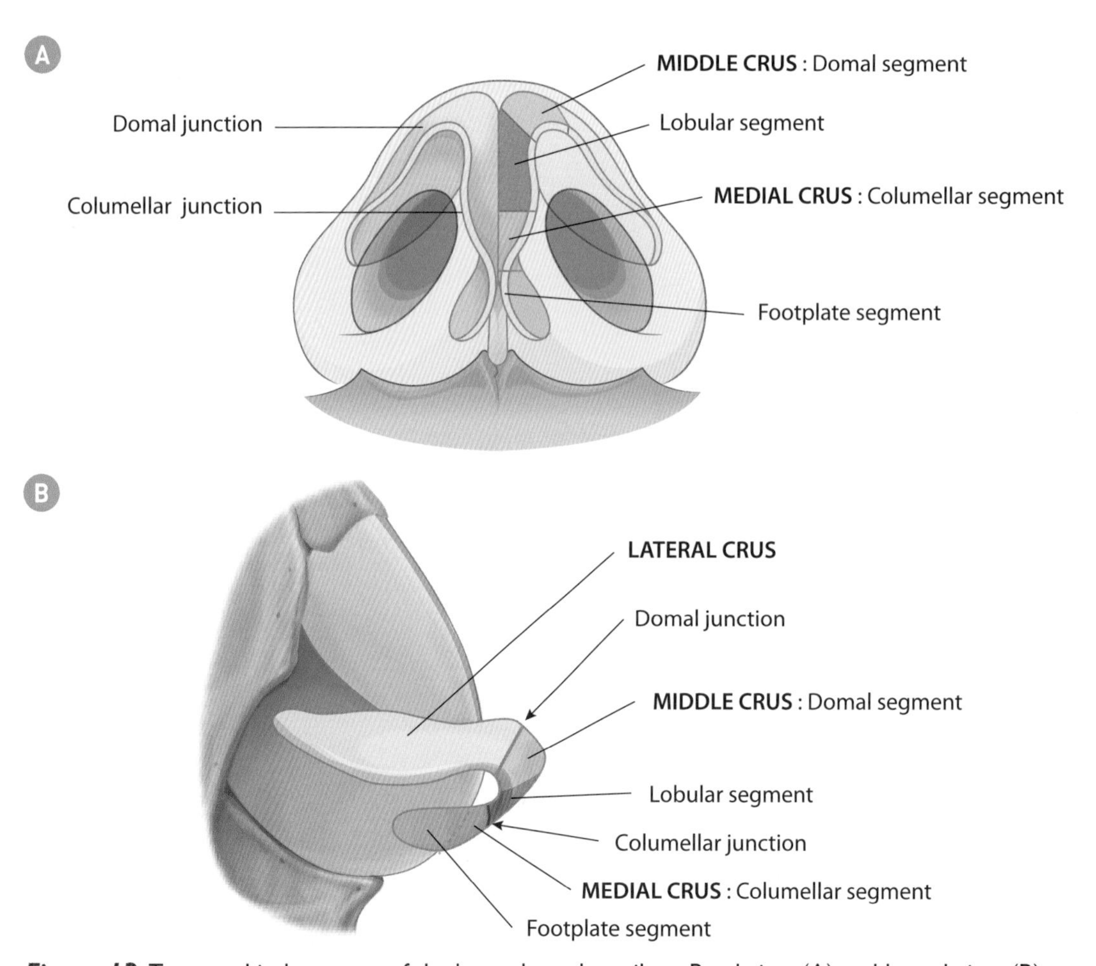

Figure 13 Topographical anatomy of the lower lateral cartilage. Basal view (A) and lateral view (B).

decides the shape of the tip and supports the skin. Resection or weakening of the lateral crus may predispose to nostril retraction and notching. Forming a well structured lateral crus is an important consideration to be made during nasal reconstruction. The angles of the septal cartilage (anterior septal angle, middle septal angle, and posterior septal angle) can greatly influence the external appearance of the lower lateral cartilages *(Figure 14)*. The lower lateral cartilages are divided by the various amounts of fibroareolar tissue. The lateral crus of the lower lateral cartilage proceeds from its junction with the middle crus in a postero-lateral direction. The nostril rim is composed mostly of soft tissue. Around the vicinity of the dome, where the middle and the lateral crura meet, is the soft triangle that is partially lacking in cartilage. Incisions made on this triangle can bring about notching of the alar margin and therefore must be carefully performed.

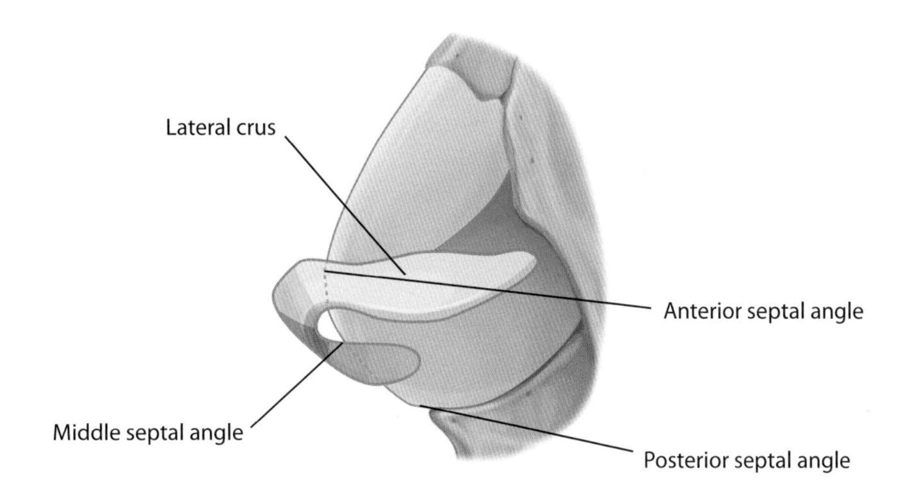

Figure 14 Angles in the quadrangular cartilage.

References

1. Bernstein L. Applied anatomy in corrective rhinoplasty. Arch Otolaryngol 1974; 99: 67-70.
2. Bernstein L. Surgical anatomy in rhinoplasty. Otolaryngol Clin North Am 1975; 8: 549-58.
3. Cho GS, Kim SH, Yeo NK, Jang YJ. Nasal skin thickness measured using computed tomography and its effect on tip surgery outcomes. Otolaryngol Head Neck Surg 2011; 144: 522-7.
4. Kim JS, Khan NA, Song HM, Jang YJ. Intraoperative measurements of harvestable septal cartilage in rhinoplasty. Ann Plast Surg 2010; 65: 519-23.
5. Lane AP. Nasal anatomy and physiology. Facial Plast Surg Clin North Am 2004; 12: 387-95.
6. Natvig P, Sether L, Gingras R, Gardner N. Anatomical details of the osseous cartilaginous framework of the nose. Plast Reconstr Surg 1971; 48: 528-32.
7. Oneal RM, Beil RJ Jr, Schlesinger J. Surgical anatomy of the nose. Clin Plast Surg 1996; 2: 195-8.
8. Wang JH, Park SK, Lee BJ, Jang YJ. Measurement of aesthetic proportions in the profile view of Koreans. Ann Plast Surg. 2009; 62: 109-13.

Physiology of the Nose

Yong Ju Jang · Nam-Kyung Yeo

The nose is an important organ that facilitates breathing and the sense of smell. Although rhinoplasty is a surgery that seeks to change the shape of the nose, attempts to alter the external shape of the nose can influence its functional aspect as well. In addition, patients undergoing rhinoplasty want to correct not only the shape but also the function of the nose. Thus, surgeons performing rhinoplasty must also have an in-depth understanding of the various physiological functions of the nose.

I. The Function of the Nose

The process of filtration, purification, heating, and humidification takes place at the mucosa, the starting point of the respiratory organ. The filtration and purification process initially takes place at the vibrissae of the nostril while the secondary process involves the mucus covering the mucosa capturing dust and microorganisms, as well as preventing them from entering the lung. Another important function of the nose involves humidifying the inhaled air so that, regardless of how dry the inhaled air is, it contains around 90% humidity by the time it reaches the lung. On average, although it varies from person to person, an individual secretes around 1 liter of mucus per day and the mucus travels towards the larynx at the speed of 1 cm/min. The nasal cavity also performs the function of controlling the temperature of the inhaled air and this process begins at the turbinate mucosa. By the time the inhaled air reaches the nasopharynx, its temperature will range between 31°C and 37°C regardless of outside temperature. Besides the above-mentioned basic physiological functions, one nasal function that must be given serious consideration is its function of controlling the flow of inhaled air. When this function fails, patients complain of nasal obstruction.

II. Nasal Obstruction

1. The Physiology of Nasal Obstruction

Nasal obstruction is an abnormal condition that not only occurs when the resistance to airflow in the nasal cavity is increased but it is a symptom that can also manifest under normal physiological conditions.

1) The Characteristics of Nasal Airflow and the Regulation of Nasal Airflow by the Nasal Mucosa

There are two types of airflow, laminar and turbulent flow. The direction and speed of air in laminar flow is identical. Turbulent flow in the nasal cavity can reduce the efficiency of breathing and increase nasal obstruction. Resistance to airflow is in inverse proportion to the diameter of the respiratory tract. The diameter of the nasal cavity, however, is irregular, and therefore resistance to airflow varies greatly between different positions in the nose. In addition, the level of resistance in the nasal cavity respiratory tract varies from person to person and can also differ according to posture and physical conditions. Nasal obstruction, despite being a subjective sensation, increases with the rise of airflow resistance. The interior structures of the nose which are most important to the regulation of airflow are the turbinates and the thick mucosa covering the septum. Located within this mucosa is a system of blood vessels called capacitance vessels *(Figure 1)*. These have a large capacity to store blood and therefore can expand its size, or shrink in volume due to changes in blood flow. Capacitance vessels in the nose are made up of interconnecting venous sinusoids and the amount of blood at this area is a critical factor in determining the size of the nasal airway and corresponding resistance to airflow. Sympathetic nerves are abundantly distributed in these vessels. These sympathetic nerves act upon the nasal mucosa to constrict the capacitance vessels which leads to the reduction in the size of the mucosa, while enlarging the cross sectional area of the nasal airway. In cases where there is chronic infection in the nasal mucosa, its ability to regulate the tone of the capacitance vessels is lost, leading to sustained hyperemia of the mucosa

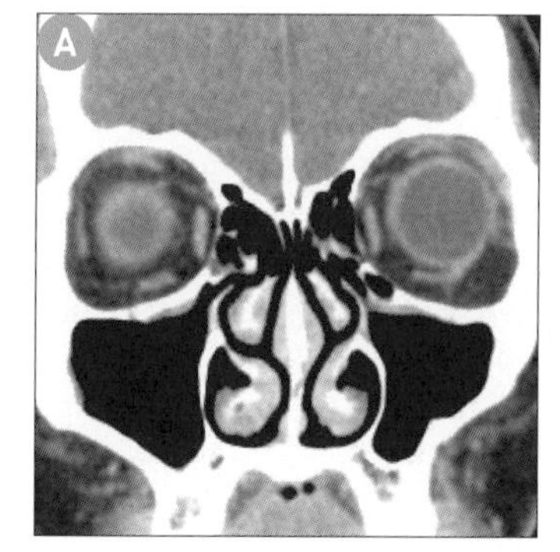

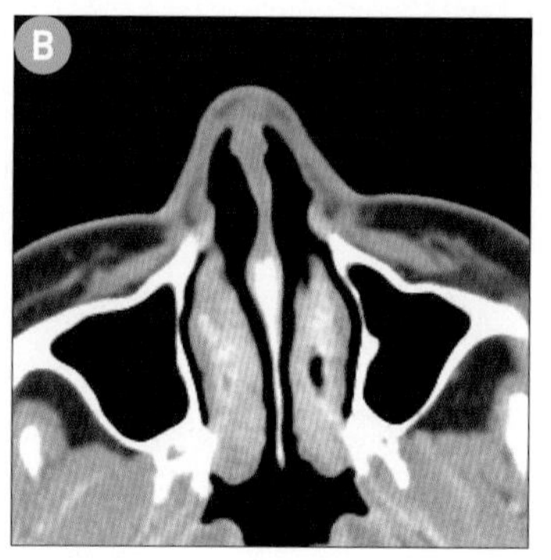

Figure 1 The capacitance vessels seen on PNS CT scans (A). These vessels in the thick turbinate musoca cause the findings of contrast-enhanced turbinate mucosa in the PNS CT scans (B).

and nasal obstruction. On the other hand, the increased parasympathetic activity in the nasal mucosa, instead of narrowing the nasal air passage, stimulates submucosal secretory glands, causing the secretion of nasal mucus to increase. Within the mucosa of the nose, periodic congestion and decongestion called the nasal cycle takes place. This cycle in which congestion and decongestion of the mucosa occurs in average cycles of 4-12 hours on both sides of the nasal cavity. This condition arises because of the increase and decrease in the amount of blood within the capacitance vessels and is regulated by the autonomic nervous system. Variations in the nasal cycle affect the level of resistance in the nasal cavity. Many factors affect the nasal cycle. Drugs that can affect the autonomic nervous system can also alter the normal nasal cycle. Temperature and humidity can also influence the nasal cycle, and the intensity of the nasal cycle increases in the reclining position. People with a healthy nasal cavity will not feel changes in the mucosa brought about by the nasal cycle. However, those with a structural disorder such as a septal deviation will experience alternating nasal obstruction that corresponds to changes in the nasal cycle.

2) Anatomical Subsites Responsible for Nasal Obstruction

Nasal obstruction is felt when nasal resistance is markedly increased within the nasal cavity. The related areas from the nasal entrance onwards will be discussed in the order; nasal ala, nasal valve, and the nasal cavity.

(1) Nasal Ala (External Valve)

This is the area where the external valve is located; the nasal ala is an area covered with skin from the nostrils to the caudal edge of the upper lateral cartilages *(Figure 2)*. A relative negative pressure is generated during inhalation which may lead to the collapse of this area. This phenomenon is rarely observed in normal adults but is a more frequent among infants. A hypertrophic scar can form over the marginal incision after rhinoplasty and can lead patients to complain of nasal obstruction. In cases of facial nerve paralysis, nasal obstruction can arise from

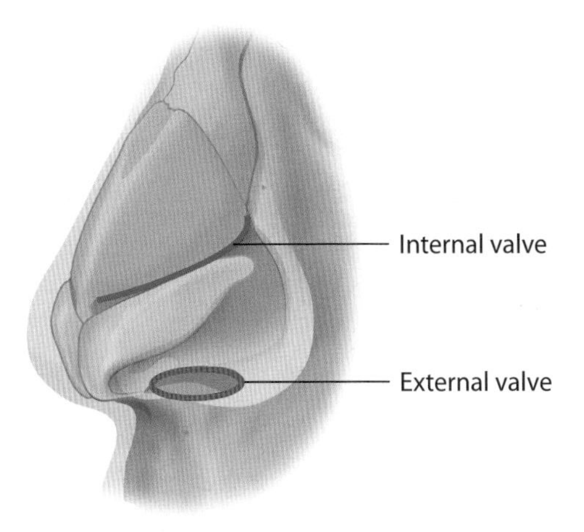

Figure 2 The location of the external and internal valves.

the dysfunction of the dilator naris affecting the function of the nasal ala. Some patients show very small nostrils caused by flaring of the footplate of the lower lateral cartilages with subsequent widening of the columellar base *(Figure 3)*. When these patients complain of nasal obstruction and their nasal obstruction is resolved by narrowing the columella by pinching it, nostriloplasty can be helpful. Patients with displacement or dislocation of the caudal septum also complain nasal obstruction and show nostril asymmetry causing external valve obstruction *(Figure 4)*.

(2) Nasal Valve (Internal Valve)

The definition of the nasal valve, also known as the internal nasal valve, differs among medical literature. However, it is appropriate to understand it as a functionally complex and dynamic structure. The opening of the nasal valve begins from the caudal edge of the upper lateral cartilage, cartilaginous septum, and the base of the nasal cavity. Functionally, the nasal valve consists of an area a few millimeters in length, starting from the triangular entrance into the nasal cavity and

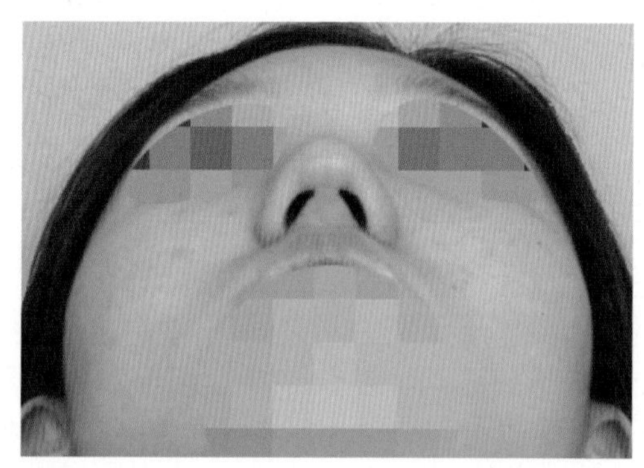

Figure 3 A patient with very small nostrils due to flaring of the footplate of lower lateral cartilages, and widening of the columellar base.

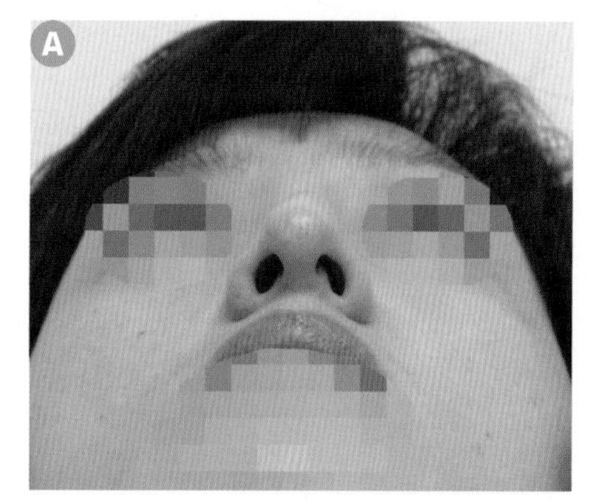

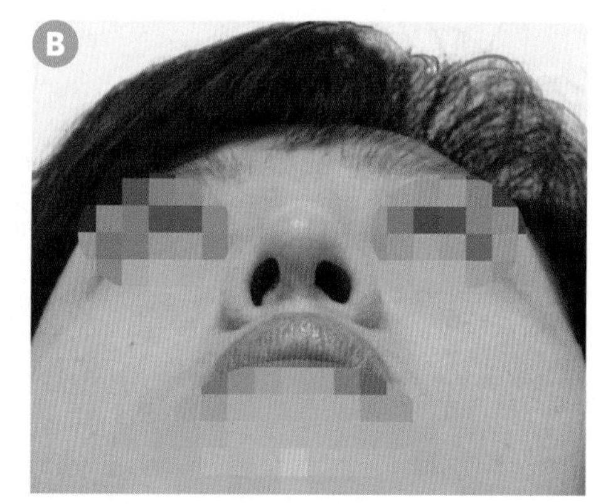

Figure 4 A patient who complained of left-sided nasal obstruction caused by dislocation of caudal septum to the left (A). After rhinoplasty, the patient complained of right-sided nasal obstruction caused by the unilateral septal extension graft on her right nasal cavity (B).

ending at the point where the inferior turbinate begins. This area is bordered by the flexible alar wall, the erectile mucosa and the septum. The angle formed by the upper lateral cartilages and the septum is called the valve angle and nasal obstruction can result if the valve angle becomes excessively acute *(Figure 5)*. Any abnormality of the nasal septum, hypertrophy of the turbinate, and deficiency, hypertrophy, deflection, or displacement of the upper lateral cartilage will cause the internal valve to narrow, causing nasal obstruction. Convexity of caudal septum without displacement can also induce nasal obstruction. Caudal septal deviation is one of the most common causes of nasal obstruction, and it affects both the external and internal valves. Therefore, it is not easy to determine which valve causes nasal obstruction in cases with caudal septal deviation. Most of caudal septal deviation patients show both a high septal deviation and valve angle narrowing *(Figure 6)*.

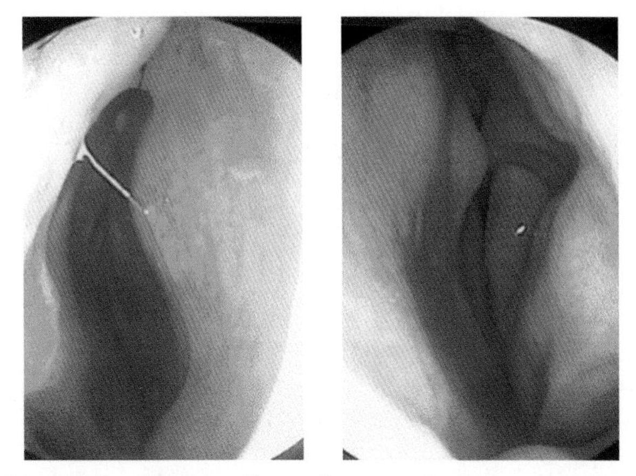

Figure 5 Nasal endoscopic finding of a patient suffering from nasal obstruction caused by the narrowing of the valve angle in the right nasal cavity due to septal deviation.

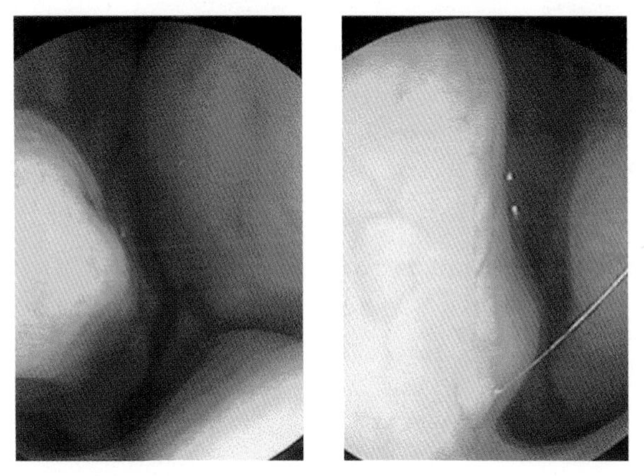

Figure 6 Nasal endoscopic finding of a patient suffering from nasal obstruction caused by the narrowing of the internal valve area due to the caudal septal deviation to the left side.

(3) Nasal Cavity

The internal valve area plays an important role in the development of nasal obstruction. The nasal cavity, an area between the internal valve area and the nasopharynx, and located further interior, also frequently plays a role in constricting the nasal airway. This in turn contributes to the development of nasal obstruction.

Most rhinologists often consider collapse or stenosis of the anterior part of nasal cavity, especially the internal nasal valve area, as the most important cause of subjective nasal obstruction. However, some patients have nasal obstruction despite of having wide internal valves, so there are clearly other causes of subjective nasal obstruction. In our study, there was a correlation between subjective nasal obstruction and abnormalities not only in the anterior part of nasal cavity including the nasal valve but also in the posterior part of the nasal cavity. To identify the narrow portion of the nasal airway, we used axial CT scans to classify patients into three groups based on the shape of the nasal septum: Group I - Anterior Deviation (narrow segment is located at the anterior part of nasal cavity); Group II - Posterior Deviation (narrow segment is located at the posterior part of nasal cavity); and Group III - Mixed Deviation (narrow segment is located at the anterior and posterior parts of nasal cavity) *(Figure 7, Table 1)*, and we compared the degree of nasal obstruction in these three groups. The conclusion was that the three groups showed similar degrees of nasal obstruction, and both the anterior and posterior anatomic characteristics were associated with the subjective severity of nasal obstruction. In other words, the patients with posterior deviation of the nasal septum also had a similar degree of nasal obstruction compared with patients with caudal septal deviation.

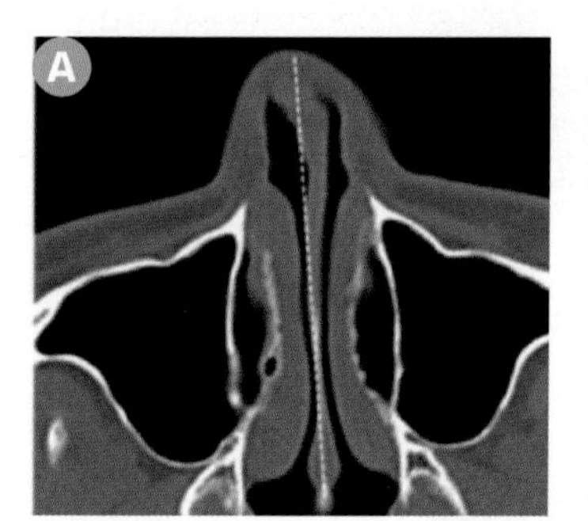

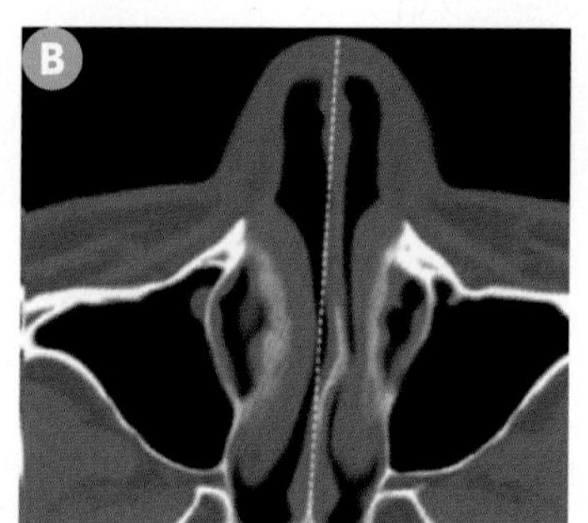

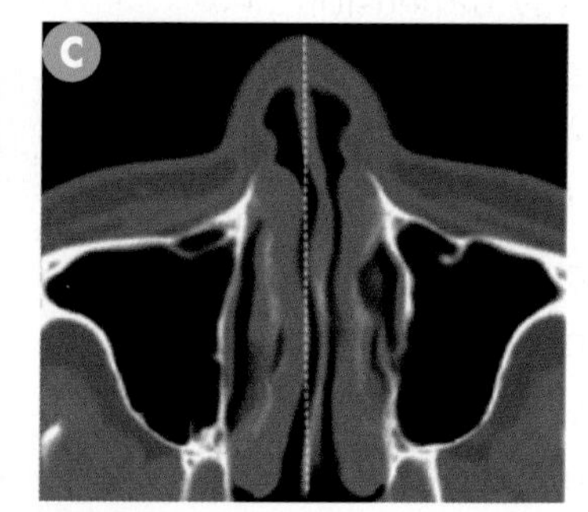

Figure 7 Three types of deviated nasal septum (anterior deviation (A), posterior deviation (B), mixed deviation (C)). Patients with posterior deviations of the nasal septum have the same degree of nasal obstruction compared to patients with anterior deviation.

Table 1 Distribution of types of deviation causing nasal obstruction (n = 71)

	Group I	Group II	Group III
Type of deviation	Anterior	Posterior	Mixed
Number of patients	32 (45.1%)	24 (33.8%)	15 (21.1%)
VAS score	6.1	5.6	6.4

Nasal obstruction associated with pathological conditions such as bony deviation of the nasal septum, chronic sinusitis, different kinds of rhinitis including allergic rhinitis and vasomotor rhinitis, nasal polyps, nasal tumors, etc. can result in the narrowing of the nasal cavity. Alcohol, use of vasodilators, antihypertensive medications, or oral contraceptive pills can result in nasal obstruction mediated by mucosal congestion in the nasal cavity. Nasal obstruction can also result from anxiety, hypothyroidism, and the early stages of pregnancy. Finally, nasal obstruction can also be brought about by atrophic rhinitis or empty nose syndrome, which is characterized by too wide a nasal cavity.

2. Diagnosis of Nasal Obstruction

1) Symptomatic Characteristics of Nasal Obstruction

Nasal obstruction is a subjective complaint that sometimes has an enigmatic and incomprehensible aspect. Nasal obstruction generally results from narrowing of the nasal cavity. If a patient has a definitely narrower nasal airway on one side compared with the other in either of the external valve, internal valve, or nasal cavity; and the patient complains of increased nasal obstruction in the constricted side, then, the narrow area can be considered as the cause of the nasal obstruction. However, in some cases, patients complain of nasal obstruction in the wider rather than the narrower side of the nose. This phenomenon can be attributed to the large difference in nasal airway dimension between the congestion and decongestion phases of the mucosa at the wider side of the nasal cavity in the nasal cycle. In such cases, treatment should be focused on reducing the hypertrophy of the mucosa with the use of a radiofrequency device or microdebrider. Another factor that makes nasal obstruction a difficult subject is that the degree of nasal obstruction is not frequently in proportion to the extent of narrowing. A frequently asked question during consultation is "Does the nasal constriction revealed in the endoscopy warrant a surgery for me?" The answer to such a question is that the need for surgery cannot be determined by the extent of constriction and that it must be made based on the seriousness of the symptoms. In treating nasal obstruction, we must attempt to understand the characteristics of the obstruction, listen carefully to the patient's clinical history, and perform a thorough examination in order to make a proper diagnostic judgement on the cause of this puzzling symptom. In evaluating nasal obstruction, diagnostic methods such as thorough history taking, endoscopic examination of the nasal cavity, objective airway testing, imaging, etc. are indispensable tools for making a comprehensive judgement on the cause or causes of the ailment. In particular, the preoperative documentation using objective examination such as endoscopic examination, nasal function testing, or radiologic examinations can help resolve complaints of patients with persistent nasal obstruction postoperatively.

2) History Taking

If a patient suffers from frequent nasal obstruction with accompanying symptoms such as runny nose, sneezing, itchy nose and eyes, the surgeon should suspect the diagnosis of allergic rhinitis, eosinophilic rhinitis or vasomotor rhinitis. If the nasal obstruction is accompanied by headache, there is a high probability of chronic rhinosinusitis or septal deviation. Besides these symptoms, patients suffering from chronic rhinosinusitis also complain of discomfort from secretion with high viscosity and discoloration. The use of medications such as antihypertensive agents, topical mucosal decongestants, oral contraceptive pills, hormone replacement therapy, etc. can also lead to nasal obstruction, and therefore, during the history taking, efforts must be made to determine whether or notthese medications are being taken. Endocrine abnormalities such as hypothyroidism or exposure to chemicals can also lead to nasal obstruction.

3) Physical Examination

If a deviated nose is seen, it would be reasonable to assume that the underlying problem would be either a septal deviation, constriction of the internal nasal value due to deformity of the upper lateral cartilage, or the constriction of the nasal cavity *(Figure 8)*. According to research done by the author, about 80% of patients with a deviated nose complain of nasal obstruction.

The first area of interest is the internal valve which has the smallest cross-sectional area in the nasal cavity. The Cottle maneuver, a test of nasal valve integrity, can be performed by retracting the cheek laterally, pulling lateral nasal wall from the septum and widening the internal nasal valve angle *(Figure 9)*. If the patient's symptoms are relieved with this maneuver, this suggests the cause of the nasal airway obstruction is related to the nasal valve area. However, this test is inaccurate because it is non-specific for any one valve, as examining thumb is as wide as the entire nasal

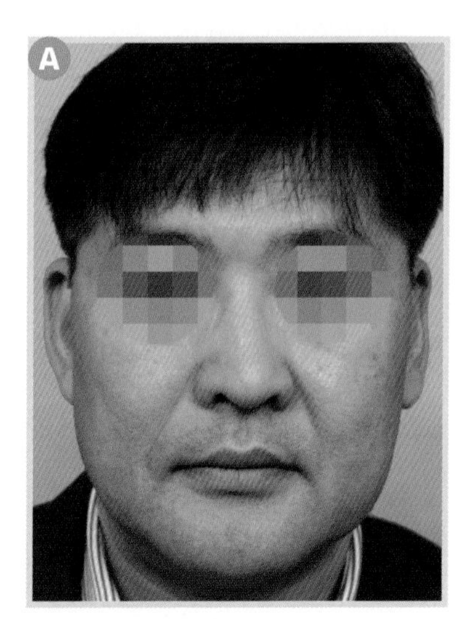

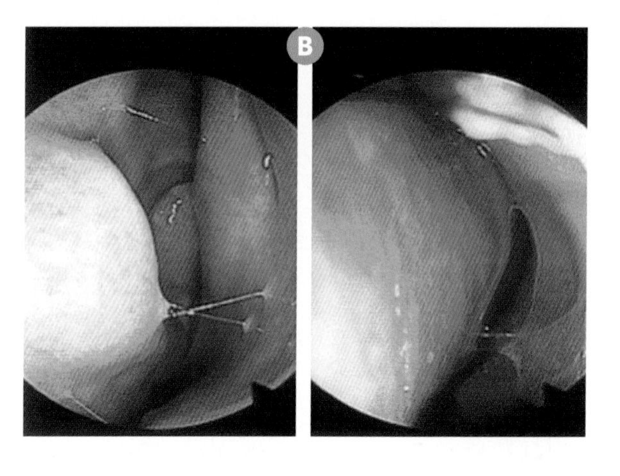

Figure 8 Patient with a deviated nose to the left (A) shows severe deviation of the septum in the same direction as seen on endoscopy (B).

wall. The modified Cottle test, which involves insertion of a cotton applicator or an endoscope inside the nose to elevate the lateral nasal wall, is a much improved version of the original test in that it can be specific for one side or the other, and be specific for the internal or external nasal valve as well *(Figure 10)*. However, it is an uncomfortable test for evaluating the valves, especially the internal valve. Like the Cottle test, it is not quantitatively accurate in that the result is dependent on the pressure exerted by the examiner. Recently, to make up for these shortcomings, a study was performed using nasal dilator strips for nasal function testing. A nasal dilator strip is placed at the lower third of the nose in the region of the lower lateral cartilages, including the alar rims. The

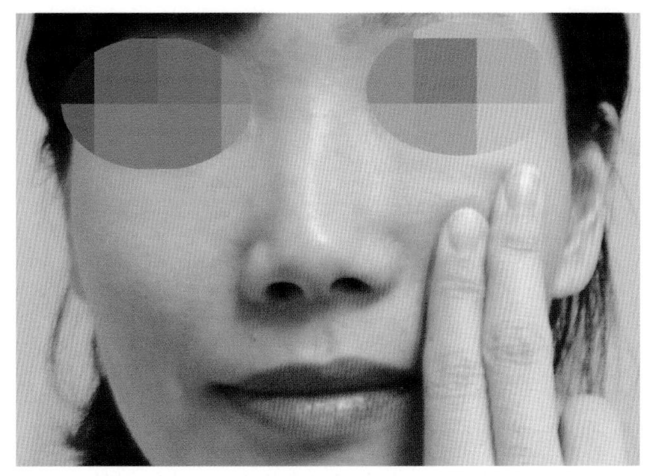

Figure 9 The Cottle maneuver, a test of nasal valve integrity, can be performed by retracting the cheek laterally, pulling lateral nasal wall from the septum and widening the internal nasal valve angle.

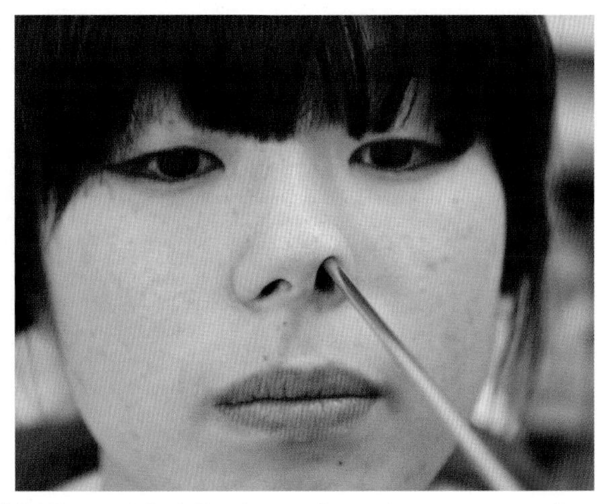

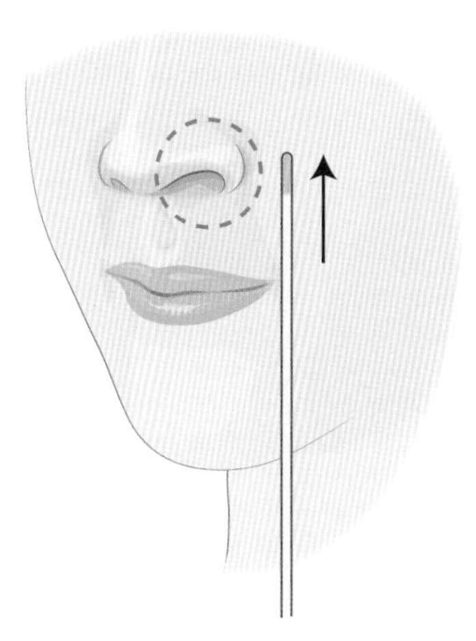

Figure 10 The modified Cottle test. It involves insertion of a cotton applicator or an endoscope inside the nose to widen the internal or external nasal valves.

patients are then asked whether the nasal dilator strip provided a better airway, a worse airway, or no change. The strip is then removed, and a new one is applied to the middle vault just caudal to the nasal bones in the region of the upper lateral cartilage *(Figure 11)*. This test is more specific and powerful than the Cottle test to evaluate the external and internal valves.

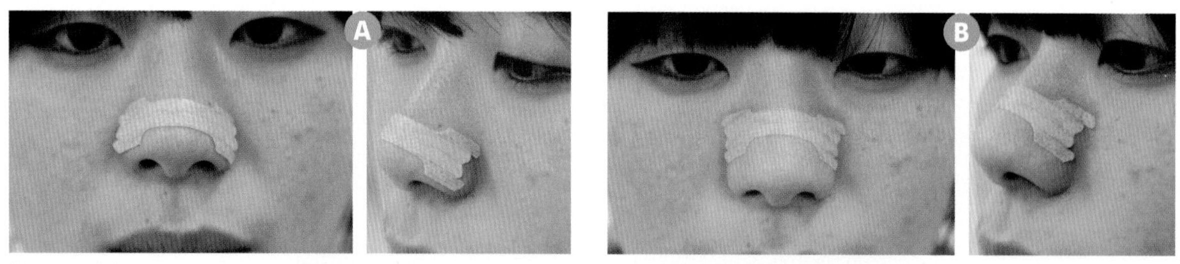

Figure 11 A nasal dilator strip is applied to the lower third of the nose in the region of the lower lateral cartilages, including the alar rims (A). The strip is removed, and a new one is applied to the middle vault just caudal to the nasal bones in the region of the upper lateral cartilages (B). The patients are told to state whether the nasal strip provided a better airway, a worse airway, or no change.

It is recommended that both the endoscope and nasal speculum, together with proper illumination be used in examining the inside of the nose. Relying only on endoscopic examination can make it difficult in identifying the general configuration of the nasal valve area. One must first examine the nasal ala and the valve area using a head mirror or headlight and nasal speculum. Next, an endoscope should be inserted to examine the valve angle, turbinate, the shape of the septum, and the cross sectional area of the valve area. The endoscope is then inserted posteriorly towards the nasopharynx to examine the possible existence of a polyp, tumor, or deformity in the posterior part of the septum. There are two types of endoscopes available, the rigid endoscope and the flexible nasopharyngoscope. For the rigid endoscope, two types are available: the 4 mm and 2.7 mm diameter scopes. Because of its size, it is difficult to access narrow areas using a 4-mm endoscope. Also, as the endoscope's field of view easily gets fogged, in order to examine deep inside the nasal cavity, it is frequently necessary to constrict the mucosa of the nasal cavity. On the other hand, the thinner 2.7 mm endoscope provides the convenience of making it possible to examine the nose all the way to the back without causing great discomfort to the patient *(Figure 12)*. If, as a result of the endoscopic examination, mucosal disorders such as rhinitis or sinusitis is suspected, additional tests such as plain X-ray, CT scan, and allergic skin test can be added.

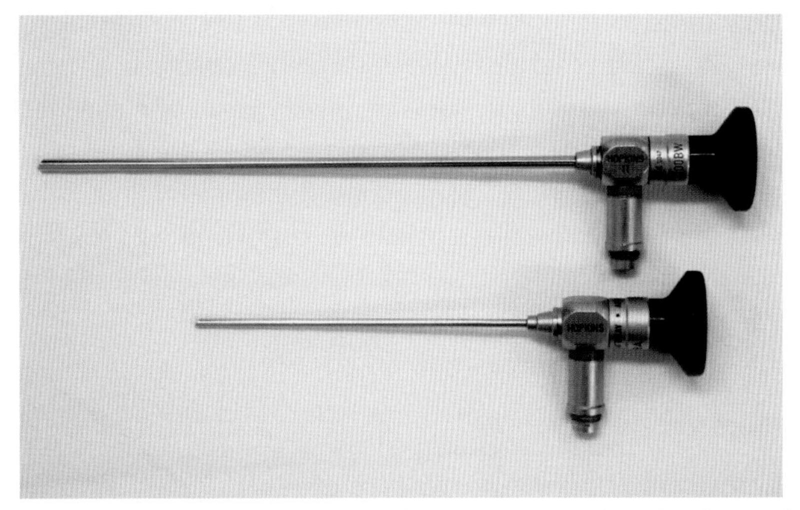

Figure 12 Rigid endoscopes. The endoscope above is a 4-mm diameter scope, and endoscope below is a 2.7-mm diameter scope.

4) Nasal Airway Testing

(1) Acoustic Rhinometry

Objective nasal airway measurement using acoustic rhinometry allows for the measurement of the cross sectional area or the volume of the nasal airway. Acoustic rhinometry analyzes reflected sound waves in order to estimate the structure of the nasal cavity and give a cross sectional area of the nasal cavity in the form of a graph. The use of acoustic rhinometry also allows for the quantitative analysis of the contribution made by the structural and the mucosal factors. The disadvantage of acoustic rhinometry is that it is unable to accurately measure beyond a narrow aperture, (i.e. the nasal valve), and is less accurate in the posterior aspect of the nasal cavity. It is not helpful in localizing nasal obstruction in cases where there is an external valve problem, because it is hard to insert the nosepiece. In addition, since the insertion of the nosepiece can expand the external valve area, it is not easy to accurately document the severity of caudal septal deviation which is one of the most common causes in nasal obstruction.

(2) Rhinomanometry

Rhinomanometry is a functional assessment of airflow and involves the measurement of transnasal pressure and airflow. The most common method in this examination is active anterior rhinomanomerty using a face mask. Transnasal pressure differences and nasal airflow are recorded at the same time for each side and the dynamic changes of airway resistance are assessed. The resulting plot, with the x-axis representing the pressure differential and the y-axis representing airflow, produces a S-shaped curve. The more obstructed the airway, the greater the pressure required to generate a certain flow. The accepted standard for displaying the pressure-flow curve is to plot pressure on the x-axis and airflow on the y-axis. With this arrangement, the greater the pressure-to-flow ratio (resistance), the closer the curve is to the pressure axis *(Figure 13)*. Thus, curves representing a more obstructed airway lie closer to the pressure axis.

The disadvantage of rhinomanometry is that it can make the facial outline distorted by using a facial mask and the pressure can be changed according to the size of the face mask. Therefore, rhinomanometry is less frequently used than acoustic rhinometry. In addition, some studies reported that the results of both objective tests had no correlation with the subjective symptom scores. However, it is meaningful for objective documentation of nasal breathing and can be useful in resolving medico-legal problems postoperatively.

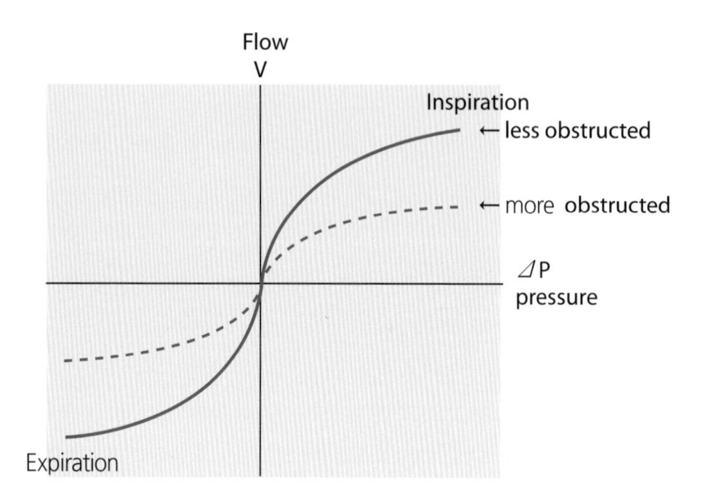

Figure 13 Results of anterior rhinomanometry. The pressure-flow curve for a nasal airway that is more obstructed will be closer to the pressure axis than the curve for a nasal airway that is less obstructed(ΔP, transnasal pressure; v, flow).

3. Treatment of Nasal Obstruction

1) Medical Treatment

If the cause of nasal obstruction is a nasal mucosal disorder such as rhinitis or sinusitis, medical treatment is tried first. For patients suffering from allergic rhinitis or nonallergic rhinitis, antihistamines or mucosal decongestants can be prescribed. Topical steroids can be used to reduce the inflammatory reaction and alleviate the nasal obstruction. In cases where the cause of nasal obstruction is chronic rhinosinusitis, symptoms can be alleviated by antibiotics, mucosal decongestants, mucolytics, and normal saline irrigation. When patients suffer from atrophic rhinitis, the nose should be kept clean through normal saline irrigation and prescribing antibiotics when necessary.

(1) Topical Steroids

Topical steroids can be prescribed for rhinitis or sinusitis patients suffering from nasal obstruction. There are several different kinds of topical steroids available including, triamcinolone acetonide (Nasacort®), fluticasone furoate (Avamys®), mometasone furoate (Nasonex®), ciclesonide (Omnaris®), etc. They can be administered once or twice a day. To administer the medication, the patient needs to hold his/her breath and lean forward so that the direction of the spray becomes parallel to the nasal cavity or points towards the lateral canthus of the ipsilateral eye, and spray as directed by the physician. As the optimal effect from the medication appears in 5-7 days, the patient must be educated on the need for regular and diligent spraying of the medication.

(2) Antihistamines

Antihistamines can be prescribed for allergic rhinitis patients. Antihistamines are effective for relieving the symptoms of sneezing, runny nose and itchiness but have minimal effects on nasal obstruction. Second generation antihistamines have some effects on nasal obstruction, namely cetirizine (Zyrtec®), loratadine (Claritin®), ebastine (Ebastel®), azelastine (Azeptin®), ketotifen (Zaditen®), etc. These can taken once or twice per day. Third generation antihistamines such as levocetirizine (Xyzal®), fexofenadine (Allegra®), desloratadine (Clarinex®) show the same effects on allergic symptoms with lesser side effects compared to second generation antihistamines.

(3) Decongestants

The typical oral mucosal decongestant is pseudoephedrine. This drug has the effect of alleviating nasal obstruction by reducing congestion in the nasal cavity by means of constricting the blood vessels of the nasal cavity. However, since this not only affects the blood vessels of the nasal cavity mucosa but the cardiovascular system as a whole, care must be taken in prescribing it to patients suffering from hypertension or cardiovascular disease. In particular, utmost caution must be exercised in elderly patients. Compared to oral decongestants, topical mucosal decongestants work quicker so that nasal obstruction can be alleviated within 2-5 minutes of application. However, if it is used continuously for more than 1 week, side effects such as rhinitis medicamentosa, characterized by worsening mucosal congestion with associated reduction in response to the topical decongestant can result. Thus, care must be exercised in prescribing topical decongestants. Among the topical mucosal decongestants being used today are epinephrine, phenylephrine, oxymetazoline, xylometazoline, and naphazoline.

(4) Leuokotriene Receptor Antagonist

Leukotriene receptor antagonist (or modifiers), such as montelukast (Singulair®), zafirlukast (Accolate®), and pranlukast (Onon®) can be used to treat allergic rhinitis. Even though they are less effective than topical corticosteroids when taken alone, combination therapy (leukotriene antagonist plus antihistamine) is a more effective strategy on nasal obstruction compared with monotherapy with a leukotriene antagonist or antihistamine in the treatment of allergic rhinitis.

2) Surgical Treatment

Septoplasty and turbinoplasty are surgeries commonly performed to improve nasal obstruction and will be discussed further in another chapter. Problems in the nasal valve can be corrected using spreader grafts. In cases of alar collapse, alar batten grafts can be placed using septal cartilage or auricular cartilage. Septal perforations can also be a cause of nasal obstruction. Standard medical treatments for this include irrigation of the nasal cavity, application of ointments and antibiotics. However, when the effect is unsatisfactory, surgical treatment may be necessary. The aim of surgical treatment in atrophic rhinitis or empty nose syndrome is to reduce the size of the nasal cavity. Surgical techniques treating empty nose syndrome will be introduced in another chapter.

4. Newly Discovered or Deteriorating Nasal Obstruction Subsequent to Rhinoplasty *(Table 2)*

It is unfortunate for both the patient and the surgeon to have nasal obstruction occur after rhinoplasty. Evaluation of nasal obstruction developing after rhinoplasty must begin with an examination of the symptoms. The time of occurrence, characteristics, severity of the nasal symptoms as well as the factors that worsen or improve the symptoms must be asked. Initial nasal obstruction subsequent to surgery generally is linked to postsurgical swelling or preexisting rhinosinusitis. Patients exhibiting these symptoms need to be assured that the postsurgical

Table 2 Newly discovered or deteriorating nasal obstruction subsequent to rhinoplasty

Nasal obstruction after operation			
Classification		Characteristic and Etiology	Treatment
Mucosal disease		Alternating, intermittent, and fluctuating symptoms accompanying rhinorrhea and postnasal drip	Medication
Anatomical problem	Septum	Remnant septal deviation Septal extension graft Narrow and weak L-strut Septal perforation	Revision septoplasty Conservative treatment Perforation repair
	Upper lateral cartilage (middle vault collapse)	Collapse of upper lateral cartilage due to excessive dorsal hump reduction Avulsion of upper lateral cartilage after rasping	Reconstruction for restoration of structure
	Nasal bone	Collapse of sidewalls after osteotomy	Reconstruction for restoration of structure
	Turbinate	Hypertrophy of inferior turbinate Excessive turbinate reduction (empty nose syndrome)	Turbinoplasty or RFTVR* Conservative treatment Endonasal microplasty

* Radiofrequency turbinate volume reduction

swelling will subside and that nasal obstruction will disappear. However, if the nasal obstruction alternates left and right, occurs intermittently, is extremely variable, or is linked to nasal discharge or postnasal drip and facial pain, then, mucosal disease should be suspected and medical treatment needs to be considered. Symptoms that appear after a certain period of time, months or years after surgery generally is linked to mucosal disease or anatomical problems. Preexisting conditions that were overlooked, for instance anatomical factors such as septal deviation, can contribute in causing postoperative nasal obstruction. Nasal obstruction that consistently occur on one side have a particularly high probability of being a problem that is linked to an anatomical abnormality. If only simple dorsal augmentation was performed during rhinoplasty, there is a low likelihood of nasal obstruction occurring after surgery. However, if techniques such as manipulation of the septal cartilage or upper lateral cartilage or osteotomy were performed, there is a high probability of nasal obstruction occurring. If turbinate reduction was performed excessively, secondary atrophic rhinitis can develop. The dimension of the nasal cavity in these patients may have been enlarged. Patients may experience an inexplicable nasal obstruction due to variations in structure involving changes in the nasal mucous and nasal cavity resistance. Treatment in such cases is particularly difficult. Using an endoscope, the remnants of a pre-existing septal deviation can be observed. If the symptoms of the patient are severe, secondary surgery needs to be considered. If it is determined that hypertrophy of the inferior turbinate is the main cause of nasal obstruction, turbinoplasty can be performed to treat the problem. Nasal obstruction can occur following lateral osteotomy. This is brought about by the narrowing of the cross-sectional area of the nasal cavity at the nasal valve and pyriform aperture following the osteotomy. Also, an improperly corrected deviated nose or septal perforation can bring about nasal obstruction. In some cases, damage to the upper lateral cartilages can be a cause of nasal obstruction. Such situations are the result of excessive dorsal hump reduction in which the upper lateral cartilages collapse towards the septum after the hump is removed. Occasionally, a middle vault collapse can be caused by the avulsion of the upper lateral cartilages due to rasping. The risk of this happening becomes greater if the nasal cavity mucosa is damaged during hump reduction. Solving the above problems involve performing reconstructive surgery in order to repair the damaged structures.

III. Olfaction

Comprising one of the five major human senses, olfaction is a very important sensation. The loss of olfactory function would not only expose the patient to the danger of not being able to detect a fire but the very quality of life would decline substantially due to the deterioration in the sense of smell and taste. All forms of nasal surgery carry the risk of inducing dysosmia, and the rhinoplasty surgeon must be careful not to overlook the possibility of inducing dysosmia through surgery. Furthermore, all patients facing nasal surgery must be warned of the possible development of olfactory dysfunction as a potential complication of nasal surgery.

1. Anatomy and Physiology

The sense of smell is detected primarily through the olfactory nerve (CN I). However, it can also be felt through the trigeminal (CN V), glossopharyngeal (CN IX), and vagus (CN X) nerves. The trigeminal nerve, which has a receptor for stimulative smell, is distributed around the nasal cavity and the pharynx. The glossopharyngeal and vagus nerves, located at the pharynx, have a supplementary chemical sensory function. The ciliated olfactory receptor of the olfactory nerves is located at the olfactory epithelium. The anatomical locations where the olfactory epithelium are distributed are the superior nasal septum, superior/supreme turbinate, supero-lateral nasal wall, and part of the middle turbinate, each distributed around the nasal cavity with an approximate area of ≦ 2 cm^2 *(Figure 14)*.

The cell body of the primary olfactory neuron is located within the olfactory epithelium. The axons (olfactory filament) from these neurons pass through the 15 to 20 cribriform plate holes up to the brain to form the synapse at the olfactory bulb. It is known that there are approximately 6 million olfactory axons in an individual. Besides the bipolar olfactory neuron receptor, the olfactory epithelium possesses the microvillar cell, supporting cell, basal cell, and Bowman gland duct cell. The transmission and perception route of olfaction is complex and involves a multilevel process. For any particular molecule to be perceived by the olfactory receptor, it must first reach the olfactory cleft. This process is brought about by the respiratory air current. Between about 10-20% of the nasal cavity air current reaches the olfactory cleft. Once the odorant molecule reaches the olfactory epithelium, it adheres to the mucus covering the mucosa and gets dissolved. The resulting chemical information is transformed into an electrical potential. The electrical

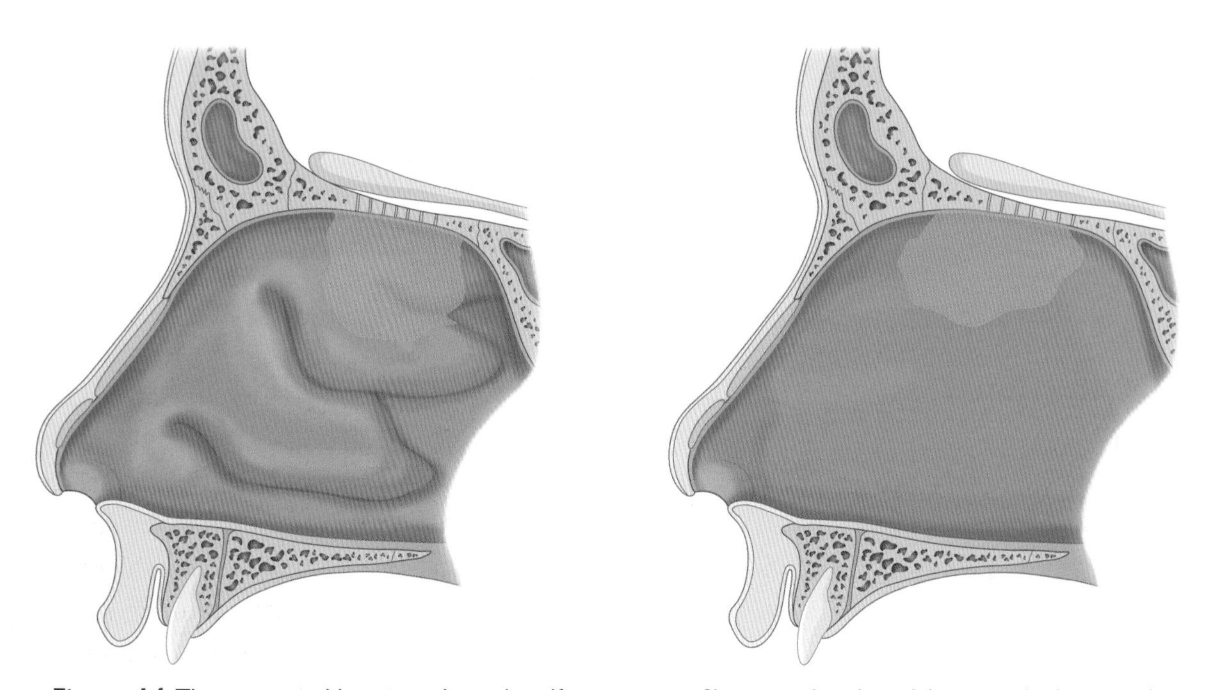

Figure 14 The anatomical location where the olfactory nerve fibers are distributed (area marked in green).

potential originates from the olfactory receptor area where the bipolar olfactory receptor, a first order afferent neuron, is located. The first order neuron synapses with the second order afferent neuron at the olfactory glomerulus, specifically between the mitral cell within the olfactory bulb and the dendrite of the tufted cell. The electrical signal is then conveyed to the olfactory cortex along the olfactory tract *(Figure 15)*. The olfactory epithelium is characterized by its ability to regenerate. All olfactory epithelial cells regenerate from the basal cells after being damaged or in the is natural regenerative process. A person's olfactory neuron is regenerated every 3 to 6 months and this process is continued as long as the basal cells remain healthy.

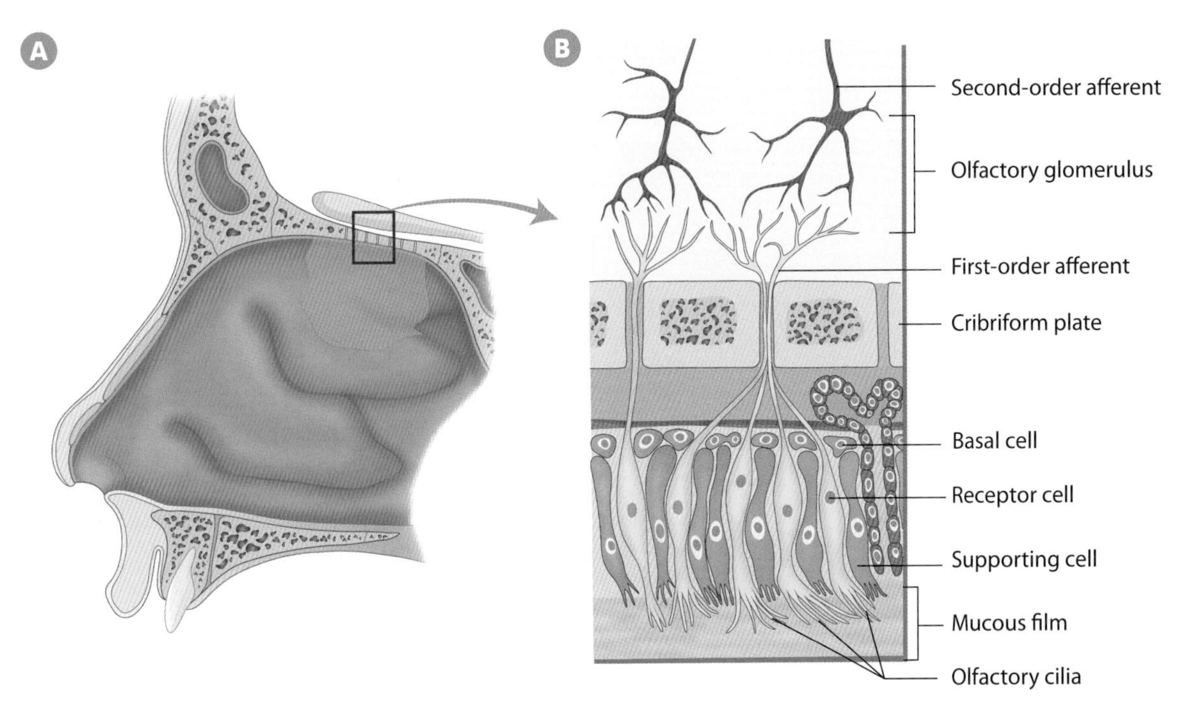

Figure 15 The structure and location of the olfactory epithelium and olfactory bulb.

2. Clinical Evaluation of Olfactory Function

1) History Taking

The first and most important step for evaluating a patient suffering from olfactory dysfunction is obtaining a thorough history. Most patients experiencing dysosmia also complain of dysgeusia. Patients can distinguish between the sweet, bitter, sour, and salty tastes but complain of not being able to appreciate the flavor of food. In most cases, not being able to detect the flavor of food is a phenomenon resulting not from dysgeusia but olfactory dysfunction. During the history taking of the dysosmic patient, the doctor must ask the patient certain details in the clinical history such as a history of head trauma, onset of symptoms, exposure to toxins, and infections of the upper respiratory tract. The olfactory dysfunction resulting from a viral infection of the upper respiratory tract is the most common cause of dysosmia and is difficult to treat. If dysosmia is accompanied by a unilateral nosebleed or nasal obstruction, a tumor of the nose can be suspected. A cyclical improvement and worsening of anosmia can be found among rhinosinusitis and nasal polyp patients. In addition, care must be taken during the history taking to ascertain the existence of allergy, change in eyesight, symptoms regarding the central nervous system, delay in puberty, endocrine disorder (i.e. hypothyroidism), etc.

2) Physical Examination of the Nose

Endoscopy of the nasal cavity is especially helpful in discovering the cause of conductive olfactory dysfunction. When conducting nasal endoscopy, the patency of the olfactory cleft and middle meatus must be carefully observed. Possible abnormalities requiring careful attention include polyps, tumors, rhinosinusitis, synechia, postoperative changes, crusts, etc. *(Figure 16)*.

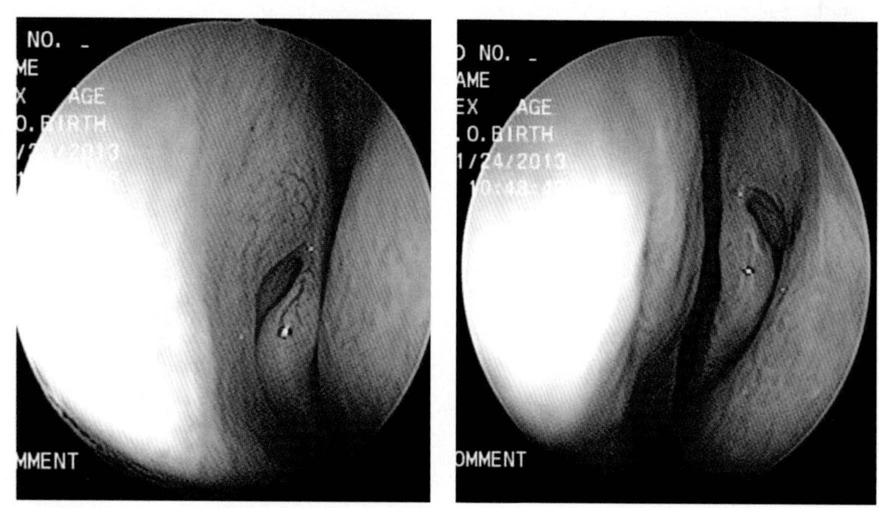

Figure 16 Nasal endoscopic findings of patent olfactory clefts and middle meatus in both nasal cavities.

3) Radiological Examination

It is extremely rare for a brain tumor to display olfactory dysfunction as the only symptom. Thus, the need to conduct a radiologic exam specific to the brain of an olfactory dysfunction patient is very low. However, if the nasal obstruction derives from an anatomical abnormality, tumor, or polyp, a sinus CT scan is needed *(Figure 17)*. If the existence of a tumor within the nasal cavity is confirmed, a MRI should be then taken to ascertain if it has invaded intracranially.

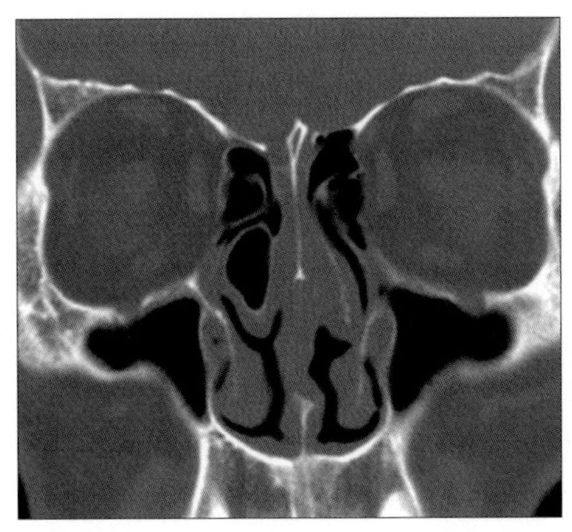
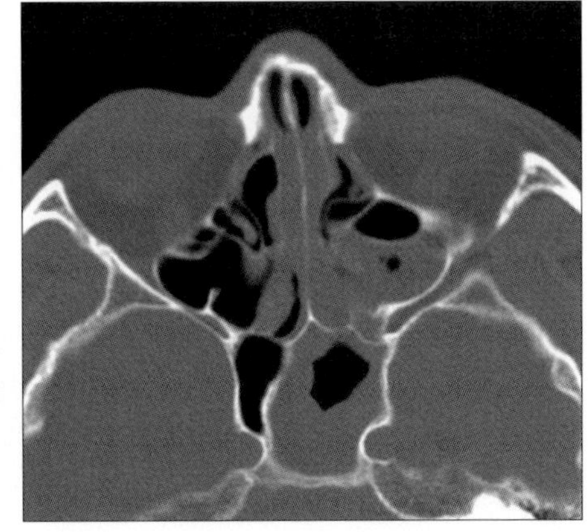

Figure 17 Obstruction of both olfactory clefts observed in PNS CT scans. Both olfactory clefts are totally obstructed by concha bullosa and polypoid mucosa of the middle turbinates.

4) Olfactory Testing

Conducting an olfaction test for a patient showing symptoms of dysosmia is an extremely essential step in the diagnostic procedure. Most olfaction test examine for the detection threshold towards a certain odorant or the ability to distinguish between various odorants. The problem with olfaction testing, however, is that it utilizes a subjective system of exam that relies on the patient's judgment and that a practical and objective exam method has not yet been established. In case the patient's dysosmia becomes a legal matter, the difficulty involved in objectifying and standardizing the extent of disorder is a limiting factor in offering medical consultation. The University of Pennsylvania Smell Identification Test (UPSIT) is an olfaction recognition test method that is universally used today. This test involves scratching 40 odorants within a mini-capsule with a pencil and having the test subject smell it in order to have them choose the correct answer from the four sample answers given. The correct answers are then calculated against the centesimal scale, taking into consideration the age and sex factors, in order to evaluate the patient's identification capabilities. The more simplified version of the UPSIT, the CCSIT (Cross-Cultural Smell Identification Test) which uses 12 odorants familiar to various cultures is also widely used. Depending on how many types of smell were correctly identified, the patients are then evaluated on a scale of 0-12; 0-5 points corresponds to anosmia, 6-10 points corresponds to hyposmia, 11-12 is judged to be normal. Olfaction threshold testing using butanol utilizes 4% 1-butanol that is diluted in multiplies of 3 in order to create a 9-12 concentration of diluted solutions. The test begins with the lowest concentration moving on to a higher concentration with every incorrect answer. When the patient provides the correct response to the concentration four times, that level is determined to be the olfaction threshold.

3. Treatment

Causes of olfactory dysfunction can be largely divided into two different categories;

- Conductive loss: occurs when the air current to the olfactory cleft is blocked. For instance, this is a dysosmia that arises from chronic rhinosinusitis, allergic rhinitis, polyp, or tumor.
- Sensory/Neural loss: occurs when any part of the olfactory neurotransmission pathway from the olfactory receptor to the olfactory bulb to the brain is damaged. Congenital anosmia, dysosmia following viral upper respiratory tract infection, head trauma, toxins, dementia, and multiple sclerosis all belong in this category.

Conductive loss has a high probability of responding to treatment. However, olfactory dysfunction from sensory/neural loss does not generally respond to treatment.

1) Instructions for Dysosmic Patients

All patients complaining of dysosmia must be given detailed warnings regarding safety. They must equip their homes with a fire and gas warning system. As long as the trigeminal nerve function is intact, efforts need to be made to develop the appetite by using stimulating spices liberally in dishes. To avoid inadvertent food poisoning, food must be stored in the refrigerator or freezer and patients should be advised to consume only food that display the expiration date.

2) Medical Treatment

Olfactory dysfunction due to nasal obstruction and infection is a relatively highly treatable condition. Methods in treating dysosmia due to nasal obstruction involves restoring the air current to the olfactory cleft. For patients suffering from allergic rhinitis or chronic rhinosinusitis, treatments such as the use of steroids, mucosal decongestants, antibiotics, antihistamines, allergy immunotherapy, and saline irrigation to reduce the edema of the mucosa and alleviate the infection, will help improve the olfactory function. Steroids are commonly used in treating dysosmia patients. Because systemic steroids have anti-inflammatory effects, it is useful for treating dysosmia by reducing the swelling in the nasal cavity and paranasal sinuses. This drug is also known to have a direct effect on olfactory epithelial cells. However, there are as yet many more unknowns regarding its function. Systemic steroids can also be effective against sensory/neural olfactory dysfunction such as dysosmia resulting from a viral upper respiratory tract infection, or dysosmia of unknown cause. Topical steroids are less effective compared to systemic steroids. The dosage and administration for the use of oral steroids in treating olfactory dysfunction is not yet clearly defined. Using prednisolone as an example, administration of 0.3-1 mg/kg/day for 1-2 weeks with 3-4 days of tapering is recommended. Using prednisolone for more than one month is undesirable due to uncertainty of effectiveness as well as a higher risk of steroid side effects. Prescribing steroids for one cycle is recommended. If the result is unsatisfactory, steroids can be prescribed repeatedly for short periods with 3-month intervals for additional effects. Besides steroids, it is reported that strychnine, zinc, theophylline, alpha-lipoic acid, and vitamins A and B are helpful in treating dysosmia. In the author's experience, alpha-lipoic acid is used as a second line maintenance drug after induction treatment with systemic steroids in the treatment of postviral anosmia. However, research into the effectiveness of these substances is as of yet inadequate.

3) Surgical Treatment

There is currently no known surgical method that can directly cure dysosmia. However, if the primary nasal cavity disorder is satisfactorily treated through septoplasty or endoscopic sinus surgery, secondary olfactory improvement may be achievable through surgery.

4. Rhinoplasty and Olfactory Dysfunction

If synechiae form between the middle turbinate and the septum following surgery within the nasal cavity, airflow to the olfactory cleft can be blocked and this in turn can lead to olfactory dysfunction. Furthermore, if the superior or middle turbinate is excessively removed during surgery or the olfactory epithelium of the upper septum is stripped off, olfactory dysfunction can develop. However, olfactory dysfunction can still manifest even though none of the above situations had occurred during rhinoplasty. In such an occasion, it is difficult to uncover the reason why the olfactory dysfunction had developed. The risk of olfactory dysfunction resulting from rhinoplasty has been reported in literature. In one study of 200 cases of rhinoplasty, 22 cases (10%) reported temporary anosmia lasting between 6-18 months, and there was one reported case of anosmia lasting for three years. Another study examined 97 patients before and after rhinoplasty reported that 3 patients (3%) developed hyposmia but that there were no long-term cases lasting for more than 2 months. Recently, a study reported that 88% of the patients who underwent aesthetic open rhinoplasty had anosmia at postoperative one week, resolved and converted to various levels of hyposmia at postoperative 6 weeks, and almost recovered to the preoperative levels at postoperative 6 months. As shown by the aforementioned paper, the aesthetic open rhinoplasty may be accompanied by some degrees of postoperative olfactory dysfunction, which may be temporary or persistent. Therefore, it is important to discuss the possibility of postoperative olfactory dysfunction to rhinoplasty candidates. When packing or silastic septal splints are left in the nasal cavity after rhinoplasty, temporary olfactory dysfunction can result from nasal blockage caused by these foreign substances. If such a dysfunction occurs after rhinoplasty, the surgeon needs to first assure the patient and ask if the patient had an upper respiratory tract infection. However, if the patient complains of dysosmia even after the nasal obstruction or edema has improved, tests such as the CCSIT needs to be conducted and systemic steroids must be prescribed. Most patients recover their olfactory function as a result of these measures. In cases where endoscopy reveals the development of a distinct synechia at the roof of the nasal cavity, it must be addressed.

References

1. Canakcioglu S, Tahamiler R, Saritzali G, Isildak H, Alimoglu Y. Nasal patency by rhinomanometry in patients with sensation of nasal obstruction. Am J Rhinol Allergy 2009; 23: 300-2.
2. Cho GS, Kim JH, Jang YJ. Correlation of nasal obstruction with nasal cross sectional area measured by computed tomography in patients with deviated septum. Annals Otol Rhinol Laryngol 2012; 121: 239-45.
3. Gruber RP, Lin AY, Richards T. Nasal strips for evaluating and classifying valvular nasal obstruction. Aesthetic Plast Surg 2011; 35: 211-5.
4. Gillespie MB, Osguthorpe JD. Pharmacologic management of chronic rhinosinusitis, alone or with nasal polyposis. Curr Allergy Asthma Rep 2004 ; 4: 478-85.
5. Hamdan AL, Sabra O, Hadi U. Prevalence of adenoid hypertrophy in adults with nasal obstruction. J Otolaryngol Head Neck Surg 2008; 37: 469-73.
6. Joe SA. The assessment and treatment of nasal obstruction after rhinoplasty. Facial Plast Surg Clin N Am 2004; 12: 451-8.
7. Lal D, Corey JP. Acoustic rhinometry and its uses in rhinology and diagnosis of nasal obstruction. Facial Plast Surg Clin N Am 2004; 12: 397-405.
8. Litvack JR, Mace JC, Smith TL. Olfactory function and disease severity in chronic rhinosinusitis. Am J Rhinol Allergy 2009; 23: 139-44.
9. Pade J, Hummel T. Olfactory function following nasal surgery. Laryngoscope 2008; 118: 1260-4.
10. Ryu CH, Lee BJ, Jang YJ. Nasal obstruction in patients with deviated nose. J Rhinology 2007: 14; 88-91.
11. Shemshadi H, Azimian M, Onsori MA, Azizabadi Farahani M. Olfactory function following open rhinoplasty: A 6-month follow-up study. BMC Ear Nose Throat Disord 2008; 8: 1-6.
12. Wrobel BB, Leopold DA. Clinical assessment of patients with smell and taste disorders. Otolaryngol Clin N Am 2004; 37: 1127-42.

Chapter 03

Anesthesia

Seung Woo Ku

The nose is a part of the respiratory tract – and thus, never is the cooperation and communication between the surgeon and anesthesiologist more important than during airway surgery. Rhinoplasty can be performed through general anesthesia, wherein a safe airway is guaranteed by intubation. It can also be done through monitored anesthesia care (MAC) or local anesthesia, wherein the airway is not secured. Once the surgery has started, the anesthesiologist faces restrictions in the form of having to step away from the airway and manage both the anesthesia and the airway. Thus, it is of great importance that ventilation is well maintained, especially if rhinoplasty is performed without intubation.

I. General Anesthesia

1. Preoperative Considerations

The preoperative evaluation for general anesthesia usually involves assessment of the airway (including the teeth), blood tests, ECG, and an examination of previous medical records. Patients who are to receive local anesthesia or MAC are also applied the same standards. Breathing difficulties are common after nasal surgery due to packing, thus patients with sleep apnea or adenoid hypertrophy must be closely watched to avoid respiratory complications after surgery, while patients with prior medical history of ischemic heart disease or arrhythmia must be monitored for hypoventilation or aggravated symptoms caused by subcutaneous injections containing epinephrine. Special care is also required for patients that exhibit sensitivity to non-steroidal antiinflammatory drugs (NSAIDs) like aspirin. Samter's triad, the association of NSAID sensitivity in patients with asthma and nasal polyposis, who may experience severe life-threatening bronchospasm, should be kept in mind. Patients who take aspirin to prevent blood clots should be advised to stop taking the medication temporarily for at least a week prior to the operation. On the other hand, it is helpful to let patients continue taking their antihypertensive medications (taken with a small sip of water) even on the day of the surgery to keep their blood pressure low, preventing bleeding during and after surgery.

With general anesthesia, including MAC, fasting for at least eight hours has been the previous recommendation. But now, in the current guidelines, ingesting clear liquids is allowed for up to two hours prior to surgery *(Table 1)*.

Table 1 Fasting Guidelines

Age (in months)	Non-clear liquids and solids (hours of fasting)	Clear liquids (hours of fasting)
< 6	4-6	2
6-36	6	2-3
>36	6-8	2-3

2. Maintaining Anesthesia, Awakening, and Complications

Inhalation is the most widespread method of maintaining anesthesia. But recently total intravenous anesthesia (TIVA) combining propofol and remifentanil has been increasing in usage. If the anesthesia is going to be delivered through an endotracheal tube, it is best to use tubes that resist bending or kinking. It is helpful to use RAE tubes *(Figure 1)* that do not block the surgeon's view. Laryngeal mask airways (LMA) can also be used, but always keep in mind the possibility of aspiration. Choosing the anesthetic and the endotracheal tube for rhinoplasty depend on the anesthesiologist's experience, duration of surgery, and patient condition.

A "Coroner's clot" refers to blood clots from surgery that are not removed and settle in the nasopharynx. This clot is at risk of being aspirated into the airway following extubation, causing acute upper airway obstruction. Placement of gauze as pharyngeal packing before starting the surgery not only prevents the blood clots from being swallowed, but also facilitates the removal of blood clots after surgery. Meticulous postoperative inspection of the upper airway, including the oral cavity, for blood clots helps prevent acute airway obstruction due to a Coroner's clot.

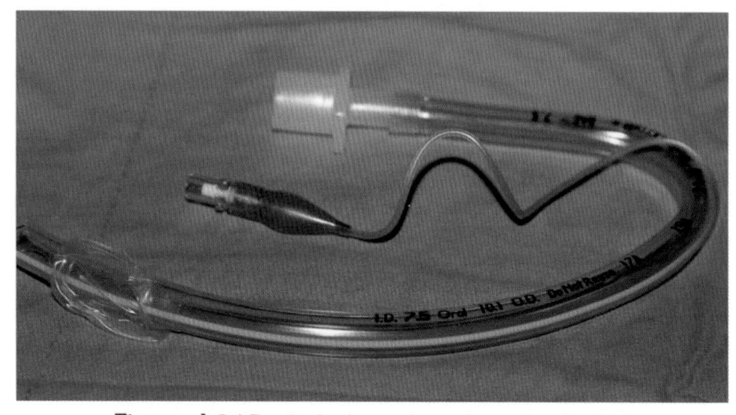

Figure 1 RAE tube(right angle endotracheal tube).

II. Monitored Anesthesia Care (MAC)

MAC refers to the state wherein the patient, either under diagnostic or surgical procedure, is administered local anesthesia, supplemented by sedatives or pain killers, while the anesthesiologist is monitoring the patients vital signs as if under general anesthesia. MAC is a deeper state of sedation and pain relief, thus requiring an anesthesiologist. MAC can be used in diagnostic procedures which could cause discomfort for patients, and could be more acceptable to both the doctor and the patient. However, due to issues with medical insurance costs and lack of interest and manpower in anesthesiology, MAC has only recently becoming popular, with very hopeful prospects ahead. Statistically, minor complications occur less frequently in MAC than in general anesthesia, but major complications occur at similar rates, thus patient monitoring and anesthesia management should follow the same standards as in general anesthesia. The most common yet lethal complications are respiratory complications. Since drugs that have depressive effects on the respiratory system are administered without intubation it is crucial that the patient's ventilation is monitored thoroughly during surgery.

1. Levels of Sedation

Sedation is classified into the three levels: minimal sedation, moderate sedation, and deep sedation. The deeper levels can be called general anesthesia *(Table 2)*. Moderate sedation maintains the patient's consciousness and can respond appropriately to the surgeon's instructions, thus this is also called conscious sedation. Sedation is a concept that is a spectrum, thus it is difficult to distinguish each level of sedation and the clear distinction between each level tends to be ambiguous. In other words, even if the procedure commences with moderate sedation in mind, it is always possible for the patient to fall into deep sedation and even general anesthesia, thus whoever is conducting the sedation must always be able to maintain breathing and deal with cardiovascular and respiratory instability.

Table 2 Levels of Sedation

	Minimal sedation (Anxiolysis)	Moderate sedation (Conscious sedation)	Deep sedation	General anestheisia
Responsiveness	Normal response to verbal stimulation	Purposeful response to verbal or tactile stimulation	Purposeful response after repeated or painful stimulation	Unarousable, even with painful stimulation
Airway	Unaffected	No intervention required	Intervention may be required	Intervention often required
Spontaneous ventilation	Unaffected	Adequate	May be inadequate	Frequently inadequate
Cardiovascular function	Unaffected	Usually maintained	Usually maintained	May be impaired

2. Monitoring Patients Under Sedation

The following principles must be adhered to in relation to sedation:

① Qualified, medical personnel must be available at all times to monitor the patient (i.e., anesthesiologist).

② Oxygen saturation, ventilation levels (such as respiratory rate), and blood pressure must be monitored regularly, and depending on the patient, electrocardiography or capnography may be useful. When measuring oxygen saturation by pulse oximetry one must record the numbers shown on the display when pulse patterns become periodic or regular (as seen on the waveform or plethysmograph of the pulse oximeter). This must be distinguished from artifacts that appear due to contact failure, patient movement, or use of electrocautery. Capnography can detect hypoventilation symptoms the quickest; pulse oxymetry can detect hypoventilation 30-40 seconds after it occurs.

③ Oxygen, oxygen supplying devices, masks, ambu bags, intubation equipment and supplies, emergency medication, defibrillators and the like must be prepared beforehand to be used whenever necessary.

④ In case of respiratory depression due to oversedation, one must awaken the patient through stimulation while conducting maneuvers to secure the airway *(Figures 2, 3)*. If the respiratory depression is persistent, perform bag valve mask ventilation using an ambu bag with an oral or nasal airway, and perform intubation if necessary.

3. Assessing Sedation Depth

1) Subjective Assessment of Sedation Depth: Sedation Scale and Scoring

Using a sedation scale is currently the most common method. Ramsay, et al. published a

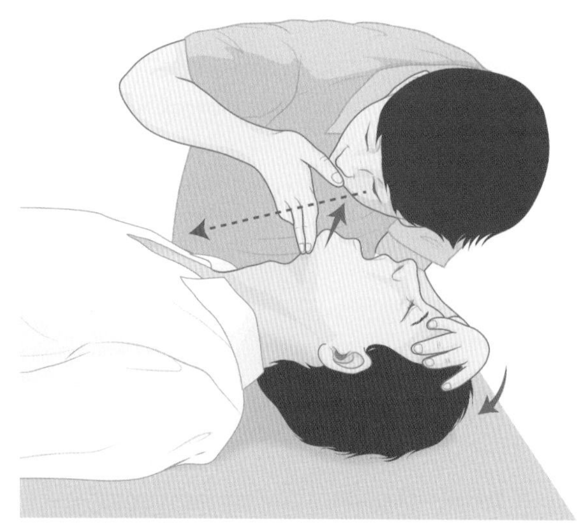

Figure 2 Head tilt-chin lift maneuver.

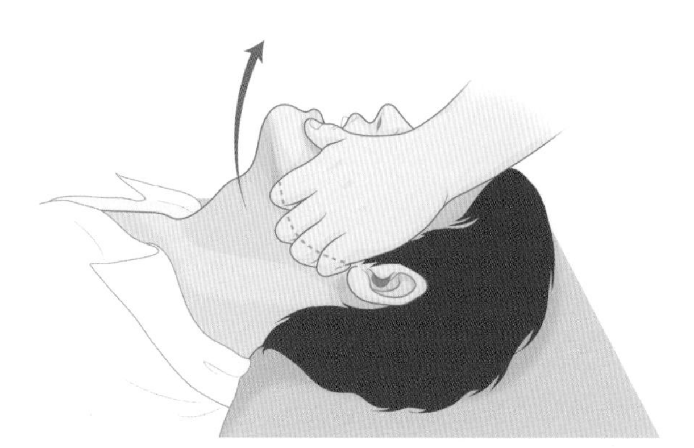

Figure 3 Jaw thrust maneuver.

sedation scoring system in 1974. Since then, many other scales have been proposed, but a common flaw is that the way in which the assessor evaluates the standards is too ambiguous, thus lowering consistency among evaluators. The Observer's Assessment of Alertness/Sedation Scale (OAA/S scale) has been validated, but it still has points of controversy and is more complicated, thus making the simpler Ramsay scale *(Table 3)* more popular. Most sedation procedures should have a score on the Ramsay scale between two and four.

Table 3 Ramsay sedation scale

Awake Levels	Patient anxious or agitated or both	1
	Patient cooperative, oriented and tranquil	2
	Patient responds to commands only	3
Asleep Levels	A brisk response to a light glabellar tap	4
	A sluggish response to a light glabellar tap	5
	No response	6

2) Objective Assessment of Sedation Depth

A call for a more objective assessment method to overcome the problems of consistency between evaluators is not a new one, but we currently lack methods and equipment to precisely measure sedation and anesthesia levels due to the fact that mechanisms behind consciousness degradation following anesthesia are not yet fully revealed. The 95% spectral edge frequency (SEF 95), median frequency, entropy methods, bispectral index (BIS), and auditory evoked potentials (AEP) are newly rising methods – and out of these BIS is the most commonly used due to convenient measurement and easy interpretation.

The BIS is based on the distinct changes in the amplitude and frequency of brain waves in awakening and loss of consciousness: as consciousness degrades, the frequency decreases and amplitude increases *(Figure 4)*. These measurements and changes can be quantitatively displayed, indicating the level of consciousness. The most awake state is a 100, while a 0 indicates that

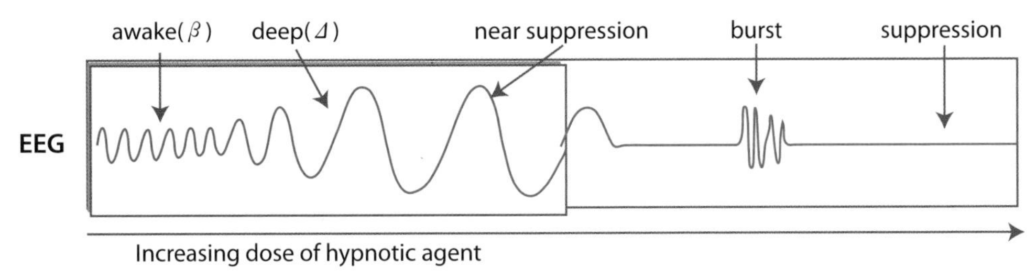

Figure 4 Change of EEG patterns at increasing doses of hypnotic agents.

there are no brain waves – as the sedation becomes deeper the score decreases. The appropriate value to be maintained for general anesthesia is between 40 and 60, and for moderate sedation is between 70 and 80. At first it was understood that BIS numbers could tell the absolute state of consciousness, but it has been revealed that such is not the case. At present however, there is no objective method more convenient or accurate than BIS, thus it is widely used in TIVA.

4. Drugs Used for Sedation

The prime principle in using sedatives is to understand the drug's characteristics and use the minimum amount required for the procedure. Since each patient reacts differently, the minimum amount is administered first, then based on the patient's response decide whether to administer additional dosages or not.

Sedatives can be classified into two major groups. The first group are drugs intended to sedate and degrade consciousness, such as benzodiazepines like midazolam, barbiturates like thiopental, and propofol. The other group are opioids intended to relieve pain. With increasing dosages of these drugs, the possibility of side effects such as hypoventilation and hypotension increase along with sedation and pain relief levels. One exception is ketamine, which can cause both pain relief and loss of consciousness without lowering blood pressure or breathing levels.

If the procedure is not expected to be very painful and is not affected by minor patient movements, it is optimal to use midazolam or propofol alone; but in most procedures a combination of these two drugs is administered. In such cases, one must keep in mind that the drugs have a synergistic effect thus must lower their respective dosages appropriately. Recently, a combination of propofol and remifentanil is becoming more popular in MAC.

1) Midazolam

Midazolam has a short half-life (1.5-2.5 hours) and does not have major respiratory depression effects or hemodynamic changes, thus is the most popular sedative for endoscopy procedures. Furthermore, it causes amnesia, thus patients cannot remember the procedure, but can cause adverse effects like disinhibition and anxiety in the elderly. Dosages should be at 0.5-2.0 mg infused slowly, and the same amount may be administered again if necessary, normally reaching amounts of up to 5 mg.

2) Propofol

Propofol is a drug that acts (within seconds) and recovers (within 10 to 15 minutes of stopping administration) quickly, both sedating and causing amnesia in the patient. Because the drug solution contains bean and chicken egg proteins, it has a high rate of bacterial infection; therefore drugs that have been unsealed for over six hours should not be used. It also has the disadvantage of being painful to the patient while being infused. Compared to midazolam, propofol induces a much stronger level of sedation, thus makes it easier to manage the sedation. However, it is strongly associated with respiratory depression and cardiovascular changes, thus highly experienced medical personnel should administer the drug. Clearance of the drug mostly involves the liver and kidneys but occurs completely from the plasma, thus making prolonged administration safe from cumulative effects. This property makes continuous intravenous infusion or target controlled infusion (TCI) a common option for propofol. Dosages are 20-50 mg administered for 5-10 minutes if administering all at once, and 25-75 μg/kg/min for continuous intravenous infusion.

3) Ketamine

Ketamine has a wide range of effects, including analgesia, anesthesia, hallucination, hypertension, and bronchodilation. Ketamine is a dissociative anesthetic developed in 1963 to replace phencyclidine (PCP), and is currently being used in human anesthesia, as well as in veterinary medicine. Ketamine functionally "dissociates" the thalamus (which relays sensory impulses from the reticular activating system to the cerebral cortex) from the limbic cortex (which is involved with the awareness of sensation). Clinically, this state of dissociative anesthesia causes the patient to appear conscious (i.e., with eye opening, swallowing, muscle contraction), but unable to process or respond to sensory input. Ketamine does not cause hypoventilation, thus is commonly used for procedures that can cause pain, minor procedures that require local anesthesia, and for children, who rarely exhibit the postoperative mental effects seen in adults. Due to its characteristics, ketamine may be dangerous for patients with a history of coronary artery diseases or arrhythmia. Nonetheless, if administered appropriately with midazolam or propofol, it is possible to maximize the advantages of both drugs. The standard dosage for infusion is 0.5-2.0 mg/kg, and the effects occur within 30 to 60 seconds after administration, lasting for 10-15 minutes. If injected into the muscle in amounts of 2-4 mg/kg, effects manifest within 3-4 minutes and last for 15-25 minutes.

4) Opioids

Benzodiazepines or propofol lack or have weak painkilling effects, thus when the patient complains of pain, it is wise to not increase their dosage but add opioids instead. Combining opioids and sedatives keeps the patient more stable and comfortable and is more advantageous in terms of amnesia. But such combinations also cause hypoventilation and cardiodepression, and as such must be used carefully. Pethidine (Demerol®) was once used widely, but drugs with shorter action times such as fentanyl, alfentanil, and remifentanil have taken its place.

5) Dexmedetomidine

This α_2-adrenergic agonist agent is under the same category as clonidine, but has eight times the selective effect on α_2 than clonidine does, making it possible to obtain stronger sedative effects without the cardiovascular effects caused by α_1 stimulation. If used alone, patients are sedated with relatively stable breathing levels, but are easily awakened with minor stimulation. Dexmedetomidine lowers the required levels of sedatives and painkillers it is administered with, has anxiolytic effects, but does not cause amnesia (in low doses). Dexmedetomidine as a sedative has several favorable properties which include: it has a relatively short half-life (2 hours), it not only sedates but also relieves pain (albeit less so than the aforementioned drugs) relatively maintains cardiac and respiratory functions (only minimal depression), and has a reversal agent like atipamezole. Its use is currently on the rise in intensive care units and similar areas.

6) Reversal Agents

An antidote to benzodiazepines is flumazenil, while the antidote to opioids is naloxone. A preparation of 0.2 mg of flumazenil is given intravenously every minute until the patient reaches the desired level of reversal (up to 2 mg in total) and has a duration of action of about 60 minutes. Naloxone is injected intravenously after diluting one ample containing 1ml (0.4 mg/ml) of naloxone with 9 ml of normal saline to produce 10 ml of naloxone solution. Doses given are at 0.5-1.0 μg/kg every 3-5 minutes until the appropriate reversal is seen. Duration of action is around 30-45 minutes. Intramuscular injections require twice the dosage of intravenous injections.

Both drugs must be injected slowly over 15-30 seconds, and if injected too quickly, the sudden reversal of sedation could cause tachycardia, hypertension, arrhythmia, agitation, and nausea. Furthermore, if the sedative a longer remaining duration of action than the reversal agent, the remaining sedative could re-sedate the patient. Therefore, it is best to avoid injecting reversal agents to awaken the patient quickly after surgery, and once injected, the patient's vital signs must be monitored longer than the reversal agent's duration of action.

III. Local Anesthetics

1. Mechanism of Action

Pain stimulation occurs due to the transmission of electrical impulses across nerve cell membranes, facilitated by the movement of sodium and potassium ions across the cell membrane. Membrane potential differences between decrease as a result of nerve stimulation, which trigger depolarization, and creates the action potential. The membrane potential difference cause one segments' depolarization to be transmitted to an adjacent non-depolarized segment, thereby carrying the action potential through the entire nerve fiber. In depolarization, the membrane potential difference change of the nerve cell is caused by sodium ions moving from outside the cell to the inside through a sodium channel, and the potassium ions move from inside the cell to the outside. Local anesthetics block the movement of the sodium ions, suppressing depolarization of the nerve cell membrane, blocking nerve conduction, thus cutting off the transmission of pain.

2. Types and Characteristics of Local Anesthetics

Local anesthetics are generally classified into two, based on chemical structure: esters have ester bonds and amides have amide bonds. Esters include cocaine, procaine, chloroprocaine, and tetracaine. Currently, the most commonly used local anesthetics are of the amides, which include lidocaine, bupivacaine, and ropivacaine.

1) Lidocaine

Anesthesia using lidocaine occurs quickly, does not have local stimulation, stronger than procaine, but weaker than cocaine. Lidocaine is an amide, slowly metabolized in the liver by microsomal enzymes, thus has a longer duration of action and is potentially more toxic than esters that are metabolized in the plasma through hydrolysis. Local anesthetics are affected by the patient's age and health, thus its half-life is 81 minutes for patients between 22 and 26, but increases to 139 minutes for patients between 61 and 71. Furthermore, since it is metabolized in the liver, when the patient has decreased blood flow in the liver due to congestive heart failure or has liver disease, blood concentrations of amide anesthetics rises, and the half-life could increase several times.

2) Bupivacaine

This has moderate action, lasts for a relatively long time, and is powerful. Depending on the type of block, bupivacaine exhibits a duration of action between 3-10 hours. Unlike other local anesthetics, it hardly blocks motor nerves in low concentrations and selectively blocks sensory nerves. These characteristics enable this drug to be used widely in obstetric anesthesia and pain management. However, bupivacaine has a greater myocardial depressant effect than other local anesthetics, thus has a relatively high chance of causing cardiotoxicity.

3) Ropivacaine

Ropivacaine has a similar structure to bupivacaine, has a similar onset of action to bupivacaine, but has lesser motor nerve blocking activity and a slightly shorter duration of action. Its myocardial depressant effect is greater than that of lidocaine but weaker than that of bupivacaine, thus is used as an alternative to bupivacaine in cases that require longer local anesthesia time than lidocaine.

3. Toxicity of Local Anesthetics

1) Central Nervous System Toxicity

Local anesthetics affect the central nervous system greatly, thus toxicity can happen in concentrations lower than the levels in which cardiovascular toxicity can be seen. The spectrum of symptoms include mild headaches, dizziness with blurred vision, hearing disturbances, numbness around the mouth and tongue, and tinnitus. Subjective symptoms include loss of orientation, lightheadedness, chills, muscle spasms, twitching across the face and extremities, ultimately leading to a generalized seizure. This is due to disinhibition in the cerebral cortex, leading to a relative stimulation state. The initial agitation or stimulation of the central nervous system occurs through the inhibitor circuit's selective blockade, but at higher blood concentrations of local anesthetics, both the stimulator and inhibitor circuits are blocked, leading to hypoventilation and apnea. The potency of local anesthetics has a direct correlation with the ability to stimulate the central nervous system. The relative toxicity of bupivacaine and lidocaine, when compared, has a ratio of 4:1, which is similar to the relative strength of anesthesia achieved by each drug in local anesthesia.

2) Cardiovascular Toxicity

Cardiovascular toxicity occurs in higher concentrations than toxicity in the central nervous system, which makes it both rare and difficult to treat. Initial symptoms are hypertension and tachycardia, but as toxicity progresses the patient exhibit hypotension, bradycardia, and ventricular arrhythmia. Local anesthetics interfere with the passage of sodium ions in the ventricular muscle, suppressing depolarization which affects the myocardium's mechanical activity. This gives local anesthetics negative inotropic properties proportional to dosage. Such negative inotropic effects also increase in proportion to potency, thus myocardial suppression is greater when using bupivacaine compared to lidocaine. The smooth muscle of peripheral blood vessels exhibit two-sided responses, with vasoconstriction in low concentrations and vasodilation at higher levels.

3) Vasoconstrictors Used with Local Anesthetics

Vasoconstrictors such as epinephrine are used to decrease the absorption of local anesthetics. Thus larger amounts of anesthetic can reach the tissues, increasing its potency and duration of action while acting as an indicator if injected inappropriately into a vessel. Epinephrine added to lidocaine for injection into the nasal mucous membranes exhibits the best effects weighed against side effects in 1: 20,000 (5 μg/ml) concentrations, and is sometimes replaced with norepinephrine or phenylephrine. Even when local anesthetics are injected intravenously along with epinephrine, in most cases the doses are not that high, thus causing only a temporary rise in blood pressure and heart rate. However, when high doses are administered, initial symptoms are hypertension and tachycardia, followed by hypotension and arrhythmias. This is due to the sudden elevation in blood pressure and heart rate caused by intravenous injection of epinephrine, which abruptly loads the heart, leading to acute heart failure caused by catecholaminergic cardiomyopathy or stress cardiomyopathy.

For surgeries on the nose, not only do surgeons inject in the nasal mucous membranes but they also use gauze soaked in lidocaine with epinephrine for nasal packing. For nasal packing, there are no set guidelines for the concentration of epinephrine on the gauze, thus making surgeons use high concentrations of epinephrine in many cases. According to a recent clinical report from the Korean Society of Anesthesiologists, a patient underwent nasal packing (with gauze soaked with lidocaine combined with epinephrine at 1:5,000 without a mucosal injection) and developed acute heart failure. Considering this case report and the concentration of lidocaine sprays (at 10% concentration, about 5 times higher than lidocaine used in intravenous injections), there seems to be no need for the epinephrine concentration for nasal packing gauze to be higher than 1:10,000-20,000.

4. Prevention and Treatment of Local Anesthetic Toxicity

1) Preventing Toxicity

The best way to avoid toxicity is to inject the minimum amount *(Table 4)* of drugs in the precise location. When injecting local anesthetics in nasal mucous membranes, it is best to inject intermittently while checking to see if the patient's blood regurgitates into the syringe. To check for regurgitation accurately, one should pull the syringe's handle slowly and softly. When pulled too quickly and with force, even if the needle is placed in a blood vessel, the blood vessel will collapse due to negative pressure and keep the blood from regurgitating. If one injects the drugs slowly and intermittently while checking the patient for signs of central nervous system toxicity and inadvertent injection into the blood vessels, it is possible to stop the further administration of anesthetic by immediately detecting the early signs of toxicity before larger doses are administered. If one avoids injection into blood vessels and using too much anesthetic, toxicity will be rare and, and even if side effects occur, immediate treatment will ensure minimal sequelae.

Table 4 Local Infiltration Anesthetics

Drug		Concentration (%)	Plain Solution		Epinephrine-Containing Solution	
			Maximum Dose (mg)	Duration (minutes)	Maximum Dose (mg)	Duration (minutes)
Short Duration	Procaine	1.0-2.0	500	20-30	600	30-45
	Chloroprocaine	1.0-2.0	800	15-30	1000	30
Moderate Duration	Lidocaine	0.5-1.0	300	30-60	500	120
	Mepivacaine	0.5-1.0	300	45-90	500	120
	Prilocaine	0.5-1.0	350	30-90	550	120
Long Duration	Bupivacaine	0.25-0.5	175	120-240	200	180-240
	Ropivacaine	0.2-0.5	200	120-240	250	180-240

2) Treating Toxicity

When symptoms occur in slow injections, in most cases stopping the injection, monitoring the blood pressure, administering oxygen, and patient reassurance will improve matters since the drug is redistributed rapidly and its blood concentration decreases quickly. If symptoms start to appear after administration of the entire dose, there is a danger of the local anesthetic's blood concentration continuing to rise. In such cases, one can check the patient's blood pressure and monitor ventilation while administering oxygen, give a small amount of thiopental or benzodiazepine, and assist spontaneous respiration by performing maneuvers to secure the airway (head tilt-chin list maneuver or jaw thrust).

Patients who exhibit severe or prolonged symptoms should be treated like patients who have had seizures. When the patient has a seizure or apnea, one must rapidly use airway-securing methods in order to ensure adequate ventilation; and if the patient's spontaneous respiration is insufficient, assisted ventilation must be done through an oral airway or through endotracheal intubation. Agitation can be treated by a low dose of barbiturates or benzodiazepines, and hypotension can be managed by epinephrine (dilute 1 ampule of 40mg/ml to make 8 ml and inject intravenously 1-2 ml at once) or phenylephrine (100 μg) initially, administering additional doses if necessary. One can use other vasopressor drugs (like dopamine) based on the patient's reaction. In cases of potentially lethal heart failure from an arrhythmia, use a defibrillator.

Barbiturates and benzodiazepines that are used in the management of toxicity in the central nervous system are drugs to treat seizures and agitation, not reversal agents of local anesthetics. It is important to keep in mind that they may induce hypoventilation, thus one must always ensure sufficient ventilation or respiration. In order to fully cure the toxicity of local anesthetics, there needs to be time for the drug to be metabolized and cleared, time during which the goal of treatment is to secure and maintain the airway and preserve hemodynamic stability.

References

1. American Society of Anesthesiologists Task Force on Sedation and Analgesia by Non-Anesthesiologists. Practice guidelines for sedation and analgesia by non-anesthesiologists. Anesthesiology 2002; 96: 1004-17.
2. Barash Paul G. Clinical anesthesia. 6th ed. Lippincott Williams & Wilkins 2009.
3. Kim JE, Kountakis SE. The prevalence of Samter's triad in patients undergoing functional endoscopic sinus surgery. Ear Nose Throat J 2007; 86: 396-9.
4. Morgan G, Edward Jr. Clinical Anesthesiology 4th Ed. McGraw-Hill 2005.
5. Ronald D. Miller. Miller's Anesthesia. 7th international ed. Churchill-livingstone 2009.

Section 02

Inside of the Nose

Turbinate Surgery

Yong Ju Jang · Ji Heui Kim

The inferior turbinates are mainly responsible for regulating airflow, conditioning the air through humidification and temperature regulation, and protection from inhaled particles. Hypertrophy of the inferior turbinate is a common cause of nasal obstruction, which can interfere with quality of life. This may occur as compensatory hyperplasia in patients with a deviated septum, or secondary to inflammatory conditions such as allergic rhinitis or vasomotor rhinitis.

Although septoplasty is the most important aspect in functional nasal surgery, turbinate surgery, although a relatively minor procedure, has great significance for the improvement of nasal obstruction. Several studies reported that the intranasal air temperature and humidity regulation, as well as nasal breathing function, improved after turbinoplasty combined with septoplasty or rhinoseptoplasty.

Hypertrophy of the inferior turbinate can be classified into mucosal hypertrophy and bony hypertrophy. Mucosal hypertrophy can be addressed with a decongestant, whereas bony hypertrophy cannot. Differentiating mucosal hypertrophy from bony hypertrophy can easily be made using acoustic rhinometry. If there is a notable change in the nasal volume or cross-sectional area after the decongestion, mucosal hypertrophy is strongly suspected. The diagnosis of allergic rhinitis using a skin test or blood test should be confirmed in patients with severe inferior turbinate hypertrophy.

I. Turbinate Surgery

It is preferable for inferior turbinate hypertrophy to be treated first with medications such as antihistamines, anticholinergics, corticosteroids, or sympathomimetics before attempting surgical treatment. It must be noted, however, that most medications that are effective against sneezing, itching, or rhinorrhea have limited efficacy when the main pathology is hypertrophy of the turbinate associated with nasal obstruction. There are various surgical treatment methods available in treating hypertrophied turbinates, including steroid injections, electrocautery, cryotherapy, laser vaporization, radiofrequency volume reduction, turbinate outfracture, inferior tubinectomy, and inferior turbinoplasty. If both the mucosa and bone of the turbinate are hypertrophied, conventional turbinoplasty or partial turbinectomy can be performed. If the condition is merely mucosal hypertrophy, microdebrider-assisted turbinoplasty, radiofrequency turbinate volume reduction, or laser turbinoplasty are usually recommended.

1. Lateralization by Outfracturing the Turbinate

This is a relatively simpler procedure compared to the other surgical techniques. It involves locating a Joseph elevator, knife handle, or Freer elevator at the lateral wall of the inferior turbinate and applying pressure to it to produce in-fracture (medial fracture). Then the elevator is relocated to the medial wall of the inferior turbinate and pushed toward the lateral wall so that the turbinate would be displaced toward the lateral wall of the nasal cavity (outfracture) and thereby create space within the nasal cavity. When the mucosal hypertrophy of the inferior turbinate is severe, this surgical technique is difficult to use alone. Thus, it is used as a supplementary technique during inferior turbinectomy or turbinoplasty *(Figure 1)*. One must note that this can result in delayed arterial bleeding.

2. Total or Partial Turbinectomy

This is a surgical procedure in which the inferior turbinate is totally or partially resected *(Figure 2)*. Total or partial turbinectomy should not be performed except for tumor surgery because it has a high risk of severely deteriorating the nasal function. The nasal manifestation secondary to turbinectomy is called atrophic rhinitis, wide nasal cavity syndrome, or empty nose syndrome.

3. Submucosal Resection of the Turbinate (Turbinoplasty)

This procedure involves partial resection of the anterior portion of the turbinate bone and lamina propria. It has the advantage of allowing the preservation of most of the mucosa, thereby maintaining a more physiologically normal nasal cavity *(Figure 3)*, and of having fewer complications such as postoperative crusting or bleeding than inferior turbinectomy.

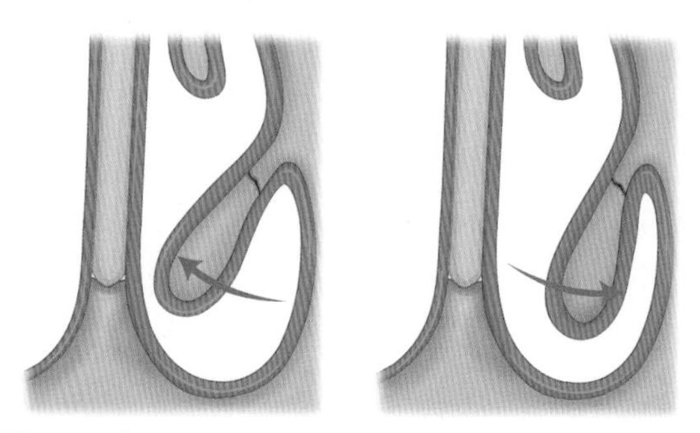

Figure 1 Lateral outfracture of the inferior turbinate.

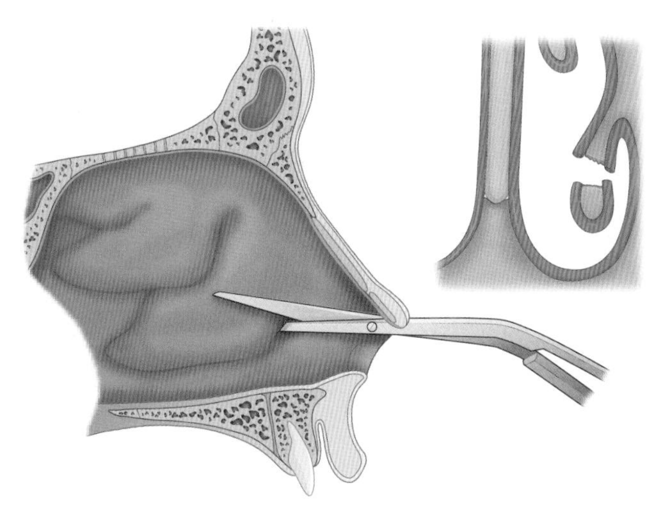

Figure 2 Inferior turbinectomy. This technique has a great potential to cause severe complications.

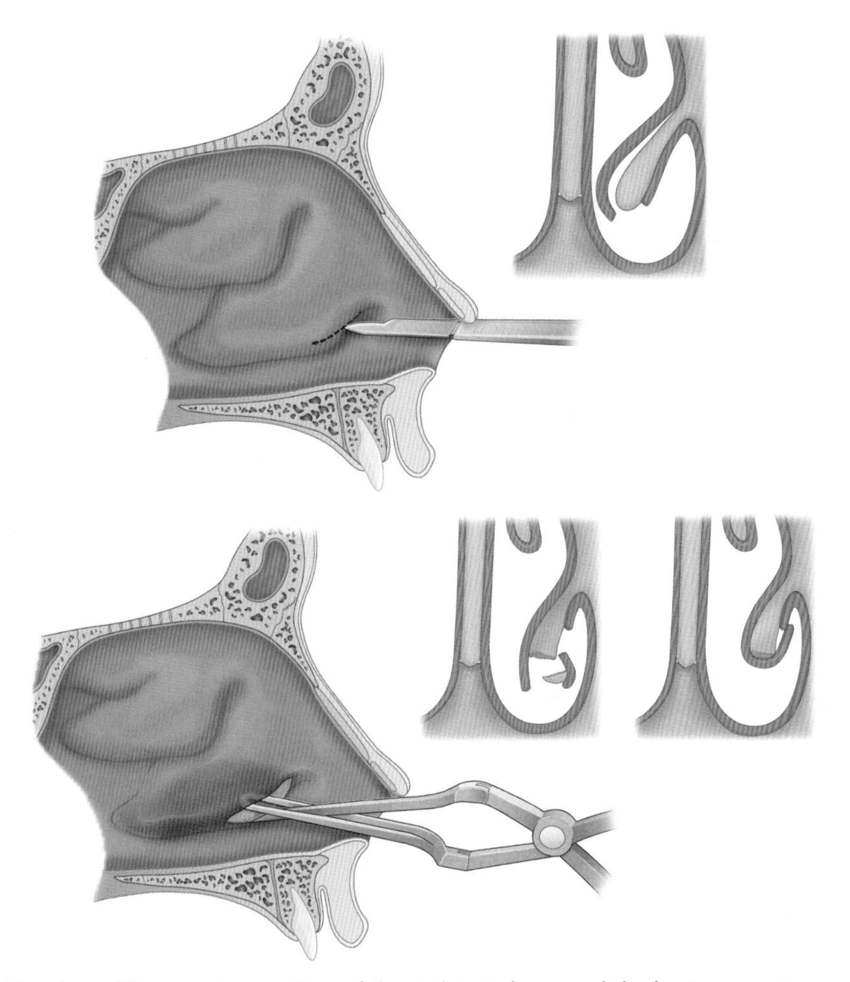

Figure 3 Turbinoplasty. The anterior portion of the turbinate bone and the lamina propria are partially resected after elevation of the medial mucosal flap. The exposed bone is covered using the remaining mucosa. Excision of the bone and mucosa should be minimized.

Turbinoplasty is usually performed in the following sequence:

① A local anesthetic agent is injected into the inferior turbinate and lateral nasal wall. Then a pledget saturated with local anesthetic is placed between the septum and inferior turbinate after decongestion. If needed, medial fracture of the inferior turbinate can be performed.

② Using a #15 blade, a vertical incision is made 1.5-2.0 cm along the antero-inferior margin of the inferior turbinate, reaching almost the turbinate bone. The 6 to 7 o'clock position is appropriate.

③ Using a Freer elevator, the mucoperiosteal flap is elevated to expose the turbinate bone.

④ Using a pair of cutting forceps or conchotomy scissors, the hypertrophic turbinate bone is removed. Then the medial mucosal flap of the inferior turbinate is conservatively resected. The remaining mucosa of the medial mucosal flap is rolled towards the lateral direction until it covers the exposed turbinate bone. As empty nose syndrome can be caused by excessive turbinoplasty, conservative turbinoplasty should be performed.

⑤ The posterior inferior turbinate is outfractured.

4. Microdebrider-Assisted Turbinoplasty

Microdebrider-assisted turbinoplasty is a procedure in which the submucosal tissue is removed using a microdebrider after making a submucosal pocket intraturbinally. The inferomedial and anterior hypertrophic submucosal tissue are mainly removed using the straight 2.0 or 3.5 mm turbinate blade of the microdebrider within the submucosal pocket, which is created using #15 blade under a 0° endoscope *(Figure 4)*.

The advantages of this technique are the accurate trimming of the submucosal tissue and preservation of the mucosa. However, if the submucosal tissue is excessively removed, packing is needed to obliterate the dead space. If the tip of the blade faces the inferomedial aspect of the inferior turbinate, the mucosa can be perforated or torn. Therefore, this method is inappropriate for reduction of the volume of turbinates with thin mucosa and bony hypertrophy. Although the mucosal surface can be extraturbinally trimmed using a microdebrider, this method damages the mucosa and may cause excessive bleeding during the operation as well as delayed wound healing.

5. Radiofrequency Turbinate Volume Reduction

Radiofrequency (RF) energy agitates ions and leads to the generation of frictional heat in the tissues around the electrode. Secondary contraction and fibrosis during wound healing subsequently decrease the tissue volume. This procedure is performed by placing the RF electrode submucosally in the anterior inferior portion of the turbinate. When the mucosa becomes pale, the delivery of RF energy should be stopped so as not to damage the surface of the mucosa *(Figure 5)*. As this method can preserve the turbinate mucosa, it is useful in addressing mucosal hypertrophy. However, an overly aggressive procedure can induce necrosis of the mucosa and/or turbinate bone. Thus, the surgeon must be careful not to burn the mucosa directly. The crust can last for a relatively long period. As with the microdebrider-assisted turbinoplasty, this technique is not indicated in patients without significant mucosal hypertrophy.

6. Laser-Assisted Turbinoplasty

CO_2 (10,600nm), Diode (805/810/940nm), Argon-Ion (488/514nm), Potassium-Titanyl-Phosphate (KTP) (532nm), Neodymium (Nd):YAG (1,064nm), or Holmium (Ho):YAG (2,080nm) lasers can be used. Laser-assisted turbinoplasty can be performed by partially resecting the turbinate tissue with the laser, making crosshatching incisions on the mucosa, or by vaporizing the submucosal tissue after creating a submucosal pocket.

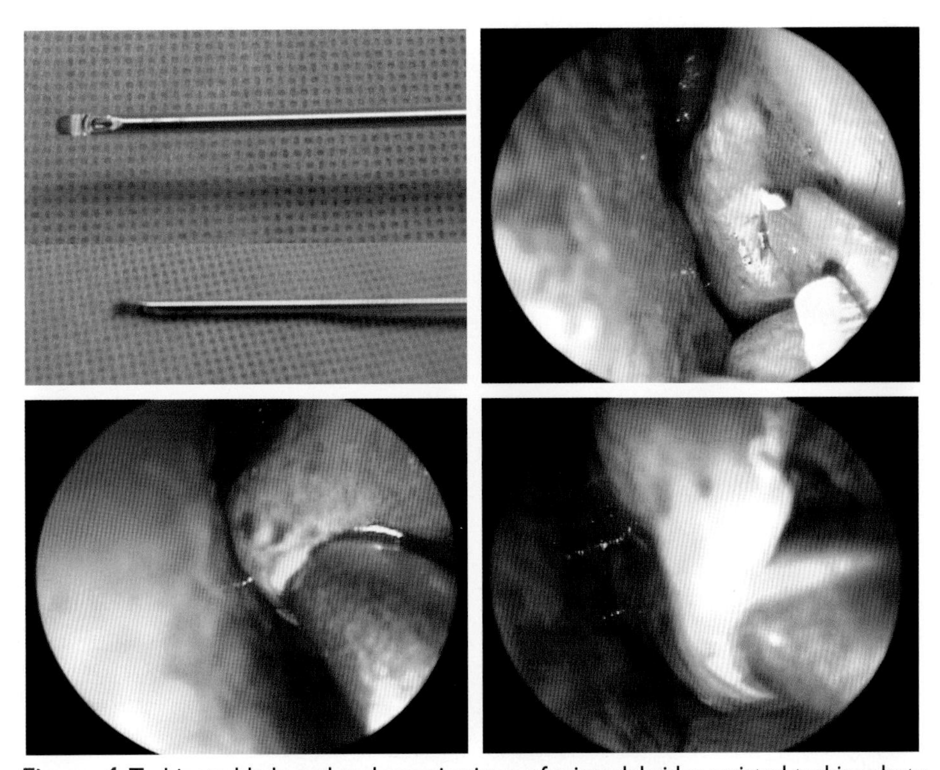

Figure 4 Turbinate blade and endoscopic views of microdebrider-assisted turbinoplasty.

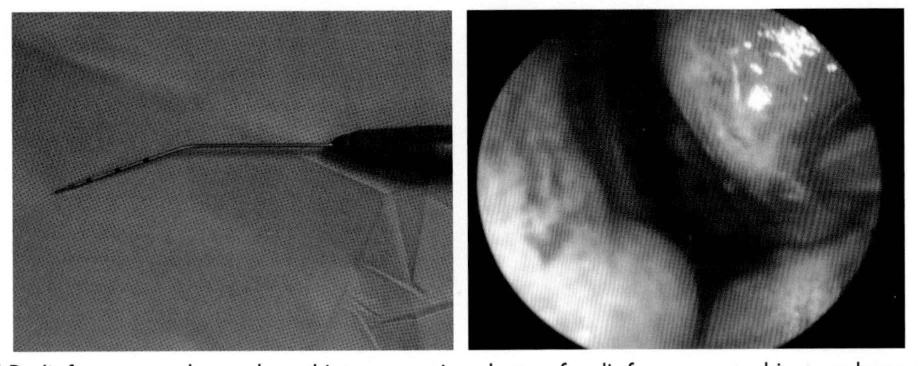

Figure 5 Radiofrequency electrode and intraoperative photo of radiofrequency turbinate volume reduction.

7. Submucosal Diathermy

A diathermy needle is inserted into the anterior end of the inferior turbinate and advanced submucosally up to the posterior end of the turbinate. Current application for 30 seconds will induce the mucosa to contract.

II. Complications of Turbinate Surgery

1. Bleeding

Bleeding is the most common early complication of turbinate surgery because of the abundant blood vessels in the inferior turbinate. Postoperative bleeding has been reported with a frequency of 3-25%. Fortunately, bleeding is often easily controlled. Because the incidence may be correlated with the degree of resection of the posterior portion, which is highly vascularized, postoperative bleeding occurs more often in turbinectomy or submucosal resection, than in other techniques. Bleeding can occur even after turbinate outfracture. Blood is supplied to the inferior turbinate mainly through the lateral branch of the sphenopalatine artery. This branch proceeds from the rear to the front of the inferior turbinate mucosa *(Figure 6)*. During surgery, damage of this branch can cause excessive bleeding.

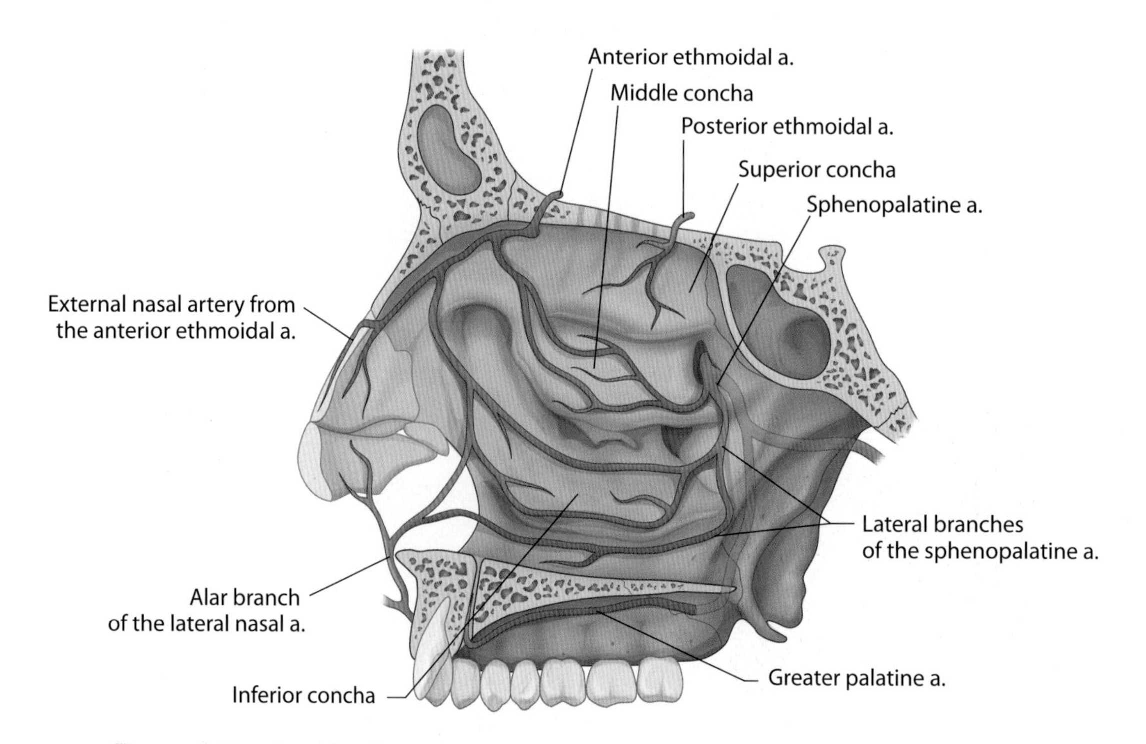

Figure 6 Abundant blood vessels in the inferior turbinate can cause postoperative bleeding.

Delayed hemorrhage may be due to dislodged clots as the packs are removed, or an inadequate excision that leaves posteriorly attached mucosal tags. This may be caused by poor technique or inappropriate pre-operative preparation using a topical decongestant.

2. Infection

Although infection very rarely occurs due to the abundant blood supply of the turbinates, postoperative infection can still occur.

3. Adhesions

Adhesions result from infection, concurrent septoplasty, or trauma to the septal mucosa leaving opposing raw surfaces.

4. Dryness and Crusting

Crusting is commonly observed in the early postoperative period, especially when the mucosa is directly damaged. Exposed bone frequently cause prolonged crusting with a foul odor. The most serious complication of turbinate surgery is empty nose syndrome, which causes long-lasting dryness and crusting.

5. Empty Nose Syndrome

Empty nose syndrome is a rare and serious iatrogenic disorder that manifests as a severely impaired nasal function caused by too aggressive turbinate reduction *(Figure 7)*. Though not all patients who had excessive turbinate resection experience debilitating empty nose syndrome symptoms, once empty nose syndrome develops, it negatively affects the normal breathing function of the nasal cavity. Patients with empty nose syndrome suffer from mucosal dryness, nasal congestion, facial pain, and headache when inhaling, and excessive crusting and discharge, as well as nasopharyngeal or chest discomfort on respiration. They usually suffer more in the dry and cold winter season than in summer.

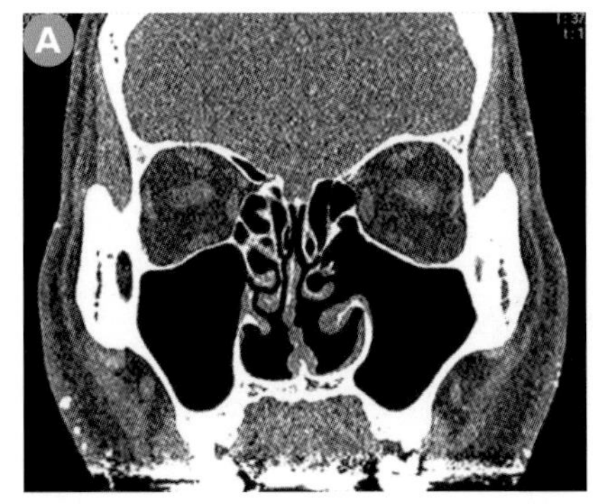

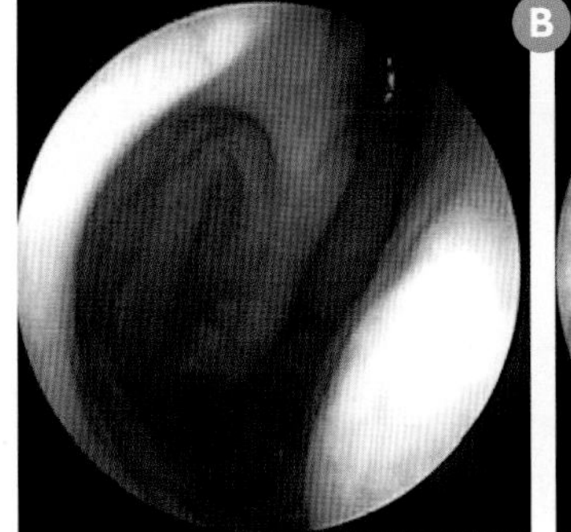
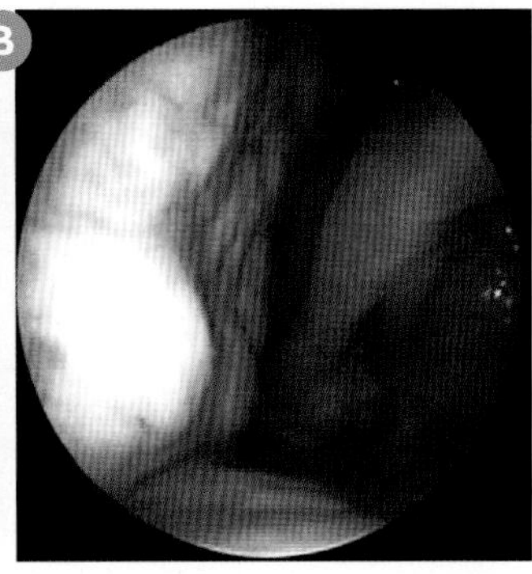

Figure 7 Coronal computed tomography scan (A), and endoscopic photographs of the nasal cavity of a patient with empty nose syndrome caused by bilateral inferior turbinectomy (B).

1) Diagnosis

Empty nose syndrome is diagnosed based on the following:

- ☑ Its characteristic symptoms, such as excessive airflow, nasal congestion, nasal or facial pain when inhaling, excessive crusting or discharge, and headache
- ☑ Partially or totally absent inferior turbinate tissue with abnormally wide nasal cavities in an endoscopic examination
- ☑ A history of partial or total turbinectomy

Excessive excision during inferior turbinectomy can reduce the regulatory capacity of the nasal cavity and expose the mucosa to dry air. This will in turn lead to an increased viscosity of mucus, crusting, bleeding, and dysfunction of the nasal mucosal ciliary movement. Furthermore, in patients with empty nose syndrome, mucosal inflammation and secondary sinusitis can develop because of the abnormally altered nasal airflow in the wide nasal cavity due to the deficient turbinate tissue, which can be seen in CT scans.

Conservative empty nose syndrome treatment includes nasal irrigation, use of nasal moisturizing ointments, and plugging of the nasal cavity. When the empty nose syndrome symptoms do not improve with conservative management, surgical treatment is indicated, in which a synthetic implant, allograft, or cartilage is submucosally implanted. Synthetic implant materials such as hydroxyapatite, or allograft materials such as AlloDerm, pose a great risk of extrusion, rejection, and infection. Cartilage does not have the disadvantages associated with synthetic implants and effectively relieves empty nose syndrome symptoms.

2) Surgical Techniques of Turbinate Reconstruction Using Cartilage

If the septal cartilage is sufficient for implantation, it is harvested, leaving at least a 1.0-1.5 cm-wide L-strut. If the patient had previously undergone septoplasty, conchal or costal cartilage is harvested *(Figure 8)*. To create a submucosal pocket, an incision is made at the inferolateral side of the lateral nasal wall, which is just at the anterior margin of the pyriform aperture. After the elevation of the mucoperiosteal flap, the pocket is filled with the cartilage implant to create a neoturbinate *(Figure 9)*. The pocket is closed with 4-0 chromic sutures to keep the cartilage implant in position, and nasal packings are placed overnight. In the authors' experience, turbinate reconstruction using costal cartilage has the best surgical outcome, because the neoturbinate can be sufficiently augmented.

6. Conchal Bone Necrosis and Sequestrum Formation

Necrosis and sequestrum formation may occur if the turbinate bone is directly cauterized or if the mucosa is seriously injured with radiofrequency.

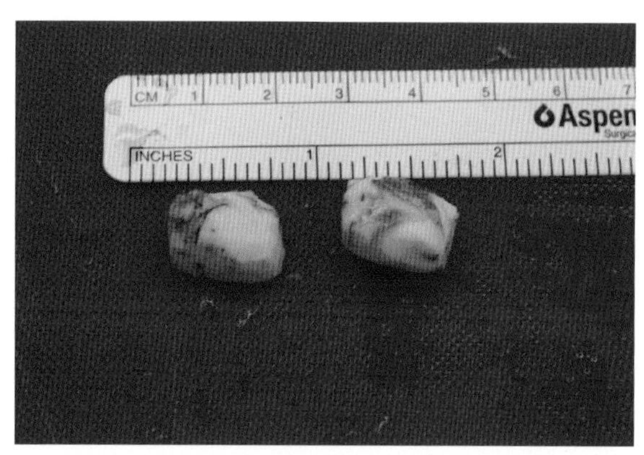

Figure 8 Harvested and carved costal cartilage for the treatment of bilateral empty nose syndrome.

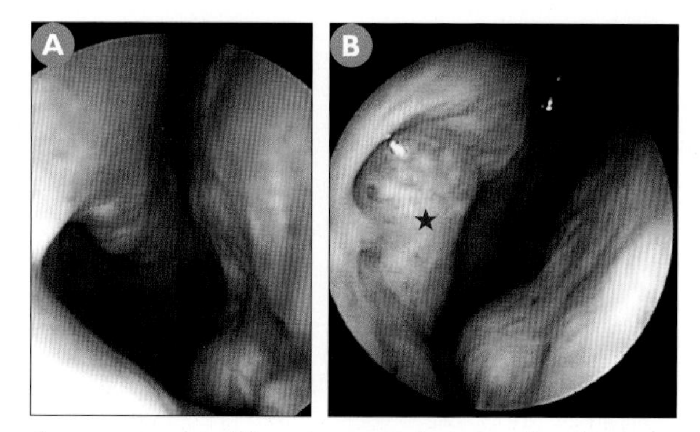

Figure 9 Preoperative (A) and postoperative (B) endoscopic findings of turbinate reconstruction using cartilage. The neoturbinate was created at the inferior side of the right inferior turbinate.

References

1. Cavaliere M, Mottola G, Iemma M.Comparison of the effectiveness and safety of radiofrequency turbinoplasty and traditional surgical technique in treatment of inferior turbinate hypertrophy. Otolaryngol Head Neck Surg 2005; 133: 972-8.
2. Cingi C, Ure B, Cakli H, Ozudogru E. Microdebrider-assisted versus radiofrequency-assisted inferior turbinoplasty: a prospective study with objective and subjective outcome measures. Acta Otorhinolaryngol Ital 2010; 30: 138-43.
3. Gupta A, Mercurio E, Bielamowicz S. Endoscopic inferior turbinate reduction: an outcome analysis. Laryngoscope 2011; 111: 1957-9.
4. Jang YJ, Kim JH, Song HY. Empty nose syndrome: radiologic findings and treatment outcomes of endonasal microplasty using cartilage implants. Laryngoscope 2011; 121: 1308-12.
5. Jung JH, Baguindali MA, Park JT, Jang YJ. Costal cartilage is a superior implant material than conchal cartilage in the treatment of empty nose syndrome. Otolaryngol Head Neck Surg. 2013; 149:500-5.
6. Liu CM, Tan CD, Lee FP, Lin KN, Huang HM. Microdebrider-assisted versus radiofrequency-assisted inferior turbinoplasty. Laryngoscope 2009; 119: 414-8.
7. Rozsasi A, Leiacker R, K-hnemann S, Lindemann J, Kappe T, Rettinger G, Keck T. The impact of septorhinoplasty and anterior turbinoplasty on nasal conditioning. Am J Rhinol 2007; 21: 302-6.
8. Wiesmiller K, Keck T, Rettinger G, Leiacker R, Dzida R, Lindemann J. Nasal air conditioning in patients before and after septoplasty with bilateral turbinoplasty. Laryngoscope 2006; 116: 890-4.
9. Van delden MR, Cook PR, Davis WE. Endoscopic partial inferior turbinoplasty. Otolaryngol Head Neck Surg 1999; 121: 406-9.

Septoplasty

Yong Ju Jang

Septoplasty is the most commonly recommended and performed surgical procedure to improve the nasal obstruction of the patients. Almost all external nasal deformities such as deviated nose, short nose, and saddle nose are associated with an underlying septal deviation *(Figure 1)*. Septoplasty is therefore a very important procedure in determining surgical success in rhinoplasty, on the other hand, poorly executed septoplasty can result in various nasal deformities.

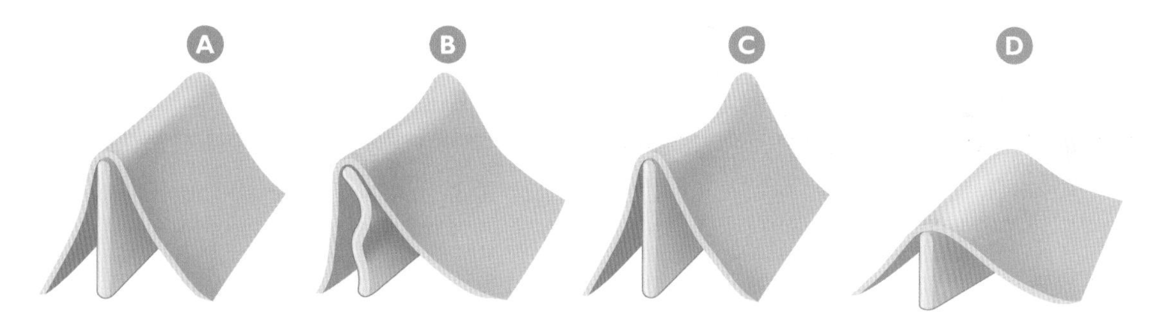

Figure 1 While a straight septum is a prerequisite for a normal looking nose (A), a deviated nasal septum can be the underlying cause of a deviated nose (B), saddle nose (C), and small nose (D) as shown above.

I. Indications for Septoplasty

During history taking, getting accurate information on the duration of the nasal obstruction is important. In patients showing severe septal deviation but complaining of acute onset symptoms, the cause of the nasal obstruction may not be due to the septal deviation, but to acute sinusitis or rhinitis. The author's indications for septoplasty are the following:

- ☑ Chronic nasal obstruction ipsilateral to the constricted side due to the deviated septum

- ☑ Alternating nasal obstruction showing septal deviation and compensatory hypertrophy of the inferior turbinate
- ☑ A patient demonstrating a septal spur or ridge which is suspicious of causing contact point headache and nasal obstruction
- ☑ Septal deviation in a patient undergoing endoscopic sinus surgery
- ☑ Septal deviation associated with an external nasal deformity

II. Preoperative Evaluation

In order to rule out a hidden paranasal sinus pathology, radiologic examinations of the sinonasal cavity such as plain films or CT scans need to be checked prior to surgery. Allergy testing must be done to diagnose allergic rhinitis. For documentation purposes, objective tests for airway patency such as acoustic rhinometry or rhinomanometry needs to be performed in the preoperative evaluation. Endoscopic photographs of the nasal cavity should be acquired before surgery, as it helps to explain postsurgical changes to the patient *(Figure 2)*. Occasionally, there are patients who complain of postoperative changes in the shape of the nose. It is therefore mandatory to take preoperative facial photographs of the patient *(Figure 3)*. For better diagnosis of caudal septal deviation, a Cottle test needs to be done at the outpatient clinic.

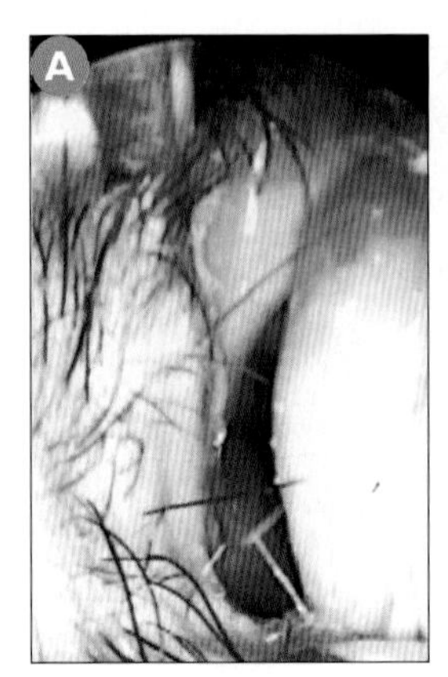

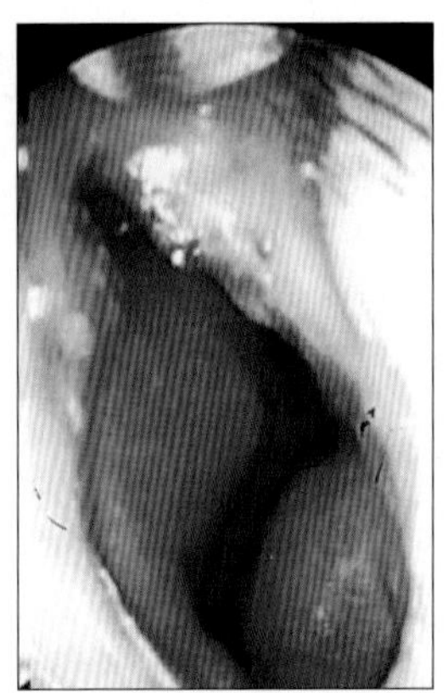
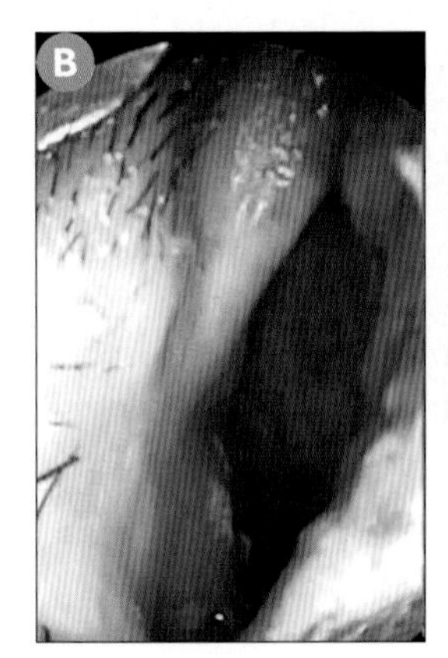

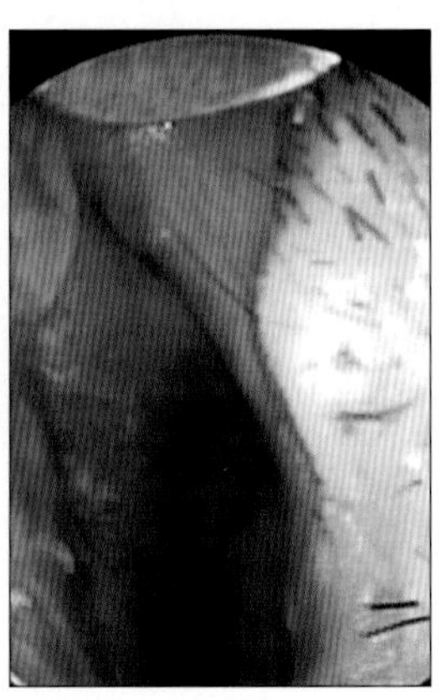

Figure 2 Endoscopic photograph of the nasal cavity showing severe caudal deviation. Before surgery (A), and after surgery (B).

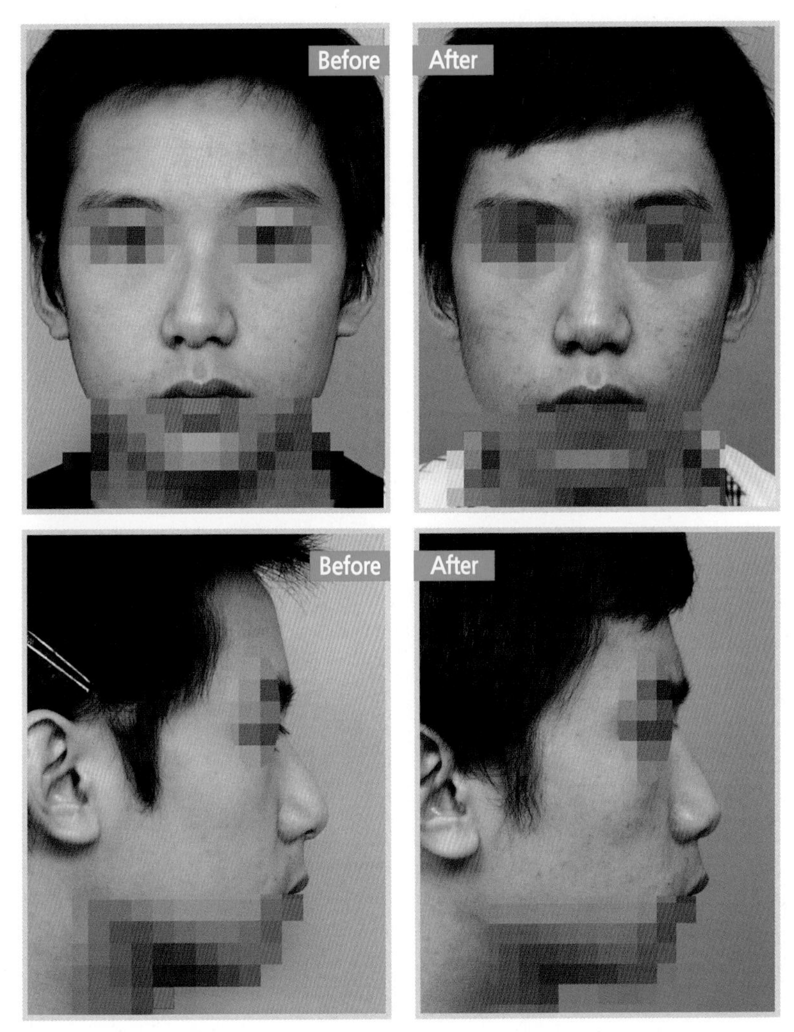

Figure 3 A patient who complained of posto-septoplasty change in the nasal shape. By the use of facial photographs, the patient was explained about the favorable changes after septoplasty.

III. Classification of Septal Deviation

The shape and direction of the septal deviation is hugely diverse, not allowing for easy and systematic classification. Each different type of septal deviation needs to be corrected by tailored surgical techniques. Based on the treatment strategy, The author classifies septal deviations into four different types and one mixed type. This classification is practical as it helps in performing the septoplasty in a more systematic way.

1. Focal Projection: Septal Deviation due to Bony Spur or Ridge *(Figure 4)*

This deviation is characterized by the presence of a bony ridge or spur in the vomer or maxillary crest, not associated with cartilaginous deviation. Septoplasty to correct this deformity can be performed by elevation of a unilateral mucosal flap on the opposite side and resection of the problematic bony structure. Endoscope guided septoplasty can also be performed through the ipsilateral side of the deviation. When performing this procedure, a mucosal incision caudal to the bony prominence is made, the mucosal flap is elevated around the spur or ridge, and the bony prominence and overlying cartilage is resected. After resecting the spur or ridge, the septal mucosal flap is redraped without suture closure. In this procedure, integrity of the contralateral septal mucosa should be preserved.

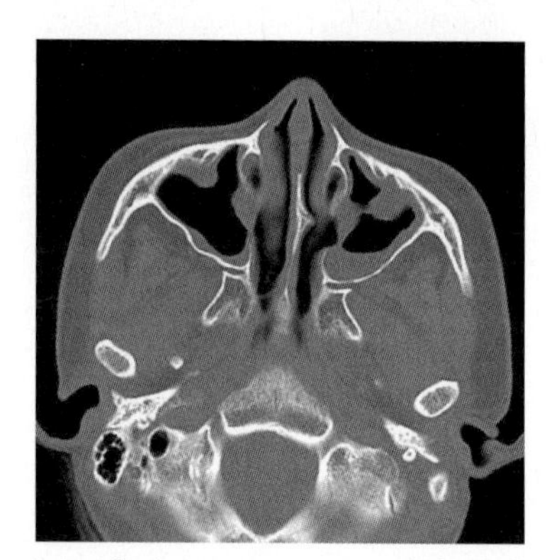

Figure 4 Focal projection of a bony spur toward the left side of the nasal cavity.

2. Deviation of Mid Part or Posterior Septum *(Figure 5)*

This type of deviation is easiest to correct. To correct the deviation, a unilateral mucosal flap is elevated usually at the concave side of the septum. Removal of the deviated bone and cartilage leaving wide enough L-strut can adequately correct this type of deviation.

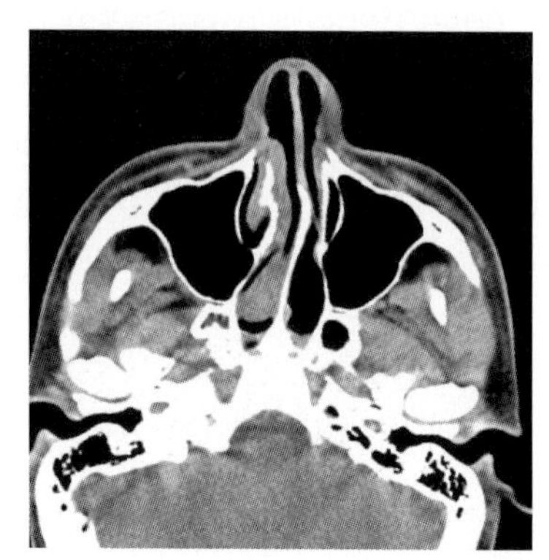

Figure 5 Posterior septal deviation due to deviated bony septum toward the left side.

3. Caudal Septal Deviation *(Figure 6)*

Caudal septal deviation is the most common and difficult to treat type of deviation causing sensation of nasal obstruction and nasal deformity. Caudal septal deviation severely limits the normal dimensions of both the internal and external valves, and is difficult to treat. The difficulty stems from the complexity in overcoming the intrinsic elastic memory of cartilage. Caudal septal deviation without an associated external nasal deformity is better managed via the endonasal approach, however if this is associated with a deformity of the external nose, the author prefers to correct this problem through an open rhinoplasty approach. Detailed treatment methods will be discussed later in this Chapter.

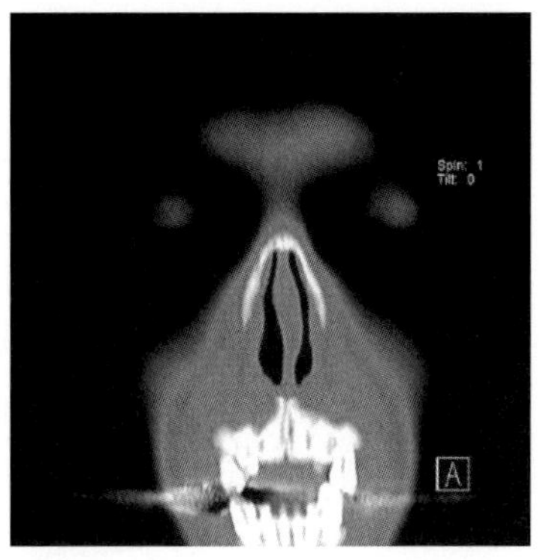

Figure 6 Typical CT scan of caudal septal deviation.

4. High Septal Deviation *(Figure 7)*

The majority of high septal deviations is a secondary phenomenon from the deviated perpendicular plate of the ethmoid. When correcting this deviation through an endonasal approach, resection of the deviated bone and adjoining septal cartilage with preservation of a generous-L-strut is best. However this technique may jeopardize the stability of septal support when there is not enough dorsal L-strut remaining after resection of the deviated portion. It is therefore extremely difficult to correct severe high septal deviation through an endonasal approach, so an external rhinoplasty approach for severe high septal deviation is justifiable because an external nasal deformity frequently accompanies this group of patients.

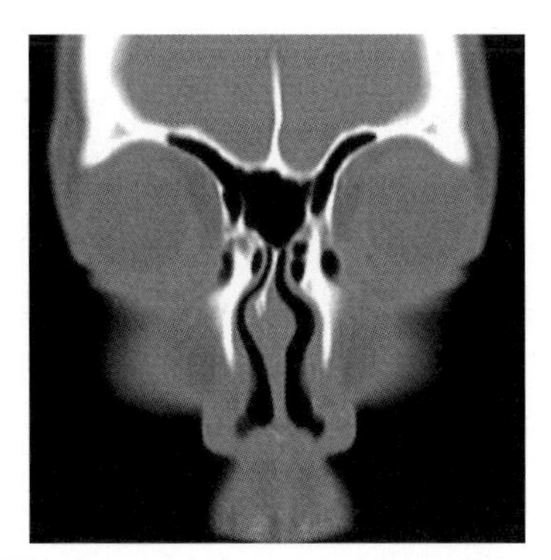

Figure 7 High septal deviation toward the right side.

5. Mixed Deviations

In clinical practice, it is sometimes difficult to make a clear distinction between the four types of deviations described above. In reality, septal deviations having mixed features of the four types is most common, and this can be classified as a mixed deviation. Combination of any of the four types is possible.

IV. Surgical Techniques

Septoplasty consists of correction of the cartilaginous and bony parts of the septum. Correction of the bony deviation usually involves direct excision of the deviated segment, or fracture-displacement into the desired position. Correction of the cartilaginous deviation is performed subsequent to bony correction. The most definitive treatment method is resecting the deviated cartilage. However, because of the importance of the septal cartilage in supporting the nose, key important areas for nasal support should be preserved in all situations. When the patient has relatively strong and thick cartilage, preserving an L-strut of 1 cm width is acceptable. However, in patients with thin and weak cartilage, it is better to preserve as big an L-strut as possible. In patients who have extremely thin septal cartilage, which is often the case in female Korean patients, it is best to preserve the entire septal cartilage and not make any incisions on the cartilage surface. For proper execution of the various septoplasty techniques, elevation of the unilateral septal mucoperichondrium in the proper subperichondrial anatomic plane is of utmost importance.

1. Conventional Septoplasty *(Figure 8)*

Septal mucoperichondrium on the concave side is elevated after making a hemitransfixion incision. After completion of the unilateral mucosal dissection, a boomerang-shaped cartilage excision is done at junctional area with the perpendicular plate of the ethmoid and the vomer. During this procedure the bone-cartilage junction at the dorsal and caudal portions are preserved. The mucosal flap covering the septal bone on the contralateral side is elevated through the chondrotomy site. After elevation of the mucosa on both sides of the septal bone, the deviated bone or bony spur is excised using bone cutting scissors and forceps. The remaining cartilaginous deviation after resection of the bony part is subsequently corrected by making crosshatching incisions on the concave side expecting it to become straight as secondary intention. This technique has commonly been used as a substitute of classical submucous resection of the septum. However, there are not enough outcome studies on the efficacy of this technique which have the inherent weakness of unpredictable surgical outcome. In the author's experience, this technique is only effective for septal deviations in which a bony deviation is the main pathology and a cartilaginous deviation is secondary phenomenon. However, this technique cannot be the panacea of all the different types of septal deviation. There is a report showing that only the removal of the bony deviation can straighten the entire septum in many cases. Expecting the septal cartilage to become straight by multiple incisions on the cartilage is unpredictable. It is practically impossible to make numerous incisions of the same depth. Furthermore, incisions on the cartilage surface have the risk of deforming the cartilage in the long run, rather than straightening the cartilage. This ill effect of crosshatching incisions can be commonly found in revision septoplasty cases where the septal cartilage is deformed and scarred with intervening soft tissue due to incisions made during the previous septoplasty *(Figure 9)*.

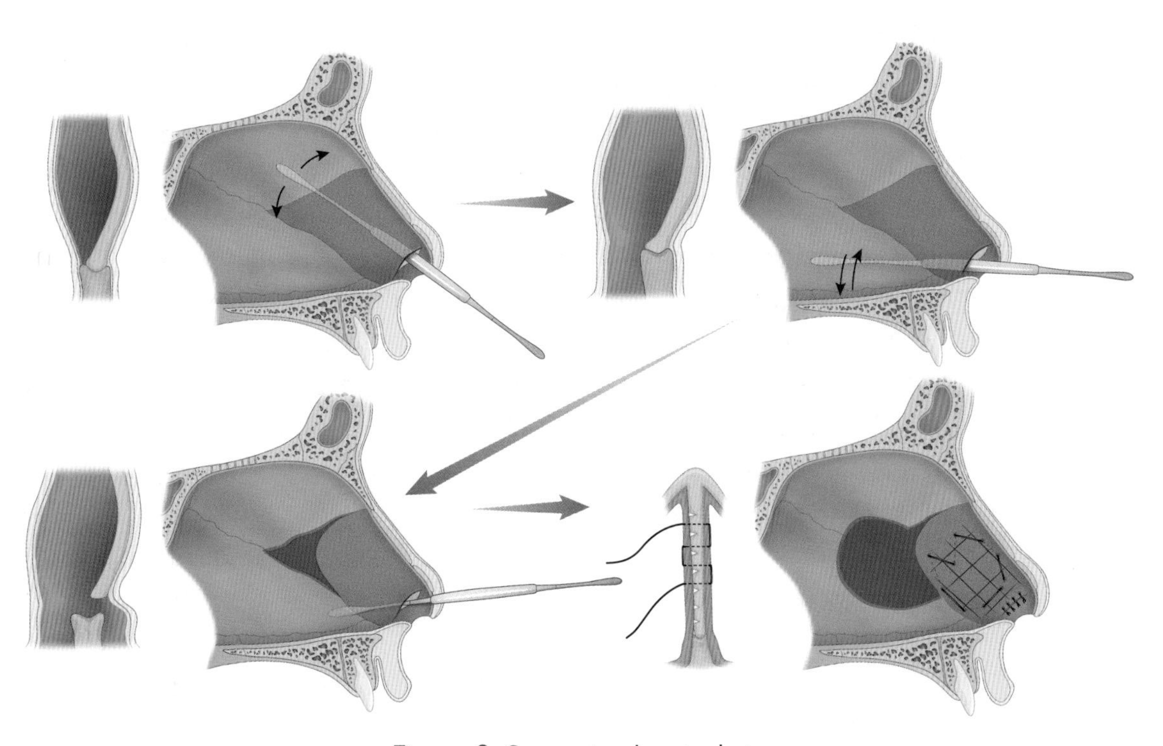

Figure 8 Conventional septoplasty.

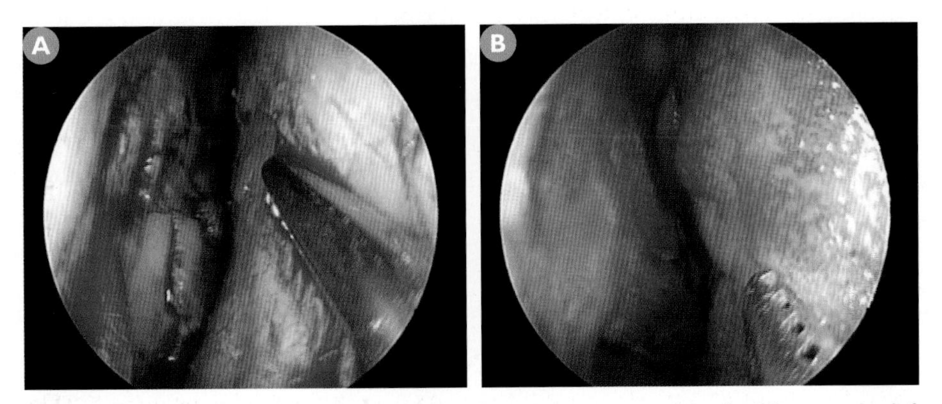

Figure 9 Detrimental effect of cross hatching incisions of a previous septoplasty. Incisions on the left-sided cartilage surface further deformed the septal cartilage as shown from the inside of the septal mucosal flap (A), and from the right nasal cavity (B).

2. Author's Septoplasty by Graduated Approach

The author experienced high failure rates in correcting the cartilaginous septal deviation by using the conventional technique relying on crosshatching incisions. Difficulty in obtaining consistent, satisfactory, and predictable outcomes using previously published endonasal septoplasty techniques led the author to seek a different approach for the correction of caudal septal deviation. Based on the author's experience, the septoplasty via endonasal approach was modified as follows *(Figure 10)*:

First, a unilateral hemistransfixion incision on the caudal margin of the septal cartilage is made on the concave side of the nasal cavity. This incision is made little more caudal than a typical hemistransfixion incision, and exposes the entire caudal border of the septum from the anterior septal angle down to the anterior nasal spine. Through this incision, a complete elevation of the ipsilateral septal mucoperichondrium all the way to the posterior part of the bony septum can be completed. Next, mucoperichondrium on the contralateral side is elevated, not by making an additional incision, but by crossing over to the contralateral side through the one incision made previously. Mucosal dissection on the convex side is performed until the point just caudal to the maximally convex part. Then, the central part of the quadrangular cartilage is resected leaving generous L-strut about 2 cm in width. Resection of the deviated perpendicular plate of ethmoid or vomer must be performed as a next step. At this stage, if there is complete correction of the septal deviation without caudal septal deviation, the procedure is terminated and the septal mucosa is closed. However, if there is persisting caudal septal deviation, additional maneuvers to correct the cartilaginous septum are done.

3. Surgical Treatment of Caudal Septal Deviation

1) Septal Batten Graft

Caudal septal deviation disturbs the normal nasal breathing because of the narrowing of the external nasal valve and the nasal valve angle. Management of caudal septal deviation is difficult because it is hard to overcome the intrinsic cartilage memory. Traditional surgical methods used for correcting caudal septum deviation include morselization, crosshatching incisions, partial thickness incision, swinging-door flap, and anchoring sutures. Although those techniques provide good immediate postoperative results, problems can emerge over time, including recurrence, saddle deformities due to L-strut weakness, and caudal septum displacement. However, caudal septal batten grafting is an excellent technique by which one can strengthen and straighten the caudal septum.

(1) Surgical Technique

A caudal septal batten graft created from the harvested septal cartilage is fitted to the desired location using counter-curvature, usually on the concave side (but may be done on both sides if there are concerns about graft tilt), and is sutured using three or four stitches. Batten grafts can

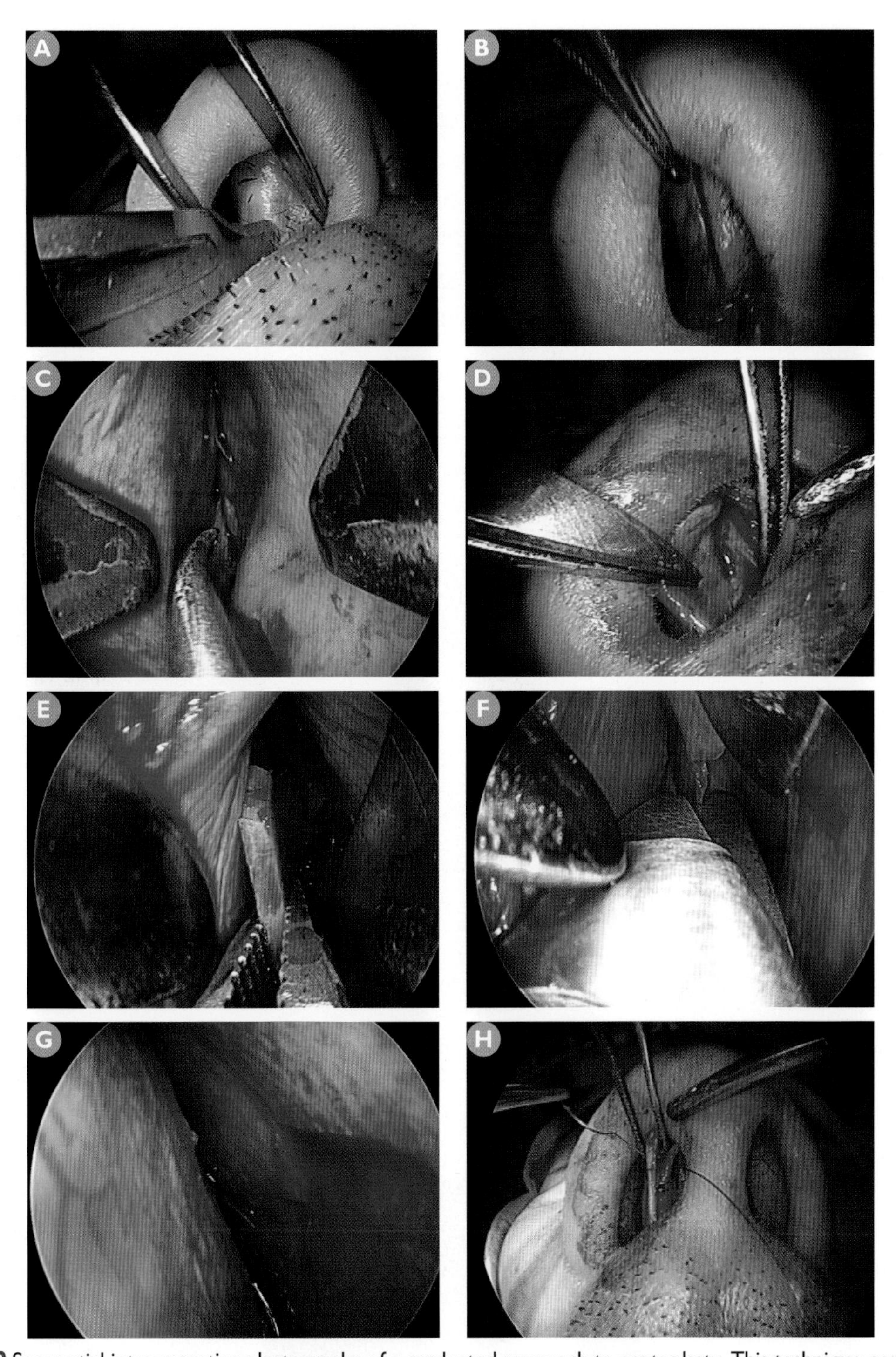

Figure 10 Sequential intraoperative photographs of a graduated approach to septoplasty. This technique consists of incision (A, B), mucosal flap elevation on the concave side (C), mucosal flap elevation on the opposite side through the same incision (D), resecting the central segment of septal cartilage leaving an L-strut (E), resecting deviated septal bone (F), septum after removal of cartilage and bone (G), and placement of caudal septal batten graft on the right side (H).

be placed with or without scoring incisions on the caudal L-strut *(Figure 11)*. The author prefers not making any scoring incisions because of concern of weakening of the caudal L-strut. The length of the septal batten graft will depend according to the size of the cartilage available, but it should cover the entire height of the caudal septum and should have a similar width with the remaining caudal L-strut. The gap between the posterior portions of the caudal septal batten graft and the caudal septum is closed using 1 or 2 through-and-through transcartilage sutures. Septal bone removed during septoplasty can also be used as batten graft material *(Figure 12)*. Because of its rigid nature, a bony batten graft can hold the curved caudal septum straight, and gives a more

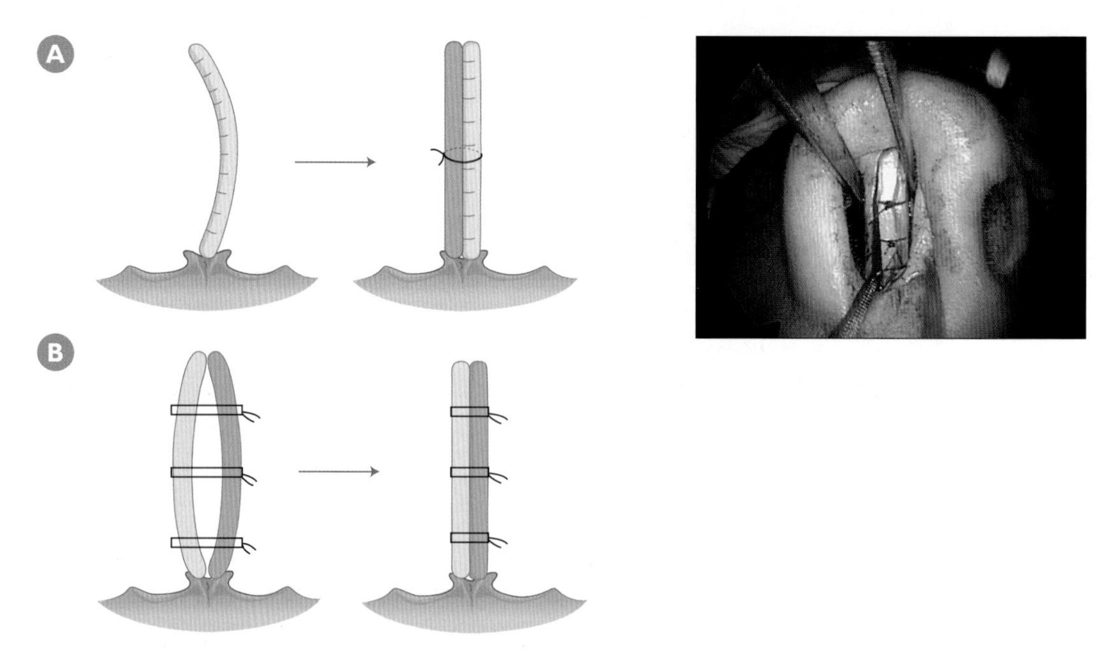

Figure 11 Septal batten graft is placed on the concave side of the caudal septum with (A) or without (B) scoring incisions on the preserved caudal L-strut.

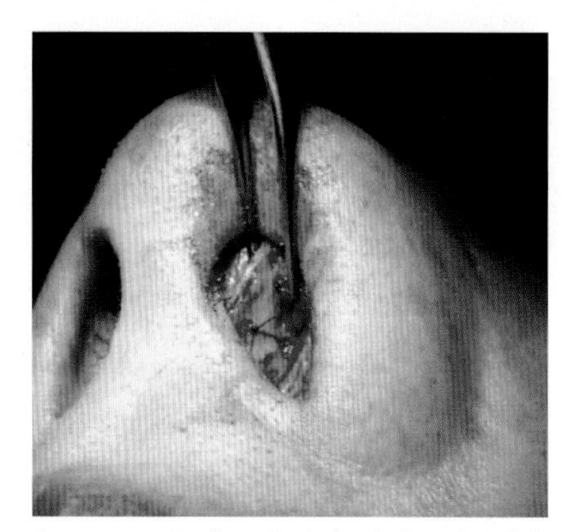

Figure 12 Bony batten graft placed at the left side of the caudal septum.

predictable result. Fixation of the bone with the caudal septum is made easier by drilling a number of holes on the bone through which suture needle easily passes. The author recommends drilling as many holes as possible for the sake of easier suture fixation with the caudal septum. In revision septoplasty where one cannot get enough septal cartilage or bone for a batten graft, conchal cartilage can be used as an alternative graft material.

(2) Advantages and Disadvantages of Batten Grafting:

Caudal septal betten grafting has following advantages:

- Intrinsic caudal septal support is maintained.
- The relationship between the caudal septum and anterior nasal spine is augmented.
- If necessary, the caudal septum can be lengthened by modification of the batten graft.
- Because the excised septal cartilage is saved, revision surgery can easily be performed using the stored cartilage if problems occur.

The major potential drawbacks of caudal septal batten grafting are:

- The contralateral nasal airway may be narrowed by the batten graft.
- The grafted batten can be bent following the curvature of the original caudal septum.

2) Cutting and Suture Technique of the Caudal Septum

(1) Theoretical Background

Caudal septal deviation can be manifest as a form of cephalo-caudal deviation and anterior-posterior deviation. In cases of deviation in the anterior-posterior direction, the caudal septum represents a C-shaped convexity, or an acute angulation less frequently. The underlying abnormality of anterior-posterior caudal deviation is usually excess septal cartilage length between the maxillary crest and the nasal roof. To straighten the cartilage, a small segment of the posterior end of the caudal septum can be resected, which can bring the caudal septum in a straight and midline position. However, the resected end needs to be reconnected with the anterior nasal spine and maxillary crest, which is difficult to reconstruct with its original strong attachment. The difficulty of reconstruction in this area is due to the complex three-dimensional relationship between the cartilage and the bony shelf; the nasal spine and the maxillary crest are tilted towards the nasal cavity. Thus, resecting the posterior end of the caudal septum carries a significant risk of inducing saddle nose deformity. The author tries to preserve strong attachment between the caudal septum and anterior nasal spine by cutting and overlapping of the convex-most part of the caudal septal L-strut that can reduce the excess length, thereby creating a straight caudal septal segment while not affecting the original tip height.

(2) Surgical Technique

After bilateral flap elevation as described before, the caudal struts is cut using scissors at the convex-most region. The excess portions of the upper and lower caudal struts are then overlapped, and the overlapping cartilages are sutured together using 3 to 4 stitches of 5-0 PDS. Straightening of the cartilage can be seen immediately after this cutting and overlapping suture maneuver. The degree of overlapping cartilage is adjusted such that the vertical height of the original caudal septum is not shortened as a result of overlapping. If the stability of the newly created caudal septum is in question, a septal batten graft made from cartilage removed from the central part is placed for further support, usually on the concave side *(Figure 13)*. Closure of the hemitransfixion incision is then performed and the surgery is concluded once straightening of the deviated caudal septum is confirmed.

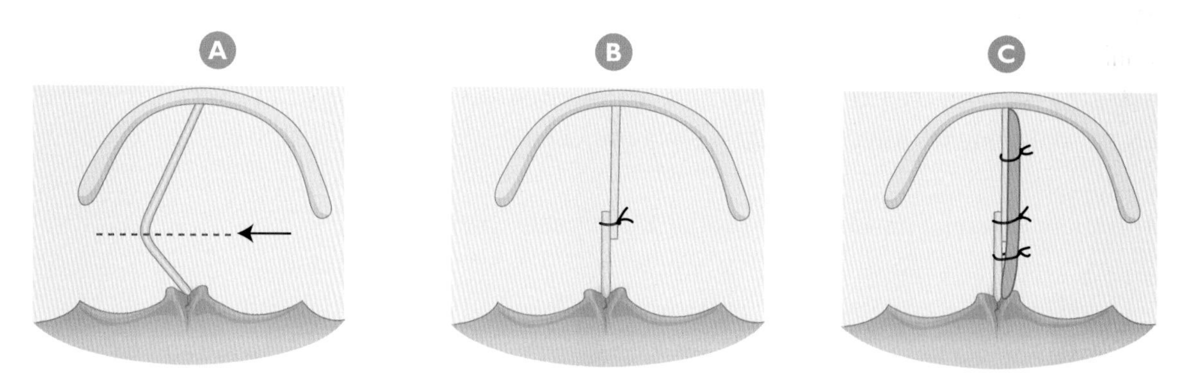

Figure 13 Cutting and suture technique of the caudal septum. An Incision is made at the convex- most part (A), cut-ends of septal cartilage are overlapped and sutured (B), and a batten graft can be placed at the concave side to provide additional support (C).

(3) Advantages and Disadvantages

The cutting and suture technique has several advantages over other corrective techniques for caudal septal deviation:

- ☑ It is useful for revision cases involving depleted septal cartilage due to previous surgery.
- ☑ It is useful for the simultaneous correction of the caudal deviation of the external nose and nasal obstruction.
- ☑ This technique completely breaks the cartilage memory for bending. An immediate intraoperative verification of straightening of the caudal septum is possible, and there is a low risk of deviation recurrence.

The cutting and suture technique has several potential drawbacks:

- Formation of the L-strut by removing the central part of the cartilage is required in every case.
- It is not applicable for linear-type caudal septal deviations with displacement from the anterior nasal spine.
- Too much overlap or loosening of the suture may shorten the caudal septal length, resulting in a saddle nose deformity.

3) Subtotal Replacement of the Caudal Septum

When the caudal septum is severely deviated or hypertrophied due to repeated trauma, no technique previously described can be applied. In this case, the severely deviated caudal septum is resected, and is replaced with straighter cartilage harvested from the central part *(Figure 14)*. This subtotal replacement technique is useful in extremely difficult caudal septal deviations.

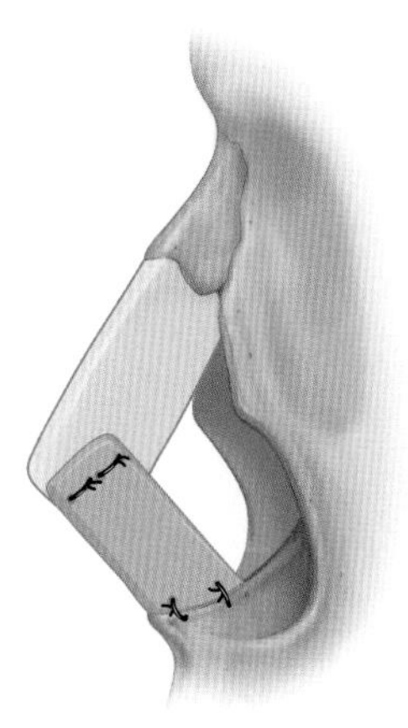

Figure 14 Subtotal replacement of the caudal septum to correct severe caudal septal deviation.

4) Treatment of Cephalo-Caudal Deviation

The caudal septum could not only show deviation towards the anterior-posterior direction, but could also show severe deviation in the cephalo-caudal direction as well. In many cases of cephalo-caudal deviation, overly developed cartilages are shown in the caudal part. In these situations, the author first cuts off the overly developed surplus cartilage in the caudal part perpendicularly. Then this excised cartilage is used as a septal extension graft graft placed on the wider nasal cavity to correct the deviation and to compensate for the shortened septal length.

This maneuver can compensate for the shortening of the caudal septum caused by the excision of cartilage *(Figure 15)*. Conducting a wedge excision on the lower part of the caudal septum is another option, which enables the surgeon to mobilize and fix the caudal septum in the desired direction and location *(Figure 16)*.

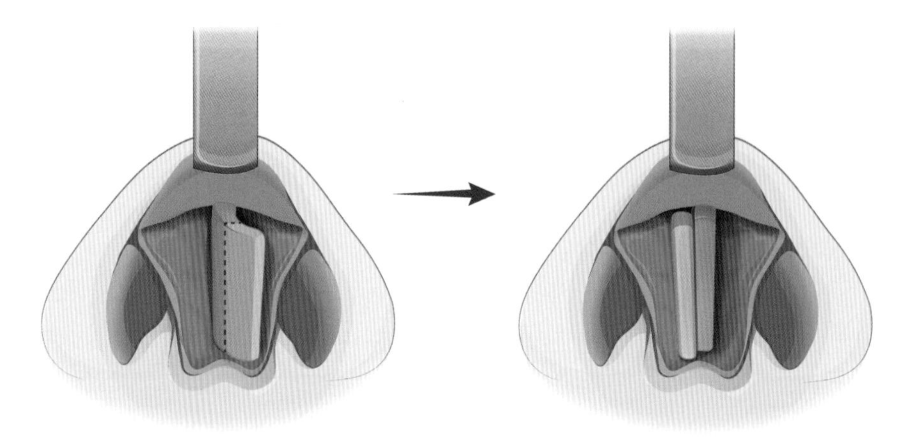

Figure 15 Excision of curved excess cartilage in the caudal part perpendicularly. This excised cartilage is used as a septal extension graft placed on the wider nasal cavity to correct the deviation and to compensate for the shortened septal length.

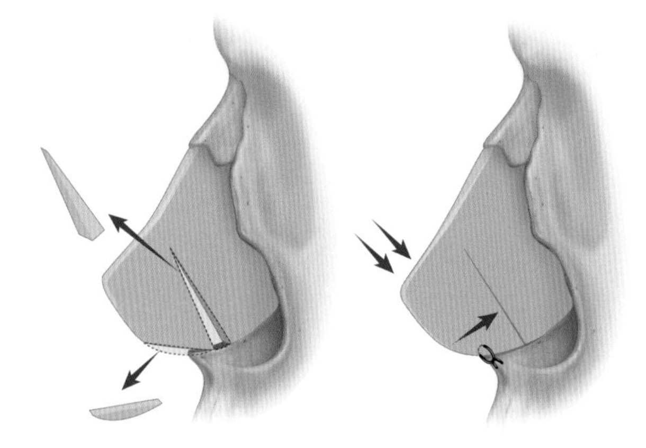

Figure 16 Wedge excision on the lower part of the caudal septum is another surgical option, which enables the surgeon to mobilize and fix the caudal septum in desired direction and location.

5) Dislocated Caudal Septum from the Anterior Nasal Spine

Excess cartilage of the displaced inferior portion should be resected. The remaining caudal septum should be carefully placed onto the anterior nasal spine and be suture-fixated with the soft tissue around the anterior nasal spine *(Figure 17)*. One should be wary that too much resection may result in shortening of the caudal height and saddle nose deformity.

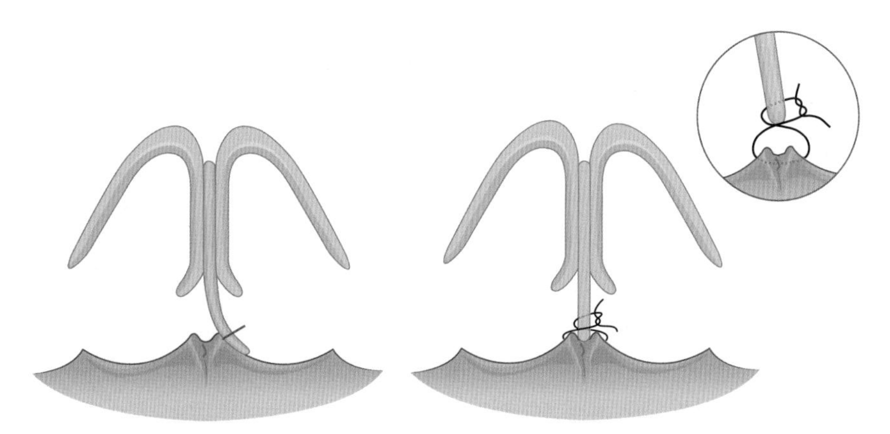

Figure 17 Excess cartilage of the displaced inferior portion should be resected. The remaining caudal septum should be carefully placed onto the anterior nasal spine and be suture-fixated with the soft tissue around the anterior nasal spine.

V. Complications

1. Persistent Nasal Obstruction (Incomplete Correction)

If the patient complains of unresolved nasal obstruction after septoplasty, the surgeon has to check whether there is undercorrection of the deviated nasal septum. If the septum looks straight, other possible causes of nasal obstruction should be looked at. Undercorrection of the septal deviation is the most common reason for functional dissatisfaction after septoplasty, however an incomplete management of compensatory turbinate hypertrophy, allergic rhinitis, or paranasal sinusitis can be the causative factors as well. Overcorrection of the septum resulting in deviation of the septal cartilage towards the opposite direction of the original deviation can also be a reason for nasal obstruction. This complication can easily take place after the conventional septoplasty using cross-hatching incisions, and tends to occur more frequently in pediatric patients. Abnormalities in the nasal valve should also be suspected when there is postoperative nasal obstruction. In the author's experience, undercorrection of the caudal septal deviation was the most common cause of unsuccessful surgical outcome.

2. Septal Hematoma

A septal hematoma is a collection of blood within the septal mucoperichondrium. Inadequate treatment of a septal hematoma may result in necrosis of the remaining septal cartilage and resultant saddle nose deformity. Hematoma of a minor degree can be absorbed spontaneously and cause fibrosis and thickening of the septal mucosa. When there is a septal hematoma following septoplasty, patients can feel persistent or even worse nasal obstruction, and tenderness and pain on the nose. Endoscopy reveals focal bulging of the septum with a round contour and fluctuation. Hematoma in the inferior part of the septal mucosa may be associated with a swollen and discolored upper lip. Once a septal hematoma is suspected, prompt drainage of the hematoma should be done. Before incision and drainage, topical anesthesia with lidocaine pledgets is done. A horizontal incision at the lower part of the hematoma pocket is made, and the blood is sucked out. Placement of nasal packing for one or two days after drainage can prevent recurrence of the hematoma. If the hematoma is very big and localized at the caudal part, the previous septoplasty incision must be opened again for complete suctioning of the accumulated blood. In severe cases, placement of a silastic splint is helpful for post-treatment management.

3. Olfactory Dysfunction

Post-septoplasty olfactory dysfunction is a not so infrequent problem, thought to be caused by hypoxic or mechanical injury to the olfactory epithelium by preoperative packing for surface anesthesia, postoperative packing for hemostasis, or by direct surgical manipulation. In most cases, olfactory dysfunction after septoplasty is hyposmic, and improves spontaneously. However, very rarely, olfactory dysfunction may persist into permanent hyposmia or anosmia. When postoperative olfactory dysfunction is found, patients need to be reassured that the prognosis is good, and a course of systemic corticosteroids for about 7 to 10 days is helpful.

4. Septal Perforation

Septal perforation is one of the common complications of septoplasty, and is mainly due to mucosal injury that occurs during surgery. Nasal mucosa may be easily torn during dissection in septal surgery, and the process requires special attention as perforations and ischemic necrosis may occur due to the deficient blood supply to the septal cartilage if both sides of the mucous membrane facing each other are torn at the same time. The first step to prevent laceration of the mucosa is to dissect and elevate it in the subperichondrial plane. The area at which mucosa is most easily torn is where cartilage or bone forms a protrusion in the form of a spine or crest, as the mucosa is extremely thin in that area. Mucosa on the opposite side of the protrusion is more easily dissected, so it is better to approach through the contralateral side of the protrusion, and carefully raise the mucosa during surgery. There is usually no problem if only one side of mucosa is torn, but if both sides are injured, even only near one another, the torn mucosa will curl up and touch the torn mucosa on the opposite side, resulting in perforations which will require treatment. If the torn part of the septal mucosa is big, it is necessary to insert interposition grafts such as autologous cartilage or fascia and make one or two stitches. If the laceration of mucosa is not that big, it will heal within a week in general. If packing exerts excessive pressure on the septal mucosa, pressure necrosis may occur on the septal mucoperichondrium and will result in perforations.

5. Infection

Some patients complain of unusually prolonged and severe pain and tenderness of the nose postoperatively indicating the possibility of chondritis. If unnoticed and improperly managed, chondritis can progress and may leave the serious sequalae of a saddle nose deformity. Typical signs and symptoms of infection are pain, tenderness, swelling, and granulation tissue formation around the incision line. Once chondritis is suspected, antibiotics should be started and opening of the mucosal flap, with debridement of the infected tissue follows, depending on the severity of the condition.

6. Unilateral Mucosal Defect with Cartilage Exposure

The causes of this uncommon complication are unilateral septal mucosal injury due to too tightly placed silastic septal splint and too tight packing especially after septoplasty using bilateral flap elevation. The initial sign is persistent crusting at the mucosa with eventual exposure of the cartilage. Small defects heal spontaneously with conservative management like the application of ointments, but a larger defect needs to be repaired by turbinate mucosal free graft or a skin graft *(Figure 18)*. To treat this problem, the author prefers to use a skin graft harvested from postauricular area.

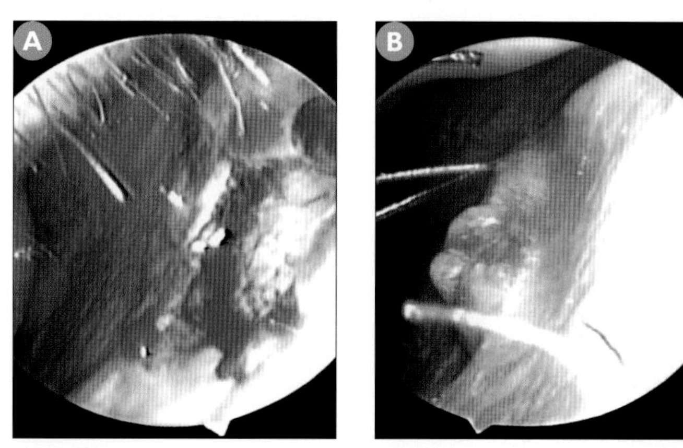

Figure 18 Unilateral mucosal defect (A), treated with skin grafting (B).

7. External Nasal Deformity

Because of the importance of the septum in the support of the nose, septoplasty inevitably can result in a change in the shape of nose. Displacement of the caudal septum from the anterior nasal spine after septoplasty may result in a deviated nose. Saddle nose, nasal tip ptosis, widening of the nasal tip, columellar retraction, and alar base widening are other aesthetic complications associated with a poorly done septoplasty. While a well conducted septoplasty can improve deviated nose, and a poorly done septoplasty can result in deviated nose. The incidence of post-septoplasty aesthetic complications is reported to be about 1-8%. In the author's research regarding postsepoplasty nasal deformities, disarticulation of the caudal strut from the anterior nasal spine, a deficient L-strut (caudal or dorsal strut), and disarticulation of the septal cartilage from the perpendicular plate at the keystone area were the reasons for external nasal deformities. In particular, a faulty postsurgical relationship between the caudal septum and the anterior nasal spine was found to be the most common pathology. This indicates that altering the normally robust relationship between the anterior nasal spine and caudal septal cartilage can simultaneously alter the nasal dorsal height, length, and direction. In addition, it can produce columellar retraction, widening, and tip deprojection. Therefore the surgeon should pay very close attention to keep the caudal septum strong and straight during septoplasty. When an immediate saddle deformity is found during septoplasty, it should be corrected by dorsal augmentation via a marginal or intercartilaginous incision before concluding the septoplasty.

References

1. Bescker SS, Dobratz EJ, Stowell N, Barker D, Park SS. Revision septoplasty: review of sources of persistent nasal obstruction. Am J Rhinol 2008; 23: 440-4.
2. Jang YJ, Kim JM, Yeo NK, Yoo JH. Use of nasal septal bone to straighten deviated septal cartilage in correction of deviated nose. Ann Otol Rhinol Laryngol 2009; 118: 488-94.
3. Jang YJ, Yeo NK, Wang JH. Cutting and suture technique of the caudal septal cartilage for the management of caudal septal deviation. Arch Otolaryngol Head Neck Surg 2009; 135: 1256-60.
4. Kim JH, Kim DY, Jang YJ. Outcomes after endonasal septoplasty using caudal septal batten grafting. Am J Rhinol Allergy 2011; 25: e166-70.
5. Karatzanis AD, Faragiadakis G, Moshandrea J, Zenk J, Iro H, Velegrakis GA. Septoplasty outcome in patients with and without allergic rhinitis. Rhinology 2009; 47: 444-9.
6. Lee BJ, Chung YS, Jang YJ. Overcorrected septum as a complication of septoplasty. Am J Rhinol 2004; 18: 393-6.
7. Yeo NK, Jang YJ. Rhinoplasty to correct nasal deformities in post septoplasty patients. Am J Rhinol Allergy 2009; 23: 540-5.
8. Yang JW, Kim SI, Kwom JW, Park DJ. Are cross hatching incisions mandatory for correction of cartilaginous septal deviation? Clin Exp Otorhinolaryngol 2008; 1: 20-3.

Septal Perforation

Jung-Soo Kim · Yong Ju Jang

Septal perforation is a disruption of the anatomic separation between the nasal cavities (i.e., due to injury or inflammation), causing symptoms such as excessive crusting, epistaxis, and nasal obstruction. Several surgical procedures have been introduced for its treatment, but repair of the nasal septum is particularly challenging because the necessary techniques such as flaps, grafts, and sutures, must be applied in the narrow nasal cavity. The most common secondary cause of perforation is complication arising from septoplasty; hence, surgeons who perform rhinoplasty must also be able to manage septal perforation.

I. Etiology

The septal cartilage is sandwiched between the blood vessels of the mucoperichondrium of the nasal septum, which provide nutrition for the cartilage. If injury occurs simultaneously on both sides of the mucoperichondrium due to surgery or any other cause, ischemic necrosis occurs in the underlying cartilage and leads to septal perforation *(Figure 1)*. If the mucosal edges of the perforation are not properly healed and become atrophied, or if inflammation occurs in the exposed cartilage, the nasal mucus becomes encrusted and the air flow around the perforation becomes turbulent, causing nasal obstruction and hemorrhage.

Another common cause of septal perforation is cauterization for epistaxis *(Table 1)*. When a patient presents with septal perforation of unknown etiology, a thorough history and physical examination must be performed to determine the cause. In particular, if there is necrosis

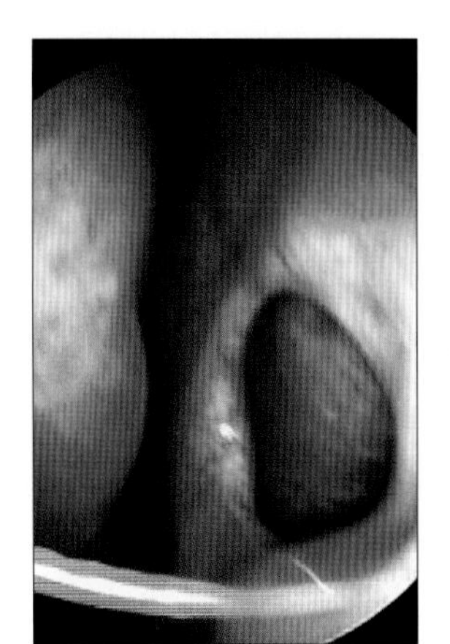
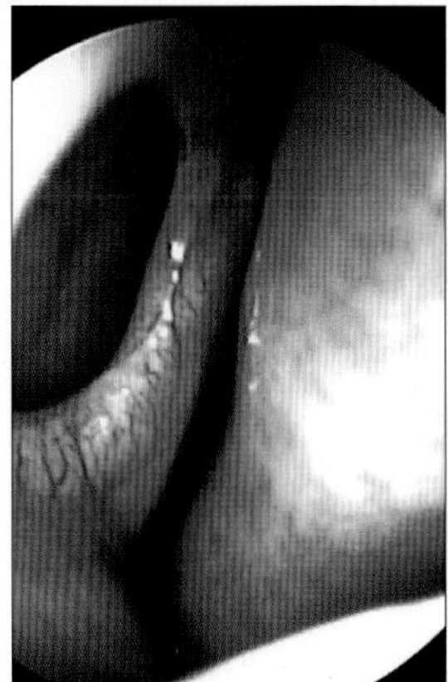

Figure 1 Endoscopic view of nasal septal perforation.

or inflammation of the mucosa in the nasal cavity other than at the perforation site, underlying medical diseases should be sought, as these findings may indicate a higher risk of recurrence of perforation, even after a successful surgery. Diagnostic evaluation should include testing for anti-nuclear antibodies (ANA) and Veneral disease research laboratory (VDRL) along with radiologic examinations, such as CT scan, as warranted. Biopsy may be required if a tumor is suspected. When biopsy is taken from the perforation margin, it is better to take the tissue sample from the posterior margin in order to prevent the perforation from extending anteriorly, superiorly, or inferiorly, which could increase the severity of the symptoms.

Table I Causes of septal perforation

Traumatic	Inflammatory or infectious	Neoplastic	Other
• Nasal surgery involving the septum • Cauterization for epistaxis • Nose picking • Nasogastric or oxygen tube placement • Button battery or foreign body in the nose	• Wegener's granulomatosis • Sarcoidosis • Systemic lupus erythromatosis • Tuberculosis • Syphilis • AIDS • Rheumatoid arthritis • Crohn's disease • Leprosy	• Carcinoma • NK T-cell lymphoma	• Intranasal steroid sprays • Cocaine • Chemical irritants : chromic, sulfuric, hydrochloric acids • Heavy metals • Chemical and industrial dusts • Renal failure

II. Symptoms

Approximately 40% of septal perforations are asymptomatic and will be missed without careful examination. Epistaxis is the most common symptom, followed by increased formation of crusts, nasal obstruction, whistling sound, and pain. Some patients may present with nasal obstruction and signs of empty nose syndrome or report pain when breathing through the nose. Symptoms are influenced by the location and size of the perforation. Small perforations are associated with a whistling sound when breathing, best heard when the surrounding environment is quiet. Large perforations are associated with extensive crust formation, possibly accompanied by nasal obstruction, pain, rhinorrhea, and frequent episodes of epistaxis *(Figure 2)*. Perforation most commonly occurs in the anterior part of nasal septum, and anterior perforations tend to be more symptomatic than posterior perforations. Pain associated with a perforation may be a sign of chondritis in the septal cartilage around the perforation, and patients who have perforation associated with marked formation of excessive crusts and accompanying mucosal inflammation in the nasal cavity must be checked for chronic inflammatory disease, lymphoma, or granulomatous disease. Patients with severe septal perforations commonly present with a simultaneous saddle nose deformity, which must be treated along with the septal perforation.

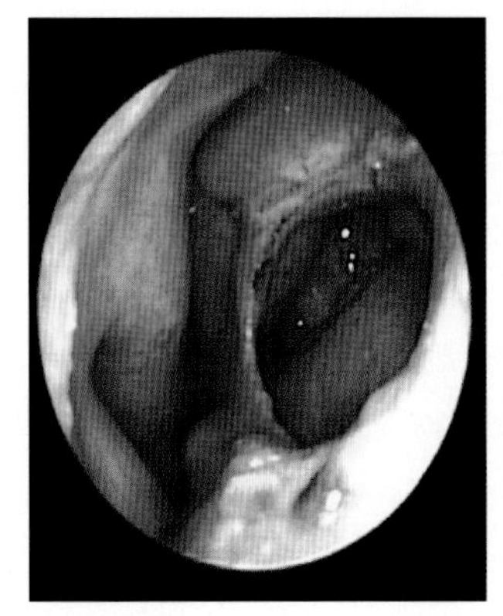
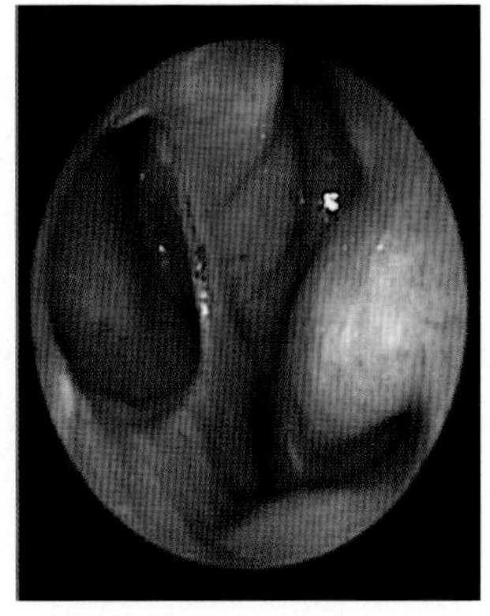

Figure 2 Endoscopic finding in a patient showing repeated hemorrhage from perforation margins.

III. Prevention and Intraoperative Treatment of Septal Perforation During Septoplasty

The nasal mucosa may be easily torn during dissection at septal surgery, and dissection must be performed with special attention to the risk of septal perforation and ischemic necrosis that may occur if both sides of the mucosa are torn, interrupting the blood supply to the septal cartilage. In order to help prevent lacerations, the mucosa should be dissected and elevated in the subperichondrial plane. Otherwise, if the mucosa is elevated while the perichondrium is attached to the cartilage, it can easily be torn, resulting in hemorrhage that will disturb the surgical field. It can be difficult to separate the well-developed fibrous tissue near the caudal septum from the perichondrium during surgery. In this event, the surgeon can more easily identify the smooth, white subperichondrial plane, and can separate the perichondrium more readily if the incision at the thick fibrous tissue is made with sharp scissors or a surgical knife. The mucosa is most easily torn in areas where cartilage or bone form spine- or crest-like protrusions, because it is extremely thin in such areas. The mucosa on the opposite side of such protrusions is more easily dissected, and an approach via the contralateral side of the protrusion should allow the surgeon to more carefully raise the mucosa during surgery *(Figure 3)*.

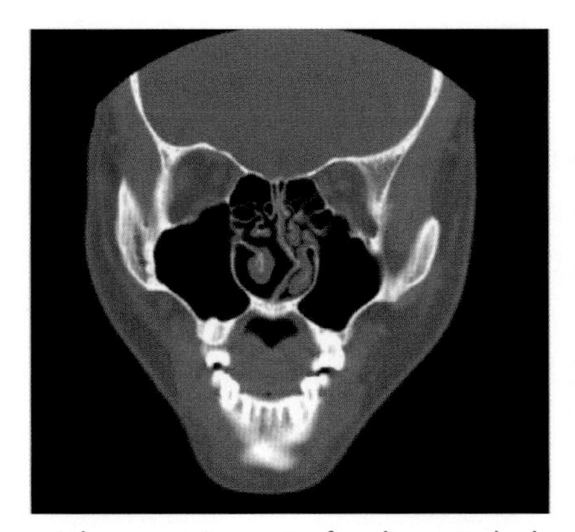
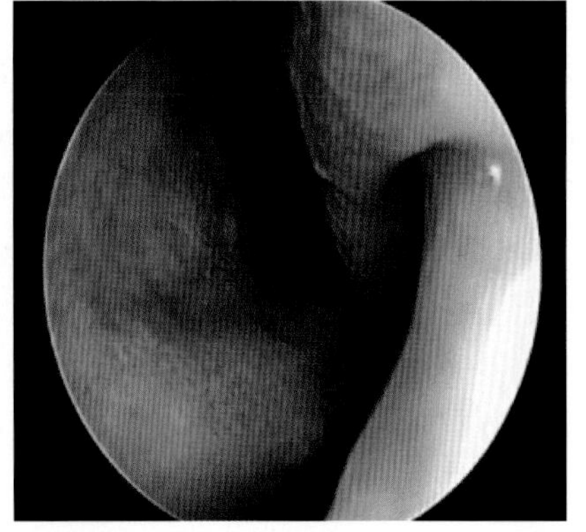

Figure 3 The septal mucosa is most often lacerated where cartilage or bone forms a spine- or crest-like protrusion.

When mucosal dissection is conducted at the convex side of a protrusion, it is impossible to see the posterior aspect of the protrusion, which leads to mucosal tears during mucosal elevation in most cases. Therefore, it is advisable to go around the protrusion and first separate the quadrangular cartilage and the perpendicular plate of the ethmoid before approaching the opposite side to dissect under the periosteum and perichondrium. Then, cut the top and bottom of the bony prominence with scissors or a chisel, keeping a portion of the mucosa in approximation with the ipsilateral side of the protrusion to be removed after securing mobility of the bony prominence. The septal mucosa at the junction between the septal cartilage and the maxillary crest can also be easily torn when dissecting because of the strong fibrous attachment, and will also require careful and meticulous dissection. If it is difficult to make a clean subperiosteal dissection, the surgeon can first elevate the mucosa from the posterior part and then move forward.

The patient should not have a problem if only one side of the mucosa is torn; however, if both sides are injured in the same area, and the injury is overlooked, even when the two sides are not directly facing each another, the injured mucosa on one side may curl up and contact the torn mucosa on the opposite side, disrupting the blood supply and leading to ischemic septal perforation, thereby requiring additional treatment. If the mucosal tear is large, it is usually necessary to insert an interposition graft of autologous cartilage or fascia and place one or two stitches. As suturing with the naked eye is a difficult procedure, the repair should be conducted under endoscopy whenever possible. Healing of torn or sutured mucosa may be promoted when silastic sheets are positioned on both sides. The silastic cover prevents the wound from direct contact with air and maintains moisture; it also aids in preventing further extension of the mucosal laceration. Smaller lacerations of the mucosa generally heal within a week.

If nasal packing exerts excessive pressure on the septal mucosa, it may cause pressure necrosis of the septal mucoperichondrium and result in perforation. Therefore, the surgeon must ensure that the packing that is not too tight in order to prevent this complication. When a perforation is discovered during a follow-up visit, an attempt to remove the dry crust around the perforation can cause extension of the perforation, it is best to moisten the crust with saline solution or ointment, which should cause it to fall off on its own.

IV. Treatment

Repair of septal perforation is one of the most difficult rhinologic surgeries, and avoiding perforation is more important than anything so that such difficulties can be avoided. If a septal perforation is very small or is grossly asymptomatic because it is in a posterior location, it is occasionally discovered only by chance during physical examination. If there are no major symptoms directly related to the perforation, additional treatment is usually not necessary, even for larger perforations. When there are symptoms, conservative treatment should be tried first and surgical treatment considered only if there is no improvement or if the patient dislikes continuous conservative treatment.

1. Conservative Treatment

Patients who have excessive crust formation should remove the crusts by washing with saline solution, and the patients must be warned that removing the crusts by force can enlarge the perforation. Applying ointment to the nasal cavity when exposed to dry climate or using an indoor humidifier may also help. A silicone obturator (button) may be applied to block the perforation in patients with severe, extremely large perforations *(Figure 4)*.

The silicone button can improve air flow in the nasal cavity and keep the margins of the perforation moist. Commercially available buttons only come in a single size. Ideally, the buttons should be customized for each patient, but this may not be possible. Silicone buttons may also increase mucus secretion and crust formation, and moreover, patients face great inconvenience in having to wash nasal cavity to keep the obturator clean, and frequently find it necessary to remove the obturator to wash. Button therapy is best considered only for patients who are poor surgical candidates, those who have large perforations of at least 4 cm in diameter, or those who do not show complete recovery after surgery. So far, in the authors' experience, most patients could not tolerate the difficulties in using the obturator and wants it removed.

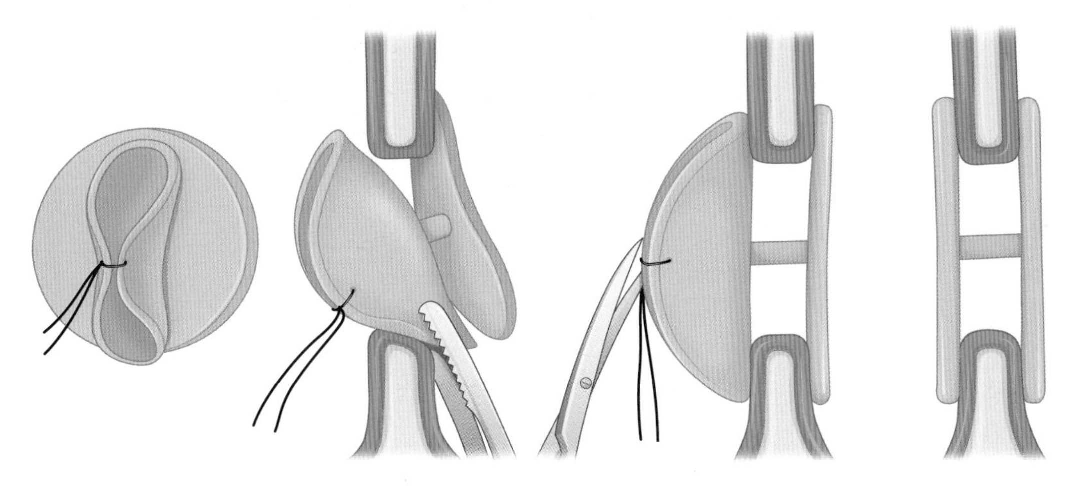

Figure 4 Silicone button placement: a conservative treatment method for nasal septal perforation

2. Surgical Techniques

The goal of surgery is to close the perforation and to restore the normal function and physiology of the nasal cavity. Various surgical approaches, techniques, flaps and grafts have been introduced for repair of septal perforations, but as yet, no single method has been shown to be the the best for successfully closing them. Perforations of 5 to 10 mm are generally classified as small. Small or medium-sized perforations can be treated solely by a local advancement flap or by advancement flap with graft (i.e., temporalis fascia). Several types of flaps and grafts have been introduced for repair of large perforations.

Mucosal flaps used for repair of septal perforations are usually moved up and down, as the superior-inferior dimension of the perforation is more important than the anterior-posterior size when considering treatment planning and prognosis. It is expected that the repair will be more difficult if the perforation is large in the vertical dimension because the available mucosa may not be sufficient for a flap *(Figure 5)*. The location of the perforation also influences the surgical planning and prognosis because repair of posterior perforations, when necessary, is usually considered more difficult, although, in general, posterior perforations have no or only minor symptoms.

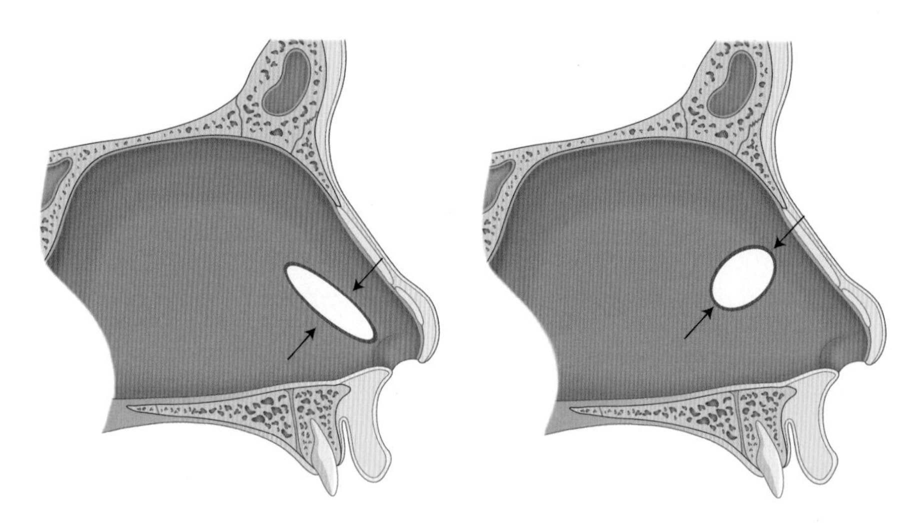

Figure 5 The superior-inferior dimension of the perforation is more important for predicting surgical success with repair based on mucosal advancement flaps than the anterior-posterior dimension. Surgery is much more difficult for perforations with a large vertical dimension.

1) Surgical Approaches

There are two approaches to surgical repair of nasal septal perforations, the endonasal approach and the external approach. Generally, the endonasal approach is preferred if the perforation is small or medium-sized, and an external approach is favored for large perforations, although ultimately, the choice of approach is determined by the surgeon's discretion, and may be influenced by factors other than the size of the perforation.

The main advantage of the endonasal approach is that it leaves no incision scar. Recent development of endoscopes that secure a better view have also made this method more preferred. Experienced surgeons who are well trained in endoscopic techniques can reconstruct even large perforations with a high rate of success, although for some large perforations, the external approach remains the technique of choice.

The advantages of the open rhinoplasty approach are a good surgical view, the ability to perform surgery with both hands, and the ability to treat any accompanying nasal deformity simultaneously. The open approach to rhinoplasty may be safer and easier when the surgeon is less experienced or not familiar with the one handed techniques of endoscopic surgery. Furthermore, suturing of the perforation margin is better facilitated during the open approach, and in some cases, an open approach can even increase the survival rate of the advancement flap by preserving the blood supply from the anterior part because it does not require a transfixion incision *(Figure 6)*. The lateral alotomy or other external approach is useful when wider exposure than that provided by an endonasal approach is necessary, even though the external approaches are accompanied by potential issues due to scarring.

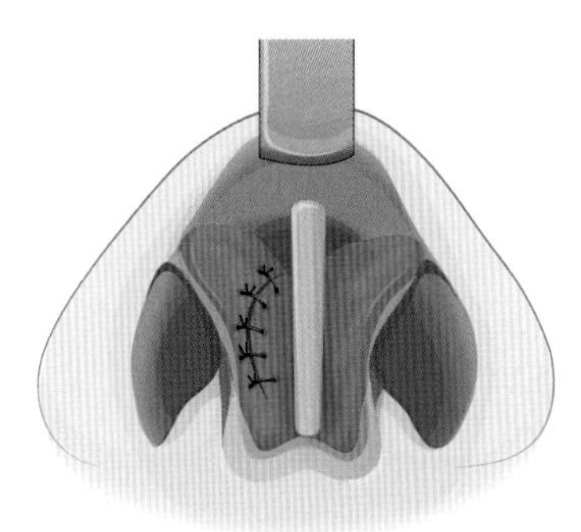

Figure 6 The open rhinoplasty approach to repair a septal perforation allows the surgeon to use both hands while performing the repair, and the open view and can allow greater ease of suturing and other surgical procedures.

2) Reconstruction of Septal Mucoperichondrium

The septal mucosa has almost no elasticity. Therefore, unlike the skin, even if a septal perforation is small, direct suturing of the perforation margins after raising the septal mucosa will have a high likelihood of failure, and the injured septum must be sutured without tension after securing mobility of the flap via sufficient dissection of the mucosa around the perforation. The types of flaps that are currently reported include the unilateral advancement flap, the bilateral advancement flap, the inferior turbinate flap, the labiobuccal flap, and skin flaps. Skin grafts, or grafts using oral mucosa do not incorporate respiratory epithelium, and are thus undesirable because they cause injury to the donor site and are accompanied by side effects such as excessive crust formation and dry nasal mucosa.

In many cases, the actual cartilage defect is much larger than the perforation. The septal mucosa immediately surrounding the perforation margin is devoid of underlying cartilage and bone, and the process of dissection of the mucosa around the perforation margin can further injure the septal mucosa, causing enlargement of the size of the perforation. Therefore it is mandatory to separate both sides of the septal mucosa very carefully. Before suturing the septal mucosa, wound tissue or granulation tissue around the edges of the perforation must be completely removed and the tissue thoroughly cleaned for better healing. When a sufficient flap size is obtained, a tension-free interrupted suture should be placed using a 5-0 cutting needle.

The most commonly used surgical techniques are the rotation flap or advancement flap of the nasal cavity floor mucosa or septal mucosa *(Figure 7)*. These methods can be applied as both a unilateral flap or a bilateral flap. Comparison of the surgical outcomes of two techniques has shown that a bilateral flap can secure more abundant blood supply and encompass all three layers of the nasal septum. This can guarantee a higher rate of success, and is more recommendable.

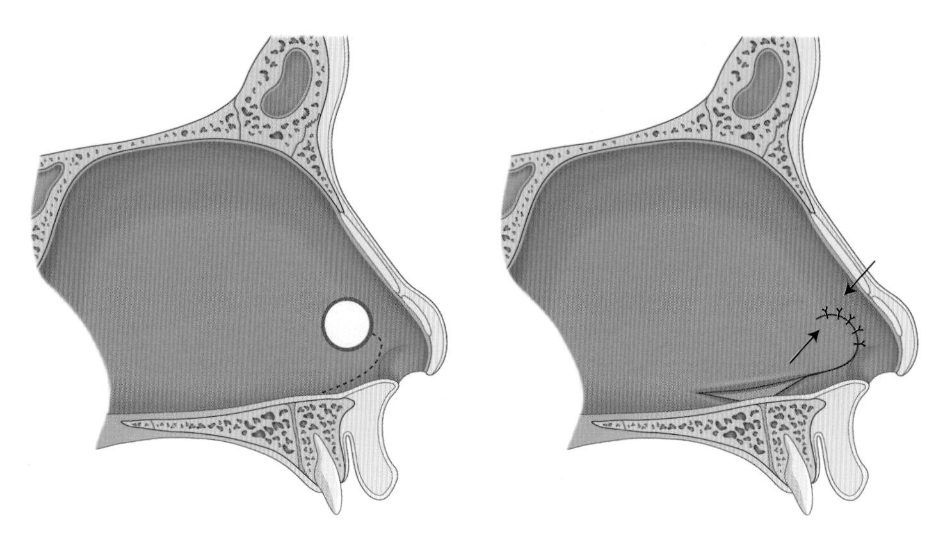

Figure 7 A rotation flap is a method of suturing after rotating the flap. It is useful when reconstructing small anterior perforations. A rotation flap can be performed on one side or both sides. When performed on both sides, one flap must be created from the top and the other from the bottom.

(1) Unilateral/Bilateral Mucosal Advancement Flap

The unilateral advancement flap technique uses a mucosal flap from the bottom and the top of the perforation on one side of the nasal cavity. The flap does not cover the contralateral side, with healing instead relying on mucosal regeneration by secondary intention *(Figure 8)*.

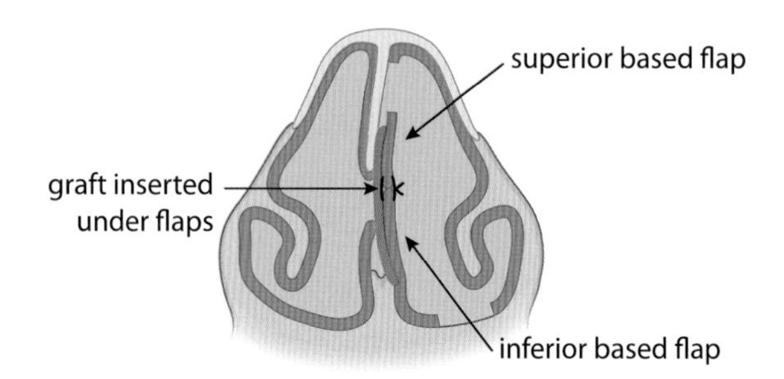

Figure 8 A unilateral advancement flap is a method of using a superior flap and an inferior flap from one side of the nasal cavity to completely close the perforation, of which flap elevation on the opposite side is not attempted because mucous membrane regeneration by secondary intention is expected.

When closing perforations from only one side, it is recommended that the exposed graft be protected from drying by keeping a silastic sheet in place for up to 3 weeks after surgery. A unilateral flap can shorten the operative time, and it can be used when the perforation is so large that the flap cannot cover the perforation simultaneously on both sides. When possible, a bilateral mucosal advancement flap remains the ideal method of reconstructing all three layers of the nasal septum by creating advancement flaps on both sides of nasal cavity *(Figure 9)*.

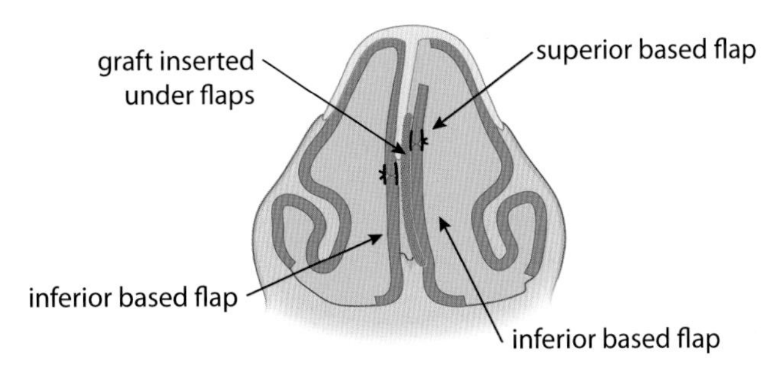

Figure 9 A bilateral advancement flap is an ideal method of reconstructing all three layers of the nasal septum by developing advancement flaps on both sides.

Mucosal advancement flaps can be classified as inferior or superior based on their location in relation to the perforation. It is easier to develop larger mucosal flaps from the inferior aspect of the perforation margin, and thus the inferior-based flaps usually play a more important role in perforation closure. To facilitate better mobilization of an inferior flap, it is better to make an incision parallel to nasal cavity at the inferior aspect of the inferior turbinate, when possible, and to dissect the mucosa off of the nasal floor in order to provide maximal mobility of the flap. If the perforation cannot be fully covered by the inferior flap, a superior based flap can be elevated *(Figure 10)*. To obtain a larger flap, the mucosal dissection can be extended toward the

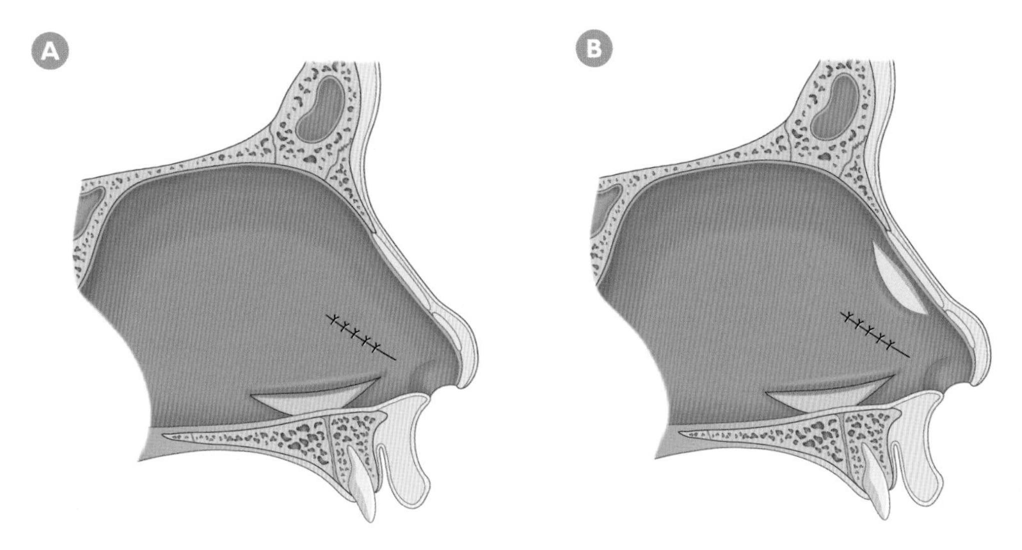

Figure 10 Perforation closure (A) using an inferior based flap, and (B) using both an inferior flap and a superior flap.

mucoperichondrium at the undersurface of upper lateral cartilage. This can be more easily done when using an open rhinoplasty approach. It is recommended that a superior flap be used on one side only. Simultaneous creation of bilateral superior flaps may cause an interruption of the blood supply on both sides, possibly creating a new perforation.

When the perforation is large, the mobility of the inferior flap can be increased by extending the incision towards the anterior part of the flap until it reaches the hemitransfixion incision. The blood supply of the flap is provided only from the posterior nasal cavity, forming a mono-pedicled advancement flap *(Figure 11)*. Using this method simultaneously on both sides requires special attention to avoid the risk of a new perforation caused by the exposure of cartilage on the antero-inferior side of the septum on both sides.

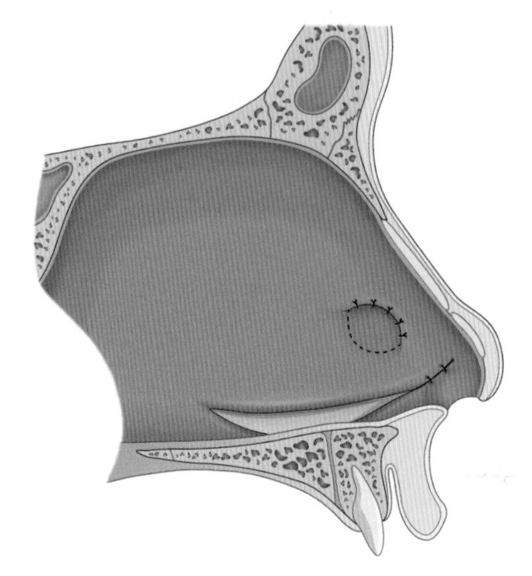

Figure 11 The incision can be extended toward the anterior part of the inferior mucosal flap until it contacts the hemitransfixion incision in order to increase the mobility of the flap.

(2) Inferior Turbinate Flap

The inferior turbinate mucosa has an abundant blood supply. An inferior turbinate mucosa flap has the advantage of being easily inserted in perforations and of containing respiratory epithelium. An inferior turbinate flap is raised in the form of anterior-based flap by dissecting off the mucosa at the posterior part of the inferior turbinate, preserving the blood supply from the anterior part. The disadvantage of this method is that it may require a secondary operation to divide the pedicle, which may cause nasal obstruction after the operation *(Figure 12)*. The size of the septal perforation

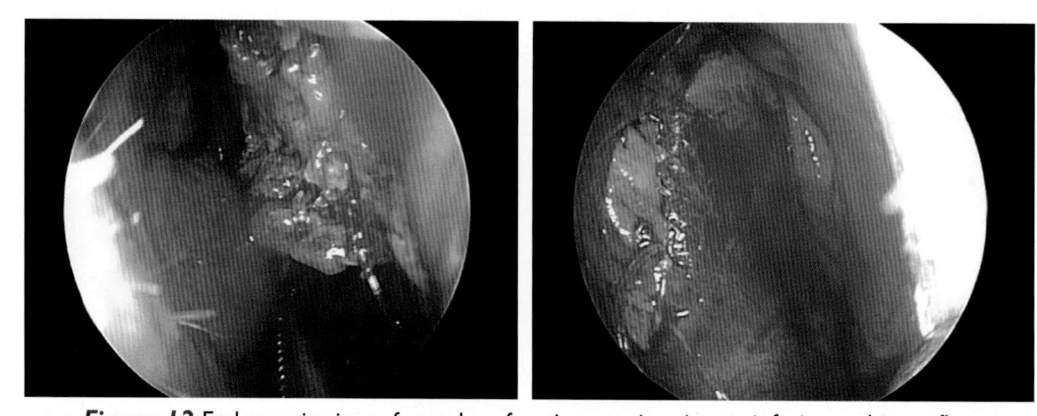

Figure 12 Endoscopic view of septal perforation repair using an inferior turbinate flap.

is an important consideration when choosing this method. It is generally recommended that inferior turbinate flaps are used for closure of perforations of ≤ 2.5 cm wide and ≤ 1.5 cm long. In the authors' experience, these flaps can be used nicely for revisions in cases where the primary operation for perforation repair has failed.

(3) Endonasal Endoscopic Perforation Closure Techniques

One of the most difficult parts of perforation closure is the suturing of the septal mucosa, and this is much more difficult in endonasal endoscopic surgery because it must be carried out using only one hand. The recommended suture for this technique is a 5-0 absorbable suture material, such as Vicryl®, with a cutting needle that can easily penetrate the septal mucosa. The needle must penetrate both sides of the septal mucosa during endoscopic suturing, and the knot is made outside the nose, after which the assistant will hold one end of the thread while the operating surgeon holds the other end, at the side of the suture needle, and together they slowly pull on both sides simultaneously. The assistant must watch the monitor to verify that the thread is being properly pulled and then tighten the knot. Subsequent knots are also formed outside the nose, but the assistant and the operating surgeon should not pull the thread simultaneously. Instead, the assistant must hold the suture thread very lightly while the operating surgeon holds uses a needle holder to pull the thread little by little inside the nose to tighten the knot. Suturing must begin in the posterior part and advance anteriorly because if the anterior part is sutured first it may block the view while suturing the posterior part. *Figure 13* shows the endoscopic findings before and after surgery as well as consecutive views of a unilateral advancement flap procedure performed under endoscopy.

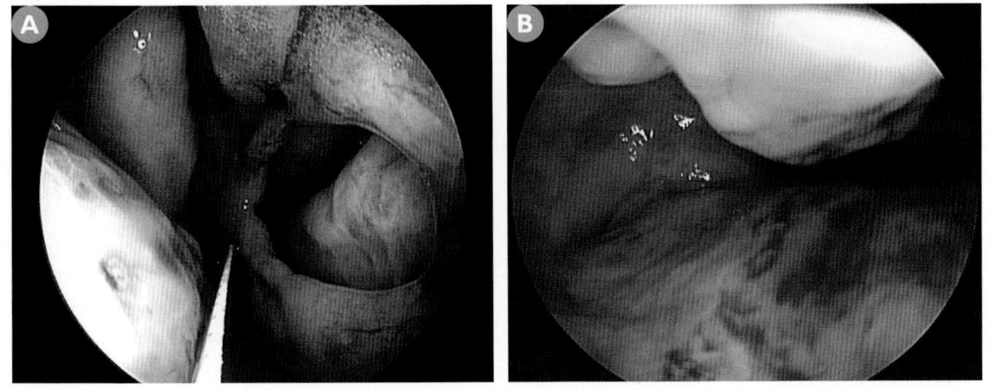

Figure 13-A Endoscopic view of a perforation before surgery (perforation size approximately 2 cm).
Figure 13-B Mucous membrane elevation to form an inferior flap. The mucosa is dissected off toward the side-wall of the inferior meatus below the inferior turbinate to enlarge the flap.

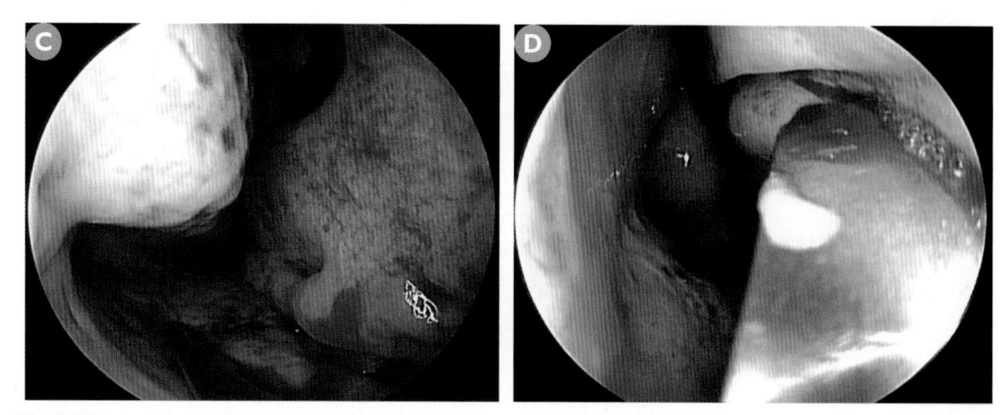

Figure 13-C The incision after inferior flap elevation may be placed near the sidewall of the inferior meatus to permit a larger flap.
Figure 13-D The incision to form a superior flap should be made as close as possible to the top of the nasal cavity, and the flap should then be raised close to the upper lateral cartilage to create a larger superior flap.

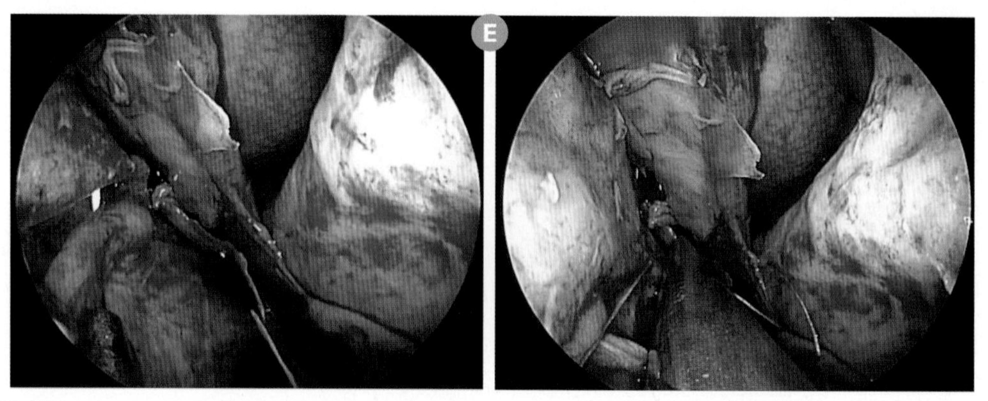

Figure 13-E Suturing with 5-0 Vicryl with a cutting needle the suture is placed under the mucosa.
Suturing the right side of the perforation from the inner side of the mucosa is easier when the operating surgeon uses the right hand; suturing on the outside of the nasal cavity mucosa is easier for the left side.

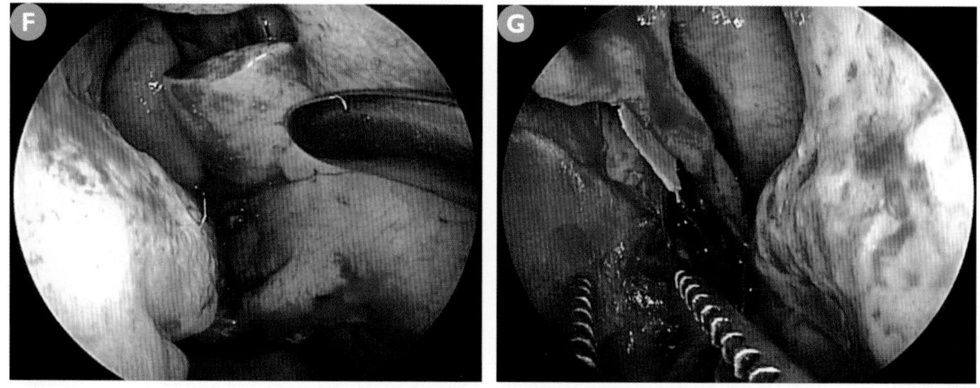

Figure 13-F Endoscopic view after suturing a nasal septal perforation. An inferior flap and a superior flap are well sutured. A mucosal defect is visible at the top of the inferior meatus due to advancement of the flap.
Figure 13-G Insertion of temporalis fascia between the septal mucosal flaps after suturing, shown through a left-side perforation that is not sutured.

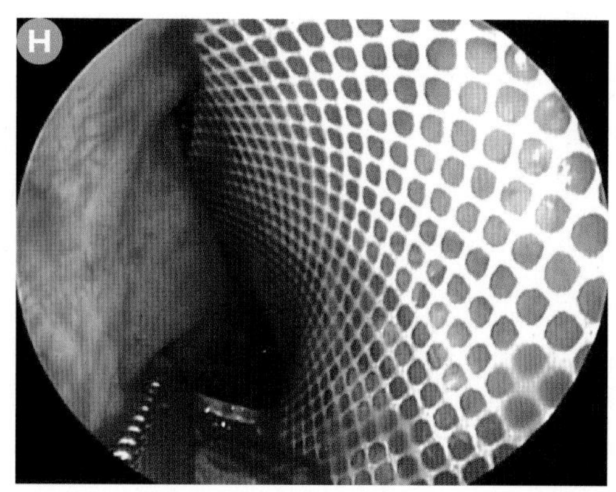

Figure 13-H Placement of bilateral silastic splints, which may be kept in place for up to 3 weeks.

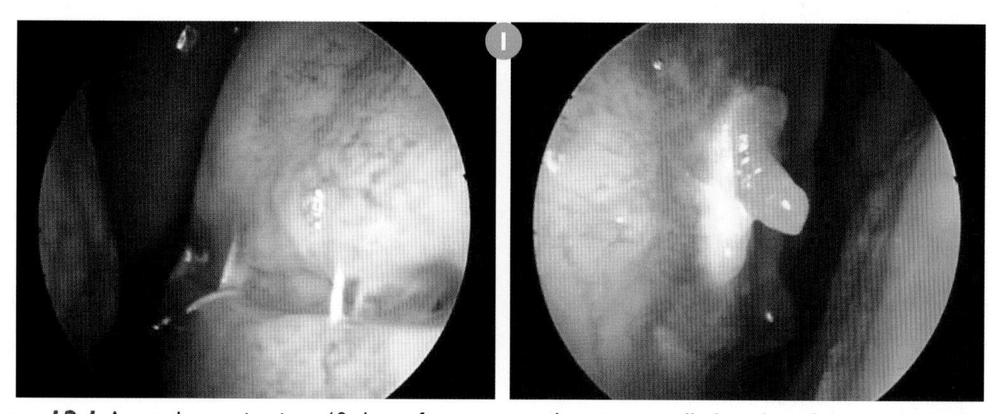

Figure 13-I An endoscopic view 40 days after surgery showing a well closed perforation on both sides.

3) Selection of Interposition Graft

Surgery is more likely to be successful if an interposition graft is inserted between the two sides of the septal mucosa after mucosal flap repair because an interposition graft will promote epithelialization of the sutured mucous membranes. Temporalis fascia is the most commonly used graft material, and homologous processed fascia can also be used, which does not show much difference from autologous fascia in terms of treatment outcomes. Other graft materials such as pericranium, mastoid periosteum, septal cartilage, septal bone, conchal cartilage, and acellular dermal allograft can also be used. When these grafts are placed between the mucosal flaps they can prevent recurrence of the perforation during the healing process and act as a support during mucosal epithelialization. Moreover, a graft can fill small gaps that occur during flap suturing, and grafts are especially useful in cases of unilateral advancement flap repair when the flap does not completely cover the perforation. In general, it is best to make an interposition graft of at least 2 cm larger than, or, when possible, twice the size of, the perforation.

3. Postoperative Care

When completing the surgery, silastic sheets should be placed on both sides of the septum to prevent the mucosal flap from drying during the healing period, and the silastic sheets can be fixed with 5-0 non-absorbable suture material. The nose should be lightly packed with gauze or gelfoam, recalling that if the packing is too tight, it may cause necrosis owing to interruption of the mucosal blood supply, resulting in surgical failure. A silastic septal splint will protect the mucosa from air currents and keep the area moist, promoting the healing process, and transparent silastic sheets will permit inspection of the repair site during postoperative follow up. When an advancement flap is used to repair a septal perforation, there may be exposed bone at the floor of the nasal cavity, and this may be associated with bloody discharge postoperatively. The patient must be informed of this in advance, and the bloody discharge should disappear within the first 24 hours after surgery. All packing should be removed on the first postoperative day, and, as mentioned, the site of the repair can be observed through the transparent septal splint when the patient comes for follow-up examinations. When both sides of the perforation are properly covered with mucosal flaps during surgery, the septal splint can be removed after 1 week. If the perforation closure is incomplete on one or both sides and there is an exposed interposition graft, it is best to maintain the splint for 3 weeks, and the patient must be instructed to use a humidifier and to apply an antibiotic ointment in the nasal cavity three to four times a day.

4. Surgical Outcomes

Factors that determine the success of septal perforation repair are the cause of the perforation, its size, whether mucosal flap was used on one side or both sides, the type of interposition graft inserted between flaps, and the technical competence of the operating surgeon. Among these, perforation size has the most significant influence on prognosis, and the rate of surgical failure increases when a perforation is ≥ 2 cm in size. The most effective surgical technique is usually one that uses interposition grafts along with bipedicled mucosal advancement flaps. The symptoms will disappear even if the perforation recurs after surgery, as the recurrent perforation will be smaller than the original defect. If it is impossible to completely close the perforation, a partial closure of the anterior portion of the perforation, repositioning the perforation more posteriorly, may be helpful for reducing the symptoms. During follow up, patients may occasionally show recurrence after a few months, even when perforations had been successfully closed during the immediate postoperative period. Thus, the ultimate success of a perforation closure should be determined by long-term follow-up.

References

1. Cogswell LK, Goodcare TEE. The management of nasoseptal perforation. Br J Plast Surg 2000;53: 117-20.
2. Eng SP, Nilssen ELK, Ranta DLOM, White PS. Surgical management of septal perforation: an alternative to closure of perforation. J Laryngol Otol 2001;115: 194-7.
3. Friedman M, Ibrahim H, Ramakrishnan V. Inferior turbinate flap for repair of nasalseptal perforation. Laryngoscope 2003; 113: 1425-8.
4. Kilty SJ, Brownrigg PJ, Safar A. Nasal septal perforation repair using an inferior turbinate flap. J Otolaryngol 2007; 36: 38-42.
5. Kriedel RW. Considerations in the etiology, treatment, and repair of septal perforations. Facial Plast Surg Clin North Am 2004; 12: 435-50.
6. Kim SW, Rhee CS. Nasal septal perforation repair: predictive factors and systematic review of the literature. Curr Opin Otolaryngol Head Neck Surg 2012: 20: 58-65.
7. Lanier B, Kai G, Marple B, Wall M. Pathophysiology and progression of nasal septal perforation. Ann Allergy Asthma Immunol 2007: 99: 473-80.
8. Lee HR, Ahn DB, Park JH, Kim YH, JS Kim. Endoscopic repair of septal perforation with using a unilateral nasal mucosal flap. Clin Exp Otorhinolaryngol 2008; 1: 154-7.
9. Watson D, Barkdull G. Surgical management of the septal perforation. Otolaryngol Clin North Am 2009; 42: 483-93.

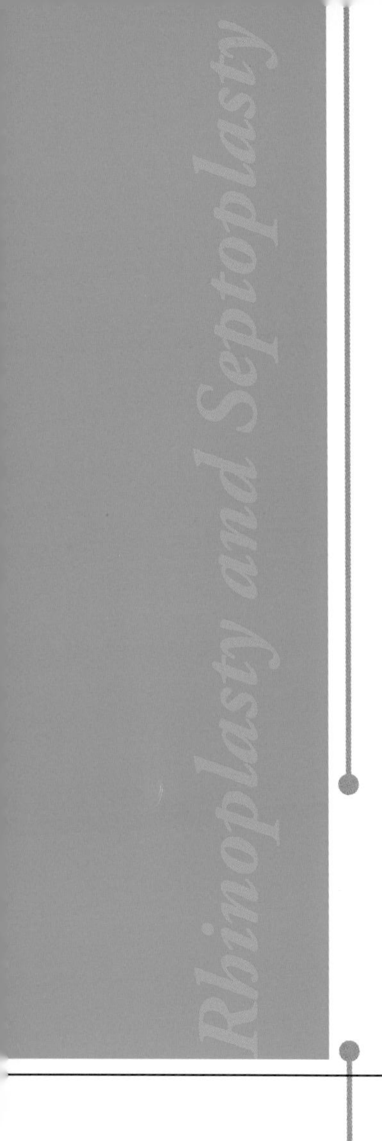

Section 03

Getting Started

Computer Simulation

Myeong Sang Yu · Yong Ju Jang

I. Usefulness of Preoperative Computer Simulation in the Rhinoplasty Patient

Photodocumentation of the patient's face in facial plastic surgery, especially in rhinoplasty, is a very crucial and necessary process. Before surgery, patients' facial photos make it possible to set up a surgical plan and explain expected results to the patients. After surgery, it can be used for objective evaluation of changes after surgery and the overall success of surgery. Recently, as acquisition of medical information through the internet or mass media is much easier, more patients who want rhinoplasty know about computer simulation and demand the simulation before surgery.

Through computer simulations on patients prior to rhinoplasty, the patient's preferred shape of the external nose can be accurately determined and communication between the patient and the surgeon can be intensified in that patient participates from the planning stage of his/her rhinoplasty process. Computer simulations also help rhinoplasty patients gain a more realistic expectation of the surgery and relieve anxiety. From an educational perspective, computer imaging makes learning easier and more effective for students.

II. Simulation Tools

Based upon the images of patients obtained from a digital camera, various plastic surgeries can be simulated using digital imaging techniques such as warping and filtering. Many kinds of software are utilized for such preoperative computer simulations *(Figure 1)*. Recently, web-based simulation programs or simulation applications that can be used in smartphones are developed, so patients themselves can figure out the shape of nose they want beforehand. Besides software developed exclusively for plastic surgery, the popular digital imaging software Adobe Photoshop® (Adobe Systems Incorporated, San Jose, CA) can be used as well. For commercial virtual plastic surgery software, they are easy to use but have a limited array of outcomes due to their sometimes inflexible systems. On the other hand, simulation through Photoshop® may be difficult for novices, but once accustomed to, it allows for more specific and realistic designs.

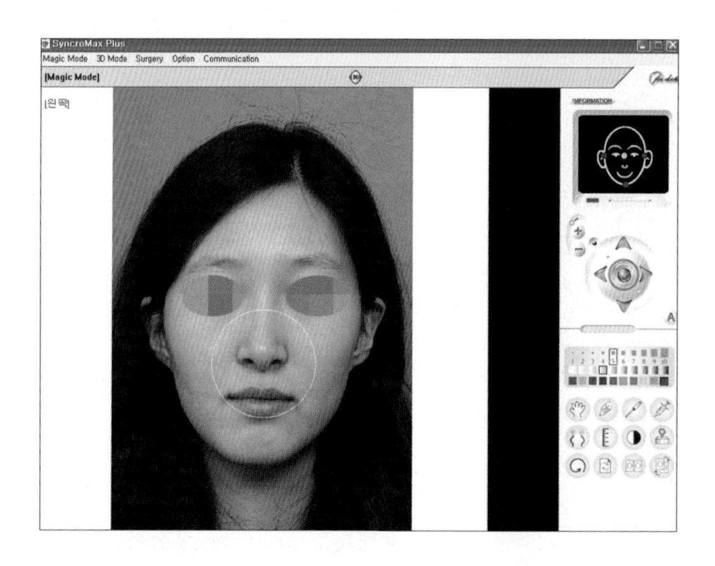

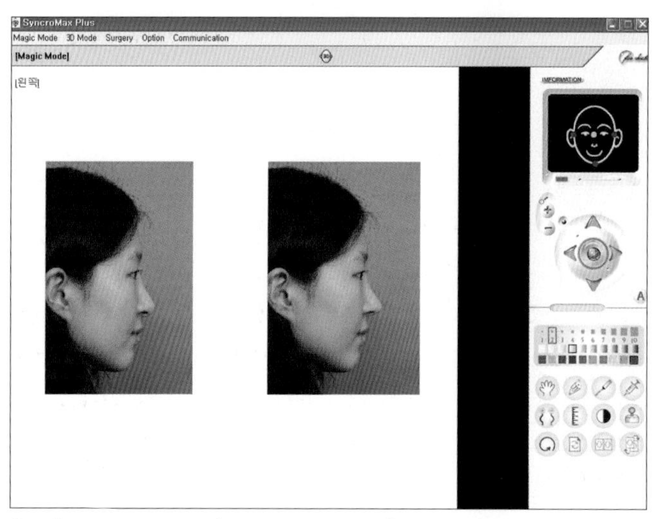

Figure 1 Example of computer simulation using simulation software (Syncromax®, version 3.0).

III. Image Warping

The most important digital imaging technique in computer simulation would be image warping. Warping is a digital technique that modifies the original image as wanted and it can give a bending effect to the image on a rubber plate by differentiating movement of each pixel. There are many types of warping such as the weight technique using line segments, the intuitive surface generation technique, and the most commonly used method of digital processing in rhinoplasty simulations, called mesh warping. Mesh warping obtains the wanted image by dividing the image into a triangular or square mesh and bending it as desired by the surgeons. Geometric changes of the mesh-shaped polygons produce smooth results *(Figure 2)*.

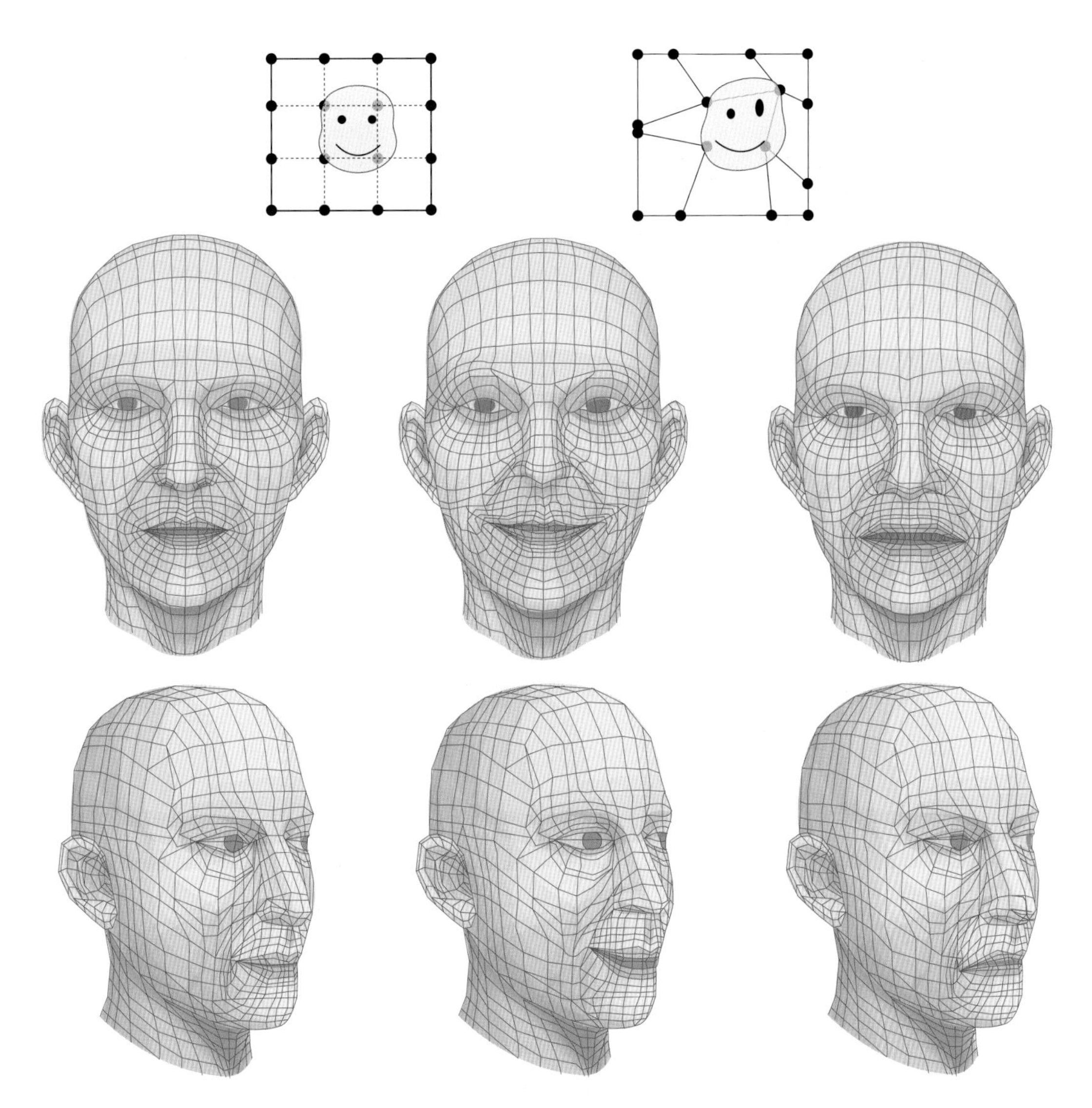

Figure 2 Example of mesh warping algorithm. Dividing the input image into small triangular or square grid (mesh) and transforming it as much as one wants to get the desired result. By performing a geometric transformation on the polygons, one is able to get a smooth output.

IV. Patient-Preferred Nose Shapes

Before conducting computer simulations on patients, understanding the ideal nose shape and anatomic proportions is mandatory. The ideal nose shape can differ based on sex, race, region, and generation, which makes it important to know the most favored shapes and types. According to research from the authors, a survey and analysis on ideal nose shapes done on patients who received preoperative computer simulations revealed that the most preferred shape of the nasal dorsum is the straight type (67.2%) followed by the mildly concave type (29.7%), with the mildly convex type being the least popular *(Figure 3)*. Preference for lateral shape of the columella limb was 51.6% and 43.8% for straight type and smooth concave type respectively, and 4.6% for the slightly convex type *(Figure 4)*. The preferred nasofrontal angle was 137.5±6.9˚, and 97.3±8.6˚ for nasolabial angle *(Figure 5)*.

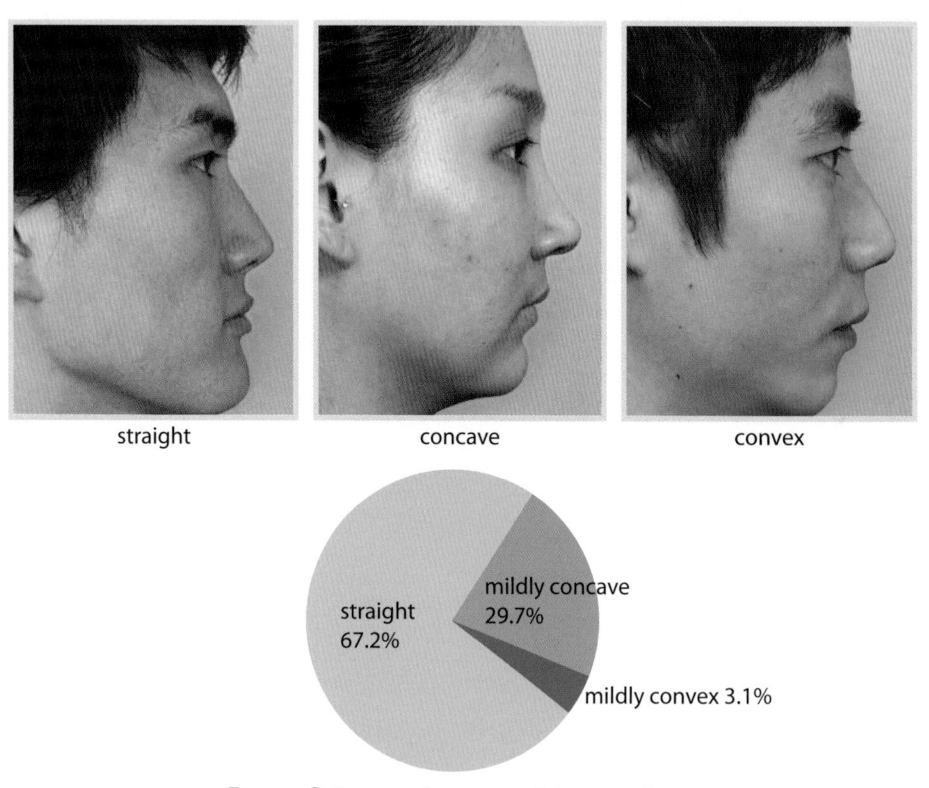

Figure 3 Most preferred nasal dorsum shape.

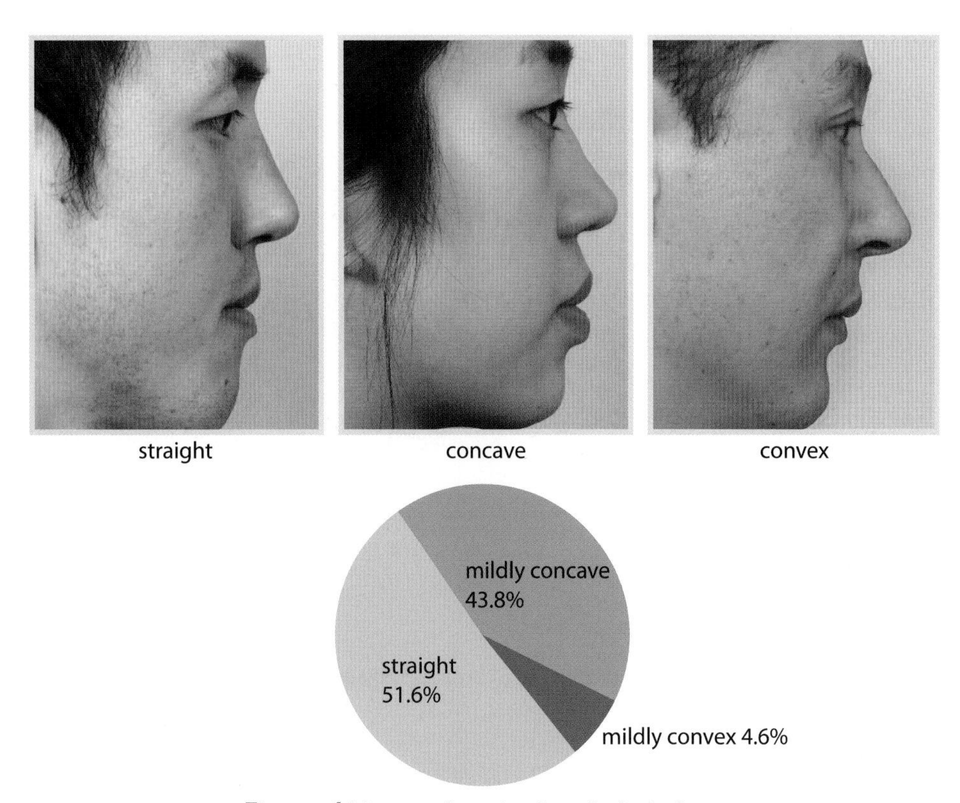

Figure 4 Most preferred columella limb shape.

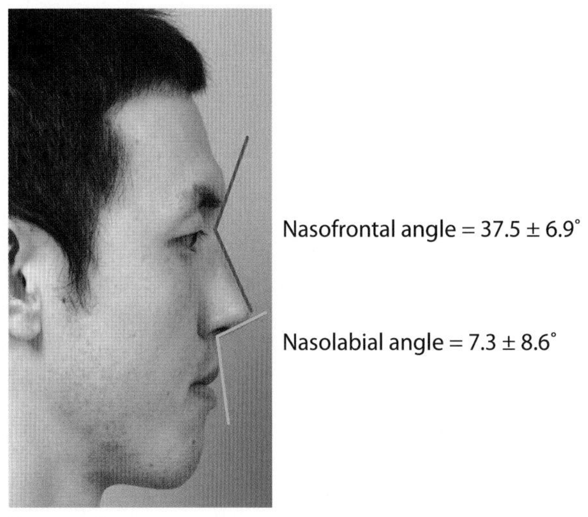

Figure 5 Most preferred nasofrontal and nasolabial angle.

IV. Simulation Process

1. Important Landmarks for Simulation

When simulation on a lateral image of a patient is performed, it must be performed based on standards such as the nasolabial angle, nasion level, rhinion height, and existence of a supratip break. Moreover, the height of pronasale, desire for columellar break points, and the patient's desired nasofrontal angle should also be points of emphasis *(Figure 6)*.

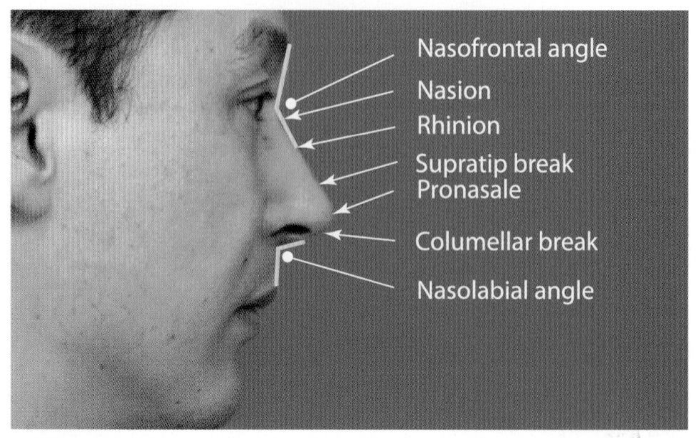

Figure 6 Important landmarks in computer simulation.

2. Examples of Simulation based on the Shape of the Nose

1) Convex Dorsum

For simulation in the profle view, the surgeon should consider not only removing the hump, but also whether additional augmentation of rthe adix and dorsum, or tip surgery should be performed simultaneously after considering the height of the dorsum after hump removal, projection of the nasal tip, rotation, and the nasofrontal angle *(Figure 7)*. It is more natural for women to have a slightly concave dorsal shape, with the dorsal line located a little lower than the line that connects the nasofrontal angle with the tip. For men, on the other hand, it is better to place the dorsal line straight or a little above the nasofrontal angle-tip line *(Figure 8)*.

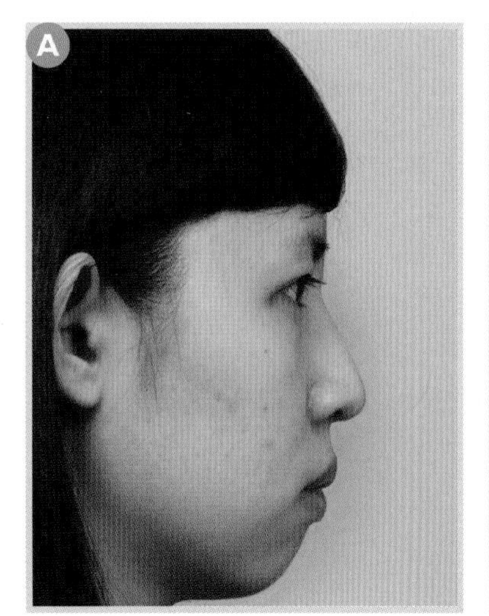

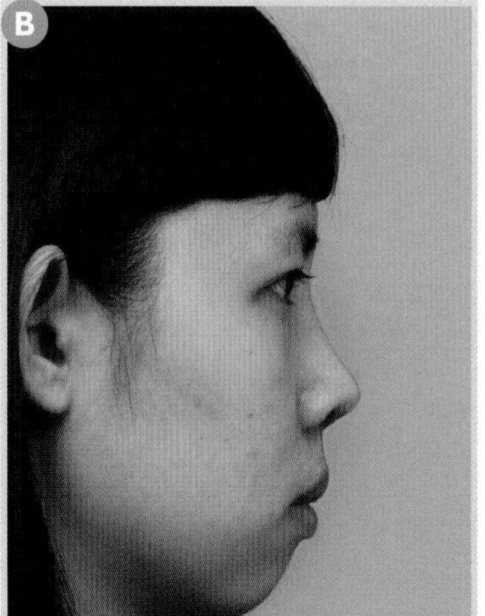

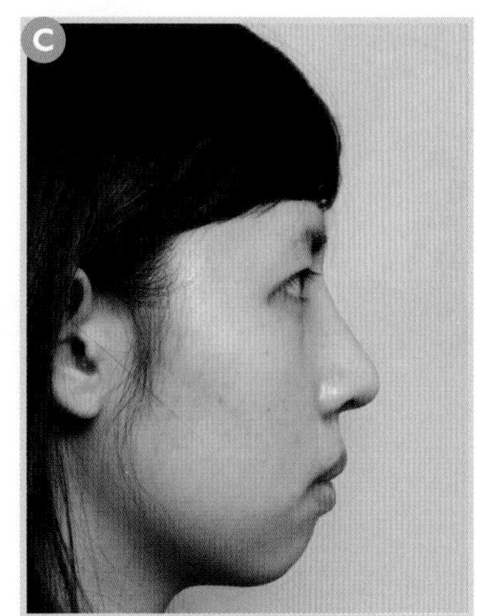

Figure 7 Before simulation (A), after simulation (B), and actual photo after surgery (C).

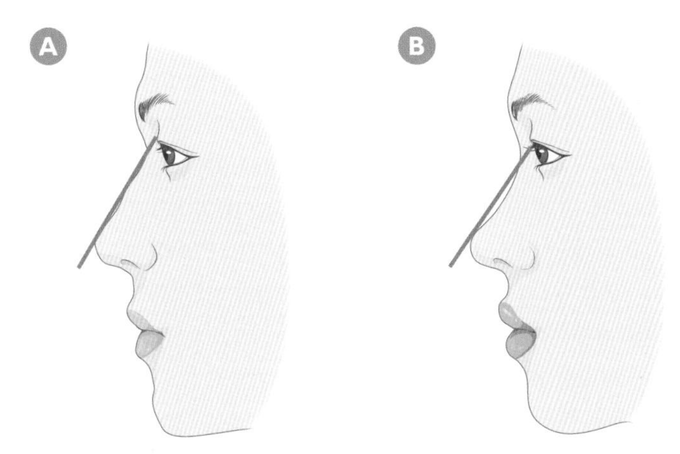

Figure 8 It is desirable that the dorsal line in men is located higher than the line connecting the nasofrontal angle and tip (A). On the other hand, in case of women, it is natural for the dorsal line to be located a little lower than the line connecting the nasofrontal angle and tip, making a mildly concave shape (B).

2) Deviated Nose

For simulation in the frontal view, to analyze asymmetry and deviation of the nasal dorsum, divide the face into three horizontal parts and assess each part's relationship with the central facial axis. In a patient with an asymmetric face, the patient can be notified at the simulation stage that once the nose is corrected by surgery, the imbalance of the overall face may get worse. The surgeon must consider during simulation the possible changes that entail each deviation correction method in order to obtain a satisfactory surgical outcome. For example, if the surgeon conducts bilateral osteotomy to correct a deviation of the bony dorsum, the bony pyramid may become narrower after the surgery. If the surgeon inserts spreader grafts on both sides to correct a deviated cartilage dorsum, the nasal dorsum may appear somewhat wider after the surgery *(Figure 9)*.

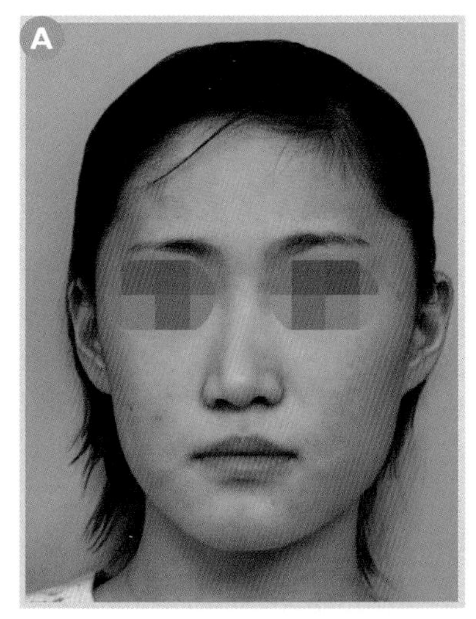

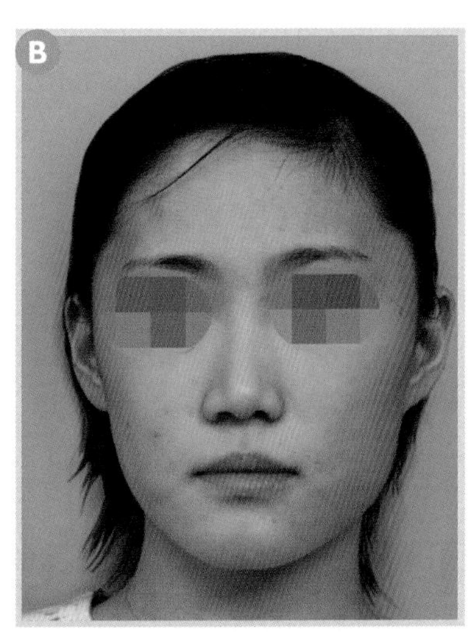

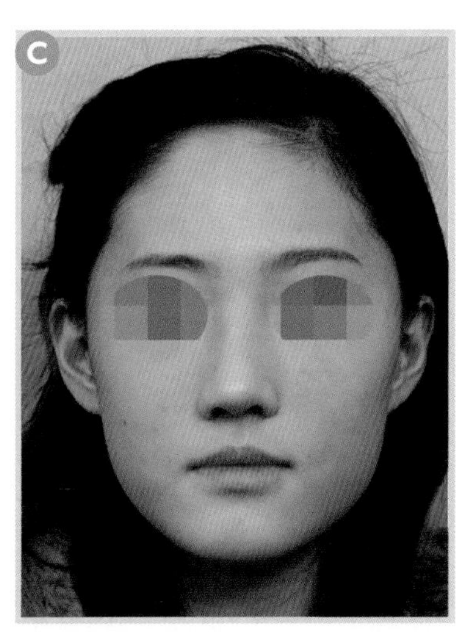

Figure 9 A patient with deviated nose. Before simulation (A), after simulation (B), and actual photo after surgery (C).

3) Flat Nose

When determining the level of projection and rotation during tip surgery, the patient's profile and basal view photos are useful for simulation. In simulations of the nasal tip, it is important to focus on the overall triangular form in the basal view, the ratio between the infratip lobule and the nostril, and the shape of the nostrils. In simulation of tip projection, if the nostril is lengthened along with the tip or if the tip is augmented without changes to the nostril, it is possible for the ratio between the infratip lobule and nostril height to become larger than the ideal 1:2 ratio or rather close to 1:1. Thus, simulation must be performed in consideration to the ideal shape of nostril and ratio between infratip lobule and nostril height *(Figure 10)*.

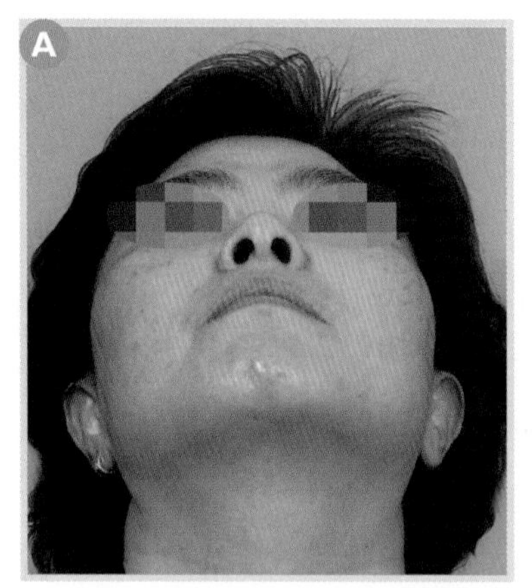

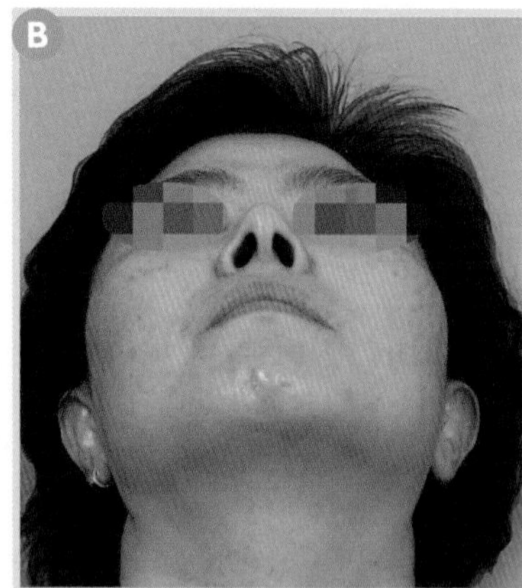

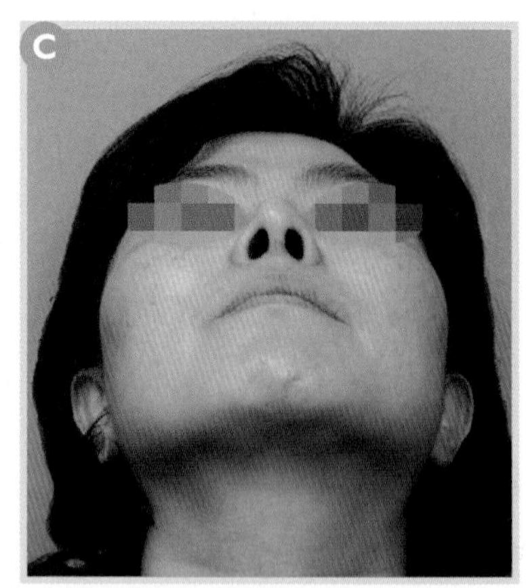

Figure 10 Before simulation (A), after simulation (B), and actual photo after surgery (C).

3. Steps of Simulation

Since the simulation process and methods are not fixed, the experience of the operator performing the simulation is the most crucial factor in deciding the quality of the simulation result. After understanding the ideal shape of the nose that the patient wants in the simulation process, the operator should decide on how much modification will be applied to original image using the warping technique, and to check if the result comes within the range of the ideal nose shape or ratio. Consistency between the actual image after rhinoplasty and the simulation image seems to depend on the operator's experience and anatomical features of the patient. Therefore, as the simulation conductor becomes more familiar with the simulation tools and gains experience, the simulation results will also improve. The conventional simulation steps for rhinoplasty patients are depicted in *Figure 11*.

V. Limitations of Computer Simulation

Despite their many benefits, computer simulation programs are costly, time and effort are required to get accustomed to the simulation software, and they require additional examination time. In addition, although computer simulation shows the height of the dorsum, contour, shape

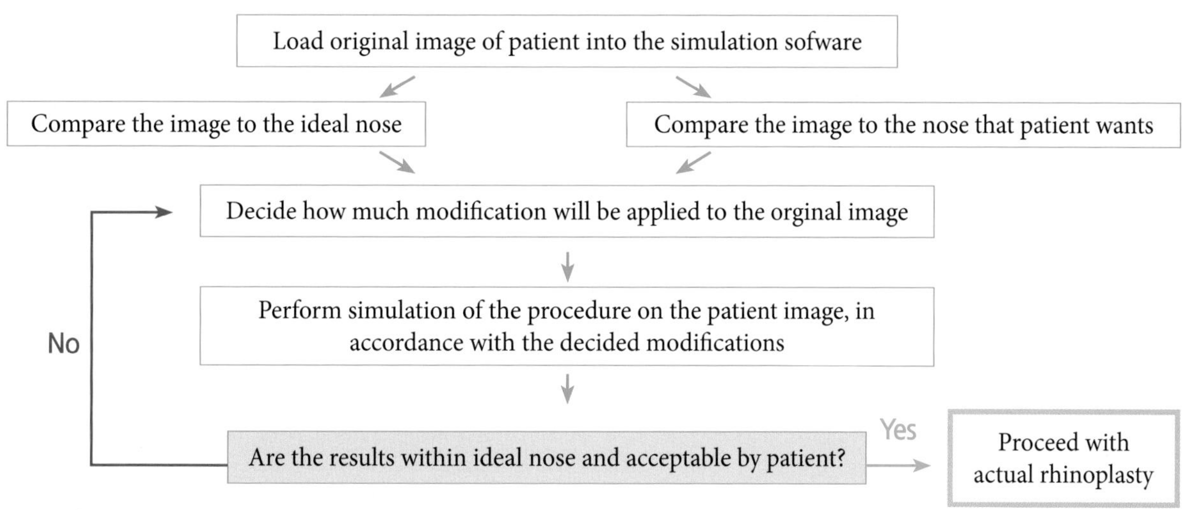

Figure 11 Algorithm on preoperative computer simulation of rhinoplasty patients.

and height of the nasal tip that the patient wants, and is a necessary step for consultation, it is not easy to create a natural-looking simulation image from the frontal photo *(Figure 12)*. Furthermore, the ethical dilemma of showing patients the ideal results and possibly coaxing them into surgery and the legal ramifications that may follow on the discrepancies between the simulation images and surgical results are yet to be resolved. Therefore, it is important that the operator knows precisely what the patient wants and helps the patient have a realistic expectation at the same time. Despite all these disadvantages, using computer simulation more actively has its advantages in that it makes the operator to pursue perfection to the result of surgery by improving the operator's eye for beauty and raising aesthetic goal. In conclusion, preoperative computer simulation may be an important factor in managing a successful rhinoplasty clinic.

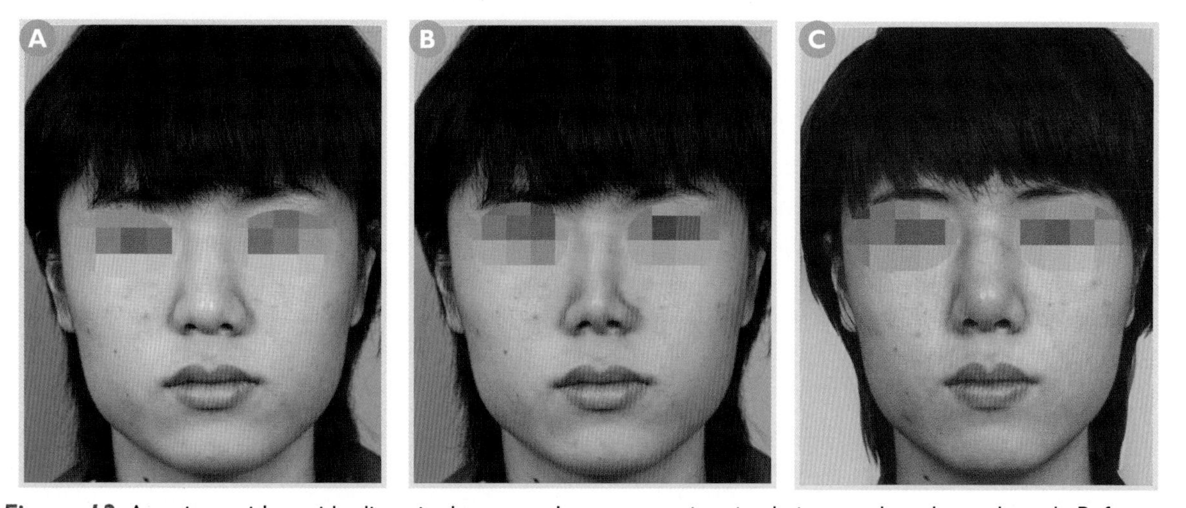

Figure 12 A patient with a wide disparity between the preoperative simulation result and actual result. Before simulation (A), simulated image (B), and actual postoperative result (C).

References

1. Anderson J.R., The dynamics of rhinoplasty, Proceedings of the Ninth International Congress of Otorhinolaryngology, Excerpta Medica 1969.
2. Wolberg G. Digital Image Warping, Wiley, IEEE Press, New York 1990.
3. Ozku.T. l, Ozkul. M.H.. Computer simulation tool for rhinoplasty planning. Computers in Biology and Medicine 2004

Incision

Yong Ju Jang

I. Significance and Classification of Incisions

The rhinoplasty begins with an incision. The success of the rhinoplasty can only be guaranteed when the appropriate incision needed for the surgery is selected and performed without causing any technical problem. Incisions made within the interior of the nose, relative to the lower lateral cartilage, include the marginal (infracartilaginous), extended marginal incision, intercartilaginous incision and intracartilaginous (transcartilaginous) incision. In addition, in performing rhinoplasty using the open approach, there is the transcolumellar incision that is made on the columellar skin. Incisions that are applied to the septum include the complete transfixion incision, the hemitransfixion incision, and partial transfixion incision. Most rhinoplasties can be performed using the above-mentioned incisions.

II. Incisions Performed on the Interior of the Nose in the Endonasal Approach

1. Marginal Incision (Infracartilaginous Incision)

1) Surgical Technique

A marginal incision, also known as the infracartilaginous incision, is placed at the caudal border of the lower lateral cartilage *(Figure 1)*. It can be made from the medial to the lateral direction in one movement. However, if this incision is selected for the delivery approach, it is recommended that the incision be made in two stages. First, begin the incision from the dome area to create the lateral limb of the incision. Since the lateral crus is located further from the nostril rim as it moves laterally, make the lateral component along the caudal border of lateral crus, which is about 15 mm from the nostril rim margin. However, in some patients the lateral crus is extremely close to the alar rim, this procedure therefore needs to be performed with great caution with constant efforts to verify the caudal margin of the lateral crus. The next step involves creating the medial limb of the incison. This medial limb must envelop the caudal border of the lower lateral cartilage (especially in the soft triangle), turning downwards to reach all the way to the middle third of the columella.

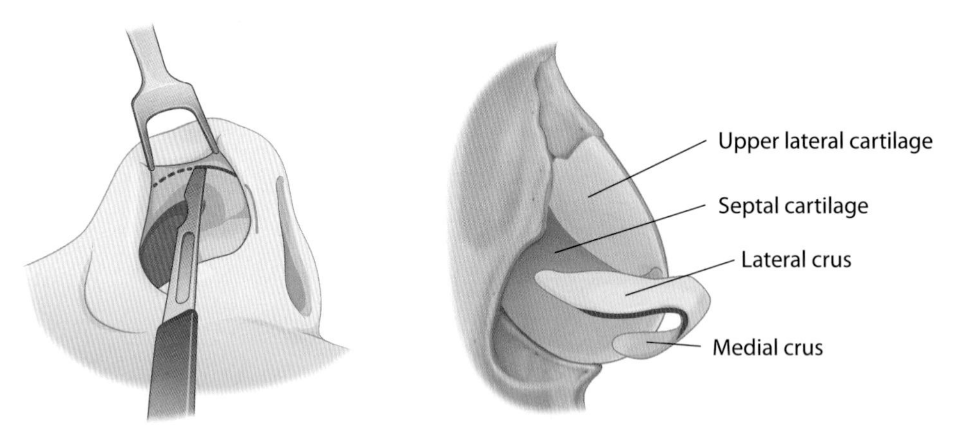

Figure 1 Marginal incision.

2) Application

More than anything else, the marginal incision is the most commonly used in rhinoplasty. Simple augmentation of the nasal dorsum using alloplastic implants can easily be done through this incision. In addition, during a closed rhinoplasty, using a limited marginal incision to place a tip onlay graft or a shield graft is a commonly used technique. In the delivery approach, this technique is used concurrently with an intercartilaginous incision.

2. Extended Marginal Incision

The lower lateral cartilages are well exposed when the marginal incision is extended to the footplate medially, and to the nostril floor laterally. When these incisions are made bilaterally, wide exposure of similar the extent with the external approach can be obtained without making a transcolumellar incision. Various procedures on the nasal dorsum can be done under good surgical view.

3. Intercartilaginous Incision

1) Surgical Technique

The intercartilaginous incision is made at the limen vestibuli or the connection between the upper lateral cartilage and the lower lateral cartilage *(Figure 2)*. Because there is a risk of damaging the nasal valve in performing this incision, the incision must be made at least 1-2 mm away from the limen vestibuli in the caudal direction. During this procedure, the cartilage beneath the incision can be partially incised. In doing this incision, the alar rim should be retracted with a double hook and gently pulled upwards as the incision proceeds laterally starting from the medial aspect using a #15 blade. During this process, the incision from the mucosa to the cartilage should be performed in one motion. If a unilateral complete transfixion incision is planned, the skin hook should be located at the medial crural footplate and pulled downward to prevent the formation of a visible scar.

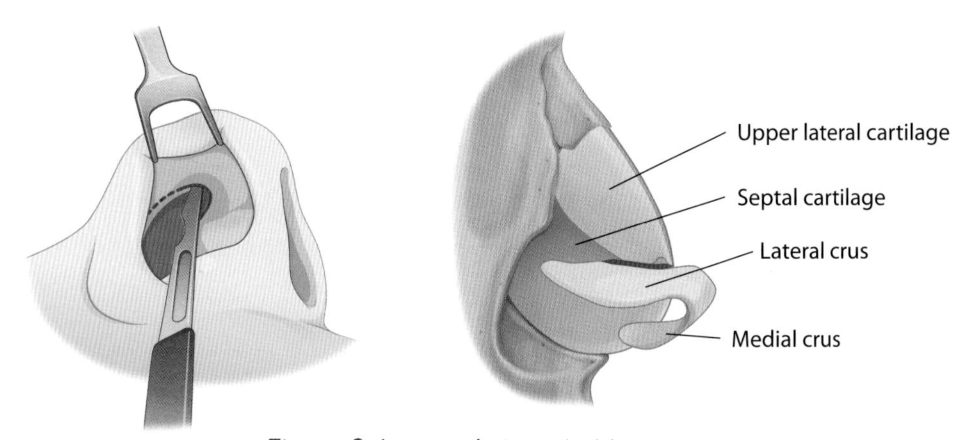

Figure 2 Intercartilaginous incision.

2) Application

This incision technique is generally appropriate for carrying out a retrograde approach by inducing eversion of the lateral crura during tip surgery, or in performing surgery using the delivery approach by adding the marginal incision. In addition, this incision is useful for accessing the osseocartilaginous vault when the incision is extended towards the medial direction to the anterior septal angle and connected to the upper part of the transfixion incision. This incision can induce tip ptosis through damage to the tip support mechanism by destroying the scroll area, as seen on long-term follow-up of patients.

4. Intracartilaginous Incision

1) Surgical Technique

This incision, also called the transcartilaginous incision, involves transecting the lateral crus of the lower lateral cartilage *(Figure 3)*. It entails making a curved incision shaped like a wing of a seagull at the cephalic location 4-6 mm from the caudal border of the lateral crus of the lower lateral cartilage. It is performed in full thickness, transecting all the layers of the cartilage.

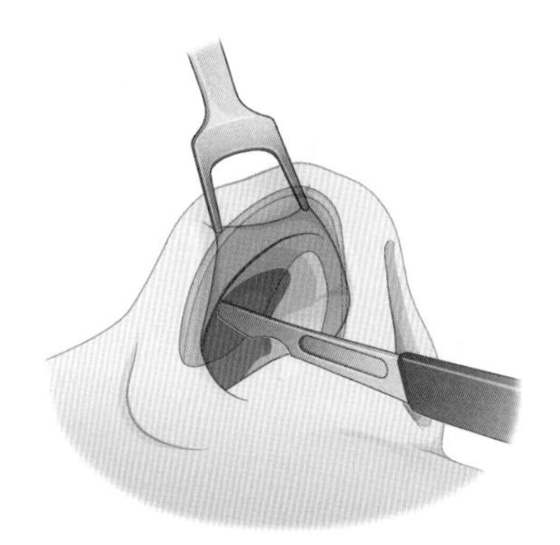

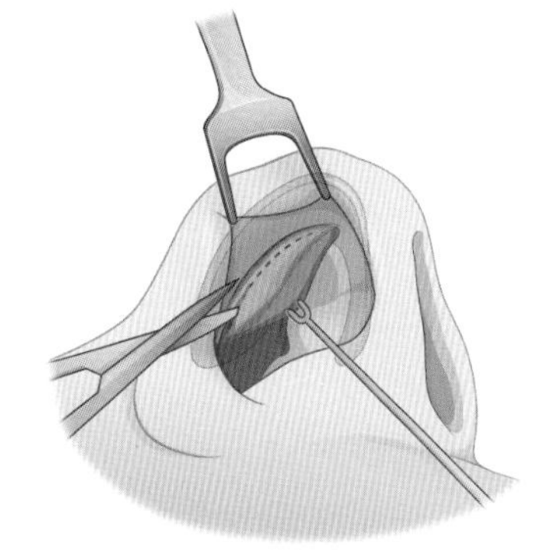

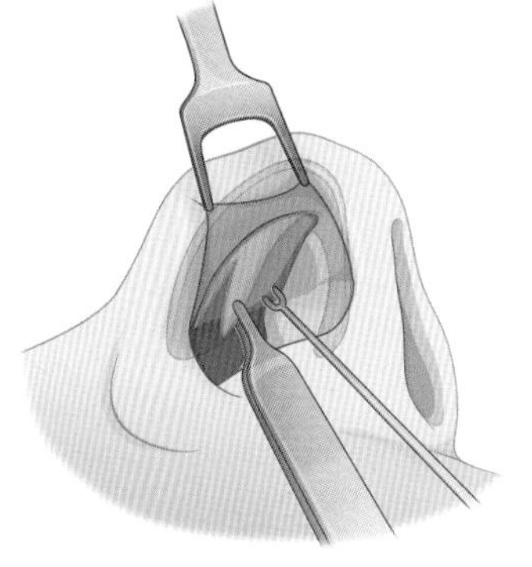

Figure 3 Intracartilaginous incision.

The resection itself is usually made after a subcutaneous dissection and shape of the cartilage is assessed by raising the vestibular skin.

2) Application

This incision is performed during the cartilage-splitting approach. During this procedure, a direct incision is made on the cartilage only to the extent where cephalic resection is possible. This incision is widely used in rhinoplasty for Caucasian noses and in operations combining cephalic resection of the lateral crus.

5. Rim Incision

This is an incision that is performed around the alar rim. In Korea, this incision has frequently been used for dorsal augmentation surgery using silicone. The inherent problem of this incision is that it can cause damage to the soft triangle on the medial side with a limited exposure of the lateral crus. Extreme caution must be taken not to induce scarring which may cause a nostril deformity.

III. Transcolumellar Incision and Marginal Incision as Applied to the Open Rhinoplasty Approach

1. Incision Technique

A transcolumellar incision, together with bilateral marginal incisions are used in the open rhinoplasty approach. A transcolumellar incision can be made in various configurations but generally the inverted V-shaped incision is preferred *(Figure 4A)*. In addition, the stair-step incision is also widely used. A V-shaped incision can also be made close to the columellar base *(Figure 4B)*. For patients with a short columella, there is a risk that one end of the stair-step incision will come too close to the soft triangle thereby resulting in an unsightly scar. Both wings of the

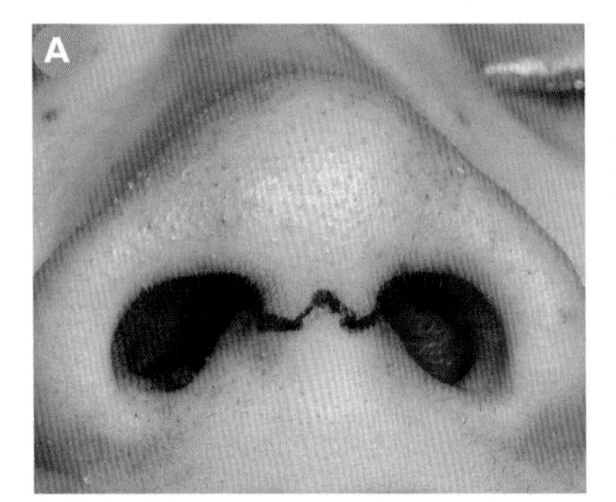

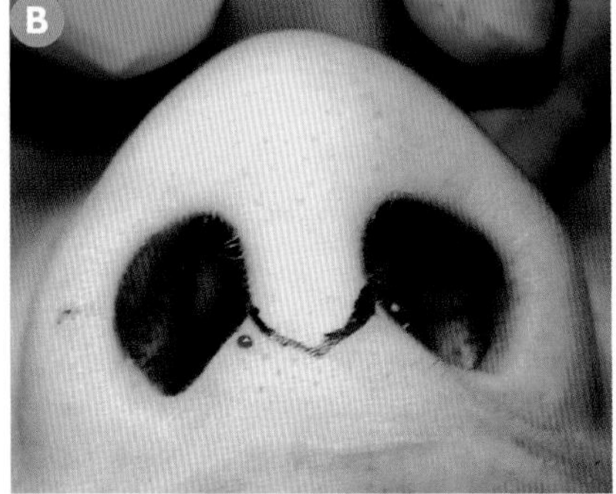

Figure 4 Inverted V- shaped incision (A), and V incision (B) for the external rhinoplasty approach.

incision line of the inverted V-shaped transcolumellar incision are located just below the narrowest region of the columella and the inverted V is extended above it for up to 2 mm.

A skin flap can also be elevated with a single V incision at the columellar base when planning a columellar flap. The columellar base or footplate can easily be accessed using this incision. According to the author's experience, the inverted V-shaped incision showed the best cosmetic outcome. In making the transcolumellar incision, first draw on the skin the desired shape of the transcolumellar incision. The biggest problem in performing the transcolumellar incision is that the skin in this region is too thin and close to the cartilage. Thus, during the incision, there are many instances where the medial crural cartilage is inadvertently cut. To avoid this, the author recommends that the medial limbs of the marginal incision be first made on both sides and a space be created between the skin and cartilage using iris scissors. The procedure is then continued towards the columella using a #15 blade after verifying the approximate boundary of the caudal margin of the cartilage at around 2 mm on the inside of the nostril rim *(Figure 5A)*. This is done on both sides. When the marginal incision is too close to nostril rim, a visible hypertrophic scar can occur at the incision site. Thus, it is important to make the marginal incision fully on the inside of the nose.

The next step is placing the scissors in the space created between the skin and the caudal margin of the cartilage and performing the transcolumellar incision using a #11 blade *(Figure 5B)*. While performing this incision, care must be exercised to make sure that the skin is incised perpendicularly instead of tilting the blade if a trapdoor deformity is to be avoided. If the above technique is followed, damage to the cartilage, a common phenomenon during the transcolumellar incision, rarely, if ever takes place.

Then, using a double hook to raise the skin flap, verify the caudal margin of the alar cartilages while extending the incision laterally. After the columellar skin flap has been raised, the columellar branch of the two superior labial arteries in front of the cartilage can become visible or, in case they are cut, bleeding frequently takes place. In this case, a bipolar cautery with a fine tip can be used to control the bleeding.

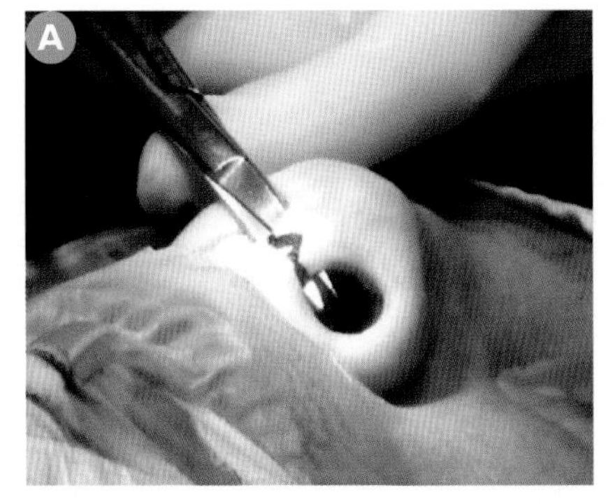

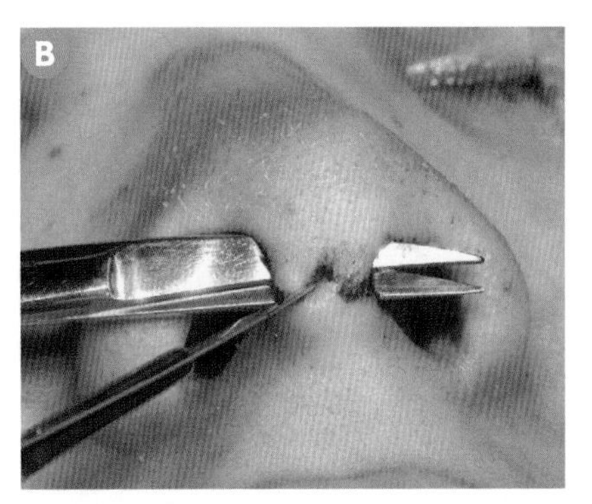

Figure 5 Photograph of a transcolumellar incision being made with a scissors inserted at the precrural space to protect the medial crus (A). Transcolumellar incision is completed using a #11 blade (B).

2. Suturing the Incision

When suturing the incision line, care must be taken to ensure that notching at the margin or other deformities are avoided. In performing the closure, the subcutaneous suture begins at the apex of the inverted V. It helps to relieve tension on the incision, so that the wound can recover without scarring. In placing the subcutaneous suture, 6-0 Vicryl or PDS is used. If there is no tension when the skin is apposed, simple interrupted sutures are placed using a 7-0 or 6-0 Nylon. The first two sutures are located on either side of the apex of the inverted V, and carried from the medial part of the lower flap to the upper flap in order to appropriately align the flap edges. In addition, the vestibular skin located in the corner of the columellar flap needs to be sutured using a 6-0 Vicryl or Chromic suture.

IV. Incisions Performed on the Septum

1. Hemitransfixion Incision

This is an incision made only on one side of the caudal septum and involves making an incision on the vestibular skin at the caudal septal edge. It is best to place the incision at a point 1 mm cephalic to the caudal margin of the cartilage. This technique allows for preservation of the basic structural integrity of the membranous septum, while adequately accessing the whole septum, including the cartilage and bony parts. In cases of severely deviated caudal septum, the author usually makes a more caudally placed hemitransfixion incision to the caudal margin of the septal cartilage for wide exposure of the anterior nasal spine *(Figure 6)*. Through this incision, a contralateral flap can be elevated on the septum without making an additional incision on the opposite side and the caudal septum can be manipulated more easily.

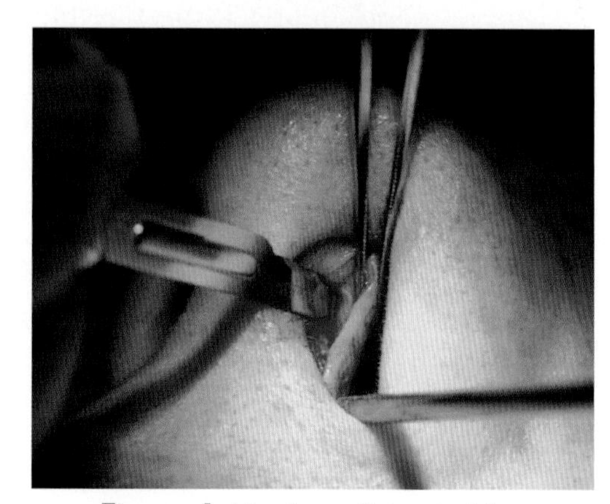

Figure 6 Hemitransfixion incision.

2. Complete Transfixion Incision

This incision starts at the membranous septum located between the caudal border of the septal cartilage and the columella and continues deep until it reaches the contralateral side of the membranous septum. This incision is generally combined with the intercartilaginous incision or the intracartilaginous incision to facilitate separation of the caudal margin of the septum from the membranous septum and the medial crura. A complete transfixion incision signifies that the posterior end of the incision had reached all the way down to the nasal spine. A problem with this incision is that it may damage the major tip support mechanisms, which consists of the medial crura and nasal septum converging to support the tip.

V. Complications

If scarring occurs at the area of the intercartilaginous incision, the nasal valve can become constricted, causing nasal obstruction. Excessive scarring can also appear in the region where the marginal incision was sutured, in which case, nasal obstruction can occur as a result of narrowing of the external valve. If suturing of the marginal incision or the rim incision in the soft triangle area isn't performed correctly, notching of this area can take place. There is a concern of obvious hypertrophic scar formation in the transcolumellar incision. However, the author has not experienced keloid or hypertrophic scar formation at the transcolumellar incision site even in patients who developed keloids at the conchal cartilage or costal cartilage harvest sites *(Figure 7)*.

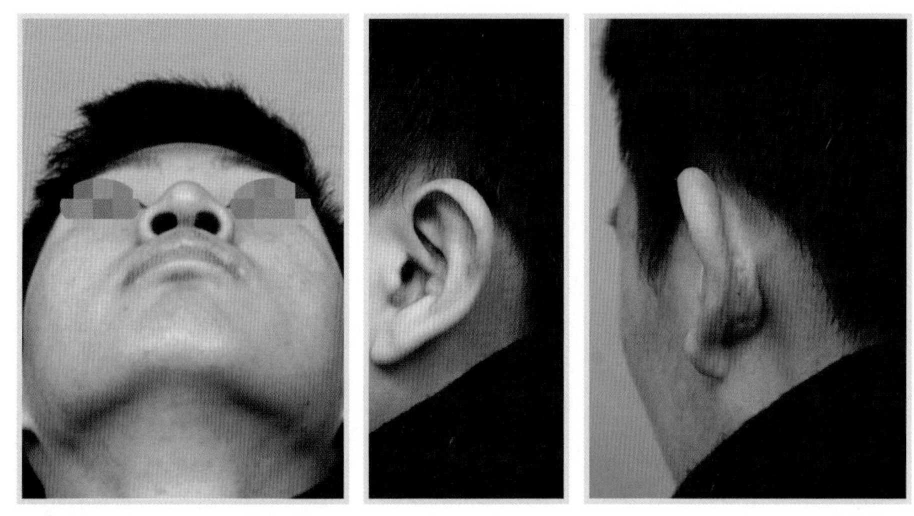

Figure 7 Even though the patient developed a keloid at the conchal cartilage harvest site, he did not show keloid or hypertrophic scarring at transcolumellar incision site.

In cases where the marginal incision is located too close to the nostril rim or wound edge, or if closure is imprecise, a hypertrophic scar can be seen. Such unpleasant scarring can develop under the following circumstances *(Figure 8)*:

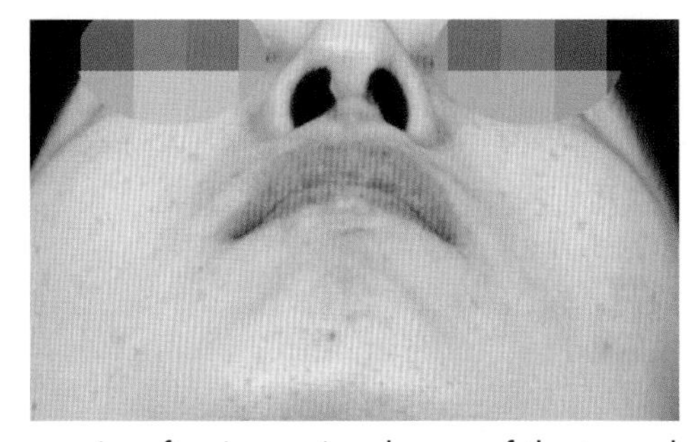

Figure 8 An unsightly scar can arise after imprecise closure of the trascolumellar and marginal incisions.

- When the suture is made too tight resulting in poor blood supply
- When the tip graft is made too large, causing excessive tension on the skin
- When there is infection in the suture area

Such complications must be avoided. And, it is quite possible to prevent such complications if the general rules of suturing and proper wound care are followed.

References

1. Adamson PA, Galli SK. Rhinoplasty approaches: current state of the art. Arch Facial Plast Surg 2005; 7: 32-7.
2. Alexander RW. Fundamental terms, considerations, and approaches in rhinoplasty. Atlas Oral Maxillofac Surg Clin North Am 1995; 3: 15-25.
3. Gamboa M, Shayani P, Schmid R, Bobadilla E, Blackwell S. Anatomic basis of notch deformity in open rhinoplasty. Ann Plast Surg 2003; 50: 282-5.
4. Kang JG, Ryu J. Nasal tip surgery using a modified septal extension graft by means of extended marginal incision. Plast Reconstr Surg 2009; 123: 343-52.
5. Mavili ME, Tuncali D. Open rhinoplasty through a forked flap incision. Aesthetic Plast Surg 1999; 23: 247-51.
6. Rohrich RJ, Muzaffar AR, Gunter JP. Nasal tip blood supply: confirming the safety of the transcolumellar incision in rhinoplasty. Plast Reconstr Surg 2000; 106: 1640-1.
7. Senyuva C, Yucel A, Aydin Y, Okur I, Guzel Z. Extracorporeal septoplasty combined with open rhinoplasty. Aesthetic Plast Surg 1997; 21: 233-9.

Osteotomy

Yong Ju Jang

Osteotomy is one of the most important surgical techniques in rhinoplasty, especially for the deviated nose, convex dorsum, and wide dorsum. However, it is also one of the most unpredictable and difficult techniques to perform accurately, as well as being the most invasive procedure. In addition, it is an important process that must be performed with utmost accuracy if a successful surgical result is to be obtained. Nevertheless, there are many technical obstacles that are needed to be overcome before osteotomy can be performed in an accurate and reliable manner. Among the various osteotomy methods, the lateral osteotomy is the most difficult to perform, because the osteotomy path is hidden under the skin. Also, the process of manipulating the bone in order for it to move to the desired position predicates the risk of weakening the supporting structures of the nose. However, these difficulties can be overcome by familiarizing oneself with the dynamics and possible complications of osteotomy. The purpose of this Chapter is to offer practical assistance on how, and in what situations osteotomy should be performed.

I. Objectives

The objectives of performing osteotomy during rhinoplasty are the following:

- ☑ Narrowing the width of a broad bony pyramid *(Figure 1)*.
- ☑ Correcting an open roof deformity created after hump resection *(Figure 2)*.
- ☑ Altering the direction of the bony pyramid while correcting the deviated nose by creating a controlled fracture at the bony pyramid.
- ☑ Correcting the concave-convex deformity of the bony pyramid.

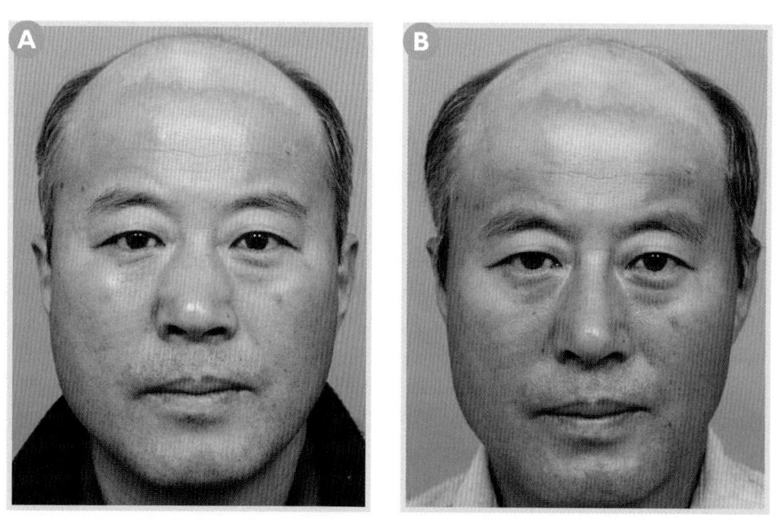

Figure 1 Before (A) and after (B) photographs of a patient displaying a wide and flat bony dorsum corrected by medial and lateral osteotomies. The dorsal aesthetic was improved.

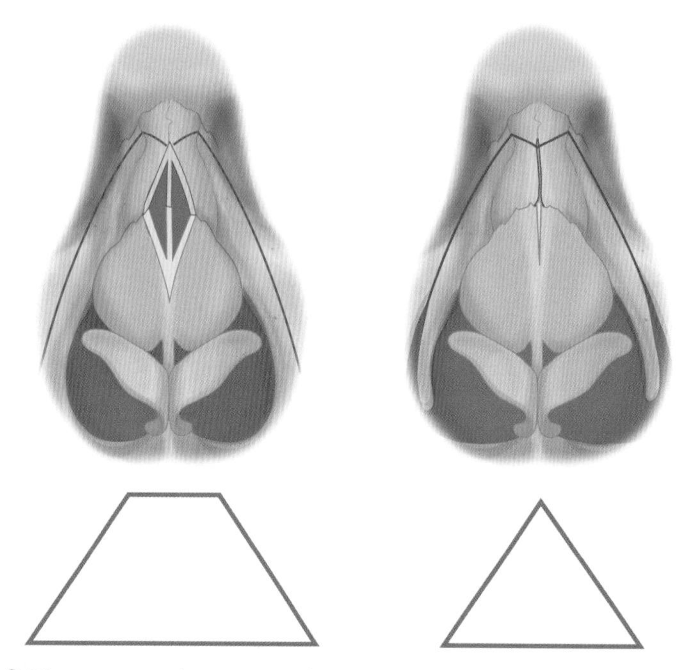

Figure 2 The process of correcting the open roof deformity through an osteotomy.

II. Classification

Osteotomy can be classified as a complete or incomplete osteotomy, depending on whether a complete incision of the bone is performed or not. An incomplete osteotomy is mostly a phenomenon that is associated with the execution of a percutaneous osteotomy, while a complete osteotomy is an osteotomy that should be created during the internal continuous osteotomy by means of an endonasal approach *(Figure 3)*. Furthermore, in accordance to which anatomical location it is performed on, it can be classified into the medial osteotomy, lateral osteotomy, and transverse osteotomy *(Figure 4)*. It can also be divided between endonasal osteotomy and percutaneous osteotomy depending on the surgical approach.

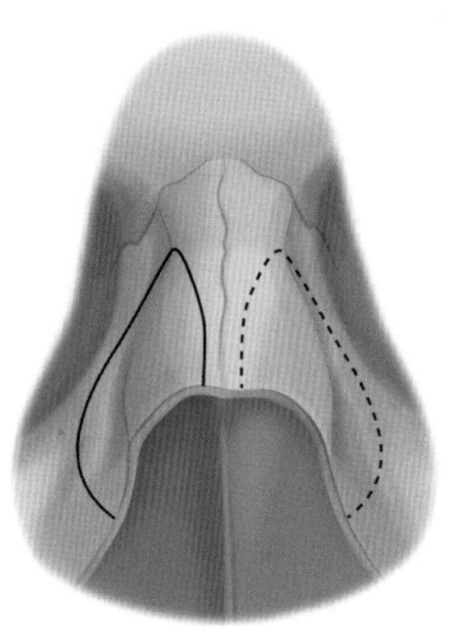

Figure 3 The continuous line on right bony dorsum shows a complete osteotomy and the dotted line on left bony dorsum shows an incomplete osteotomy.

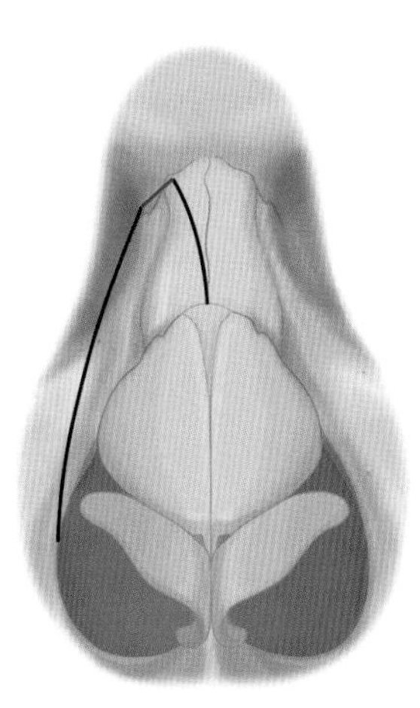

Figure 4 Connecting the medial osteotomy line and lateral osteotomy line (black lines) using a transverse osteotomy (red line).

III. Surgical Technique

1. Selection of Osteotome

Selecting the proper surgical instrument is a very important part of osteotomy. The answer to the question on what type of osteotome to select varies greatly in accordance to the individual preference of the surgeons. The smaller the osteotome, the less bleeding there is. However, the force that can be applied during the bony incision gets much smaller, thereby reducing its effectiveness. Widely used are the 3 mm and 2 mm osteotomes, and they are very helpful to precisely incise the bone *(Figure 5)*.

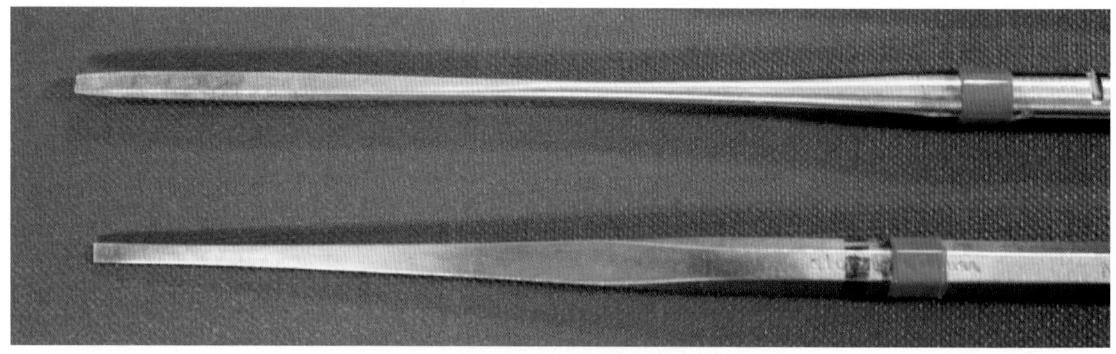

Figure 5 3 mm and 2 mm osteotomes are very helpful in performing an accurate osteotomy.

The bigger the osteotome, the easier it is to perform a complete osteotomy. However, the risk of damaging the mucosa increases in proportion, leading to a tendency for severe bleeding. The osteotome can be classified between the guarded and unguarded osteotomes. The advantages of a guarded osteotome are that it can be easily hooked to the bone, reduces slippage, and the surgeon can perform the osteotomy while palpating the advancement of the guard *(Figure 6)*. The guard attached to the guarded osteotome was originally designed to point towards the nasal cavity, thereby elevating the nasal cavity mucosa and reducing hemorrhage. Nevertheless, it is now more common to use the method of doing the osteotomy wherein the guard is directed towards the skin so that the movement of the guard is felt through the skin *(Figure 7)*. An unguarded osteotome is more difficult to handle because of the greater tendency of slippage during its manipulation. It is also possible to classify the osteotome between the curved and straight osteotome according to its shape. The curved osteotome is usually used to perform a lateral osteotomy. A straight osteotome can be used during a medial osteotomy as well as in a lateral osteotomy. For the purpose of moving the incised area of bone towards the desired location, it is more expedient to use a straight osteotome. When performing a lateral osteotomy, the author usually uses a 4 mm guarded curved osteotome. For patients with particularly thick bones, a straight osteotome, which can convey

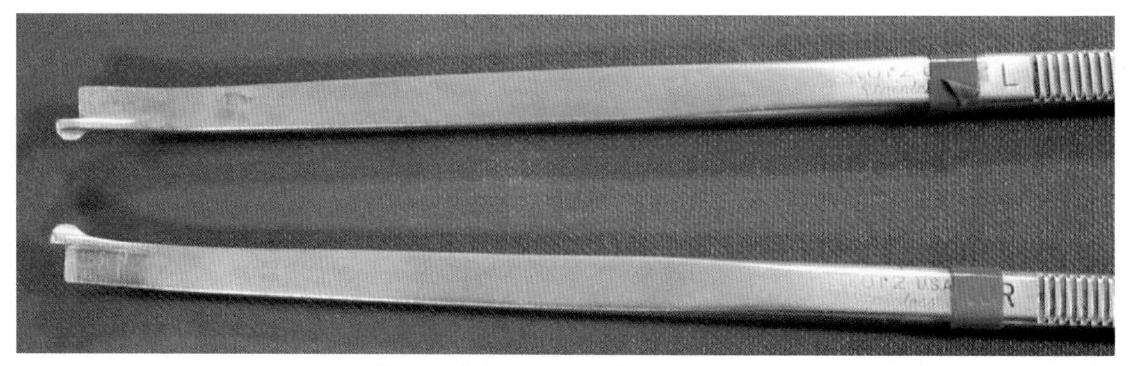

Figure 6 4 mm guarded osteotomes.

the force of the mallet more effectively, is used. For the medial osteotomy, a straight and sharp osteotome is preferred *(Figure 8)*. A 2 mm osteotome is usually used for percutaneous osteotomy.

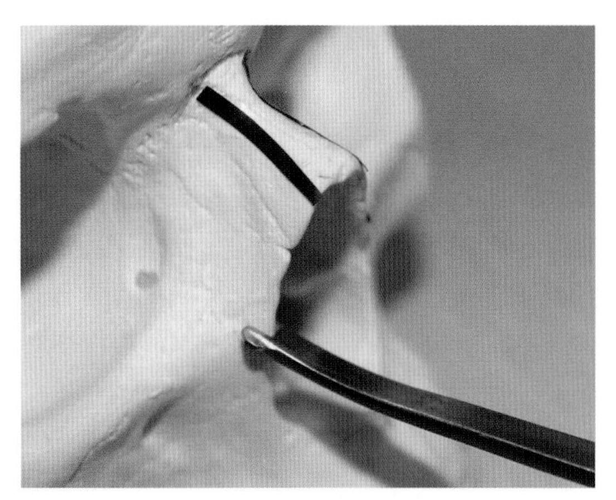

Figure 7 The method of conducting a right lateral osteotomy using a 4 mm guarded osteotome wherein the guard is directed towards the surface.

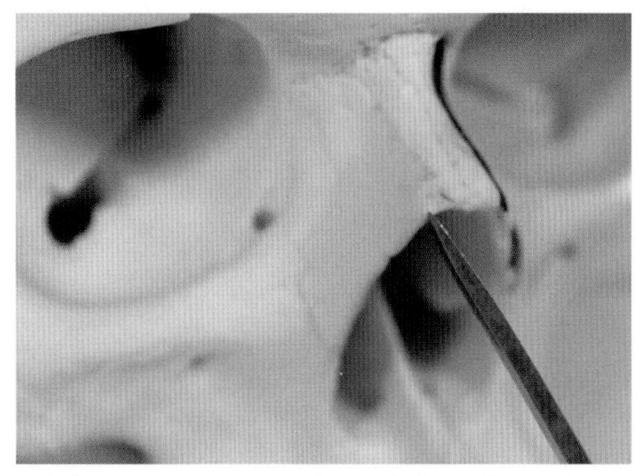

Figure 8 For a medial osteotomy, a straight and sharp 3 mm osteotome is preferred.

2. Medial Osteotomy

The medial osteotomy denotes the process of separating the bony septum from the nasal bone. Basically, it is performed to ensure that the result of the lateral osteotomy takes effect properly. As such, it is a supplementary surgical technique to the lateral osteotomy. A medial osteotomy alone cannot directly influence the correction of the shape and direction of the bony pyramid. The significance of this surgical technique, then, lies in the fact that it is a process whereby the rhinion of the bony pyramid and the bony septum connected to the cartilaginous septum is preserved while creating a bending area in advance so that the incised triangular bone fragment made after a lateral osteotomy can be manipulated to the desired area. Therefore, if a significant amount of nasal bone has been resected during humpectomy, there may be instances where the medial osteotomy may not be necessary. If a lateral osteotomy is performed prior to a medial osteotomy, as the nasal bone is already in an unstable condition, it will be difficult to perform medial osteotomy. Thus, it is preferable to perform the medial osteotomy first, followed by the lateral osteotomy. When performing a medial osteotomy through an open approach, after separating the upper lateral cartilages from the septum, the osteotome should be engaged on the caudal nasal bone and continued in an oblique direction towards the inner canthus, or in a paramedian direction almost parallel to the central line *(Figure 9)*. When performing a medial osteotomy for correcting bony deviation in cases of deviated noses, a paramedian position should be maintained to make a narrow midline bony segment. In this way, this narrow bony segment can be fractured easily by digital compression *(Figure 10)*. One must, however, be wary of the fact that if the medial osteotomy is carried too close to the paramedian location, a rocker-bottom deformity can occur when it is connected to the lateral osteotomy *(Figure 11)*. Therefore, it is best to start the medial osteotomy from the point of origin and proceed 15-25° in an oblique direction.

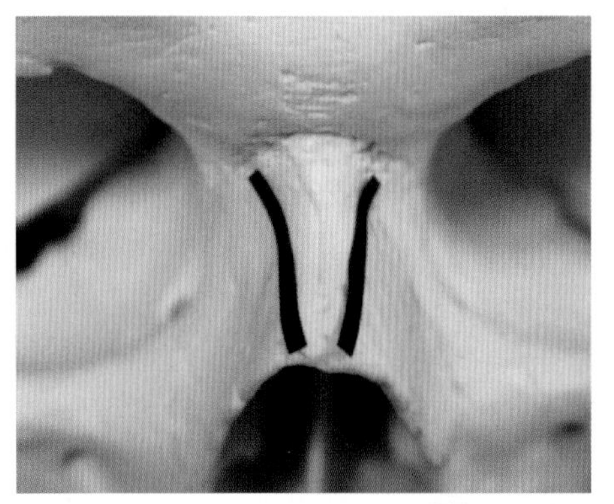

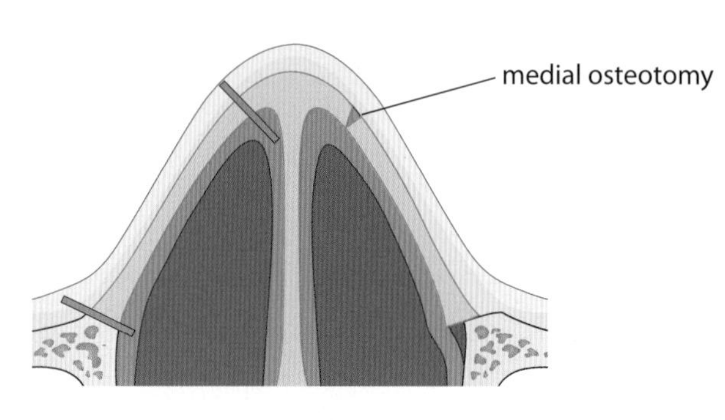

Figure 9 Typical site of medial osteotomy.

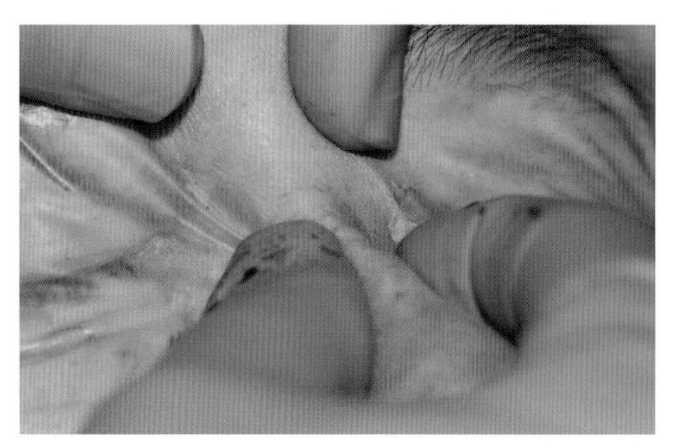

Figure 10 Further fracture of the midline bony structure can be made by digital compression after conducting medial and lateral osteotomies for deviated nose correction.

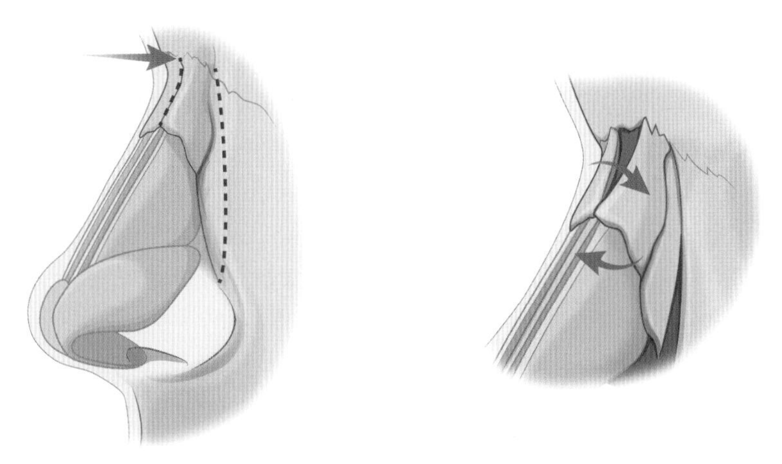

Figure 11 A rocker bottom deformity can occur when a medial osteotomy is performed too close to the paramedian location.

Because a medial osteotomy carried properly in this direction can be connected naturally with the lateral osteotomy, one need not go to extreme lengths in creating a back fracture. In patients with small nasal bones, however, bony comminution can complicate the lateral osteotomy if the medial osteotomy is performed too obliquely. In surgery that does not require the separation of the upper lateral cartilages and the septal cartilage, and rhinoplasty using the open approach isn't planned, it is possible to perform the medial osteotomy through a purely endonasal approach. This technique involves inserting an osteotome into the nasal cavity, and using the osteotome guard, create a perforation at the junction area of the nasal bone and the upper lateral cartilage. After the osteotome is engaged, one proceeds with the osteotomy from the paramedian to oblique directions (inside-out osteotomy) *(Figure 12)*.

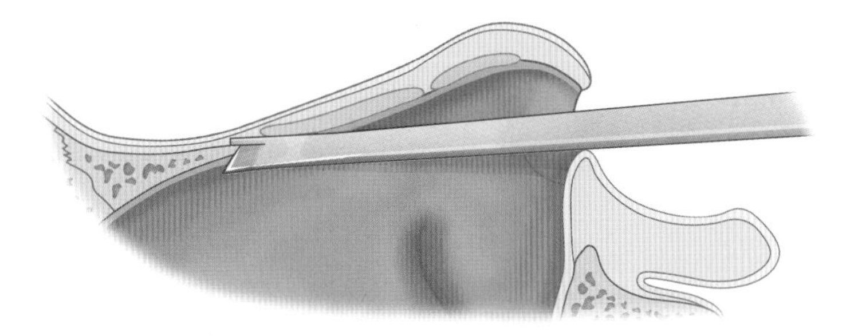

Figure 12 "Inside-Out" medial osteotomy via an endonasal approach.

A medial osteotomy can also be performed from above the upper lateral cartilage via an endonasal approach. In this method, perform dissection on the dorsum using the intercartilaginous incision and proceed further upward in the cephalic direction. One can begin performing the osteotomy, starting from the caudal margin of the nasal bone (outside-in osteotomy) *(Figure 13)*. A matter requiring special attention when performing a medial osteotomy is making sure that the starting points of both sides of the medial osteotomy are not kept too close to each other. If the starting points are located too close to each other, the keystone area can be damaged, and there is subsequent risk of inducing a saddle nose deformity *(Figure 14)*. Thus, a medial osteotomy should be performed in such a way that the bony septum, which is connected to the dorsal part of the septal cartilage, can maintain sufficient width. After medialization of the nasal bones following a lateral osteotomy, the mobilized bony segments can be asymmetric in height on the two sides, or both segments are symmetrical but higher than the midline segment. In such situations, the most prominent portion of the bony segment should be removed by bone cutting scissors to equalize the level *(Figure 15)*.

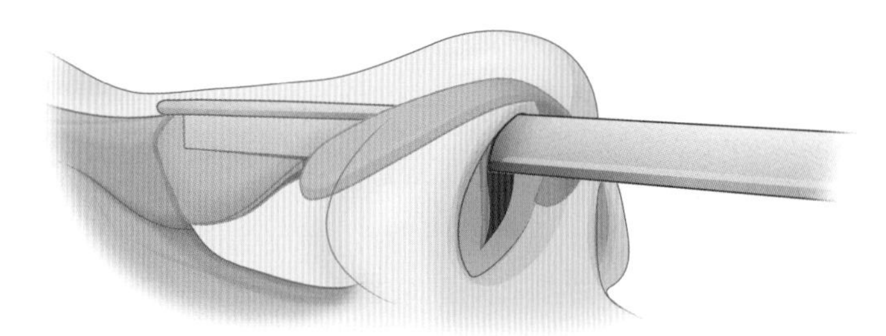

Figure 13 "Outside-In" medial osteotomy via an endonasal approach.

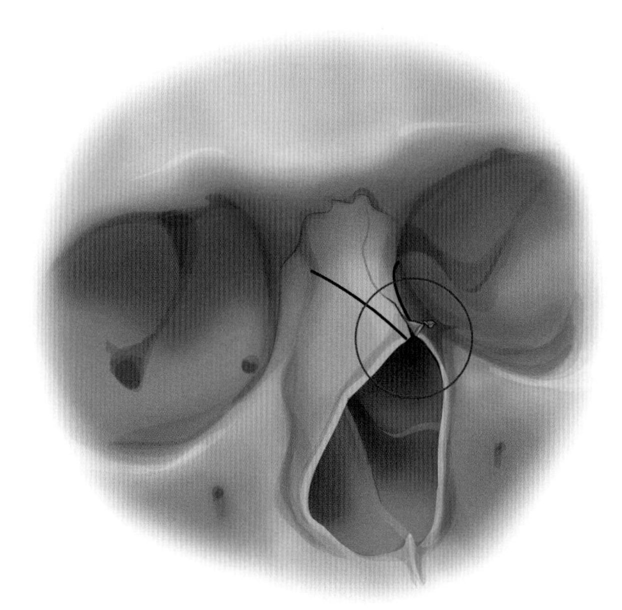

Figure 14 If the two starting points of the medial osteotomy are located too close to each other, an unwanted fracture can take place at midline bony segment.

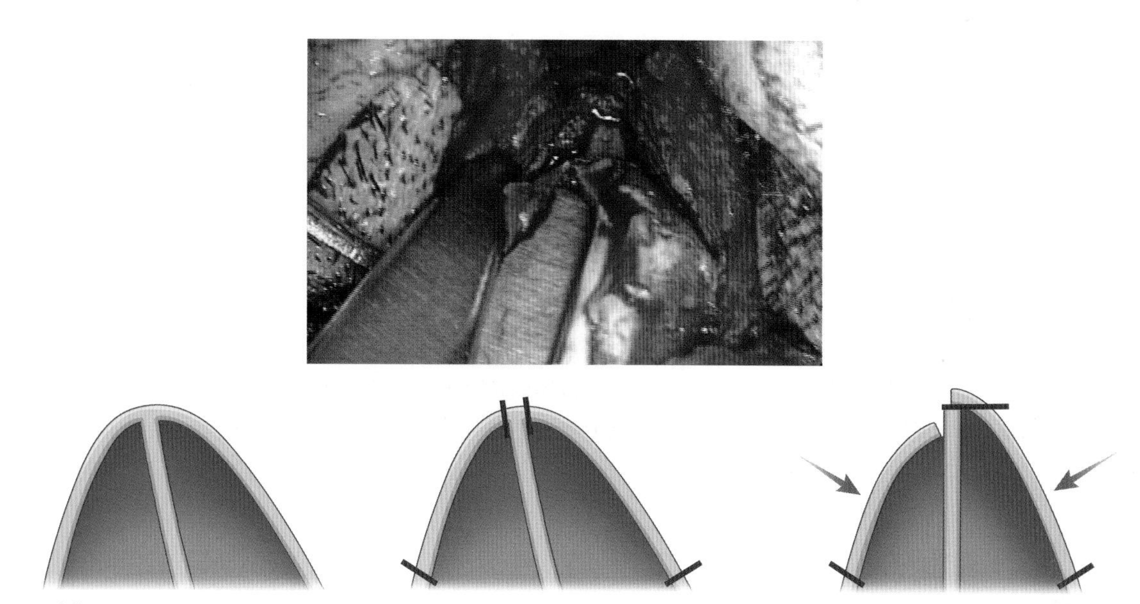

Figure 15 After medialization of the nasal bone segments following osteotomy, the mobilized bony segments can be asymmetric, or higher than midline segment. The most prominent point of the bony segment should be removed.

3. Lateral Osteotomy

1) Internal Continuous Lateral Osteotomy

This is used to incise the nasal bony sidewall in order to push it inward. At 10 to 15 minutes prior to the execution of the osteotomy, injection of a local anesthetic agent mixed with epinephrine should be infiltrated along the anticipated path of the osteotomy. Then, using a #15 blade, make an incision all the way to the periosteum at the pyriform aperture above the attachment of the inferior turbinate. Once the pyriform aperture bone is exposed, conduct the osteotomy along the planned osteotomy line using a curved osteotome or straight osteotome *(Figure 16)*.

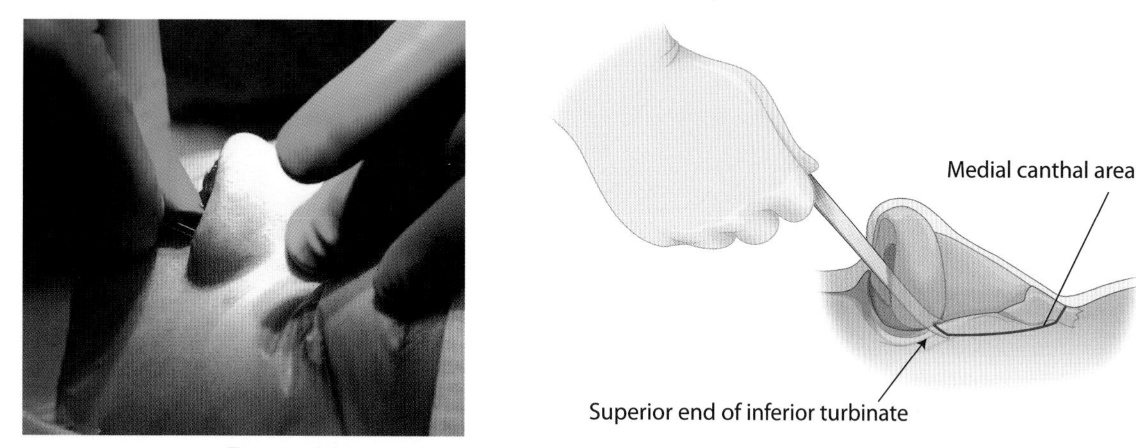

Figure 16 Internal continuous lateral osteotomy via an endonasal route.

Depending on the preference of the surgeon, there are instances where a subperiosteal tunnel is created along the incision line using a periosteal elevator. If the osteotomy commences at the bottom of the pyriform aperture, there is a risk of nasal obstruction occurring as a result of a reduction in the cross sectional area of the nasal airway when the incised bone is pushed medially. Thus, the osteotomy should be started above the attachment of the inferior turbinate. According to the vertical level of lateral osteotomy, it is described as low to low, low to high, high to high, etc. Considering the nasal dorsum as the apex, the area situated far from this apex is defined as "low" and the area close to it is defined as "high" *(Figure 17)*. When performing an osteotomy along the sidewalls of the nose, one can simply perform the osteotomy by following the nasofacial groove. Once the osteotomy gets closer to the lacrimal crest, the direction of osteotomy should be changed so that it proceeds towards the apex of the nose. Often, there are many instances of high osteotomies being formed in this area due to the excessive fear of damaging the lacrimal apparatus. However, because the bone of the lacrimal crest is very thick, it is very rare for actual damage to take place. Hence, it is necessary to perform osteotomy at the low position decisively. Furthermore, when using a curved osteotome, there is a high probability that a high osteotomy would be created if the osteotome proceeds exclusively along the thin area of bone. Should such a high osteotomy be formed, it can bring about a stair-step deformity that is both visible and palpable when cut bones are pushed inward.

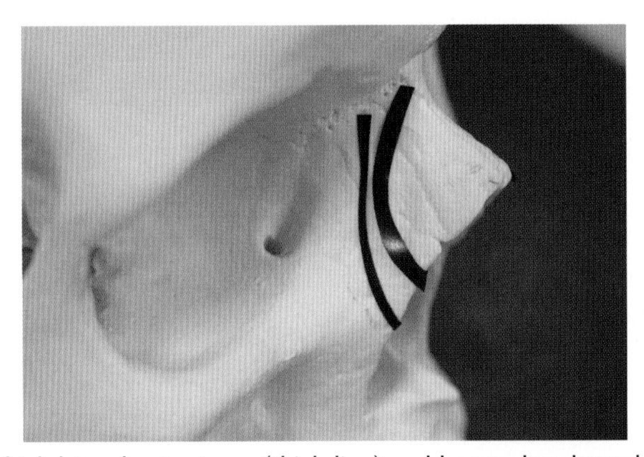

Figure 17 High-low-high lateral osteotomy (thick line) and low to low lateral osteotomy (thin line).

2) Percutaneous Lateral Osteotomy

When performing a percutaneous lateral osteotomy, using a 2 mm osteotome, an incision is made on the skin at the nasal base at about the level of the inferior orbital rim, and then the osteotome is inserted through this incision. To avoid damaging the angular artery, the incision is made slightly medial to the nasofacial groove, but the osteotomy is performed slightly lateral to the nasofacial groove by pulling the skin towards the cheek *(Figure 18)*. This is an important surgical technique to avoid injuring the angular artery.

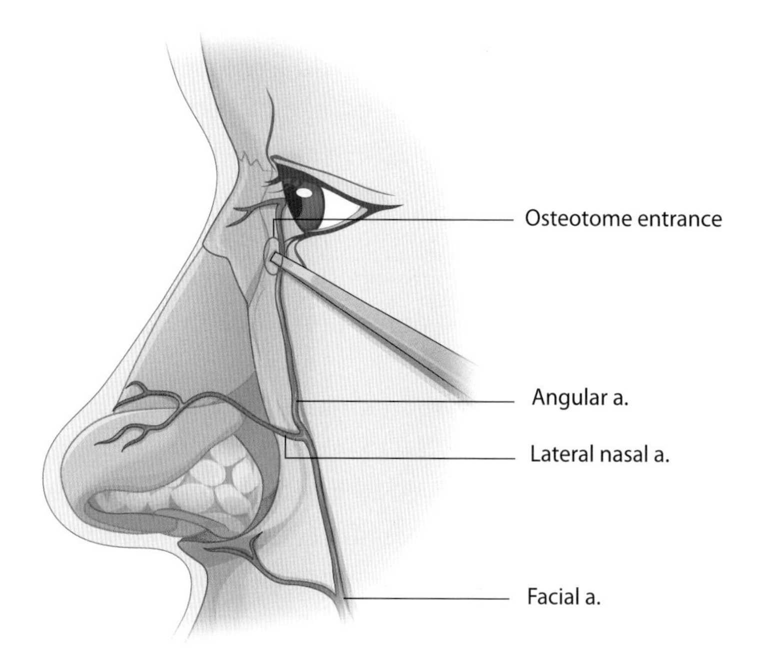

Figure 18 The percutaneous lateral osteotomy starts with an incision on the skin using an osteotome. To avoid damaging the angular artery, the incision should be performed at a slightly higher position than the actual osteotomy line and the osteotomy is performed while pulling the skin towards the cheek.

When conducting the osteotomy, the osteotome should be tilted at a 45° angle, and using a corner of the osteotome, a hole or perforation in the bone is created *(Figure 19)*. Once a hole is made, the osteotome should be slightly withdrawn and moved to an adjacent area in order to create a new hole. The purpose of this method is not creating a continuous line of incision, but creating a series of small holes *(Figure 20)*. Only a small amount of force is necessary to pierce the bone when using a 2 mm osteotome. Therefore, it is important to avoid the use of excessive

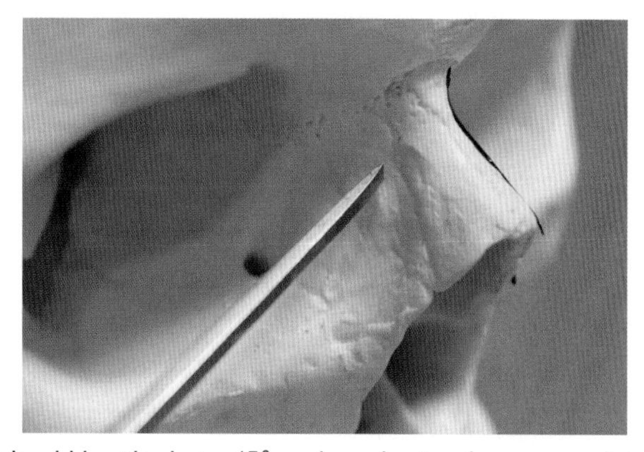

Figure 19 The osteotome should be tilted at a 45°-angle and using the corner of the osteotome, a hole or perforation in the bone is created

force. When the proper amount of force is used in this manner, damage to the mucosa within the nasal cavity can be reduced. The osteotomy should first proceed all the way to the pyriform aperture in the caudal direction. The closer the osteotomy gets to the caudal side, the thinner the bone becomes and less force is required in making subsequent perforations on the bone. Once the osteotomy in the caudal region is completed, the process is repeated to the cephalic direction, this time in the cephalo-medial direction from the skin incision and proceeds across the thick nasal bone area. Stronger force is needed when proceeding to the cephalic direction towards the nasal dorsum. The above mentioned procedures all can be performed through a single skin incision.

After doing the same procedure on the other side, pressure is applied evenly to the whole nasal bone by pressing down with a finger. The planned osteotomy is completed once the holes in the bone connect to each other. This surgical technique is reported to allow for easy visibility during surgery and reduce postoperative edema by causing less bleeding and damage to the mucosa. However, there is a technical difficulty in which the holes are difficult to create in people with thick bones. Also, because the procedure involves creating an incomplete osteotomy and then completing it by fracturing it, there is the disadvantage of not being able to make accurate adjustments of the osteotomy line. Thus, the author prefers the internal continuous osteotomy over the percutaneous lateral osteotomy.

3) Double Level Lateral Osteotomy

When performing lateral osteotomies, there are instances where the bony incisions on either side

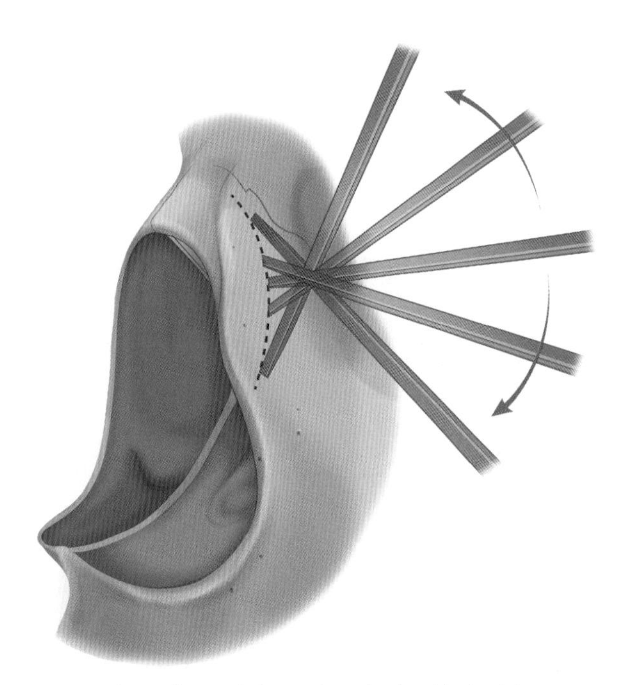

Figure 20 Percutaneous osteotomy is performed through a single skin incision to create multiple small holes.

are made at a slightly uneven level, resulting in a discrepancy between the two osteotomy lines. In such cases, a low to low osteotomy can be added from the side where the higher level osteotomy has been performed *(Figure 21)*.

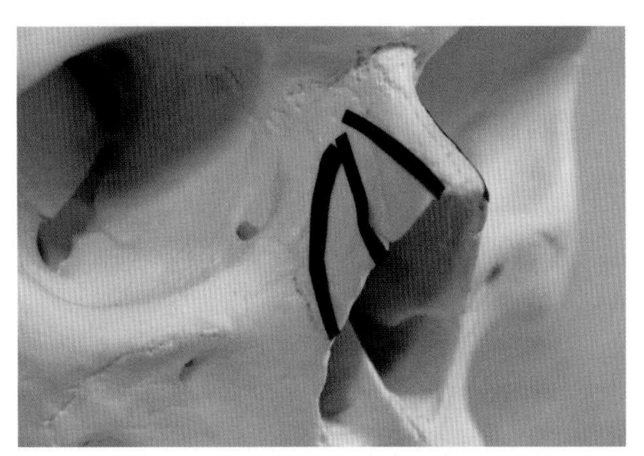

Figure 21 Double level lateral osteotomy (the lowermost and middle lines).

In doing so, the bone will be comminuted into small fragments and severe bleeding may occur. Thus, it is best to avoid this procedure. It is important to keep in mind that when performing a double level osteotomy, the higher osteotomy must be done first prior to performing the lower osteotomy in order for the osteotomy to be effective and to avoid comminution. This osteotomy is rarely performed in Korean patients as the nasal bone development is poor.

4. Transverse Osteotomy

When the medial osteotomy is performed close to the paramedian location and the lateral osteotomy is performed in a low to low manner, a transverse osteotomy can be performed to connect these two osteotomy lines *(Figure 22)*.

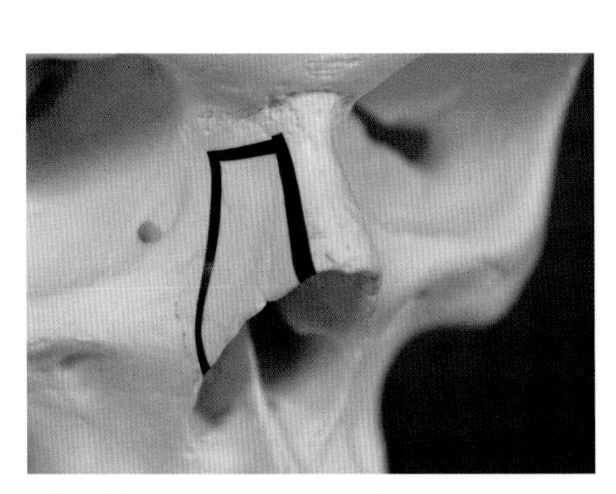

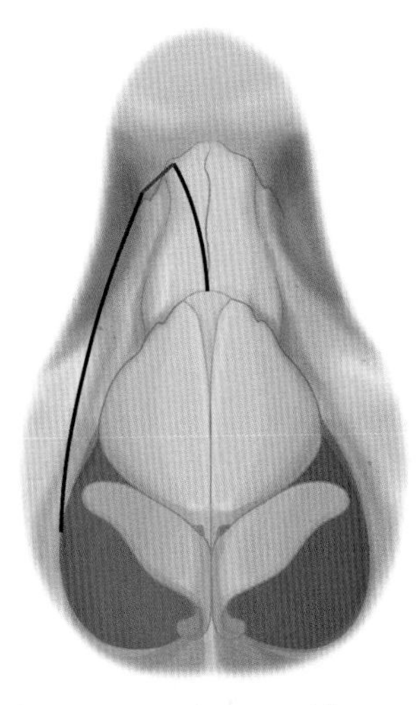

Figure 22 When the gap between the medial osteotomy and lateral osteotomy is too wide, a transverse osteotomy can be performed to connect the two osteotomies.

In the correction of a deviated nose, a medial osteotomy is performed in an oblique direction and connected to the lateral osteotomy. As such, a triangular shaped bony fragment (bony septum) will remain in the central area of the nasal bone. At this juncture, if the bony septum is deviated to one side and is left uncorrected, the overall axis of the nose cannot be relocated to the center *(Figure 23)*. In such a case, correction of this central part can be attempted by pressing down with a finger in order to induce a fracture. But this method carries the risk that the fracture may not occur at the desired location *(Figure 24)*. However, if a percutaneous root osteotomy is performed instead, the midline bony septum can be mobilized to the center. A percutaneous root osteotomy is performed at the intercanthal area using a 2 mm osteotome *(Figure 25)*. After making a partial fracture with 2 mm sharp osteotome targeting the midline bony segment, the midline bony segment becomes freely movable. The skin incision is sutured with 6-0 Nylon. This technique is useful in treating severe nasal bony deviations. As a prerequisite to this technique, the dorsal part of the cartilaginous septum must be separated from the upper lateral cartilages. A saddle nose deformity may occur after this procedure although it rarely happens if the caudal septum and the anterior nasal spine are firmly attached to each other. There are instances where the cut section collapses towards the nasal cavity following a root osteotomy. In such a case, it is recommended to perform onlay grafting using a bony fragment or cartilage, in addition to the reduction of the depressed portion by forceps through the nasal cavity.

IV. Things to be Considered During Osteotomy and Contraindications

The thickness of the bone is an important element that needs to be considered during osteotomy. The nasomaxillary complex comprising the bony pyramid is thick around the vicinity of the lacrimal crest and at the junction of the nasal bones, while it is thinnest at the caudal part, which is where the lateral osteotomy commences. In cases where the nasal bone is small but thick, instead

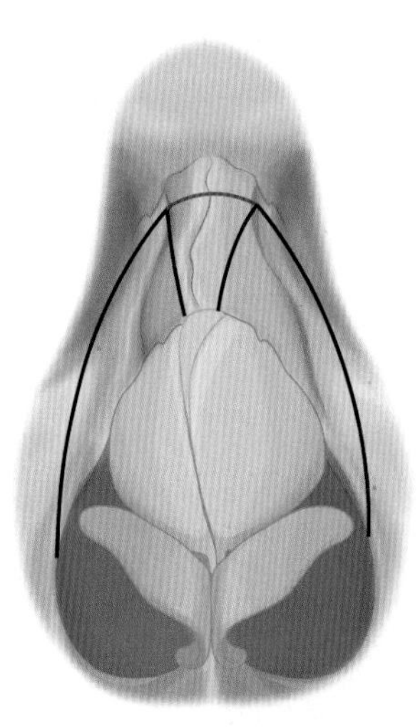

Figure 23 If the bony septum is still deviated to one side after osteotomies, central axis correction should be done to ensure successful correction of the deviated nose.

of achieving the desired incision of the nasomaxillary complex by means of osteotomy, there is a higher probability that the impact of the osteotomy will shatter the bone, fracturing it into small pieces. Thus, when the nasal bone is small and thick, it is desirable that alternative procedures such as an onlay grafting be contemplated instead of an osteotomy. Also, in cases where the patient had previously undergone a osteotomy, there is a high likelihood of inducing a comminuted fracture, instead of creating controlled fracture lines; the surgeon must be mindful of this. Once a comminuted fracture develops, it is recommended that augmentation of the dorsum be carried out. Augmentation helps prevent the irregular skeletal structure from showing through the skin. Also, because of the loss of skin elasticity in the elderly, there are instances where the transformed skeletal structure resulting from the osteotomy cannot be covered correctly. Also, among patients with excessively thick skin, the changes created by the osteotomy frequently cannot be reflected in the external appearance.

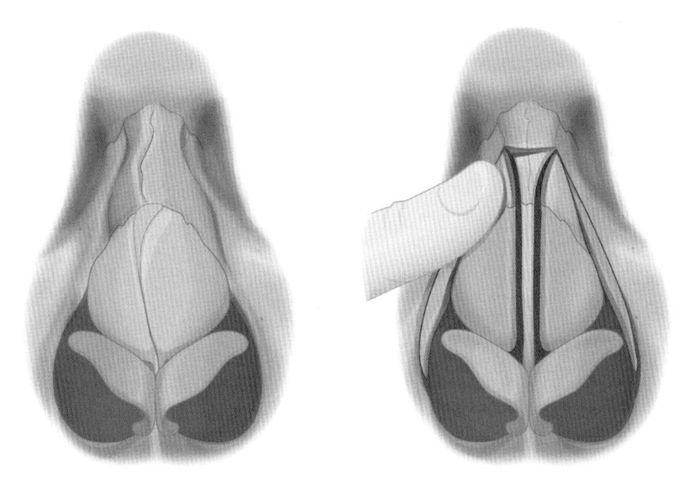

Figure 24 The midline bony septum can be fractured by digital compression.

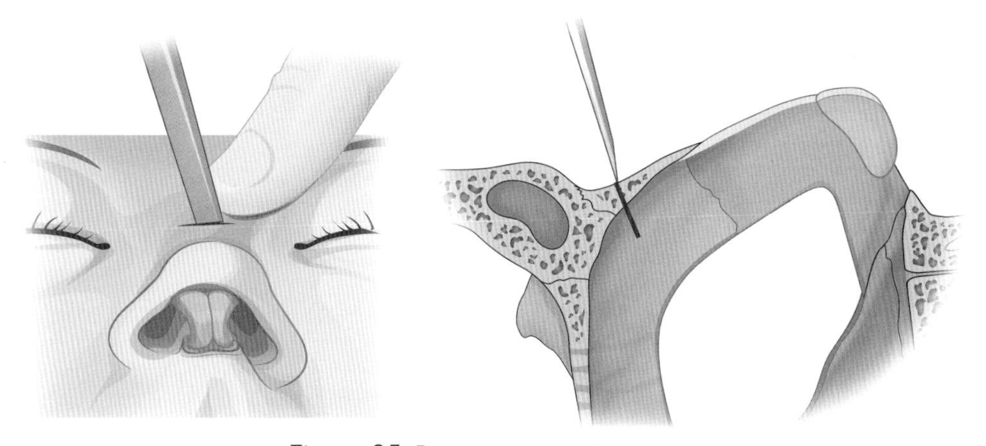

Figure 25 Percutaneous root osteotomy.

V. Complications

Among the various rhinoplasty procedures, osteotomy is the most invasive, and as such, the risk of complications is great. Possible complications are as follows:

- Hemorrhage
- Edema
- Secondary deformity: deviation, inverted V deformity, bony dorsum irregularity
- Olfactory dysfunction
- Nasal obstruction
- Damage to the lacrimal apparatus

Making use of direct hemostatic techniques such as electrocautery is impractical for managing postoperative hemorrhage. In most cases, there is no other option except applying pressure using fingers, packing or splinting in the hope that the bleeding resolves on its own. Hemorrhage usually occurs as a result of damage to the mucosa and the lateral nasal artery, and the severity increases as the surgery turns into a complete osteotomy. While performing surgery, applying proper amount of topical vasoconstrictor, using a small osteotome, and striving to maintain the attachment of the periosteum are helpful in reducing hemorrhage. Performing osteotomy near the end of the surgery and applying a splint right away can help reduce postoperative hemorrhage and edema. However, because osteotomy for deviated nose correction and dorsal hump reduction procedures must be performed in the middle of surgery so that its influence on the overall nasal shape can be judged, to advise that osteotomy be performed at the end of a surgery is impractical from the realities of rhinoplasty.

If osteotomy for correcting a deviated nose was done imperfectly, over time, the incised bony segments will return to its original location, which in turn can lead to re-deviation of the external nose *(Figure 26)*. Also, a hypertrophic change of the bone (callus) can form at the osteotomy site. Another major complication is the inverted V deformity, which occurs as a result of a depression between the nasal bone and upper lateral cartilages due to a comminuted fracture of the nasal bone. The inverted V deformity can be corrected by means of spreader grafting, cartilage onlay grafting, dorsal augmentation, and osteotomy. The irregularity of the bony dorsum resulting from a comminuted fracture of the nasal bone is probably the most commonly occurring postoperative complication. In addition, functional disorders of the nose such as postoperative olfactory disorder or nasal obstruction, as well as damage of the lacrimal apparatus can also take place.

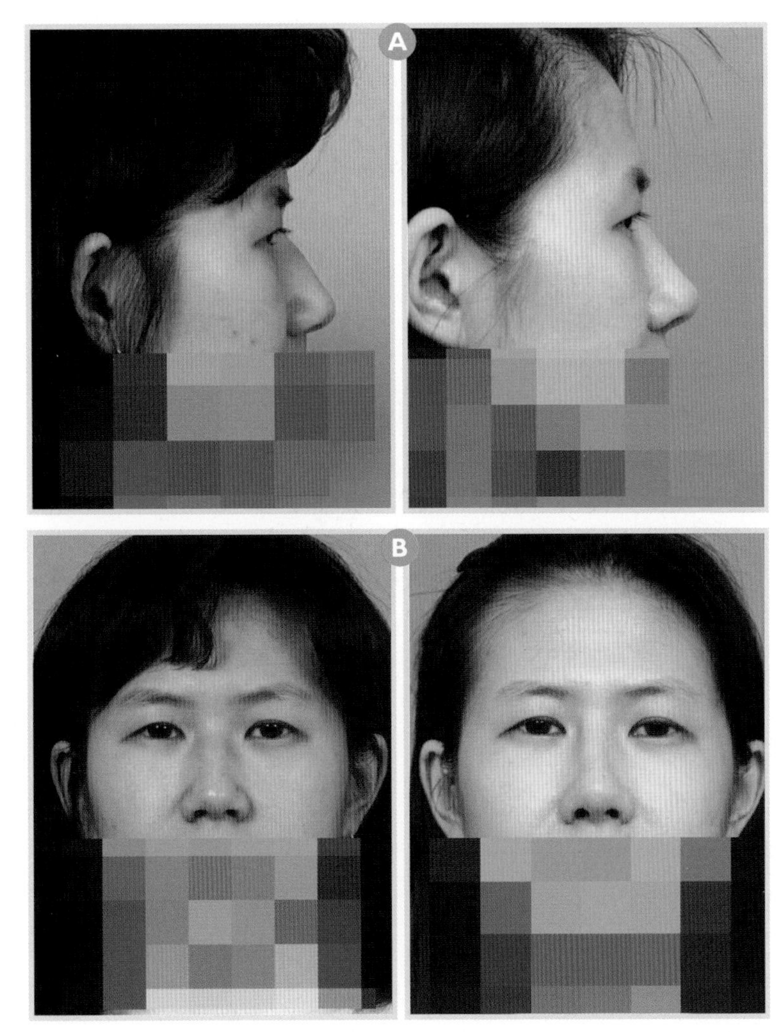

Figure 26 A patient showing satisfactory correction of a hump (A), but showing a nasal deviation (B) as a complication of osteotomy.

References

1. Becker DG, Park SS, Toriumi DM. Powered instrumentation for rhinoplasty and septoplasty. Otolaryngol Clin North Am 1999; 32: 683-93.
2. Bull TR. Percutaneous osteotomy in rhinoplasty. Plast Reconstr Surg 2001; 107: 1624-5.
3. Conrad K, Gillman G. Refining osteotomy techniques in rhinoplasty. J Otolaryngol 1998; 27: 1-9.
4. Giacomarra V, Russolo M, Arnez ZM, Tirelli G. External Osteotomy in rhinoplasty. Laryngoscope 2001; 111: 433-8.
5. Gryskiewicz JM, Gryskiewicz KM. Nasal osteotomies: a clinical comparison of the perforating method versus the continuous technique. Plast Reconstr Surg 2004; 113: 1445-56.
6. Guyuron B. Nasal osteotomy and airway changes. Plast Reconstr Surg 1998; 102: 856-60.
7. Hilton AE, Connell M. Visibility of puncture sites after external osteotomy in rhinoplastic surgery. Arch Facial Plast Surg 2003; 408-11.
8. Jang YJ, Wang JH, Sinha V, Lee BJ. Percuteneous root osteotomy for correction of deviated nose. Am J Rhinol 2007; 21: 515-9.
9. Jang YJ, Park CH. Osteotomy. In : Practical septorhinoplasty. Seoul, Koonja Publishing, 2007: 201-19.
10. McCollough. Moblizing the lateral walls : Lanteral and medial osteotomies. In Nasal plastic surgery. WB Saunders Co, 1994; 1: 137-46.

Postoperative Care

Yong Ju Jang · Jong Sook Yi

I. Conclusion of Surgery

At the conclusion of surgery, it is of utmost importance to verify that hemostasis is done properly. If bleeding persists at the osteotomy site, hemostasis needs to be performed by applying pressure on the affected area for a few minutes with a finger. Severe bleeding occurring at the soft-tissue of the skin should be controlled by bipolar cautery prior to suturing the incision. If septoturbinoplasty or osteotomy is performed as part of the surgical procedure, the nasal cavity should be lightly packed with gauze coated with antibiotic ointment near the conclusion of the surgery. If too much packing is inserted after an osteotomy is carried out, the side walls of the nose may become lateralized and this is a problem that must be avoided. In particular, there is a high probability that the use of Merocel® packing will cause this lateralization. As such, if possible, it should either be avoided or, if packing is unavoidable, it should be made slim and placed at the floor of the nasal cavity. The use of absorbable packing material can reduce patient's discomfort and problems related with excessive packing. If septoplasty is performed as a part of the rhinoplasty procedure, it is recommended that a silastic septal splint be placed *(Figure 1)*. When positioning the septal splint, a through and through suture is placed using an absorbable material such as a 4-0 PDS.

The purposes of the septal splint are as follows:

- ☑ To prevent the formation of hematoma by approximating the septal mucosa on both sides
- ☑ To help the reepithelialization of the mucosa when it is damaged during surgery
- ☑ To keep the mucosa moist during healing
- ☑ To prevent synechia formation between the septum and the turbinate.

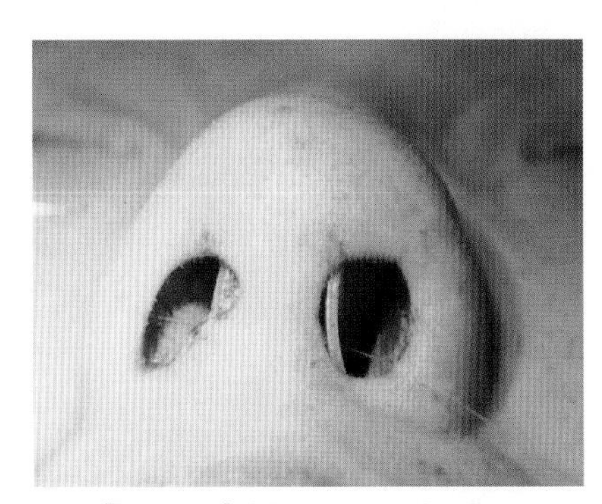

Figure 1 Silastic septal splint.

After bilateral dissection of the septal mucosa is completed and the redraping of the mucosa is being attempted at the end of the surgery, it is useful in preventing the formation of a hematoma if there is a small defect of the mucosa in one of the two sides of the septal mucosa. In cases where the mucosa is completely intact, it is recommended that a small incision be made intentionally on one side for the drainage of blood. If the silastic sheet is fixed too tightly, and kept over one week, secondary septal mucosal perforation can occur. Thus, excessive compression and prolonged placement of septal splints should be avoided.

When skin closure and nasal packing has been completed, the exterior of the nose must be stabilized using an external splint such as Plaster of Paris, Denver Splint, or Aquasplint. Before applying the splint, taping is applied to the skin, using paper tape, in order to reduce the edema of the skin and to make sure that the skin-soft tissue envelope is re-draped in the desired shape. After taping, the author applies the Aquasplint. Even when some blood is still draining from the dissection area, it usually stops once the Aquasplint has been applied. Applying firm pressure with the fingers before applying the final tape layer to secure the external splint can be of additional help in controlling bleeding. The Aquasplint becomes soft when dipped into water which is 70℃ or higher, which can then be placed at the nose and shaped into the desired form with the fingers and left to harden as it cools. Taping then can be applied over to fix the splint. The external splint prevents the formation of a hematoma at nasal dorsum and it fixes the dorsal implant in the most favored location with the most favorable shape *(Figure 2)*.

Five layers of plaster of Paris or a Denver splint can be used as an alternative for Aquasplint. A Denver splint consists of two layers, a malleable aluminum splint as the external layer and an attachable velcro as the internal layer. The advantages of this splint are that it only takes a short period of time when applying will not require hot water.

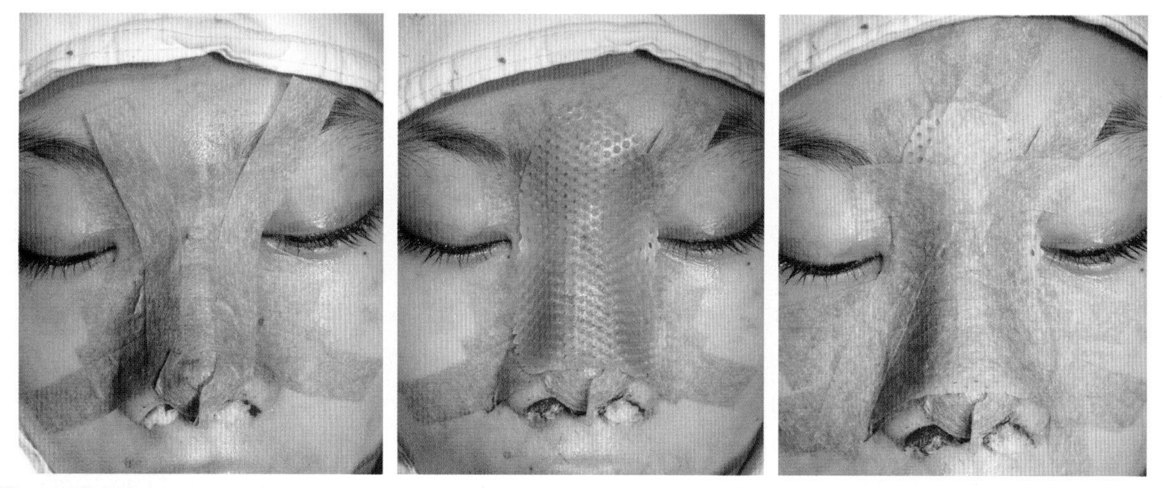

Figure 2 When positioning the external splint using Aquasplint, taping on the skin using a paper tape is performed first, and then the Aquasplint is applied in the desired shape, then taping on top is again performed.

II. The Day of Surgery to 1-2 Days after Surgery

On the first day after surgery, the patient will usually complain of bloody postnasal drip and pain. This is not a major concern if the patient can continue to spit out the blood and secretions and the pain can be adequately controlled with painkillers. A changeable drip pad is useful for the mild oozing from nasal cavity *(Figure 3)*. However, if severe bleeding occurs, the packing should be removed to be able to examine the nasal cavity, and hemostasis established using monopolar suction cautery or bipolar cautery followed by re-packing. The suction cautery, which allows for the simultaneous suction and cauterization in a patient with nasal bleeding, is a very useful surgical instrument. Most patients usually display the maximum degree of edema and ecchymosis on the first day after the surgery. These signs of edema and bleeding can upset the patient greatly. In order to prevent severe edema, the author prescribes 5 mg of intravenous dexamethasone on the day of surgery or first day after surgery. Also, if the edema is severe, massage can be administered using an ice pack. Antibiotics should be administered through an intravenous route a few hours prior to, and following surgery. An antibiotic that covers for the gram-positive organisms should be selected. The nasal packing can be removed one or two days after surgery.

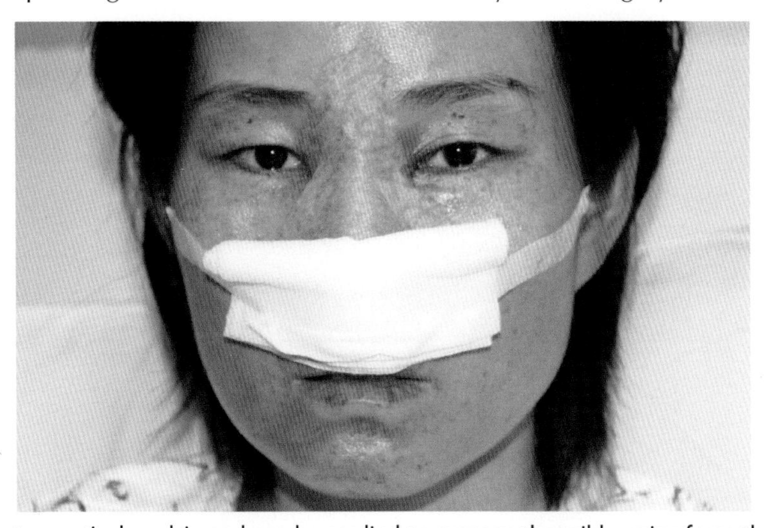

Figure 3 Postoperatively, a drip pad can be applied to manage the mild oozing from the nasal cavity.

III. Day 3 and Onwards Following Surgery

The patient can experience persistent nasal obstruction when a septal splint is left in place after surgery and thus the patient needs to be informed of this in advance. It is normal for bloody nasal discharge to occur for up to 2-4 days after surgery. The suture of the transcolumellar incision is removed 5-6 days after surgery. For the closure of the marginal incision, absorbable suture material is used and therefore the stitches do not need to be removed. As long as the sutures are in place, the patient should be made to apply an antibiotic ointment such as polymyxin or tetracycline three times a day in order to prevent the wound from drying out. It is best to abstain from blowing the nose hard for a period of three weeks following surgery. It is also recommended that antibiotics be prescribed to patients when they are discharged. Of the various oral antibiotics available, Augmentin®, which is effective against gram-positive organisms, or a cephalosporin is preferred by the author. It is rare for patients to complain of severe pain after surgery. But, until the first scheduled visit 5 to 6 days after surgery, non-steroidal anti-inflammatory drugs are prescribed to control pain and edema. For patients complaining of nasal obstruction, pseudoephedrine, a nasal mucosal decongestant, can be prescribed. It is rare to have bleeding occur after packing removal. Nevertheless, bleeding can take place around the turbinoplasty or the osteotomy sites. A case of minor bleeding can be controlled by raising the head and applying light pressure on the nostril for 15 minutes. However, when the bleeding cannot be controlled using this method, the patient should visit the surgeon who performed the operation. The author usually lets the patients visit the out-patient clinic on the sixth postoperative day at which time the suture, Aquasplint, and septal splint are removed. At this time, the patient should be asked if they have tinnitus, nausea or dizziness. If patients complain about these symptoms and develop pallor, they should be laid down in a supine position and asked to take deep breaths. This phenomenon can be induced by low cardiac output and slow heart rate when naso-cardiac reflex was activated by the severe nasal pain or lidocaine application to the nasal cavity.

When a localized edema or a protruding area is discovered after the external splint is removed, the shape can be corrected by gentle massage by the surgeon and re-taping or placing a new external splint for about 1 week. If postoperative edema persists even after two weeks, the patient is advised to apply paper tape while sleeping *(Figure 4)*.

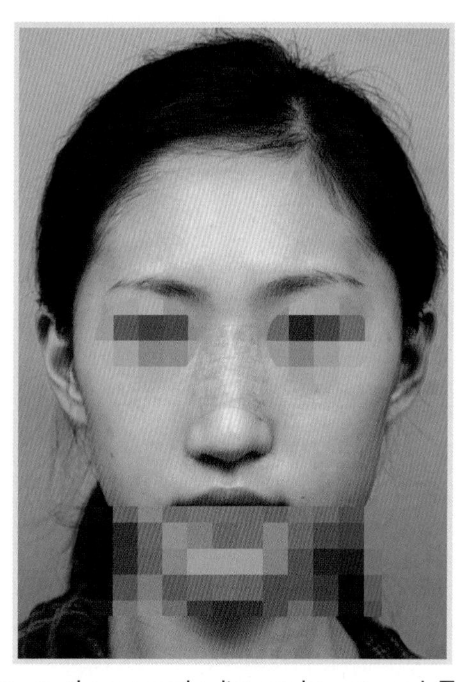

Figure 4 On the first visit after surgery, the external splint can be removed. Taping on the nasal dorsum for a few more days helps reduce postoperative edema.

The authors recommend that the patient visit the surgeon once a week during the first month after surgery and once a month for two times after that. Then, follow-up is every 3-4 months. Quite a number of patients stop visiting the surgeon when they are satisfied with the results of surgery. It can be assumed that all postoperative visits after 3-4 weeks may be the patient's last visit, and the surgeon should take steps to take as many photographs as possible. If postoperative photographs were taken around the 4th week after surgery, it can be used with the preoperative photographs to provide a comparative explanation to the patient. Most postoperative edema improves after 2 weeks but the recovery process can continue on slowly for several months thereafter, and the patient should be informed of this. There are patients who experienced ecchymosis and severe edema who develop discoloration around the eyes even after a month after surgery. Hence, patients who experienced severe bleeding around the eyes should be sufficiently informed of the possibility that such discoloration can persist *(Figure 5)*.

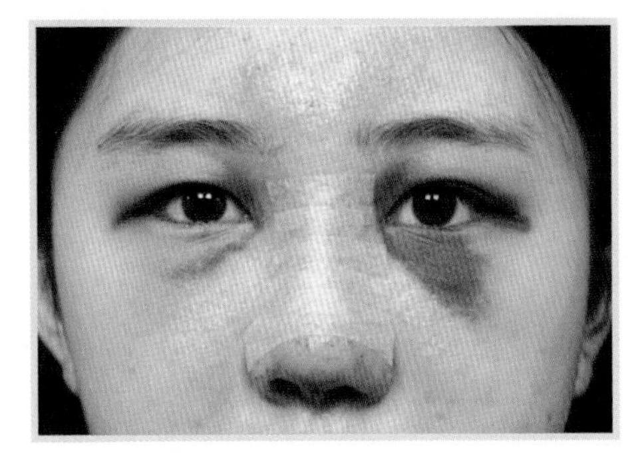

Figure 5 Patients who experience severe bleeding around the eyes should be informed of the possibility that such discoloration can persist.

Many patients may develop a red eye (subconjunctival hemorrhage) due to the migration of the blood from the operation site to the subconjunctival area *(Figure 6)*. In such a case, the patient should be reassured that it would disappear within a few weeks.

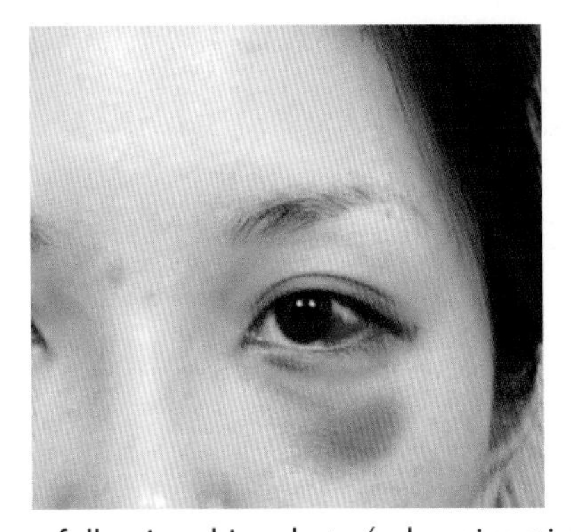

Figure 6 Red eye following rhinoplasty (subconjunctival hemorrhage).

Alcohol intake after surgery not only increases the risk of infection but also increases the risk of trauma. Therefore, the patient should be advised on the importance of avoiding alcohol. For the period of three weeks after surgery, the patient should be restricted from intense physical activities such as gymnastics or exercise. Everyday activities can be gradually increased by 2 weeks after surgery and, from the third week onwards, normal activities can be resumed. Care should be taken to avoid external trauma for the period of 6 weeks after surgery. For 4-6 weeks after the splint is removed, nothing including eyeglasses should be mounted on the nose. The nasal skin is sensitive to sunlight. Thus, exposure to strong sunlight should be avoided for 8 weeks. In areas where bleeding occurred, exposure to ultraviolet light will prolong the recovery from discoloration. The patient should wear a broad-brimmed hat and put on sunblock lotion. In order to detect the occurrence of infection early, patients who underwent dorsal augmentation using an alloplastic implant should be informed of the warning signs of infection such as pain on the nasal skin, swelling, erythema, etc. Furthermore, they should be instructed to visit the surgeon promptly when these signs develop. Some patients show telangiectasias on the skin of the nasal dorsum. These patients should be referred to a dermatologist for proper management.

IV. Hyperbaric Oxygen Therapy after Surgery

There is paucity of literature which demostrates the efficacy of hyperbaric oxygen therapy after rhinoplasty. Nevertheless, many surgeons use hyperbaric oxygen based on their personal experience. This is used by the authors in multiply revised cases in which the columellar skin has compromised circulation, or when the use of large amounts of costal cartilage grafts exert undue tension on transcolumellar incision *(Figure 7)*.

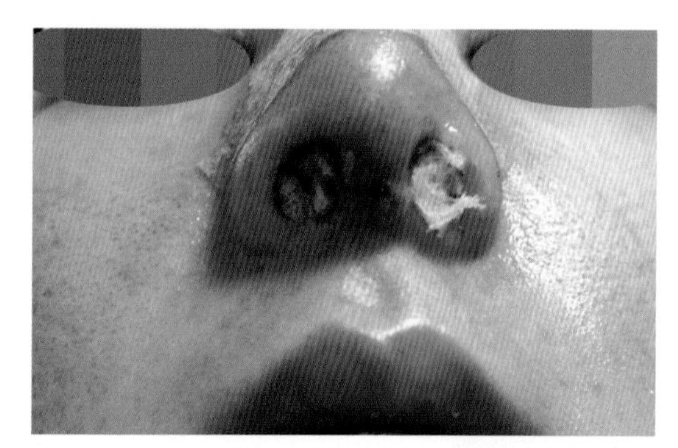

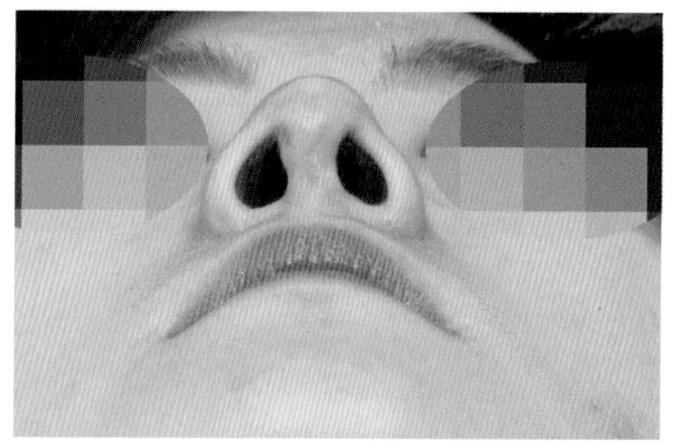

Figure 7 A patient who experienced wound breakdown at the transcolumellar incision site after revision rhinoplasty. The incision site healed well by administering hyperbaric oxygen and meticulous wound care.

1. Definition and Goal of Hyperbaric Oxygen Therapy

Hyperbaric oxygen therapy uses 100% oxygen at pressures greater than atmospheric pressure. This treatment method has been successfully used as an adjunct for better wound healing. In general, hyperbaric oxygen therapy is known to enhance cellular revitalization. Moreover, higher arterial partial pressures of oxygen facilitate angiogenesis and better wound healing.

2. Administration of Hyperbaric Oxygen Therapy

The patients can be administered 100% systemic oxygen via a hyperbaric oxygen chamber, sometimes called a pressure chamber. The air pressure inside a hyperbaric oxygen chamber is about two and a half times greater than the normal atmosphere pressure. The duration of a single treatment session varies from 60-90 minutes depending on the severity of infection or necrosis. The authors usually perform the therapy once or twice a day, for more than two weeks. However, there is no consensus on the treatment protocol for post-rhinoplasty patients. In cases of revision surgery or prior infection, some surgeons recommend preoperative hyperbaric oxygen therapy.

3. Hyperbaric Oxygen Therapy in Rhinoplasty

In the revision case, hyperbaric oxygen therapy reduces not only the risk of postoperative infection, but also the duration of wound healing. If too big an alloplastic implant is inserted exerting undue pressure on the skin-soft tissue envelope, or if ischemic injury is expected by excessive tissue manipulation, hyperbaric oxygen therapy can be considered along with antibiotics to prevent infection and necrosis. In primary rhinoplasty, postoperative edema is also decreased after hyperbaric oxygen therapy.

4. Complications

Some adverse effects may occur after hyperbaric oxygen therapy.

- ☑ Oxygen toxicity
- ☑ Barotrauma
- ☑ Cardiopulmonary injury

1) Oxygen Toxicity

Due to the increase in blood oxygen partial pressure, shortness of breath, changes in behavior, nausea, dizziness, and muscle spasms may occur.

2) Barotrauma

The pressure difference between the middle ear and the surrounding environment can lead to middle ear effusion, by which patients complain of hearing disturbance or ear fullness. Thus, tympanic membrane and eustachian tube function testing should be performed prior to starting hyperbaric oxygen therapy. Moreover, evaluation of the paranasal sinuses should be done using X-ray because of the risk of barosinusitis.

3) Cardiopulmonary Injury

Chest tightness and abnormal heart beats can occur after hyperbaric oxygen therapy. Thus, an initial electrocardiogram (ECG) should be evaluated prior to starting hyperbaric oxygen therapy to be able to compare it to the post-treatment ECG when symptoms appear. A chest x-ray helps to diagnose pulmonary edema, infection, or other lung problems when respiratory symptoms occur.

References

1. Stong BC, Jacono AA. Effect of perioperative hyperbaric oxygen on bruising in Face-lifts. Arch Facial Plast Surg 2010; 12: 356-8.
2. Diewulski P, Dujon D, Spyriounis P, Griffiths RW, Shaw JD. A retrospective analysis of the results of 218 consecutive rhinoplasties. Br J Plast Surg 1995; 48: 451-4.
3. Ellis DA, Strelzow VV. Pre- and postoperative management of the rhinoplasty patient. J Otolaryngol 1978; 7: 49-55.
4. Guyuron B. Is packing after septorhinoplasty necessary? A randomized study. Plast Reconstr Surg 1989; 84: 41-4.
5. Grundmann T, Jaehne M, Fritze G. The value of hyperbaric oxygen therapy (HBO) in treatment of problem wounds in the area of plastic reconstructive head and neck surgery. Laryngorhinootologie 2000; 79: 304-10.
6. Nolst Trenite GJ. Postoperative care and complications. In Rhinoplasty 2nd ed. Kugler Publication,1998; 31-40.
7. Rees TD. Postoperative considerations and complications. In: Rees TD(ed). Aesthetic plastic surgery. Philadelphia: WB Saunders, 1980.
8. Schwab JA, Pirsig W. Complications of septal surgery. Facial Plast Surg 1997; 13: 3-14.
9. Weber R, Hochapfel F, Draf W. Packing and stents in endonasal surgery. Rhinology 2000; 38: 49-62.

Section 04

Grafts and Implants

General Considerations in Dorsal Augmentation

Yong Ju Jang

Dorsal augmentation is the most important part of rhinoplasty for Koreans. It is also critically important not only in simple cosmetic rhinoplasty but all types of rhinoplasty for their aesthetic perfection. Aesthetic perfection of the nose is determined by the height and shape of the nasal dorsum seen from the side and front, and the harmonious alignment with the nasal tip. Thus, in order to create a beautiful nose, one must possess an aesthetic understanding of what kind of dorsum constitutes a beautiful dorsum.

I. Aesthetic Considerations

The beauty of the nasal dorsum viewed from the front is primarily determined by the dorsal aesthetic line. This line must be adequately formed in all rhinoplasty procedures. The dorsal aesthetic lines start from the supraorbital ridges, passing the corrugators, and converge at the medial canthal ligaments. Then, they diverge a little at the keystone area and go down parallel to each other and reach the tip defining points. In males, it is acceptable for the lines to connect almost parallel to the tip without the width between them changing. For female patients, however, a gentle slope from the supraorbital ridge to the tip is preferable *(Figure 1)*.

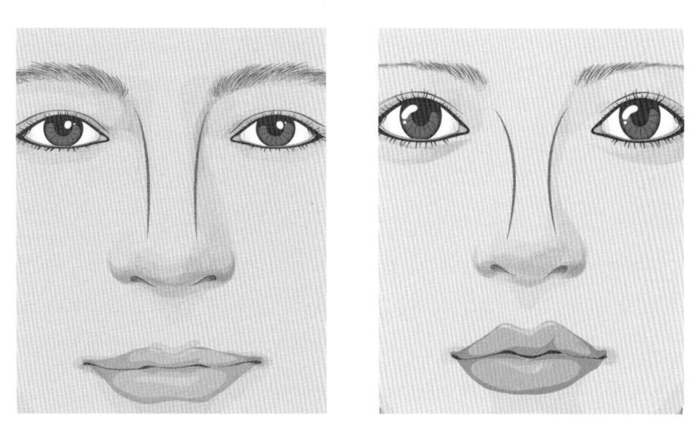

Figure 1 Ideal dorsal aesthetic line in males and females.

If the dorsal implant is too wide, the risk of displacement or implant visibility is relatively lower, but the dorsal line looks masculine, creating an aesthetically less pleasing dorsal appearance in females. If the dorsal implant is too narrow in the radix area, the risk of implant visibility or deviation increases. Therefore, the implant should be designed with an appropriate width *(Figure 2).*

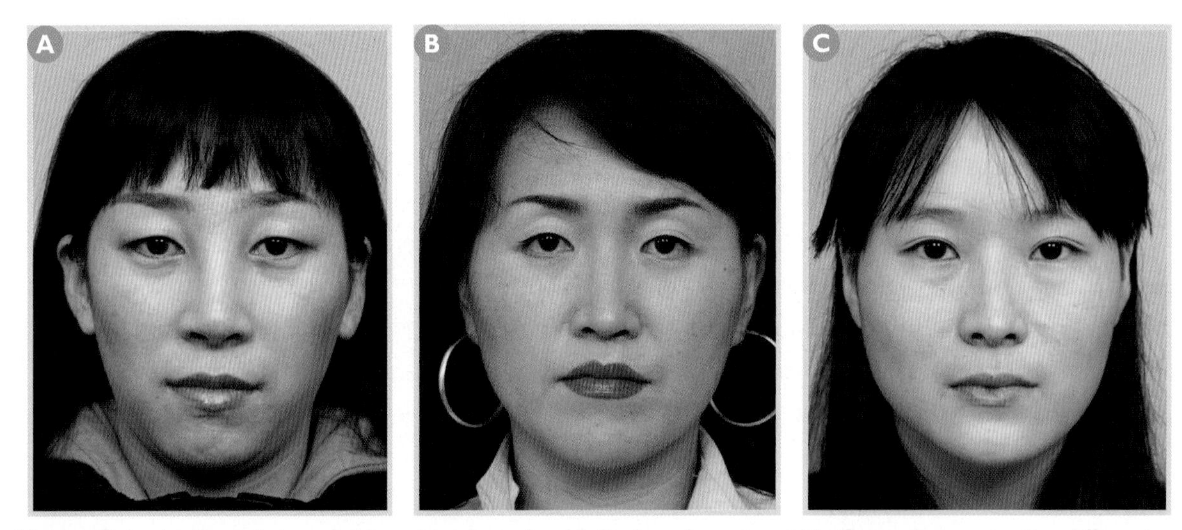

Figure 2 In the frontal view, the dorsal implant should display adequate width. Cases demonstrating different width of dorsal implants on the nose. Too wide an implant in the radix (A), dorsal implant of ideal width creating a natural looking brow-tip aesthetic line (B), and too narrow dorsal implant in the radix (C).

Female dorsal lines as seen from the side, may preferably be placed a little lower than the line connecting the nasofrontal angle and the tip, in a slightly concave shape. However, focusing too much on dorsal concavity might exhibit a washed-out appearance like saddle nose, so surgeons must be careful. In male patients, to avoid a feminine appearance, the dorsal line should be placed on or a little above the nasofrontal angle-tip line *(Figure 3).*

When observing the patient's lateral view, adequate nasofrontal and nasofacial angles are prerequisites for an aesthetically pleasing nose. The radix and nasion are reference points for nasofrontal angle *(Figure 4)*. To understand the ideal position of the radix, one must know the definition of nasion and radix. The nasion (sellion) is a term referring to the innermost point of the nasofrontal angle. The radix is an anatomic term referring to the region with the nasion as the center reaching down to the lateral canthus, and reaching upwards the same distance. In order to get good rhinoplasty outcomes, the surgeon must fully understand the concept of the appropriate position and height of the radix. The height and position of the radix can have a major influence on the degree of augmentation required during surgery.

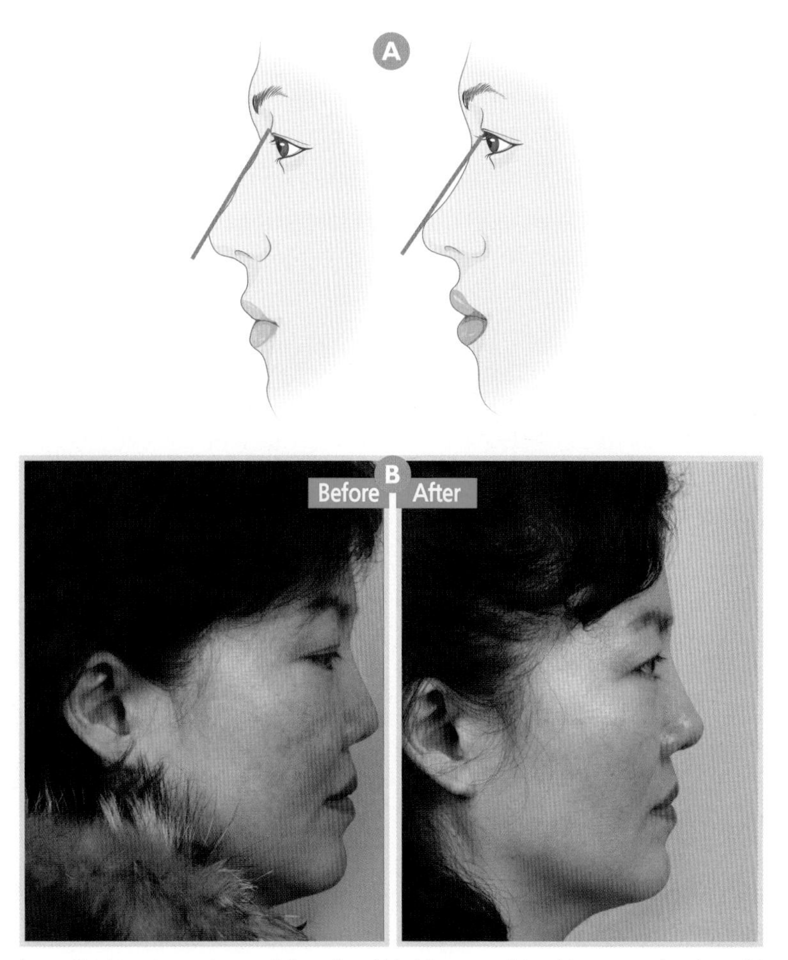

Figure 3 Ideal dorsal profile line in males and females (A). Unnatural looking straight dorsal line (left) is changed into a mildly concave dorsal line (right) by revision operation (B).

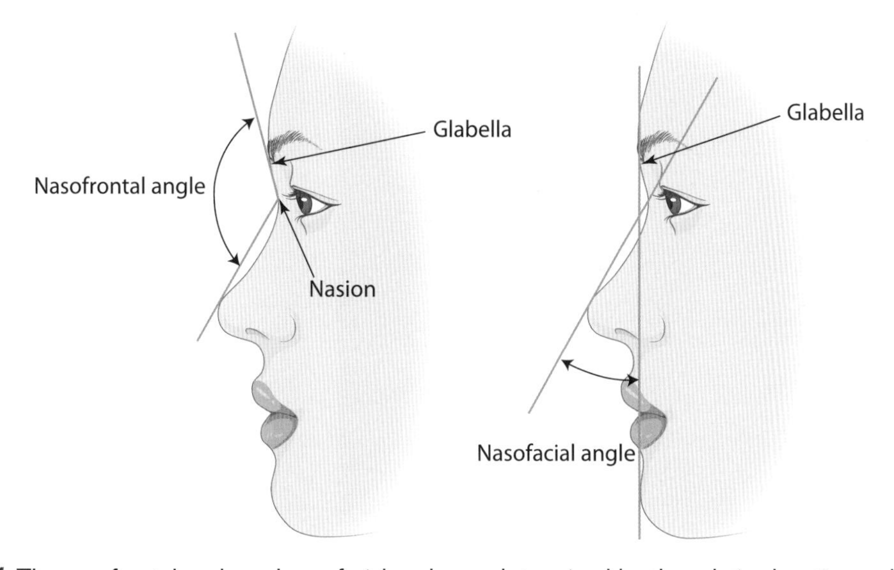

Figure 4 The nasofrontal angle and nasofacial angle are determined by the relative location and dimension of the glabella, nasion, and pogonion.

In female Korean patients, the nasion or nasal starting point's level should be placed between the mid-pupillary line and the double eyelid line, also taking into consideration the patient's preferred nose shape. For male patients it may be preferable to place the nasion a little higher *(Figure 5)*.

Surgical maneuvers on the radix can change the nasion levels. When the patient wants a smooth/soft looking nose, nasion should be placed closer to the mid-pupillary line, and a little higher for a strong/powerful looking nose *(Figure 6)*. A high nasal starting point gives a strong facial impression

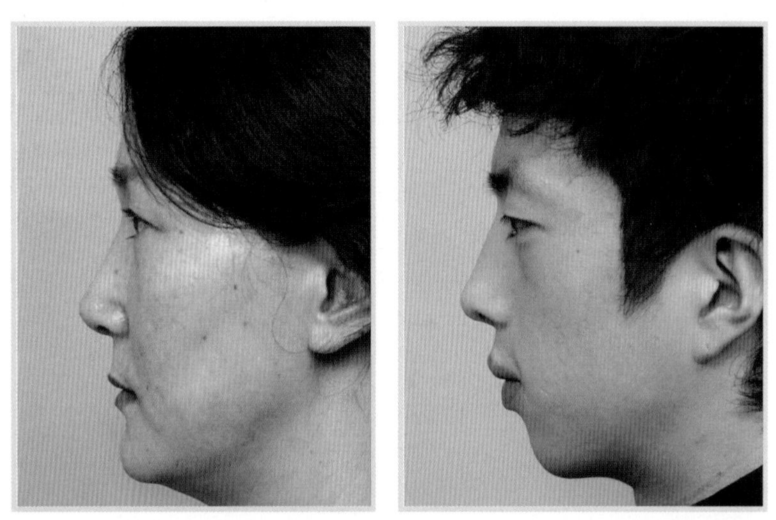

Figure 5 In female Korean patients, the nasion or nasal starting point's level should be placed between the mid-pupillary line and the double eyelid line. For male patients it may be preferable to place the nasion a little higher.

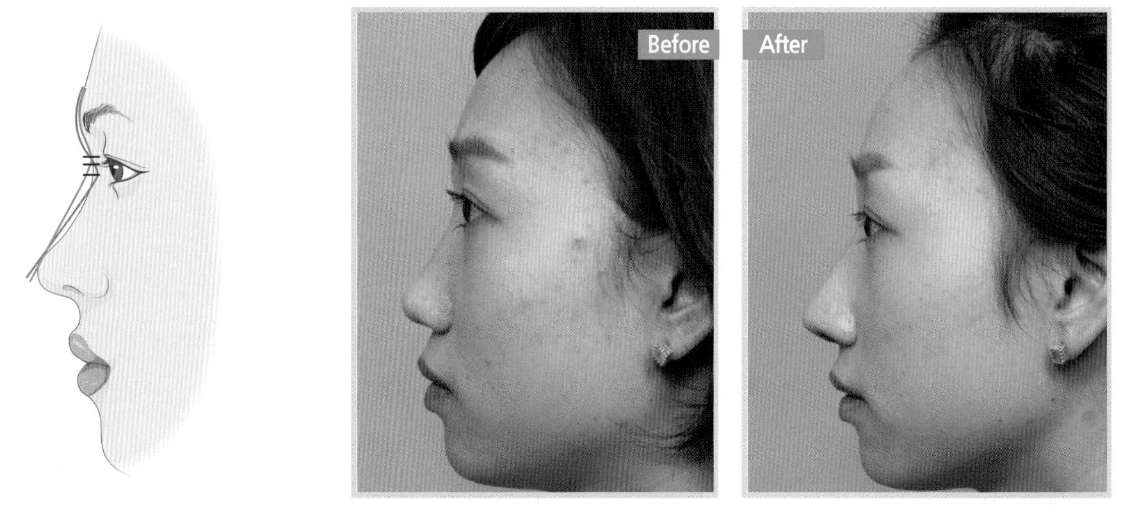

Figure 6 When the patient wants a smooth/soft looking nose, nasion should be placed close to the mid-pupillary line, and a little higher for a strong/powerful looking nose. The patient in this photograph got a stronger looking nose as a result of dorsal augmentation.

seldom preferred by female Asians. Especially for people who have poorly developed and flat foreheads, excessive radix augmentation can create an unnatural looking nose with no clear distinction between the nose and forehead *(Figure 7)*.

The level of the nasion is important, but its height is also equally important. If the patient already has his/her nasion's vertical level in an appropriate location before dorsal augmentation, the surgeon should leave the vertical level as it is and try to adjust the horizontal height *(Figure 8)*.

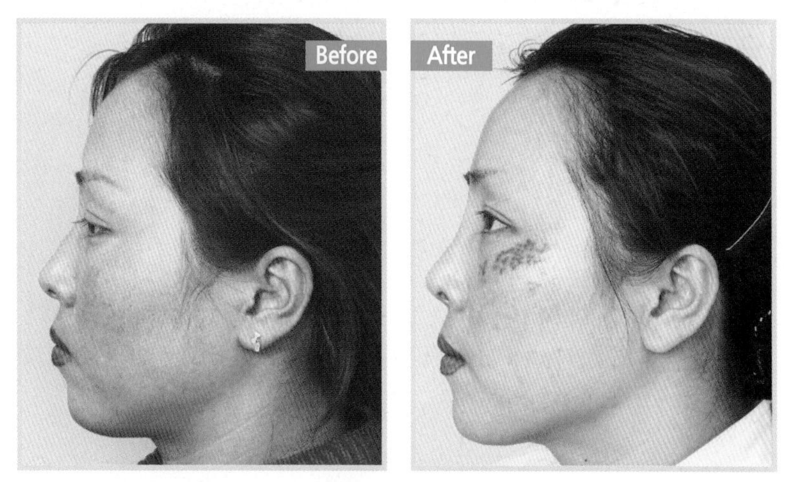

Figure 7 In a patient who has less developed and flat forehead, excessive radix augmentation can create an unnatural looking nose with no clear distinction between the nose and forehead.

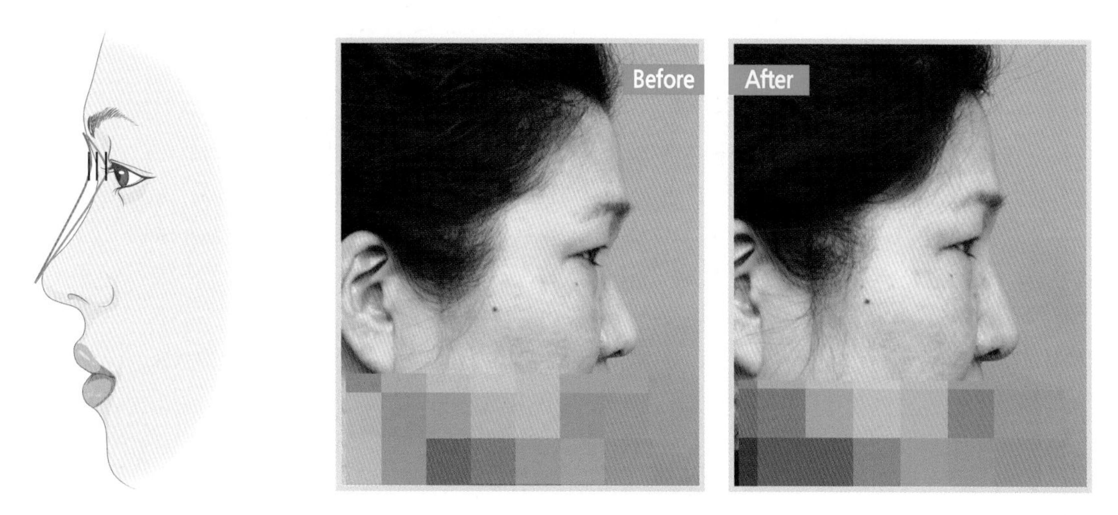

Figure 8 A rhinoplasty patient who shows only a change in the horizontal height of the radix after dorsal augmentation.

The nasofrontal angle should have a gentle curvature. But for patients who have a sunken radix, showing relatively sharp nasofrontal angles, if beveling of the implant's upper end was not performed well, the implant's cephalic margin can be conspicuous when seen from the front. This phenomenon is common among patients who have a prominent forehead. Therefore, for such patients it is important to sculpt the implant meticulously in order to keep the implant's upper margin from showing, and to create a smooth transition with the surrounding structures *(Figure 9)*.

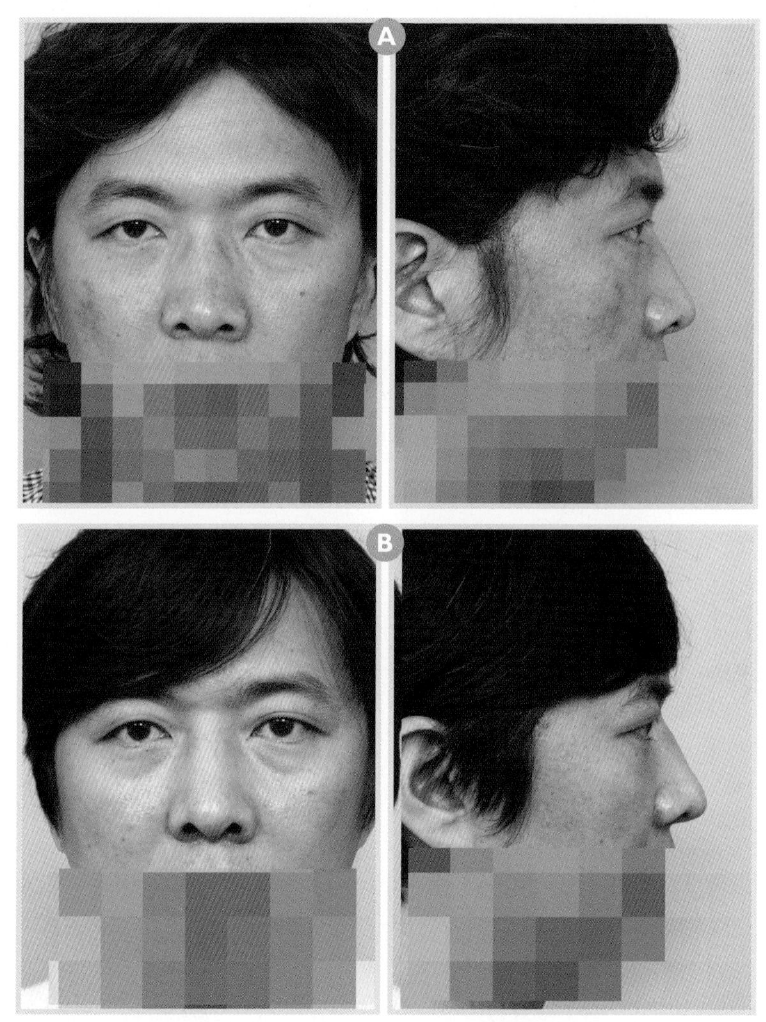

Figure 9 In a patient who has a sunken radix showing a relatively sharp nasofrontal angle, there is a higher risk of creating a nose where the implant's cephalic margin can be conspicuous when seen from the front.

To satisfy the aforementioned aesthetic elements, the surgeon must design a dorsal implant or graft of appropriate width, length, and shape. This is a difficult process that requires experience and immense effort. An implant's base should be wide, the area placed near the surface should be narrow, and it should be in good contact with the nasal dorsum to prevent implant movement. Normally, implants or grafts required for dorsal augmentation should be about 3-5 cm long and

0.7-1.0 cm wide. Placing the implant's caudal end some distance from the rhinoplasty incision site may be effective in preventing infection and inflammation. However, overly focusing on this aspect and consequently having too big a gap between the implant and the domal portion of the nasal tip or failure to perform smooth beveling of the implant's caudal end can result in visibility of the implant's edge near the nasal tip, so surgeons must be careful *(Figure 10)*. In addition, if the height of the implant's caudal end is higher than the tip height, the profile view show, an unnatural contour since the dorsum is placed abnormally higher than the tip *(Figure11)*.

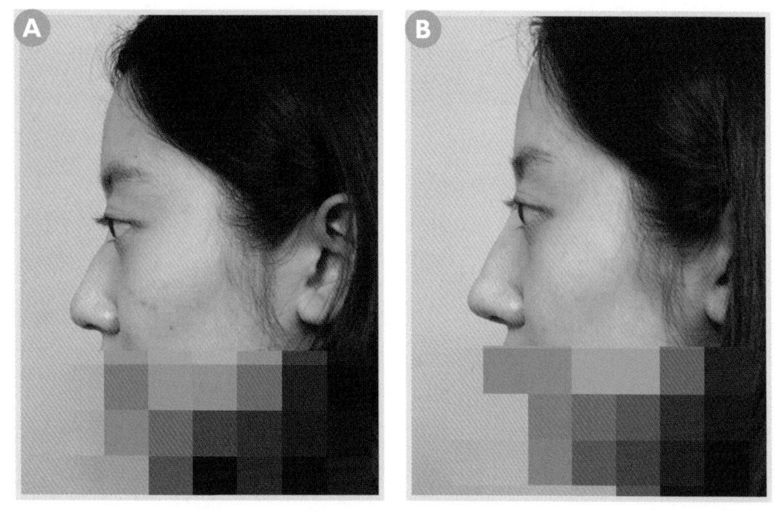

Figure 10 Having too big a gap between the implant and the domal portion of the nasal tip can result in a supra tip saddle-like deformity. Before operation (A) and after operation (B)

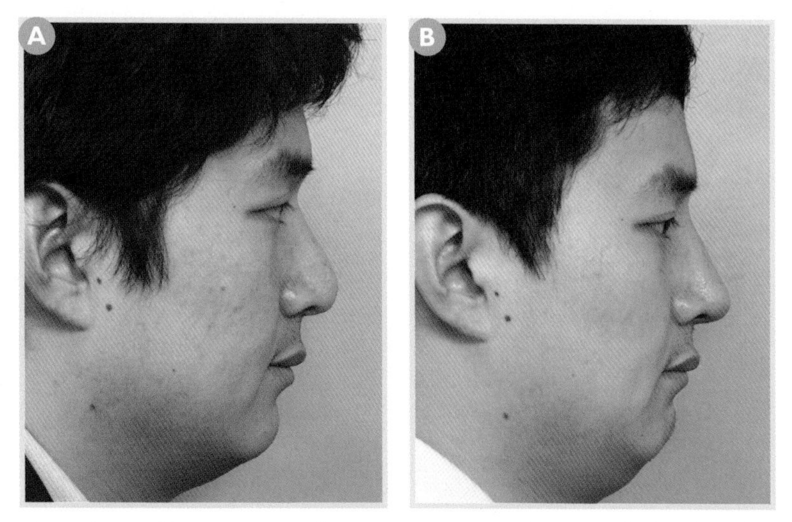

Figure 11 In this patient, the profile view showed unnatural contours because the height of the implant's caudal end is higher than the tip height. It was corrected by revision operation. Before operation (A) and after operation (B).

II. Selection of Dorsal Augmentation Material

To raise the height of the nasal dorsum, the appropriate augmentation material must be chosen. Augmentation material can be classified into biologic implants and alloplastic implants. Biologic implants include autologous cartilage, fascia, and dermofat. Homologous tissues such as costal cartilage, fascia, and dermis obtained from cadaver donors also belong to biologic implants. Biologic implants obtained from other species are also included in this category. Alloplastic implants include silicone, Gore-Tex, and Medpor. The characteristics and use of each material is covered in separate chapters. Determining the material of choice for dorsal augmentation depends on the surgeon's experience, surgical proficiency/mastery, philosophy, treatment methods, and rhinoplasty patient groups' characteristics. So far, there is no ideal dorsal implant material that can satisfy every criteria. *Table 1* compares the various materials and their advantages and disadvantages. Advice from the author, who has experience using an array of materials, is:

- ☑ It is easier to use prefabricated alloplastic implants to achieve aesthetic perfection
- ☑ Infections in the early stages of surgery are more common in biologic implants. Delayed inflammations and infections that are seen a long time after the surgery are more common in alloplastic implants, and if not treated adequately, can cause serious deformities.
- ☑ Long-term follow up of rhinoplasty patients demonstrate that aesthetic complications are more frequent in dorsal augmentation using biologic implants. These include visibility of the dorsal cartilage implant, resorption or deformation, and absorption occurring in cases using fascia or dermofat.

Inserting a foreign material between the nasal skin soft tissue envelope and the nasal framework is a procedure bound to involve unexpected complications. The surgeon must adequately explain these risks to patients and be able to handle problems appropriately when they occur.

Table I Characteristics of various graft and implant materials

Implant material	Advantages	Disadvantages
Septal cartilage	• Same surgical field with rhinoplasty	• Insufficient quantity • Nasal supporting structure can be weakened
Conchal cartilage	• Similar characteristics with upper lateral cartilage and lower lateral cartilage • Easy harvesting	• Donor site morbidity • Intrinsic curvature • Not so strong to be used as structural grafting
Costal cartilage	• Easy to carve into a various shapes • Enough cartilage for one-piece dorsal augmentation • Beneficial for structural reconstruction due to its hardness	• Donor site morbidity • Warping and resorption • Necessity of surgeon's abundant experience to form an aesthetically pleasing nose
Fascia wrapped diced cartilage	• Can create smooth dorsal line	• Donor site morbidity • Change in volume and shape over time
Homologous costal cartilage	• No donor site morbidity • Shorter operation time	• Higher absorption and fracture rates than autologous cartilage
Fascia	• Can create a soft contours	• Resorption • Not suitable for structural grafting
Dermofat	• Soft texture • Ample in quantity	• Resorption
Silicone	• Easy to handle • Cheap • Various ready-made products make application convenient • Easily removable when complications occur	• Displacement • Formation of a fibrous capsule around the implant, can deviate, and create an upturned nose • Infection, inflammation, and extrusion
Gore-Tex	• Less possibility of implant displacement than silicone • Softer texture suitable for creating natural looking dorsal lines	• Decrease in volume after insertion • Delayed inflammation
Medpor	• Easy to handle • Hardness suitable for structural reconstruction	• Unnatural shape can be made by its innate hardness • Risk of infection and inflammation

References

1. Jang YJ, Yu MS. Rhinoplasty for the Asian nose. Facial Plast Surg 2010; 26: 93-101.
2. Jang YJ, Moon BJ. State of the art in augmentation rhinoplasty: implant or graft?. Curr Opin Otolaryngol Head Neck Surg 2012; 20: 280-8.

Septal Cartilage

Yong Ju Jang

Septal cartilage is the cartilage on the caudal part of the nasal septum, acting as the central structure in supporting the structural integrity of the entire nose. It is critically responsible for the formation of symptoms of nasal obstruction. In rhinoplasty, septoplasty is frequently conducted additionally to manage nasal obstruction, calling for the removal of the middle part of cartilage as a part of the procedure. This removed part of the cartilage is an important graft material used preciously in rhinoplasty.

I. Anatomy

Normally, the septal cartilage composes half the caudal part of nasal septum. But for some patients the cartilage is very small and the septum is mainly composed of bones. According to the author's research, the dimension of the average septal cartilage harvested during external rhinoplasty, leaving an L-strut of 1 cm, has caudal length, dorsal length, and area of 15.1 mm, 18.2 mm, and 520.9 mm^2, respectively. The thickness of the septal cartilage differs greatly from patient to patient. Cartilage harvested from patients with thin septal cartilage is difficult to use for various grafting purposes. This is commonly seen in female patients with a poorly developed nasal skeleton. Grafts harvested from patients with well-developed, thick, and abundant cartilage and grafts harvested from patients with weak and small cartilage differ greatly in its quality *(Figure 1)*.

Septal cartilage is harvested through an external rhinoplasty approach or by applying a hemitransfixion incision through an endonasal approach. The sphenoidal process extending posteriorly toward the sphenoid sinus *(Figure 2)* can be obtained during the harvest procedure of the septal cartilage. In patients with weak cartilage, it is preferable to preserve over 2 cm of dorsal strut and caudal strut. On the other hand, it is best to preserve about 1.5 cm of L-strut, for patients with thick cartilage. The cartilage removed while preserving the caudal and dorsal struts is used in rhinoplasty for various purposes.

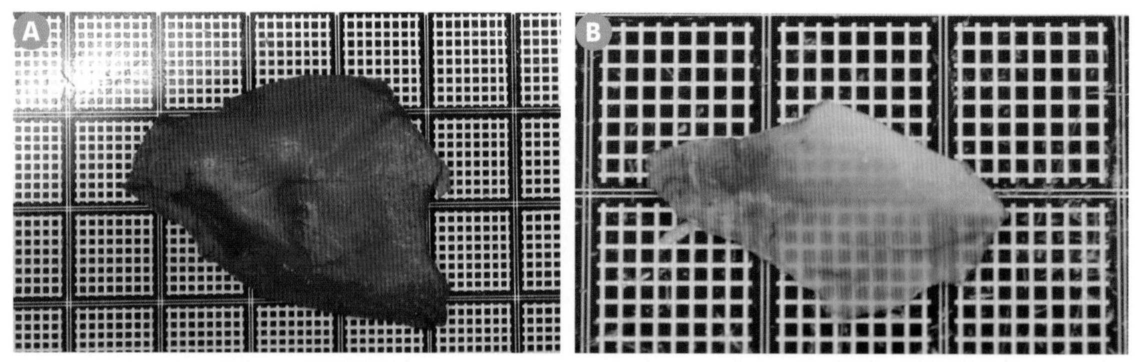

Figure 1 The thickness and size of the septal cartilage harvested after preservation of a 1.5 cm wide L-strut differs greatly between patients. Big and thick septal cartilage (A) and thin and small harvested cartilage which is not suitable for grafting purposes (B).

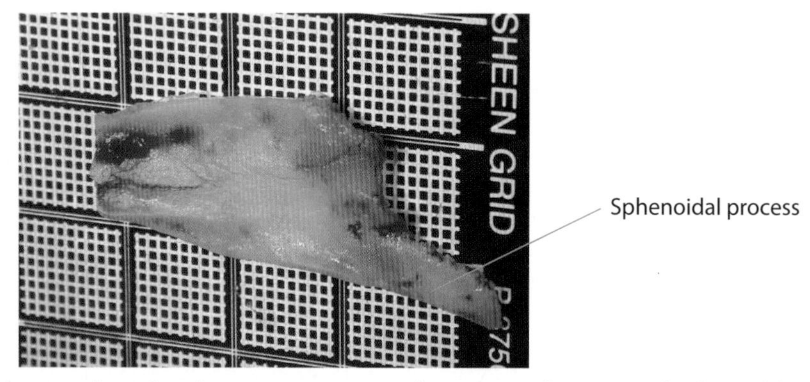

Figure 2 During septal cartilage harvest, one can get the posteriorly projected sphenoidal process of the septal cartilage.

II. How to Use the Harvested Septal Cartilage

Septal cartilage is hyaline cartilage with some degree of hardness, thus is suitable for grafting such as a columellar strut, spreader graft, septal batten graft, or septal extension graft. Aside from the aforementioned structural grafting purposes, it is also commonly used as an onlay graft, shield graft, or lateral crural onlay graft *(Figure 3)*.

If the cartilage is thick and strong enough when used for tip grafting, suture fixation of the cartilage graft to the underlying lower lateral cartilages and creation of the desired shapes and closure of the skin becomes easy. But many patients who undergo rhinoplasty have very thin and weak septal cartilage, thus making it difficult to perform the suture fixation appropriately. When trying to secure it in the desired location, the

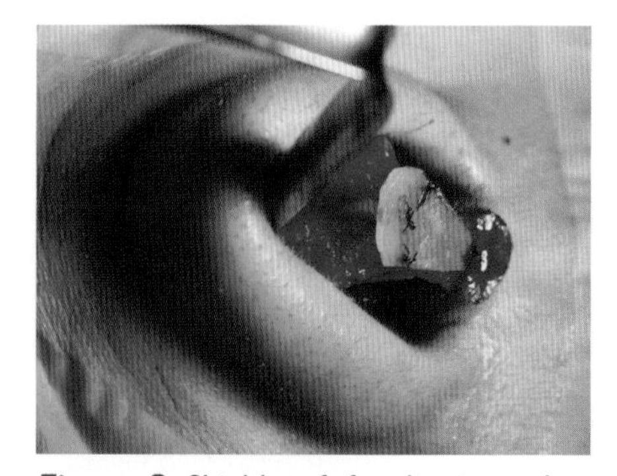

Figure 3 Shield graft for the tip made from septal cartilage.

thin cartilage gets easily torn and damaged by the suture. Moreover, the tip graft made from weak cartilage becomes deformed when covered with skin, making it difficult to create the desired tip shape. Therefore, one must understand such limitations when using weak and thin cartilage for tip graft purposes.

After using septal cartilage for the aforementioned purposes, in most cases only a small piece of cartilage remains. Very rarely, when the harvested cartilage is large and the amount used for structural grafting or tip grafting is small, it is possible that the amount of cartilage remaining can be used for dorsal augmentation. The author believes however that the use of septal cartilage for dorsal augmentation is not the ideal surgical technique. First of all, it is difficult to obtain a long enough piece of septal cartilage (3-4 cm) for dorsal augmentation. Second, using septal cartilage with an angled margin for dorsal augmentation is less aesthetically suitable compared to using alloplastic implants. Thus it is uncommon to use septal cartilage as a one piece dorsal augmentation material. Usually the piece of cartilage remaining after structural grafting or tip grafting is crushed using a cartilage crusher and used as a volume filler to correct focal depressions or uneven areas in the nasal dorsum or tip *(Figure 4)*.

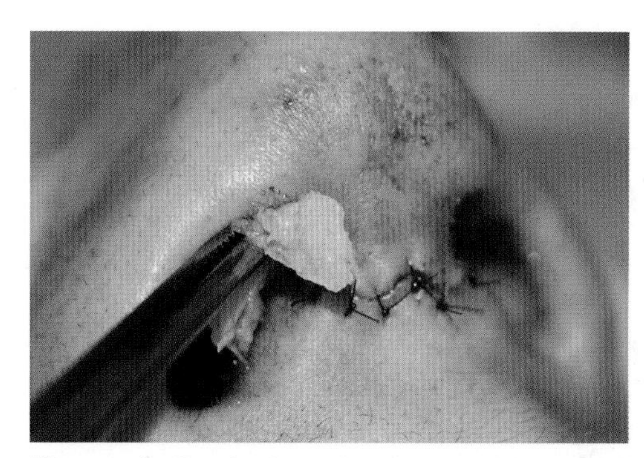

Figure 4 Crushed cartilage is a useful material to serve as a volume-filler for the nasal dorsum and nasal tip.

When excessively crushed, the septal cartilage placed on the dorsum is more easily absorbed and the dorsum sinks. On the other hand, when crushing is inadequate, uneven surfaces of the cartilage can show through the skin.

References

1. Kim JS, Khan NA, Song HM, Jang YJ. Intraoperative measurements of harvestable septal cartilage in rhinoplasty. Ann Plast Surg 2010; 65: 519-23.
2. Jang YJ, Moon BJ. State of the art in augmentation rhinoplasty: implant or graft?. Curr Opin Otolaryngol Head Neck Surg 2012; 20: 280-8.
3. Jang YJ, Yu MS. Rhinoplasty for the Asian nose. Facial Plast Surg 2010; 26: 93-101.

Conchal Cartilage

Yong Ju Jang · Hyung Min Song

The most common types of autologous cartilage used in rhinoplasty are septal cartilage, conchal cartilage, and costal cartilage. Currently in many facial plastic surgery clinics in Korea, augmentation of the nasal dorsum with alloplastic implants and using conchal cartilage in tip surgery is the most popular surgical technique. Conchal cartilage, unlike septal cartilage, has the disadvantage of leaving an additional scar during cartilage harvest, but its elasticity and softness, as well as having the most histological similarity to the lower lateral cartilage make it popular as graft material for the nasal tip. It would be ideal if one could obtain enough amounts of septal cartilage during rhinoplasty, but in Koreans, especially women, the nasal septal cartilage is often small, thin, and weak, making it common for conchal cartilage to be harvested simultaneously. Since conchal cartilage can be taken from both ears, it seemingly has a quantitative advantage over septal cartilage, but harvesting the cartilage from both ears should be carefully thought out. The reason is that conchal cartilage is not only the first cartilage used for simple rhinoplasty but also the last resort—a crucial cartilage that can reconstruct nasal shapes that other cartilage cannot do for complicated revision cases who exhibit severe contraction.

I. Anatomy

Though the pinna is comprised of one cartilage, it can be divided into different regions based on the convex and concave areas. The protruding area of the external ear is the helix, and the protruding area in front of, and bent parallel to the helix is the antihelix. The antihelix divides into two crura, and the concave triangle in the middle is the fossa triangularis. The sunken area between the helix and antihelix is the scapha. The two deep spaces divided by the crus of helix are the cymba concha (superior) and cavum concha (inferior). The protruding area anterior of the external auditory meatus is the tragus and the protrusion on the opposite side is the antitragus *(Figure 1)*.

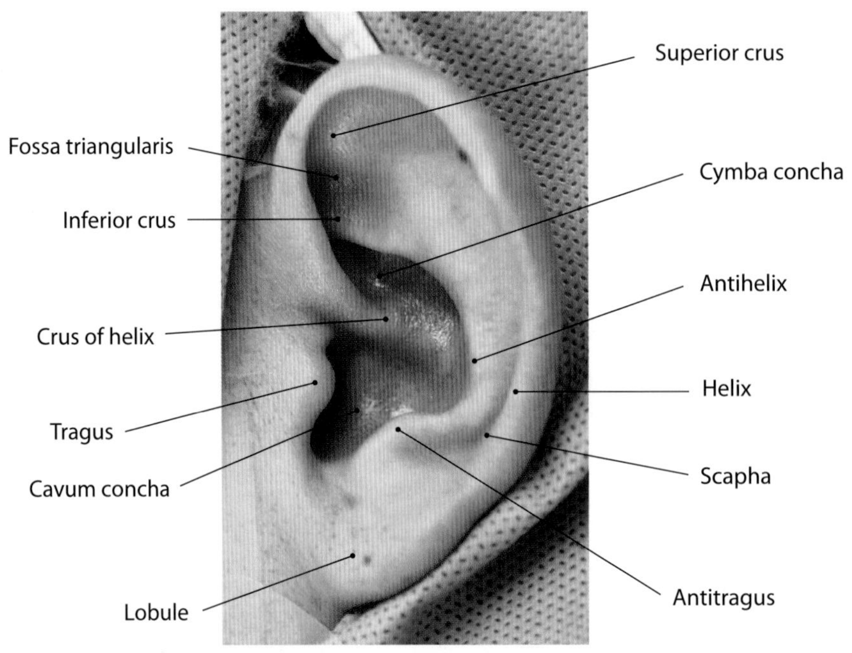

Figure 1 Surface anatomy of the ear.

Anatomical regions of the conchal cartilage used for rhinoplasty are the cavum concha, cymba concha, and tragus. The cavum concha, due to its concave shape, is useful as a tip graft. The cymba concha is shaped similarly to the lateral crus of the lower lateral cartilage, thus is useful for the reconstruction of the lower lateral cartilage. The tragus is a relatively small cartilage useful when small amounts of conchal cartilage are required *(Figure 2)*.

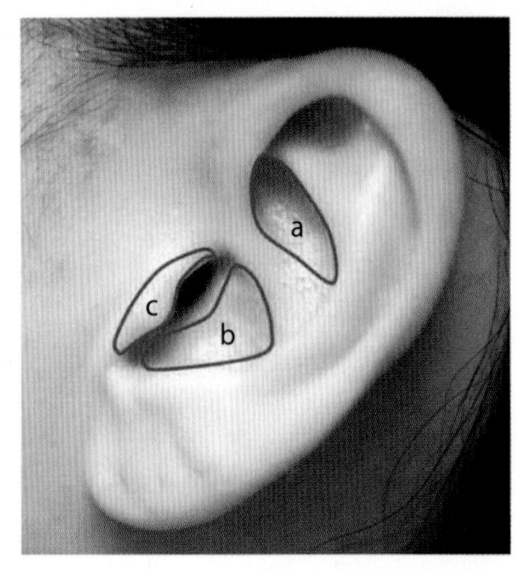

Figure 2 Anatomical regions of conchal cartilage used for rhinoplasty; cymba concha (a), cavum concha (b), and tragus (c).

Conchal cartilage does not have uniform cartilage thickness all throughout. This difference in thickness may be considered a disadvantage, but making use of it can help create grafts useful for tip surgery. The thick parts are the areas around the crus of helix and external auditory meatus *(Figure 3)*.

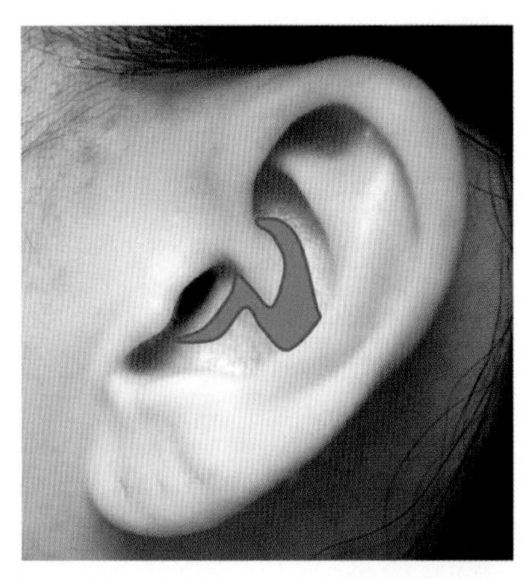

Figure 3 The thick parts of ear. The areas around the crus of helix and external auditory meatus (area marked blue).

II. Harvesting Conchal Cartilage

1. Cavum Concha and Cymba Concha

In the anterior aspect of the concha, inject 2% lidocaine (1:100,000 epinephrine) in subperichondrial plane for easy dissection. The posterior side of the ear should be injected in the subcutaneous plane according to the size of cartilage to be taken and the corresponding size of incision (2-3 cm). Important structures to be preserved to prevent ear deformation after harvesting conchal cartilage are the antihelix, antitragus, inferior crus of antihelix, crus of helix, and the part of the cavum concha adjacent to the external auditory meatus *(Figure 4)*.

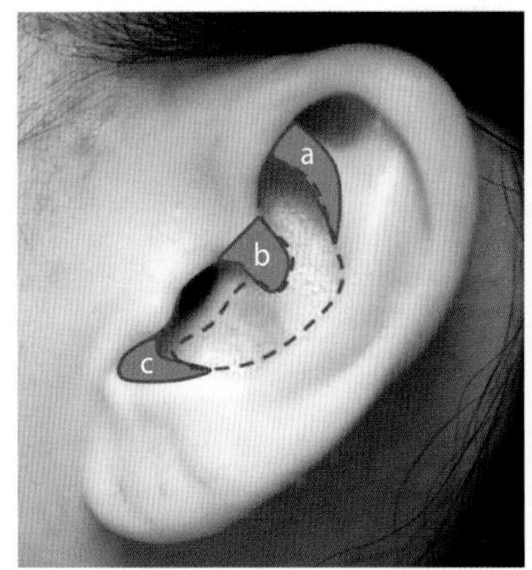

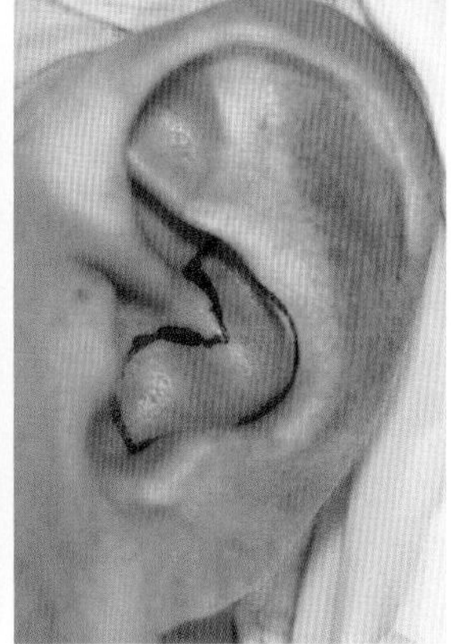

Figure 4 Important structures to be preserved to prevent deformation after harvesting conchal cartilage: Inferior crus of the antihelix (a), crus of the helix (b), and the part connecting the cavum concha to the lower part of external auditory meatus (c). In addition, the antihelix and the antitragus should be preserved. The photo on the right shows skin markings ideal for cartilage harvesting.

When harvesting cartilage either through a posterior or anterior approach, dissection should be carried out with perichondrium on one or both sides attached to the cartilage. This prevents the cartilage from breaking easily during dissection and makes it easier to suture to the lower lateral cartilage. The author prefers the postauricular approach to harvest cartilage in most cases. During conchal cartilage harvest, using the opposite hand's finger to check the location of the antihelix, make an incision of around 2 cm on the back of the conchal bowl, followed by dissection of the posterior side of the cartilage. Dissection should be limited on the cavum concha and cymba concha. Preserve the crus of the helix, making the harvested cartilage a kidney bean shape *(Figure 5)*.

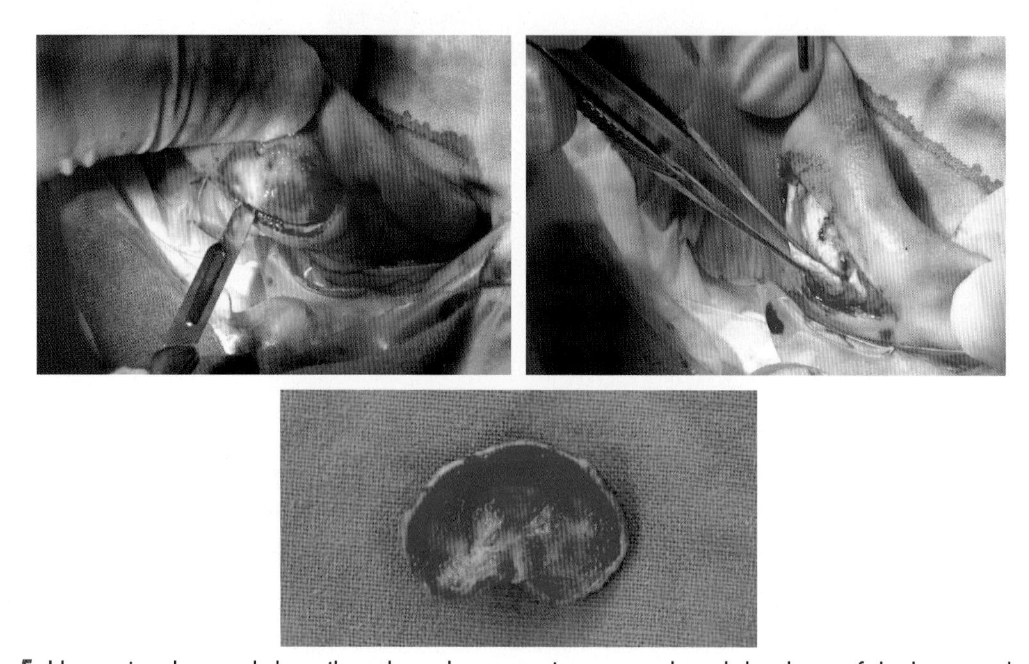

Figure 5 Harvesting the conchal cartilage through a posterior approach, and the shape of the harvested cartilage.

The surgeon should first perform subcutaneous suturing followed by cutaneous closure of the harvest site. Since some cases may develop hematoma formation at the donor site, placement of a bolster dressing is useful to prevent this complication *(Figure 6)*. The skin sutures should be removed after 7-10 days. Instead of a bolster dressing, one can apply pressure a dressing by fitting in an ear mold in the external auditory meatus. This method is less painful than a gauze bolster and keeps the skin in front of the concha smooth.

2. Tragal Cartilage

The tragal cartilage is small, but can be harvested quickly and easily in a size of about 1×1 cm. This cartilage is especially useful in minor refinements of the nasal tip. It is also useful when only a small amount of autologous cartilage is required during rhinoplasty. Before harvesting the cartilage, inject local anesthetic agent under the skin of the tragus and external auditory meatus to

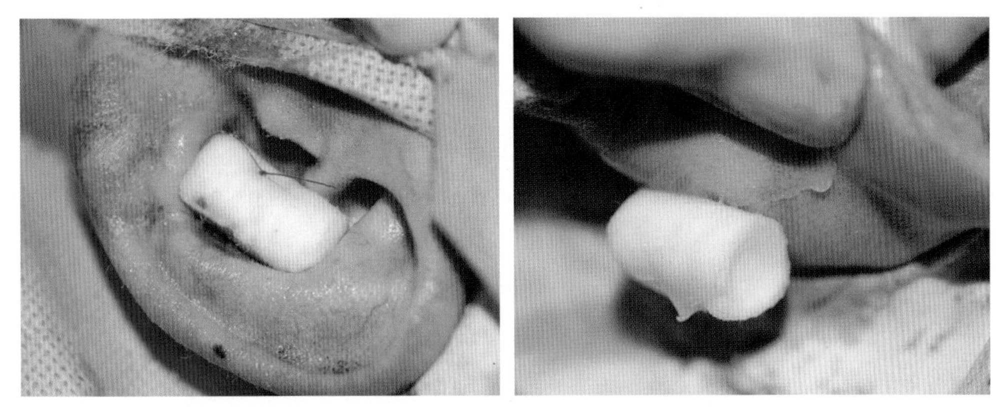

Figure 6 Placement of bolster dressing is useful to prevent hematoma formation at the donor site.

make hydrodissection easy. Make an incision about 1.5 mm from the tragal outer rim on the inside of the external auditory meatus. Unlike in the concha, subperichondrial dissection is easy, thus one should make sure to keep the perichondrium on the harvested cartilage on both sides. After removing cartilage, skin closure using 6.0 Nylon can be performed without subcutaneous sutures.

3. Composite Graft Harvesting

A composite graft—in which the skin and cartilage are harvested together—is a graft material that can be used effectively in many aspects of rhinoplasty. Composite grafts can be used for the loss of alar nasal lining due to infection, correction of nostril stenosis, and correction of alar retraction. This graft can be harvested from either the cavum or cymba concha, depending on the desired size. The anterior and posterior skin can be attached to the cartilage. If the skin paddle of the harvested composite graft is not that large, primary closure of the donor site can be done by pulling the skin. If the donor defect is large, rather than pulling the skin, reconstruct the graft-donor site by using a skin graft taken from the post-auricular region *(Figure 7)*.

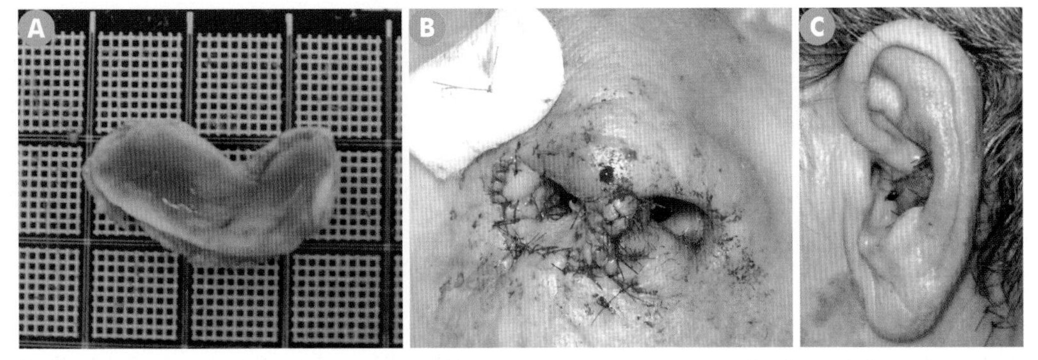

Figure 7 Composite graft of conchal cartilage (A), case using a composite graft of conchal cartilage to correct nostril stenosis (B), and postauricular skin grafting for the donor site (C).

III. Rhinoplasty Using Conchal Cartilage

1. Tip Surgery

It is easy to make a natural-looking tip using conchal cartilage due to the histological characteristics of its elastic cartilage and inherent curvature, thus making it the most commonly used graft in the nasal tip.

1) Onlay Graft

This technique is used to prevent implants for dorsal augmentation from coming into contact with the tip skin directly or used in multiple layers to make the original tip higher. In order to prevent prominent graft contour, the cartilage graft should be crushed with a morselizer or the margin should be beveled. It is good to use cartilage from cavum concha as an onlay graft *(Figure 8)*.

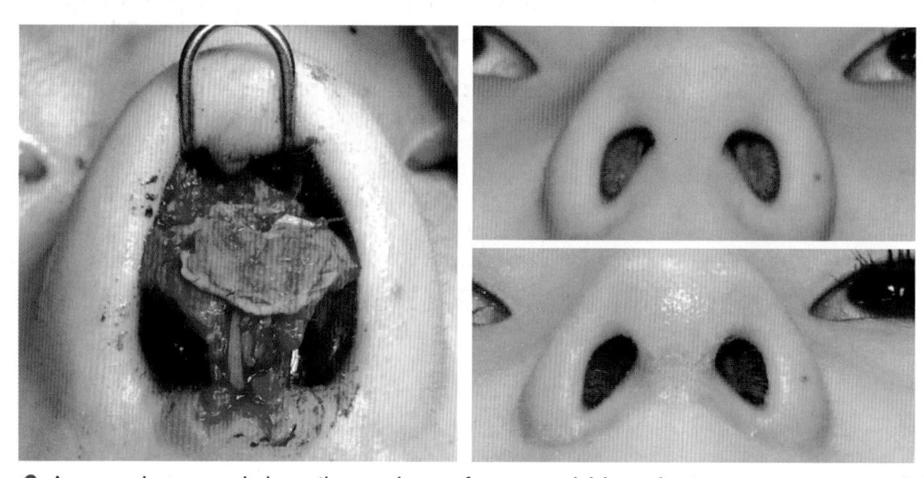

Figure 8 A case where conchal cartilage onlay graft was used. Note the improvement in tip definition.

2) Shield Graft and Multilayer Graft

When designing the shield graft out of conchal cartilage, use the part where the cavum concha meets the inferior crus of the antihelix as it goes upwards since that part is thick. Doing so will produce a graft as strong and as well-defined as septal cartilage. When using conchal cartilage for the tip, it is possible to use its inherent curvature in whatever direction the surgeon prefers. If caudal rotation of the tip is desired, making the concave part of the cartilage face caudally will give desirable shapes *(Figure 9)*. This method is appropriate for patients with thick nasal tip skin.

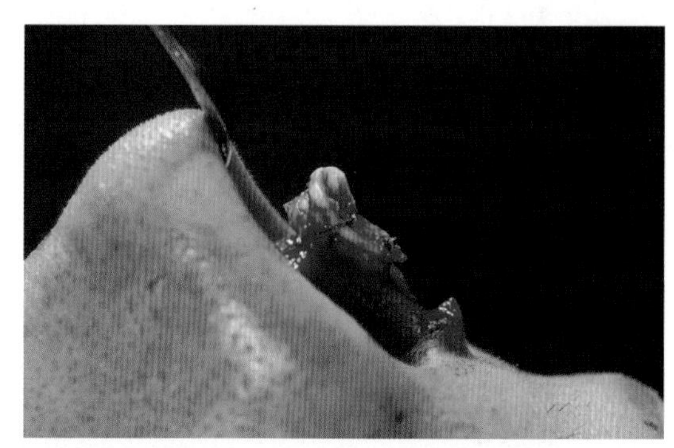

Figure 9 When placing a conchal cartilage shield graft, facing the concave part of the cartilage caudally can avoid cephalic bending and will give a natural tip contour.

In patients with thinner skin, perform morselization to keep the graft margin from showing *(Figure 10)*. Conchal cartilage has numerous advantages as multilayer tip grafting material. A detailed discussion on multilayer grafting is provided in the chapter "Tip Surgery".

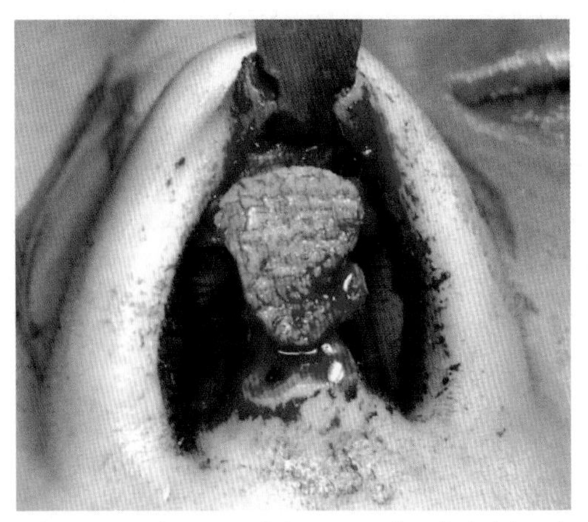

Figure 10 In patients with thinner skin, morselization of the tip graft is helpful to keep the graft margins from showing.

3) Lateral Crural Graft

When the tip graft is over 3 mm higher than the surrounding cartilage, placement of lateral crural onlay grafts is recommended to reduce the possibility of a prominent contour of the tip graft. For patients who have flat noses, pinched tips that reveal tip graft margins on each side can occur when extending alloplasic implants to the tip. In these situations, using conchal cartilage as lateral crural onlay grafts can create a much more natural-looking tip shape. Lateral crural onlay grafts can also be used to correct the short nose deformity *(Figure 11)*, and using conchal cartilage can be used to correct alar retraction.

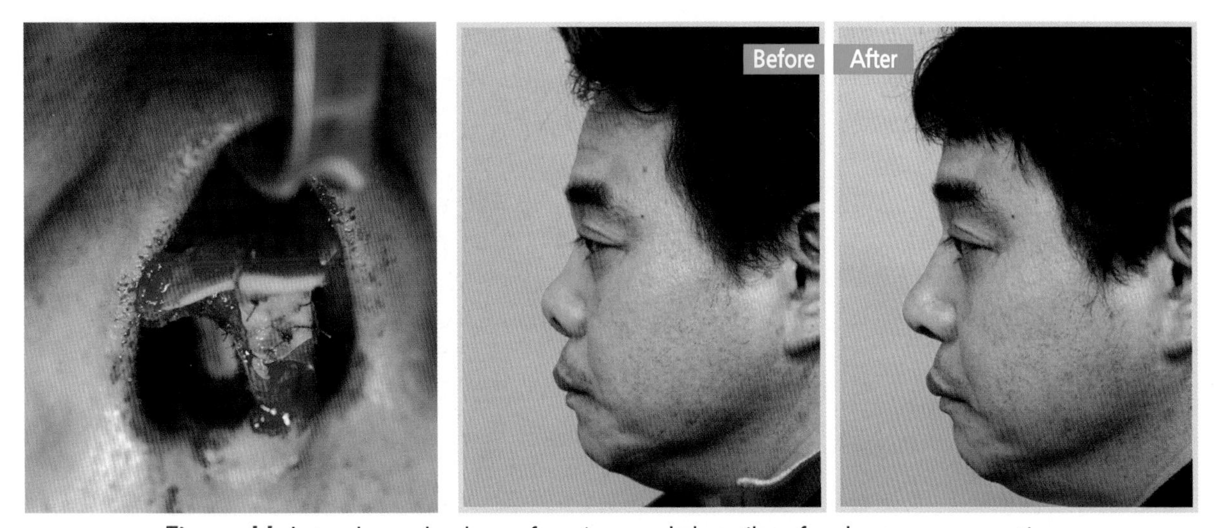

Figure 11 Lateral crural onlay grafts using conchal cartilage for short nose correction.

2. Dorsal Augmentation

Due to its intrinsic curvature and limitations in length, conchal cartilage has clear limitations as dorsal augmentation material. However, it is useful for partial augmentation. It can be used as a graft for a sunken supratip following tip surgery, or to make up for the height imbalance of the nasal dorsum following surgery on convex dorsum. For full-length nasal augmentation using conchal cartilage alone (from the radix to the tip), one must harvest a big piece of cartilage *(Figure 12)*. In such cases, its natural curvature can be eliminated by cutting it in a convex shape and stacking it into multiple layers; making it useful as dorsal augmentation material. However, dorsal augmentation using such methods increases the possibility of contour visibility of the graft through the skin over time. Therefore, it is not wise to use conchal cartilage as dorsal augmentation for severe dorsal deficiency.

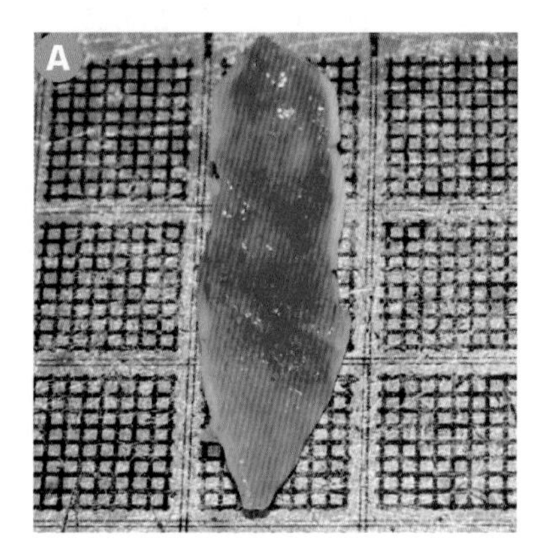

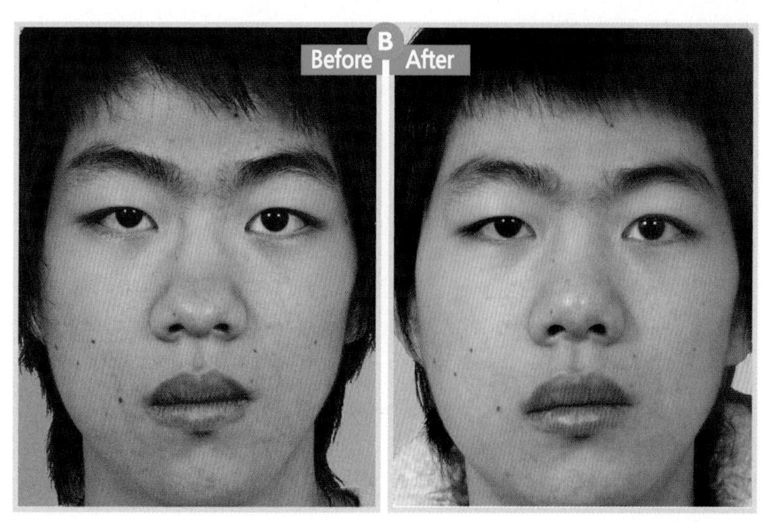

Figure 12 Due to its intrinsic curvature and limitations in length, it is not easy to harvest quality conchal cartilage which can cover the entire nasal dorsum smoothly for dorsal augmentation (A). A case of dorsal augmentation showing a good postoperative result because of a graft with good quality (B).

When there is only a partial depression or a minor saddle in the nasal dorsum, partial dorsal augmentation can be nicely achieved through making cuts in the cartilage with the perichondrium of the harvested conchal cartilage intact and still attached, making the divided pieces maintain a state of attachment with each other through the perichondrium. It is possible to avoid graft visibility through this method when used on patients with thick skin *(Figure 13)*.

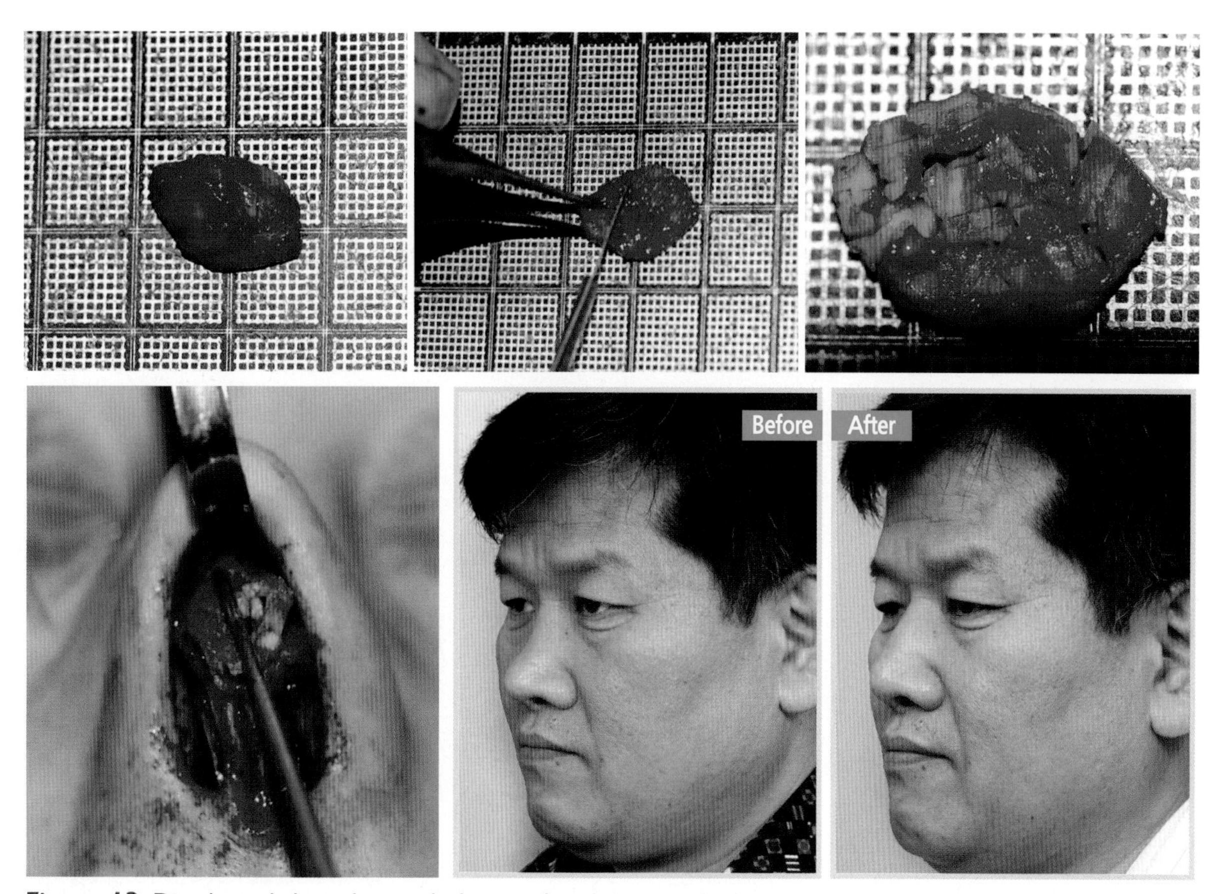

Figure 13 Diced conchal cartilage with the perichondrium attached retains its shape and can be used for partial dorsal augmentation as demonstrated in this case.

Partial augmentation can also done by dicing the cartilage into smaller pieces and using the cartilage alone, or using the pieces as part of the fascia-wrapped diced cartilage graft. When performing augmentation with diced cartilage alone, it is essential that a small skin pocket is created to prevent migration of the cartilage pieces *(Figure 14)*.

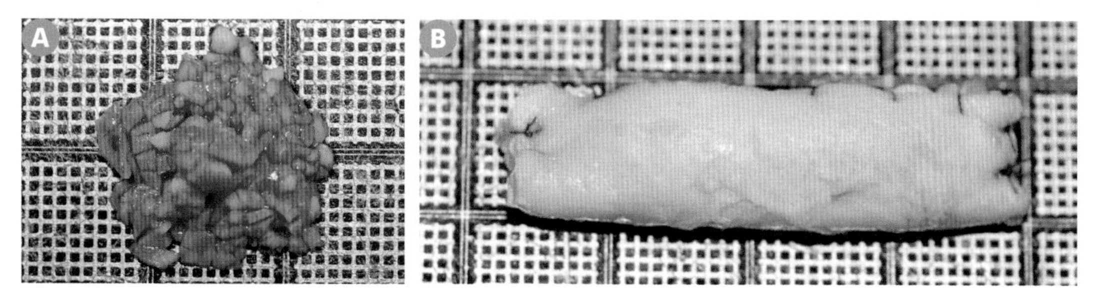

Figure 14 Diced conchal cartilage (A) and fascia wrapped diced cartilage (B) can be used as good material for dorsal augmentation.

3. Structural Graft

It is not easy to use conchal cartilage for reconstruction of the weakened septum. However, if the caudal or dorsal strut of the septal cartilage has a convexity toward one side, using the natural curvature of conchal cartilage as a batten or spreader graft in a way that straightens the convexity of the septum can be effective for septal reconstruction *(Figure 15)*. However, with its high elasticity and low rigidity, conchal cartilage often fails to provide as much strong support as costal cartilage. It is can be used on both sides for middle vault reconstruction or only on one side. Usage in the form of a butterfly graft for the improvement of nasal valve collapse can also be done.

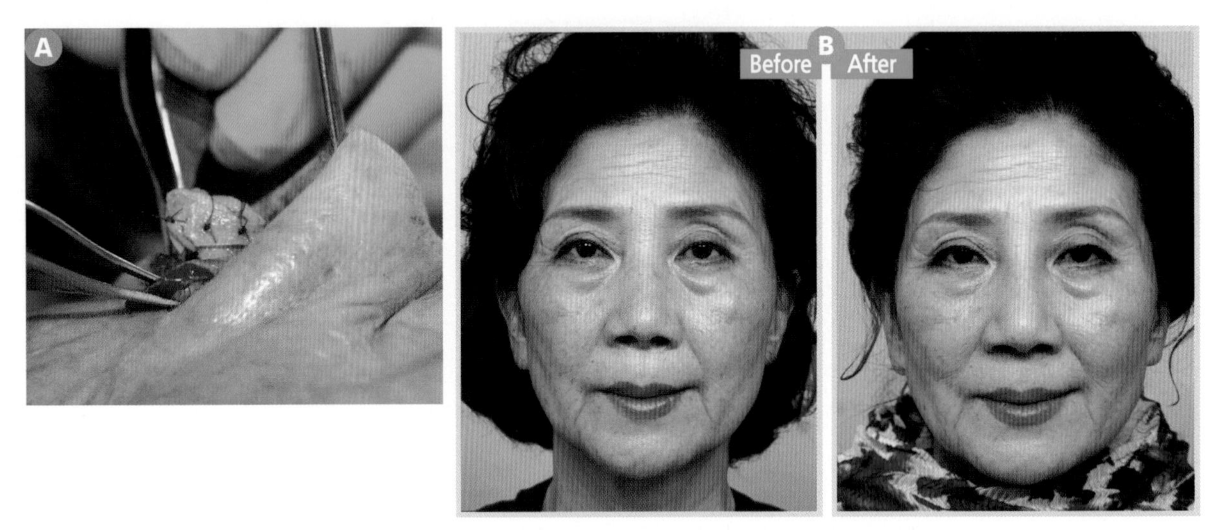

Figure 15 Intraoperative photograph of the extended spreader graft made of conchal cartilage (A). A patient showing successful derotation of the nose by the use of the extended spreader graft (B).

IV. Complications

A hematoma can occur after surgery. In such situations, partial stitch removal should be performed to evacuate the hematoma, and then pressure reapplied. When too much cartilage is removed, not leaving enough antihelix and antitragus, the ear becomes weak and deformed *(Figure 16)*. Severe keloids can form where the cartilage was harvested, thus the surgeon must explain this possibility to the patient before surgery *(Figure 17)*.

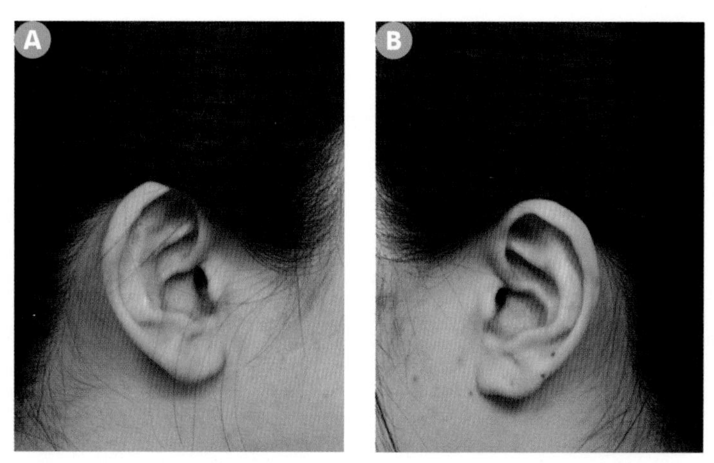

Figure 16 A deformed ear characterized by the loss of surface landmarks. This deformity was caused by an aggressive harvesting of conchal cartilage for grafting (A). Normal ear on the left (B).

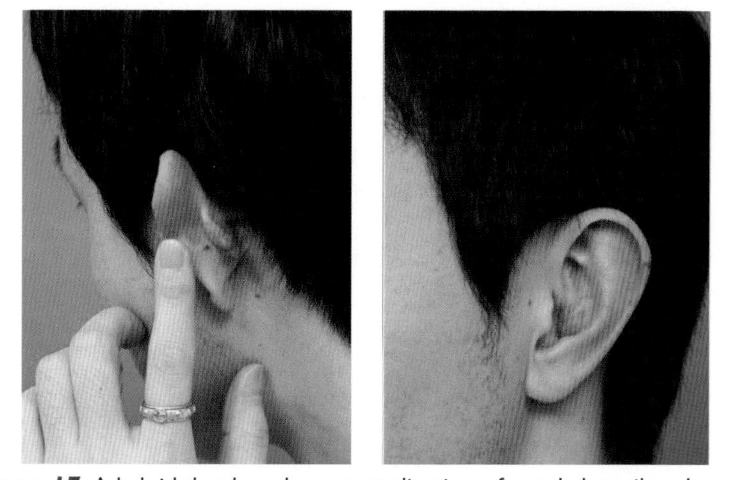

Figure 17 A keloid developed as a complication of conchal cartilage harvest.

References

1. Antohi N, Isac C, Stan V, Ionescu R. Dorsal nasal augmentation with "open sandwich" graft consisting of conchal cartilage and retroauricular fascia. Aesthet Surg J 2012; 32: 833-45.
2. Chang YL. Correction of difficult short nose by modified caudal septal advancement in Asian patients. Aesthet Surg J 2010; 30: 166-75.
3. Hafezi F, Bateni H, Naghibzadeh B, Nouhi AH, Emami A, Fatemi SJ, Pedram M, Mousavi SJ. Diced ear cartilage with perichondrial attachment in rhinoplasty: a new concept. Aesthet Surg J 2012; 32: 825-32.
4. Hagerty RC, Mittelstaedt S, Vu le P, Harmatz AS, Harvey TS. Countercurve placement of conchal cartilage grafts used for correction of nasal tip deformities. Ann Plast Surg 2007; 59: 566-8.
5. Han K, Kim J, Son D, Park B. How to harvest the maximal amount of conchal cartilage grafts. J Plast Reconstr Aesthet Surg 2008; 61: 1465-71.
6. Jang YJ, Song HM, Yoon YJ, Sykes JM. Combined use of crushed cartilage and processed fascia lata for dorsal augmentation in rhinoplasty for Asians. Laryngoscope 2009; 119: 1088-92.
7. Mowlavi A, Pham S, Wilhelmi B, Masouem S, Guyuron B. Anatomical characteristics of the conchal cartilage with suggested clinical applications in rhinoplasty surgery. Aesthet Surg J 2010; 30: 522-6.
8. Park TH, Park JH, Kim JK, Seo SW, Rah DK, Chang CH. Analysis of 15 cases of auricular keloids following conchal cartilage grafts in an asian population. Aesthetic Plast Surg 2013; 37: 102-5.
9. Wright ST, Calhoun KH, Decherd M, Quinn FB. Conchal cartilage harvest: donor site morbidities, patient satisfaction, and cosmetic outcomes. Arch Facial Plast Surg 2007; 9: 298-9.

Costal Cartilage

Yong Ju Jang

I. Characteristics and Applications

Costal cartilage is an important graft provider for rhinoplasty in that it provides large amounts of quality cartilage. Like septal cartilage, costal cartilage is a hard hyaline cartilage useful for structural grafting. Carving and trimming it well makes it applicable for both the nasal dorsum and nasal tip, justifying its value as a versatile graft material. In humans, cartilage ossifies over time, and this ossification is especially evident in costal cartilage. Young patients have a whiter and more malleable cartilage. However, the older the patient, the harder and more yellow the cartilage becomes (especially at the center); sometimes exhibiting ossified centers *(Figure 1)*.

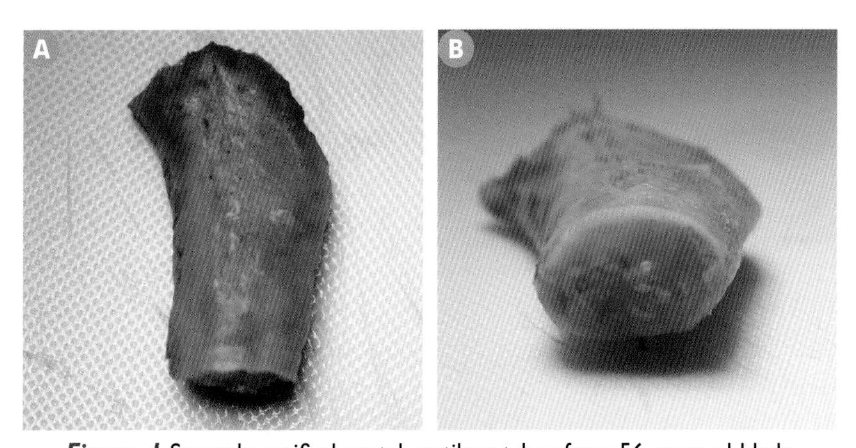

Figure 1 Severely ossified costal cartilage taken from 56-years old lady.

Though it differs among individuals, the cartilage of patients between 50 and 60 years of age is generally of poor quality. This point should be considered before surgery of older patients. However, severely ossified costal cartilage can be encountered in younger individuals as well. Prior to surgery, it is necessary to check the degree of ossification using radiologic imaging modalities.

The author uses costal cartilage for the following:

- ☑ Reconstructive rhinoplasty that requires large amounts of sturdy cartilage for nasal septal reconstruction and grafting due to severe deformation
- ☑ Saddle nose
- ☑ Short nose
- ☑ A patient who has small nose and wants major changes
- ☑ A patient with very thick skin who wants well defined and projected nasal tips with distinct contours

II. Anatomy of Costal Cartilage Harvest

Though costal cartilage is an excellent autologous implant material that can be used for saddle noses, congenital deformities, and difficult revision surgeries, insufficient understanding of its surrounding anatomy during harvest can lead to complications such as pneumothorax, hemorrhage and chronic pain. Therefore, before surgery, the surgeon must understand the anatomy surrounding the costal cartilages, and know the methods to deal with possible complications during surgery.

1. The Chest Wall

The bony thorax is composed of cartilage, the sternum, clavicles, thoracic vertebrae, and twelve pairs of ribs. The 1st-7th ribs are directly connected to the sternum, and are thus called “true ribs”, and the most commonly used 6th and 7th ribs have a connection with each other in the middle. The 8th-12th ribs are connected, through cartilage, indirectly to the sternum, and thus called “false ribs”. The 11th-12th ribs are only connected to the thoracic vertebrae, and are called “floating ribs” *(Figure 2)*.

Each rib is made up of a head, neck, and shaft. The head is connected to the vertebrae and the shaft is connected to the costal cartilage. The sternum is a flat bone of 15-20 cm in length composed of the manubrium, body, and xiphoid process, and is attached to true ribs 1st to 7th by cartilage. On each side of the sternum run vertically the internal thoracic artery and vein, which gives off the intercostal artery and vein through the intercostal space *(Figure 3)*.

The bony thorax, under the skin and subcutaneous tissue, is surrounded by three groups of muscles. These muscle layers are:

1) First muscle group: diaphragm and intercostals (external, internal, transverse, or innermost muscle)
2) Second muscle group: sternocleidomastoid and serratus posterior
3) Third muscle group: pectoralis major and minor, trapezius, latissimus dorsi, serratus anterior and posterior, levator, and external oblique abdominal.

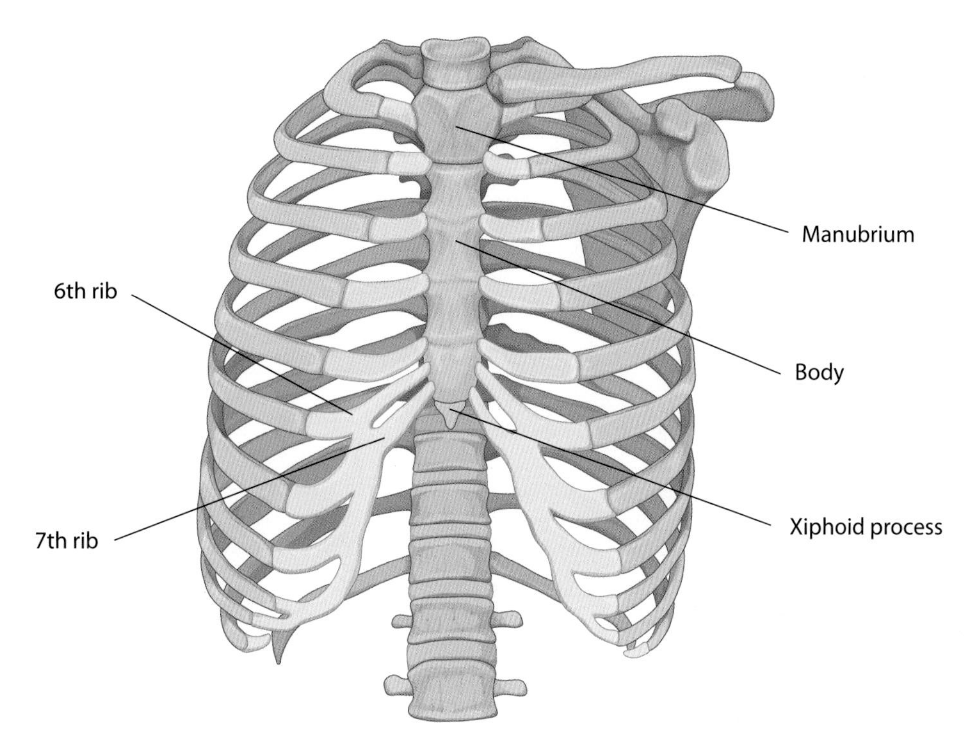

Figure 2 Rib cartilages and bones.

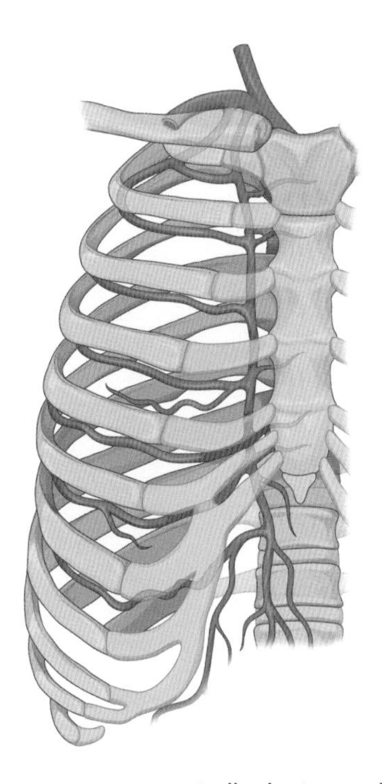

Figure 3 On each side of the sternum run vertically the internal thoracic artery and vein, which give off the intercostal artery and vein through the intercostal space

For the 6-7th costal cartilages (harvested the most for surgery), the lateral edge is below the external oblique abdominal muscle, or pectoralis minor muscle and the medial edge is below the aponeurosis of the external oblique abdominal muscle and rectus abdominis muscle *(Figure 4)*.

In each of the 11 intercostal spaces lie the intercostal bundle (vein, artery, and nerve) that run along each rib's lower margin *(Figure 5)*. The intercostal space is wider in the front, and each intercostal bundle runs along the rib's lower edge in the front and runs through the middle of the intercostal space as it progresses to the back.

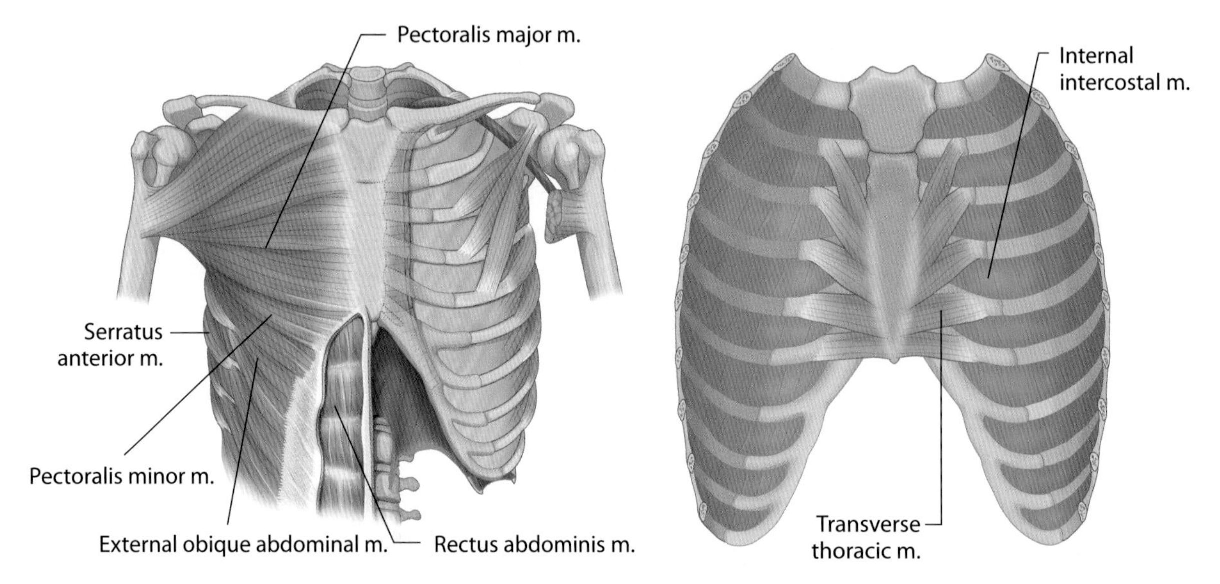

Figure 4 Muscles of the chest wall.

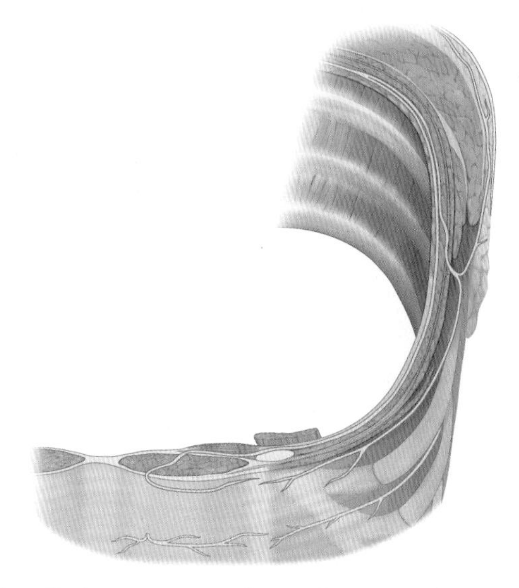

Figure 5 Intercostal bundle (vein, artery, and nerve) running along each rib's lower margin.

2. Pleura

The pleura is composed of the two layers of the parietal and visceral pleura. The space between them is called the pleural cavity. Parietal pleura is divided into four parts according to region: cervical pleura that surrounds the apex of the hemithorax to the 1st rib level, costal pleura that is attached to inner surface and chest wall of the sternum and ribs, mediastinal pleura that surrounds the pericardium and other mediastinal structures, and the diaphragmatic pleura that is strongly adherent to the central tendon of the diaphragm *(Figure 6)*. The parenchyma of the lung is adjacent to the upper part of cartilage number 6, and parietal pleura reaches down to near cartilage number 7.

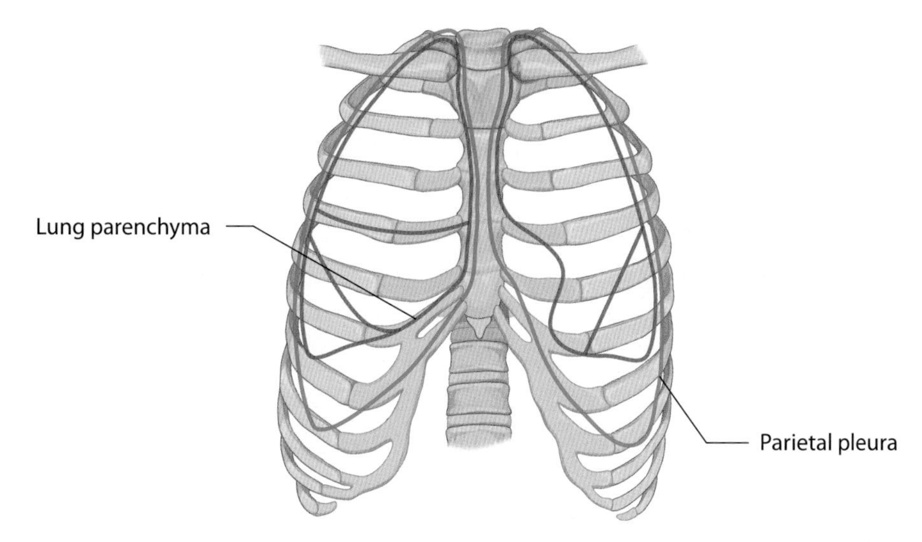

Figure 6 The parenchyma of the lung is placed up to the upper part of the 6th rib, and parietal pleura reaches down to near the 7th rib.

III. Cartilage Harvest Technique and Postoperative Management

The author usually harvests the 6-7th costal cartilages. The rib cartilage harvest steps are described in *Figure 7*. First, the xiphoid process, rib cage margin, and nipple line are marked on the patient's skin. Medial to the the nipple line, mark the lower margin of the rib cartilage that descends from the xiphoid process in a slope. Make a 3-4 cm incision about 2 cm above the lower margin of the confirmed rib cartilage *(Figure 7A)*. Incising through the fat reveals the fascia *(Figures 7B, 7C)*. An incision on the fascia is made and the muscle fibers are spread without cutting the muscle (external oblique abdominal muscle or pectoralis minor muscle).This exposes the outer surface of the cartilage *(Figure 7D)*. Inserting a retractor and pulling the muscle reveals the entire cartilage. The cartilage seen at this point is either the 6th or 7th costal cartilage *(Figure 7E)*. The 6th cartilage, in many patients, has a part showing a 90° angle or gentle slope that is fused with 7th cartilage *(Figure 8)*. The cartilage can be harvested with the perichondrium attached to the cartilage, or by performing subperichondrial dissection within the surrounding perichondrium *(Figure 9)*. The first method has a slightly higher possibility of hemorrhage during surgery or seroma formation than a subperichondrial dissection. If the perichondrium is going to be harvested, the intercostal muscle attached to the cartilage is cut using cautery and cartilage is separated. When working within the perichondrium (subperichondrial dissection), the risk of hemorrhage decreases and preservation of perichondrium deep to the cartilage is easier, lowering the possibility of pleural damage. When harvesting the cartilage in this manner, the soft tissue around the cartilage should be dissected first, then an I or H shape incision should be made on the outer perichondrium using a number 10 blade or bovie. Then, using a blade, make incisions on the upper and lower dissection planes, the deep inner part of the cartilage should be dissected

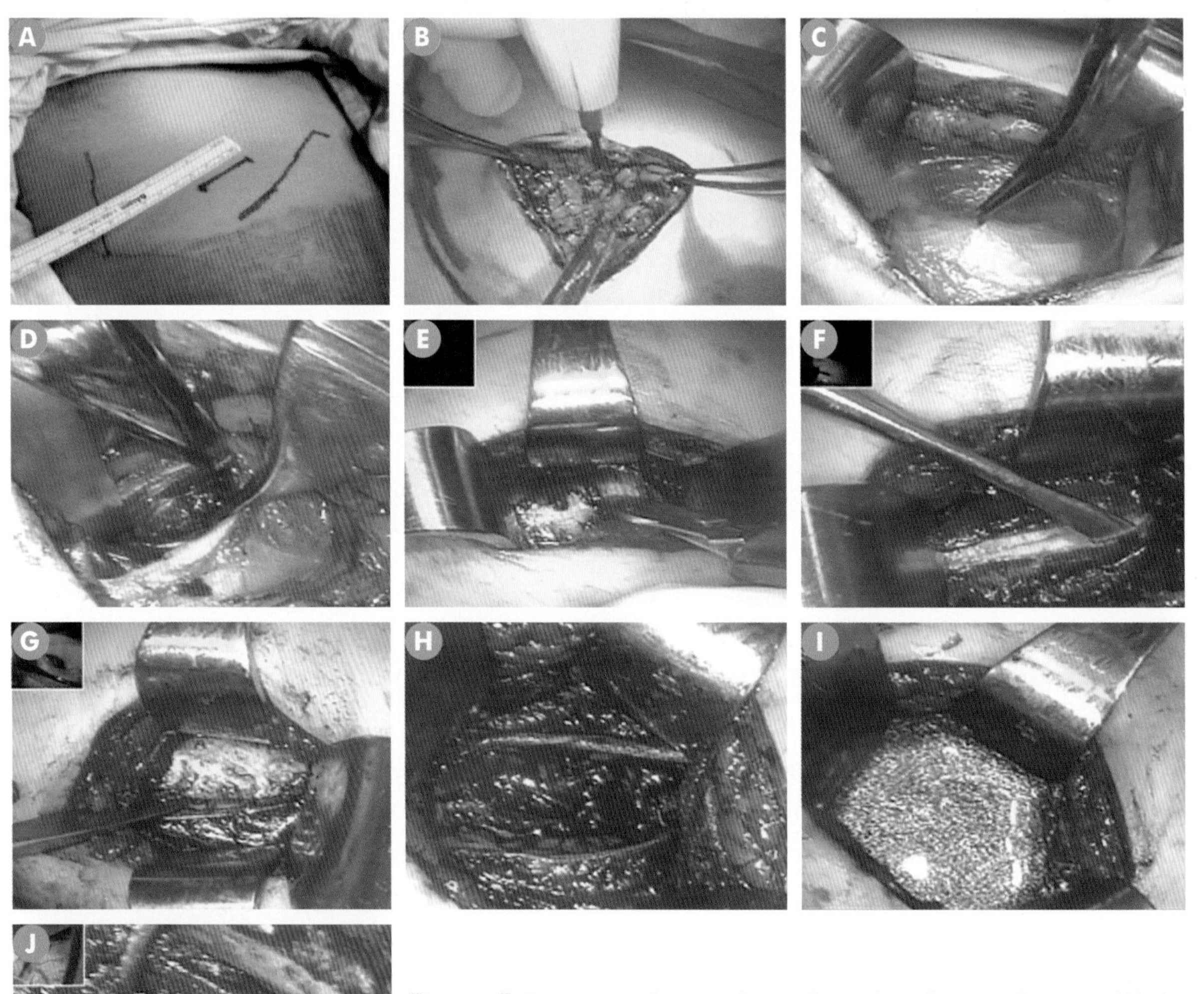

Figure 7 Operative photos of costal cartilage harvest. Incision (A), fat dissection (B), identification of muscle fascia and incision of the muscle (C), splitting the muscle layer (D), identification of the outer layer of the costal cartilage (E), incision and dissection of the perichondrium (F), dissection of the perimeter of the costal cartilage within the perichondrium (G), surgical field after delivering the cartilage (H), filling the donor site with saline to check air-leakage (I), and insertion of fat graft at the cartilage harvest site (J).

cautiously using an elevator. Dissection around the cartilage should be performed using a blunt curved elevator to carefully peel off perichondrium and lift the cartilage. The surgeon must keep the medial perichondrium from attaching to the cartilage, instead making it adhere to the deep inner soft tissue *(Figures 7G, 7H)*.

After harvesting the cartilage, fill the field with saline and request lung expansion from the anesthesiologist. If there is no pleural damage, air bubbles will not appear *(Figure 7I)*. If there is pleural damage, air bubbles can be seen every time the lungs expand, thus making pleural damage easy to detect. In cases of pleural damage, insert a thin nelaton catheter through the pleural tear, attach it to a suction, and maintain clamping until the lungs momentarily expand, at which point suction should be turned on and suture (purse string suture) should be performed carefully around the catheter. In cases of mild pleural damage, the pneumothorax can be resolved easily without using a chest tube, so one should keep calm. The parenchyma of the lung extend to the upper part of the 6th cartilage, so air leakage due to pleural damage is not common during surgery on the 7th rib cartilage. A more common complication of cartilage harvest is hemorrhage. Unintentional damage to the intercostal neurovascular bundle running horizontally below the cartilage, can happen while maneuvering a blade or elevator to cut the cartilage, thus leading to hemorrhage through the gap of in the incised cartilage. In such cases, remove the cartilage promptly to secure proper visualization and perform cauterization. The author fills the donor site with fibrin glue or fat collected from under the incised skin, and the muscle layer is closed *(Figure 7J)*. A suction drain can be placed on the outer side of the muscle layer and removed 2-3 days later. However, compressive dressing without using a suction drain is usually enough for recovery without serious complication.

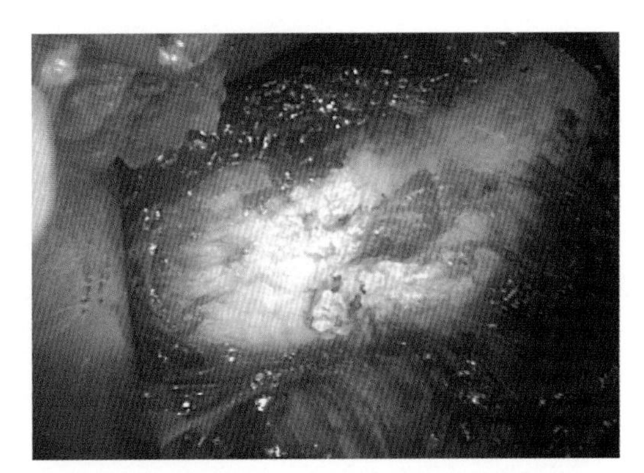

Figure 8 Confluence of the 6th and 7th ribs at the angulated portion of the 6th rib cartilage.

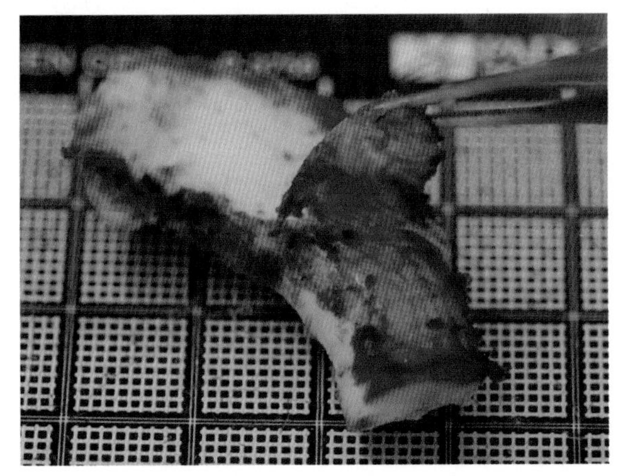

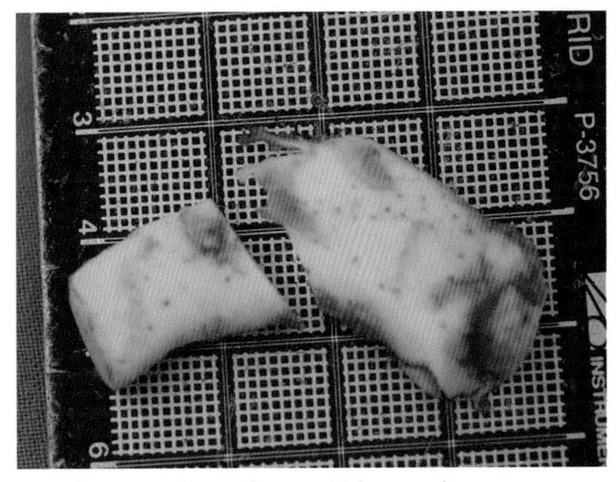

Figure 9 Perichondrium of the costal cartilage can be harvested together with the cartilage.

IV. How to Use the Harvested Cartilage

The 6th costal cartilage, in most cases, has a round cross section and has a bent shape in the part fused with the 7th costal cartilage. The 7th costal cartilage has a flatter cross section compared to the 6th costal cartilage, and has a more linear shape, thus is more appropriate for dorsal augmentation. Harvested cartilage should be further modified according to purpose. The author uses rib cartilage more often for septal reconstruction or tip surgery. If cartilage is harvested for the aforementioned purposes, use a dermatome blade to cut the cartilage into long, slender strips *(Figures 10, 11)*. This is then used for septal reconstruction or tip surgery. Reasons for using this cartilage for the above purposes will be explained in detail in each according Chapter, as this Chapter focuses on dorsal augmentation. In order to be used for dorsal augmentation, the harvested cartilage should be carved to a dimension of 3.5-4 cm in length and 0.7-1 cm in width *(Figure 12)*.

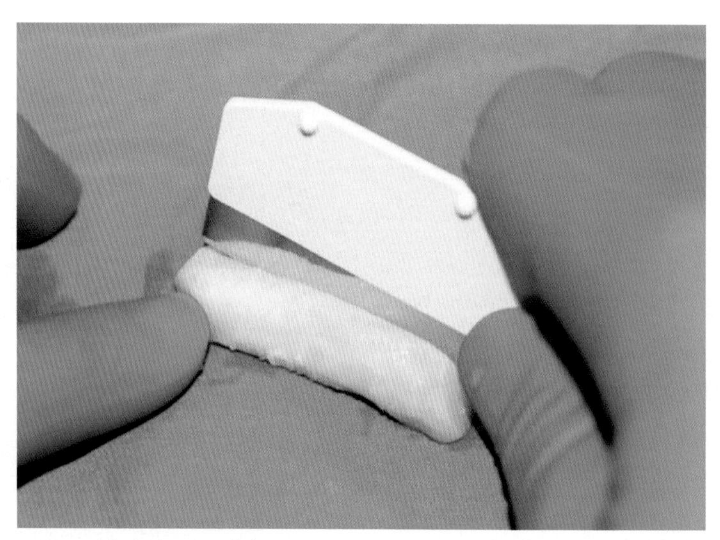

Figure 10 A dermatome blade is a useful instrument in cutting the harvested costal cartilage into strips.

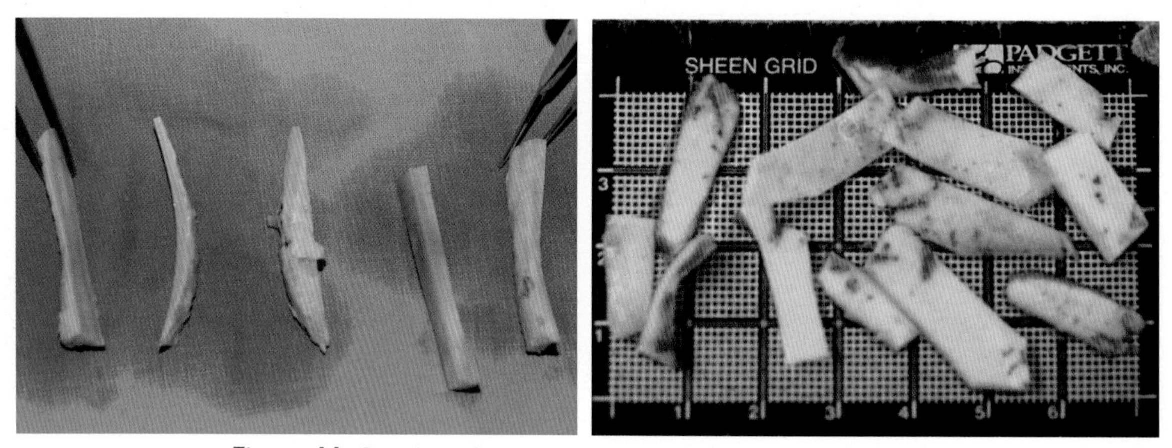

Figure 11 Costal cartilage cut into long strips and are ready for use.

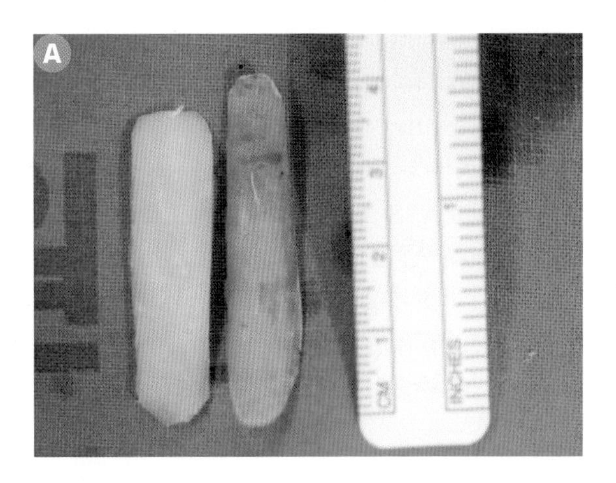

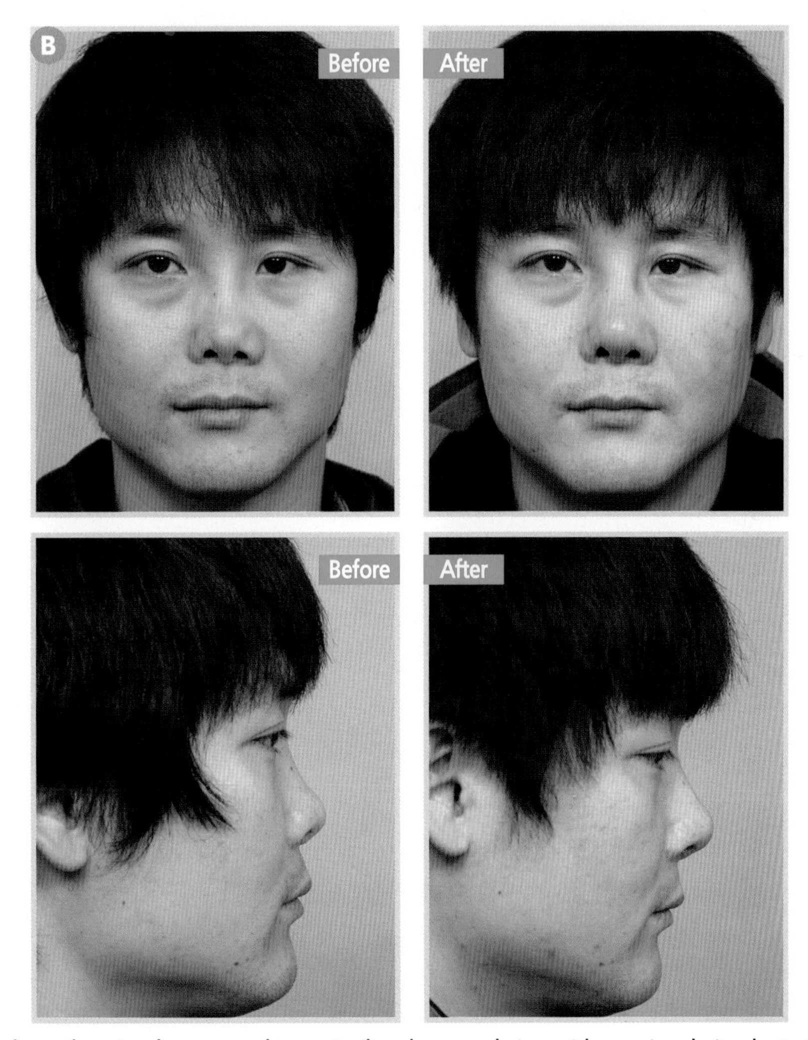

Figure 12 Costal cartilage implant carved to a similar shape and size with previously implanted silicone (A). Patient who underwent revision rhinoplasty using costal cartilage (B).

A #10 blade and drill can be used for carving, and it should be conducted free of time constraints and with immense caution. Place the carved cartilage in cold saline for initial warping to take place, and carve the cartilage again right before implantation. However, a successful one piece dorsal augmentation using rib cartilage for the entire dorsum is very difficult to create and requires a lot of experience. The author does not recommend using costal cartilage as a nasal dorsal implant unless there are no other choices. Methods such as using the core of cartilage or K-wire to prevent warping of costal cartilage have been introduced, but applying such methods does not ensure freedom from the risk of warping. Other methods to prevent warping include stacking pre-made long pieces of cartilage. This method is called laminated cartilage grafting. Based on the author's experience, applying this technique moderately lowers the risk of warping *(Figure 13)*.

There are cases when the shape or amount of cartilage remaining after septal reconstruction or

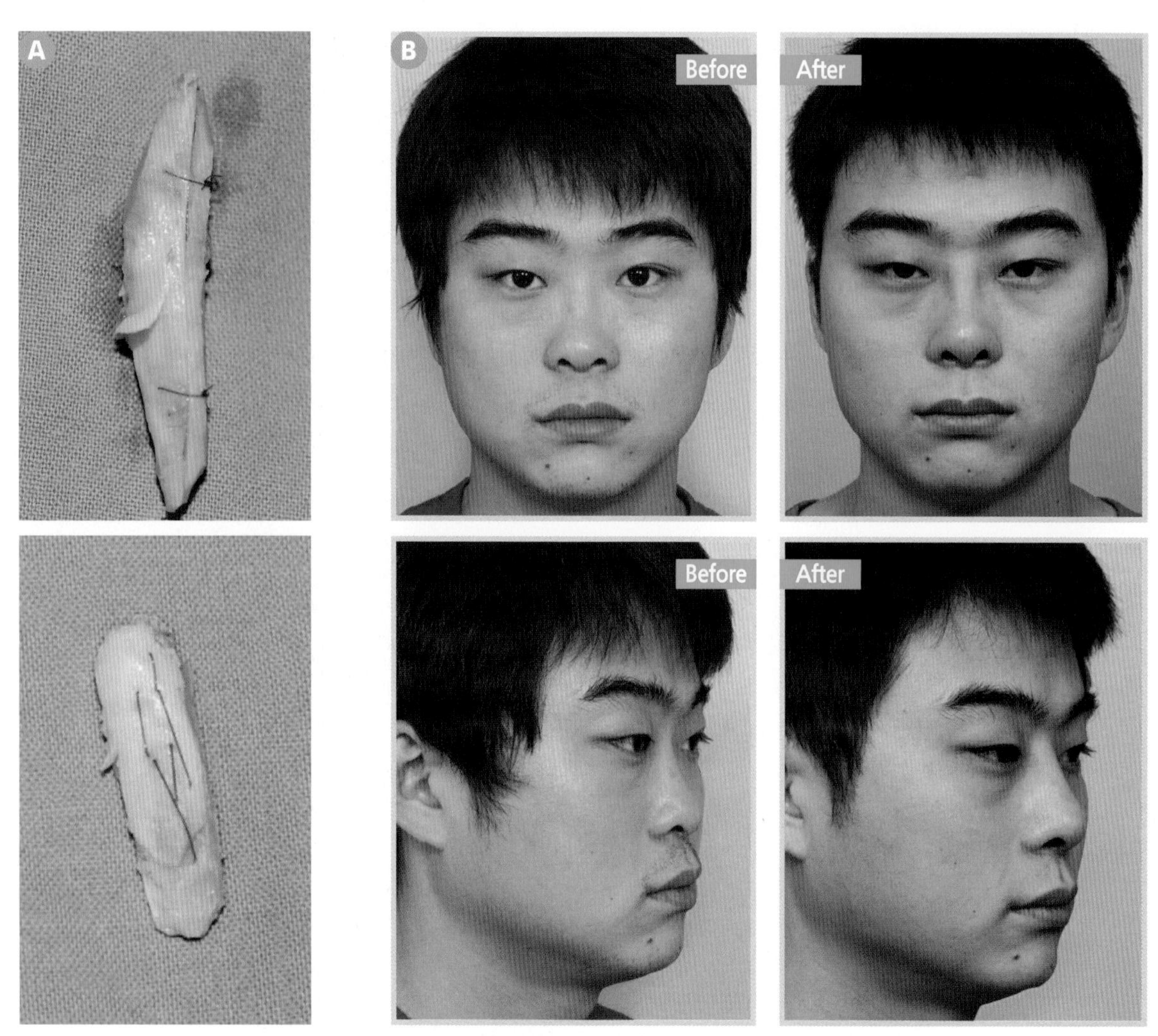

Figure 13 Laminated costal cartilage graft designed to be used as a dorsal implant (A). Patient showing a favorable surgical outcome after dorsal augmentation using laminated costal cartilage (B).

tip surgery is insufficient for dorsal augmentation. In such situations, dice or crush the remaining cartilage to make fascia-wrapped diced cartilage, or place fascia or Gore-Tex below the dorsal skin and place the cartilage fragments underneath for dorsal augmentation *(Figure 14)*.

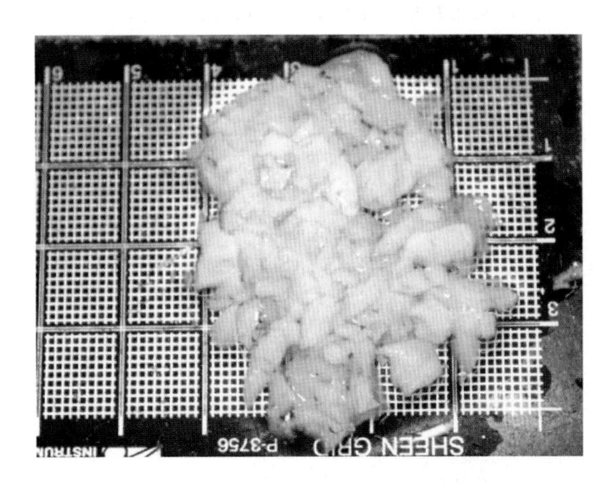

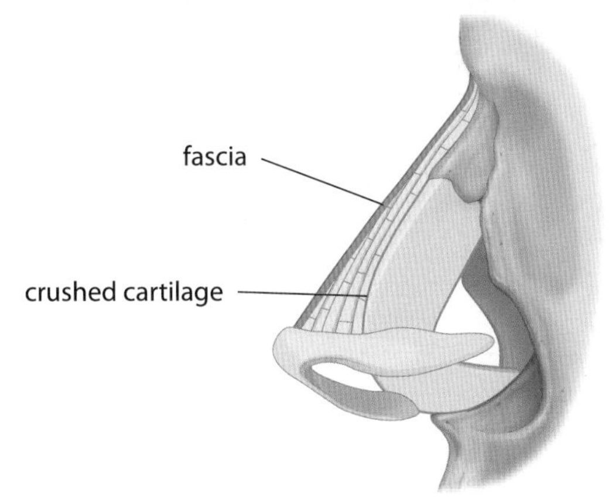

Figure 14 Combined use of diced costal cartilage with fascia for dorsal augmentation

V. Complications of Costal Cartilage Harvest

1) Donor Site Complications

Donor site complications are:

- Pleural injury
- Seroma
- Keloid
- Intercostal neuralgia

Although patients occasionally complain of pain after surgery, severe problems are rare. Signs of seroma manifest through swelling and pain of the cartilage harvest site. Fluid collection under the incision can be easily palpated. When one suspects seroma formation, repeated aspiration with a needle and compressive dressings with elastic bandage and gauze usually is enough. Keloids on the skin incision site are a relatively common complication, and the possibility should be explained to the patient before surgery *(Figure 15)*. Although it is very rare, the patient may suffer from intercostal neuralgia at the harvest site for a prolonged period after the surgery.

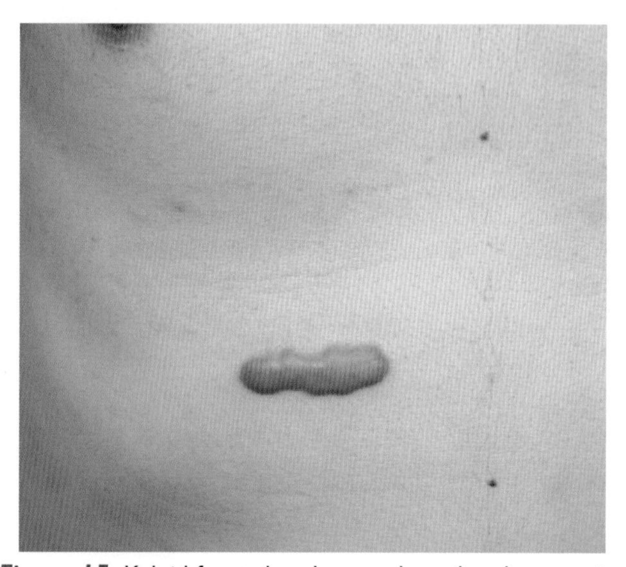

Figure 15 Keloid formed at the costal cartilage harvest site.

2) Recipient Site Complications

Complications in noses with costal cartilage grafts are:

- ☑ Graft visibility
- ☑ Warping
- ☑ Absorption
- ☑ Infection

Using costal cartilage as augmentation material for the nasal dorsum has a lower risk of delayed infection and inflammation when compared to alloplastic implants. However, the risk of aesthetic complications is higher. In patients with thin skin, the graft becomes visible after a long period of time, exhibiting an unnatural shape. Warping is also a common problem *(Figure 16)*. Cartilage can be absorbed to a certain degree, causing aesthetic changes. Many believe that using autologous cartilage for rhinoplasty rarely causes infection or inflammation, but this is not the case. Patients for whom costal cartilage is used during rhinoplasty have often been through multiple previous surgeries, and thus have a high chance of insufficient blood supply to the cartilage. The use of excessive suture materials when using costal cartilage as nasal tip graft, and increased risk of dead space formation following the use of thick angulated cartilage could be factors underlying infection. Infection as a complication of the costal cartilage grafting may manifest in the form of secondary infections, which is preceded by an initial inflammation from cartilage necrosis due to the insufficient blood supply to the cartilage. For the implanted cartilage to survive, blood supply is required not in the form of blood vessels directly growing into the cartilage, but through diffusion. This gives a thick costal cartilage a higher risk of necrosis due to insufficient nourishment.

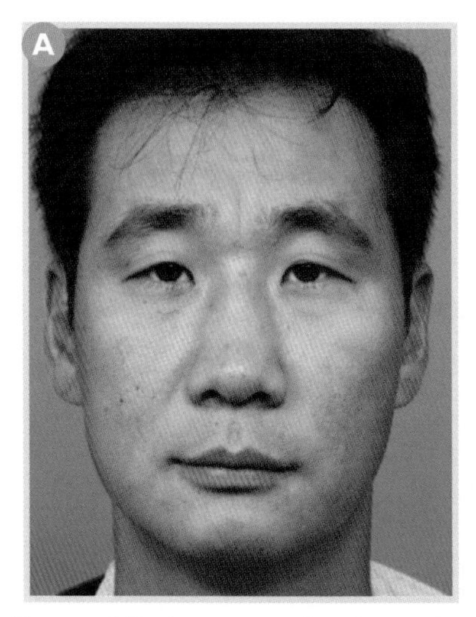

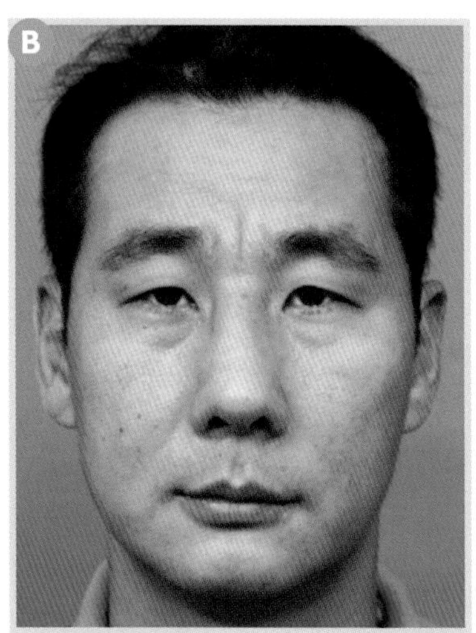

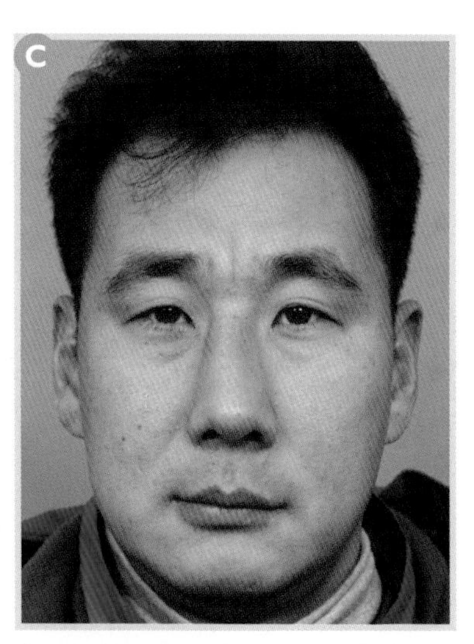

Figure 16 A patient who showed warping of the implanted costal cartilage 6 months after rhinoplasty. Before surgery (A), 1 month after surgery (B), and 6 months after rhinoplasty (C).

VI. Homologous Costal Cartilage

This graft material is created by applying various tissue processing methods to cartilage harvested from cadavers in order to make it safe for use in other patients' surgeries *(Figure 17)*. Processing methods may differ from each tissue bank, but most methods include gamma radiation processing (15-24 kGy for 1.5-2.0 hours), osmotic destruction, and freeze drying. One advantage of using homologous cartilage in rhinoplasty is being able to avoid donor site morbidity. However, reports frequently indicate that homologous cartilage is often more easily absorbed than autologous cartilage, and the author has had a similar experience. Furthermore,

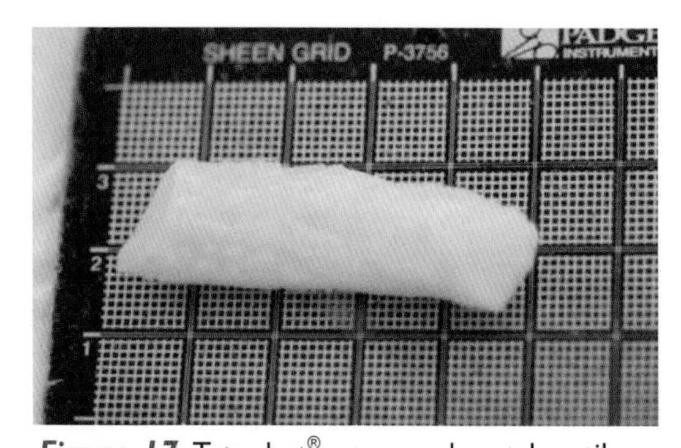

Figure 17 Tutoplast®-processed costal cartilage.

since cartilage differs in physical characteristics based on tissue processing methods, and the cadavers who provide the cartilage are of different age groups, it is hard to expect consistent quality of cartilage from these implants. The author has abundant experience using Tutoplast®-processed costal cartilage. According to the author's experience, this cartilage is generally useful for septal reconstructon or tip surgery *(Figure 18)*. However, when used for the nasal dorsum, complications like resorption, fracturing, and deformation were somewhat frequent. The author has concluded that this is not the optimal cartilage to be used as dorsal implantation material *(Figures 19, 20)*. However this material is still useful for the patients who require ample graft

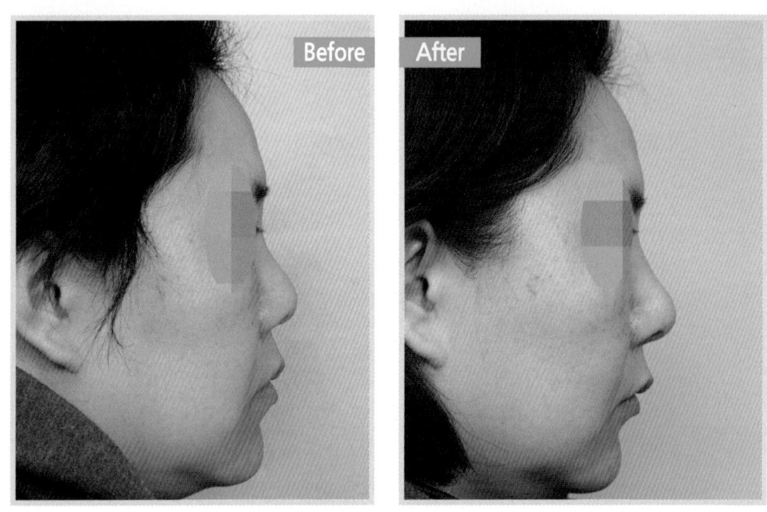

Figure 18 A typical example of a good surgical outcome of rhinoplasty using Tutoplast®-processed costal cartilage. Dorsal augmentation and tip derotation were achieved.

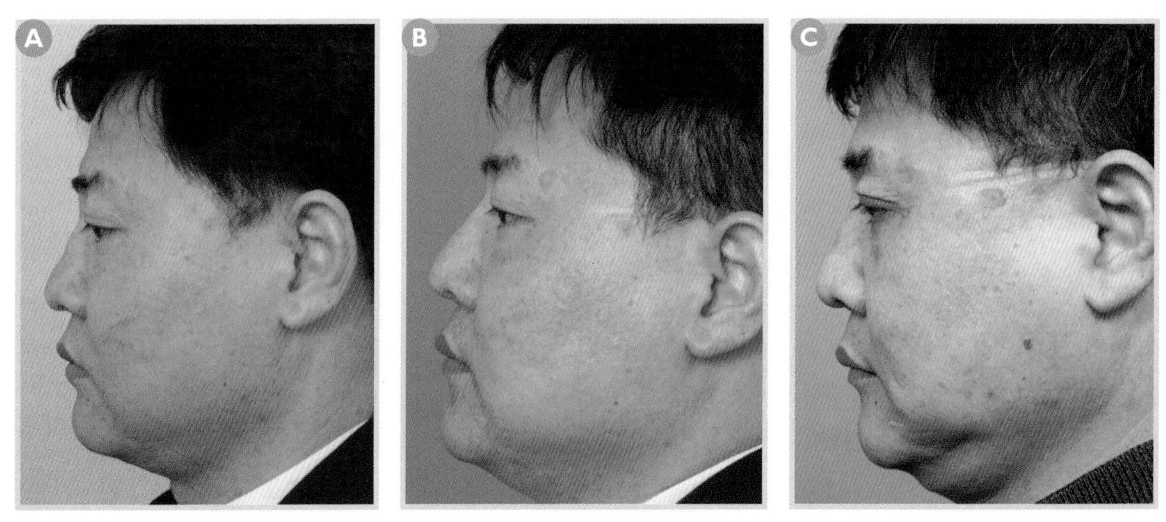

Figure 19 A patient showing cartilage resorption and recurrence of saddle nose 9 years after dorsal augmentation using Tutoplast®-processed costal cartilage. Before operation (A), 2 years after operation (B), and 9 years after surgery (C).

material, whom autologous costal cartilage cannot be harvested. Patients who do not want a harvest site scar and older patients showing extensive ossification of costal cartilage can be ideal candidates for using homologous costal cartilage.

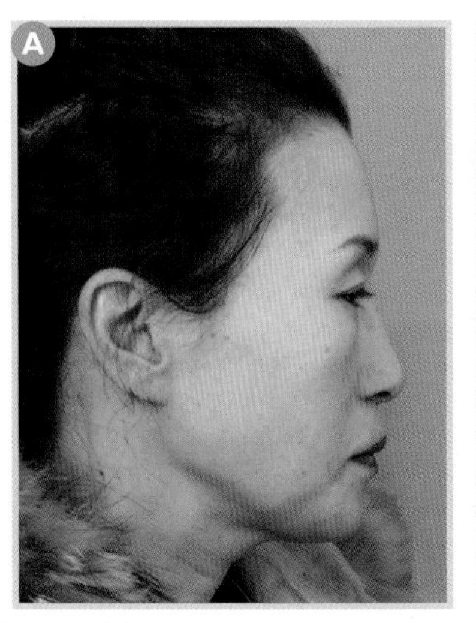
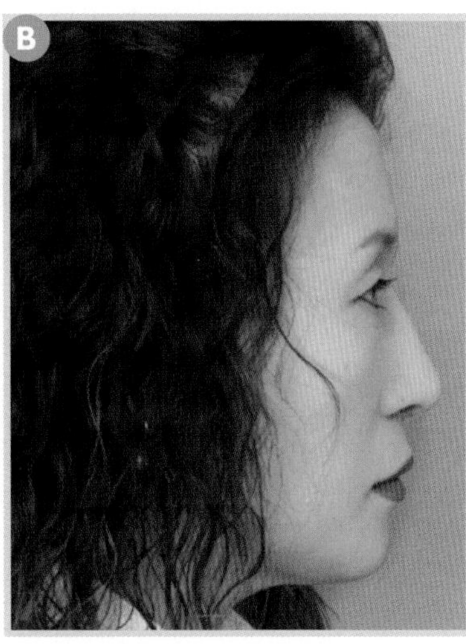
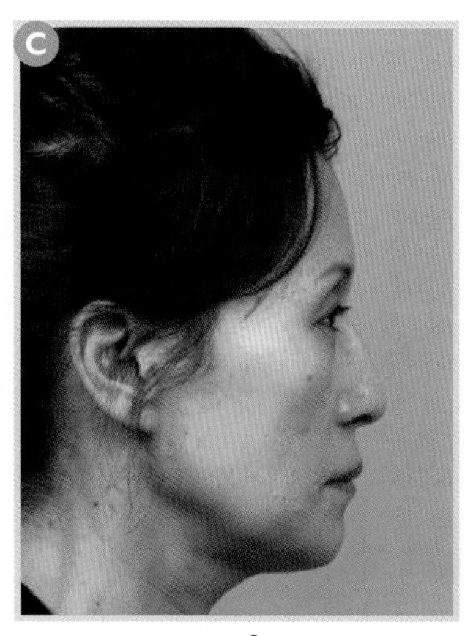

Figure 20 A patient showing dorsal convexity 4 years after dorsal augmentation using Tutoplast®-processed costal cartilage. Before operation (A), 1 year after surgery (B), and 4 years after surgery (C).

References

1. Daniel RK. Rhinoplasty and rib grafts: evolving a flexible operative technique. Plast Reconstr Surg 1994; 94: 597-609.
2. Demirkan F, Arslan E, Unal S, Aksoy A. Irradiated homologous costal cartilage: versatile grafting material for rhinoplasty. Aesthet Plast Surg 2003; 27: 213-20.
3. Kridel RW, Ashoori F, Liu ES, Hart CG. Long-term use and follow-up of irradiated homologous costal cartilage grafts in the nose. Arch Facial Plast Surg 2009; 11: 378-94.
4. Moon BJ, Lee HJ, Jang YJ. Outcomes following rhinoplasty using autologous costal cartilage. Arch Facial Plast Surg 2012; 14: 175-80.
5. Song HM, Lee BJ, Jang YJ. Processed costal cartilage homograft in rhinoplasty: the Asan Medical Center experience. Arch Otolaryngol Head Neck Surg 2008; 134: 485-9.
6. Swanepoel, PF. Fysh R. Laminated dorsal beam graft to eliminate postoperative twisting complications. Arch Facial Plast Surg 2007; 9: 285-9.

A 50-year-old male visited for a deviated nose and low nasal bridge with nasal obstruction.

Analysis

Frontal: Deviated nose, wide dorsum, poor tip projection
Basal: Nostril asymmetry, low tip projection, tilted columella
Lateral and Oblique: Saddle nose, poor tip definition

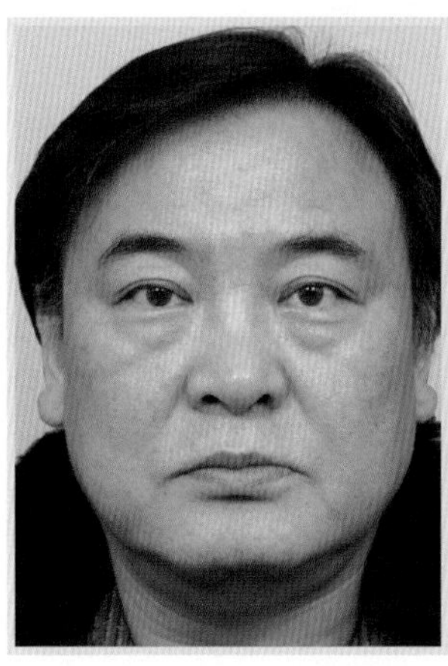
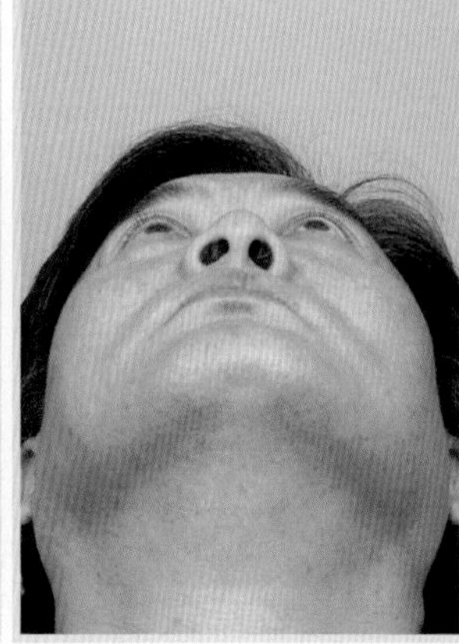
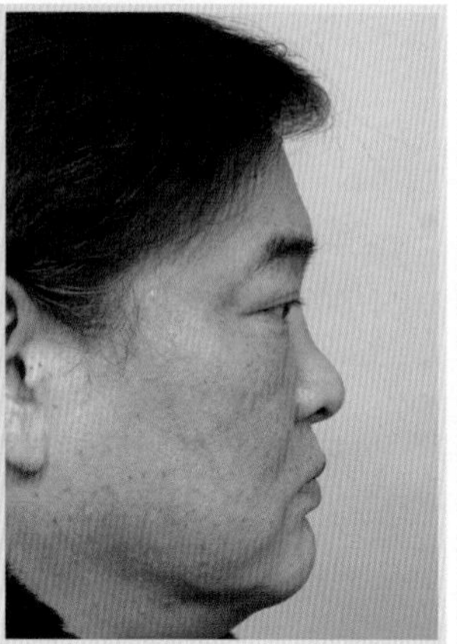
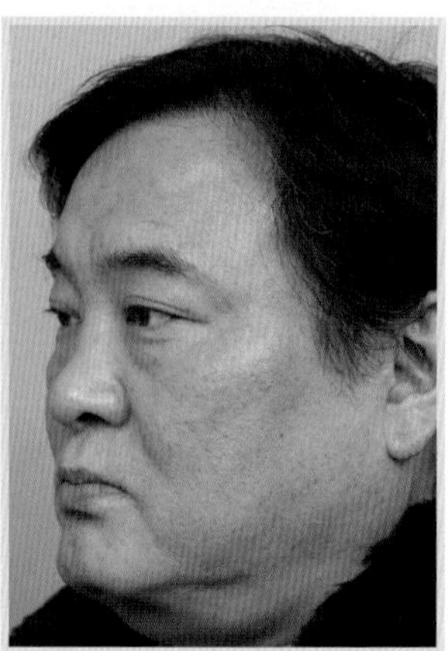

Operative Procedures

Open rhinoplasty approach
Septoplasty and harvest of septal cartilage and bone
Costal cartilage harvest
Caudal septal extension grafting using costal cartilage (bilateral)
Multilayer tip grafting
Dorsal augmentation using costal cartilage and processed fascia lata

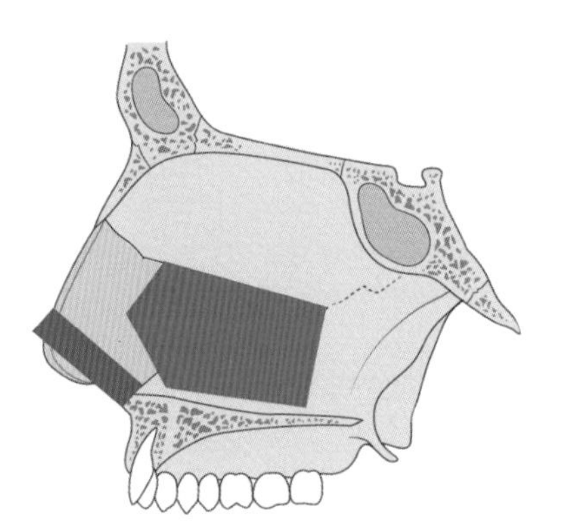
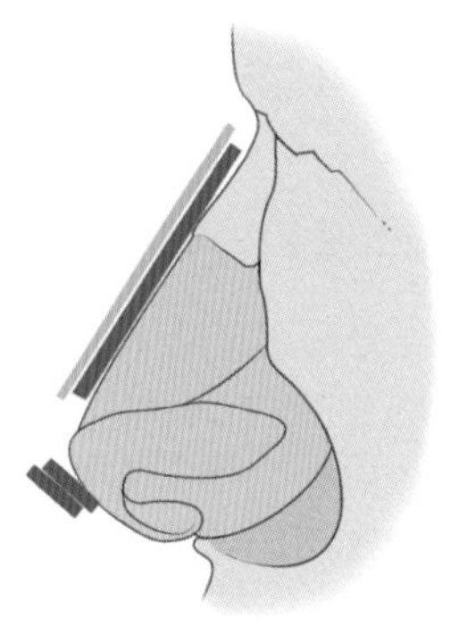

Postoperative Changes

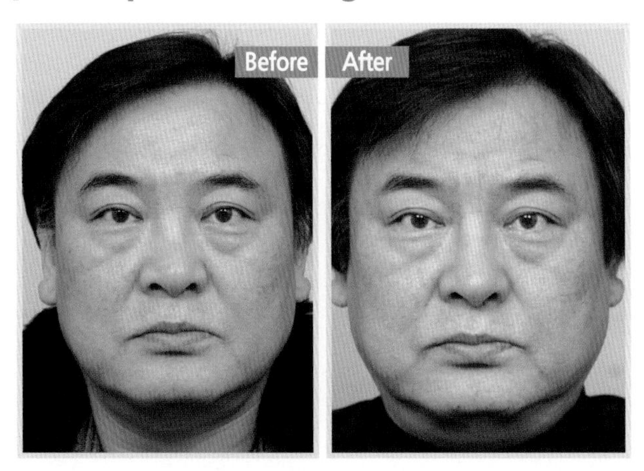

Frontal: Dorsal deviation was improved. Augmented dorsal height gave the dorsum a proper aesthetic line.

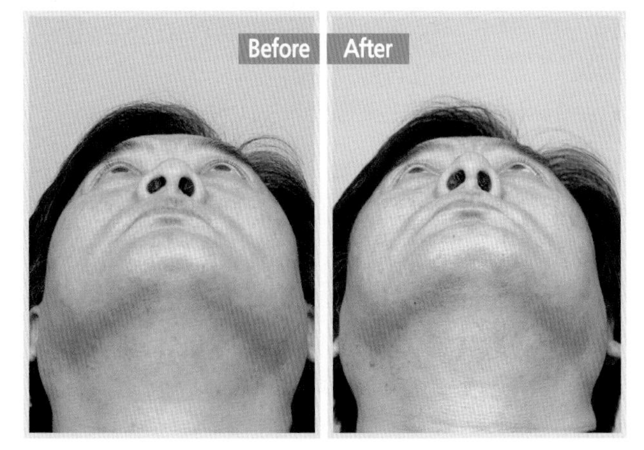

Basal: Tip height was improved significantly. Tilted columella was straightened. Nostril asymmetry was incompletely corrected.

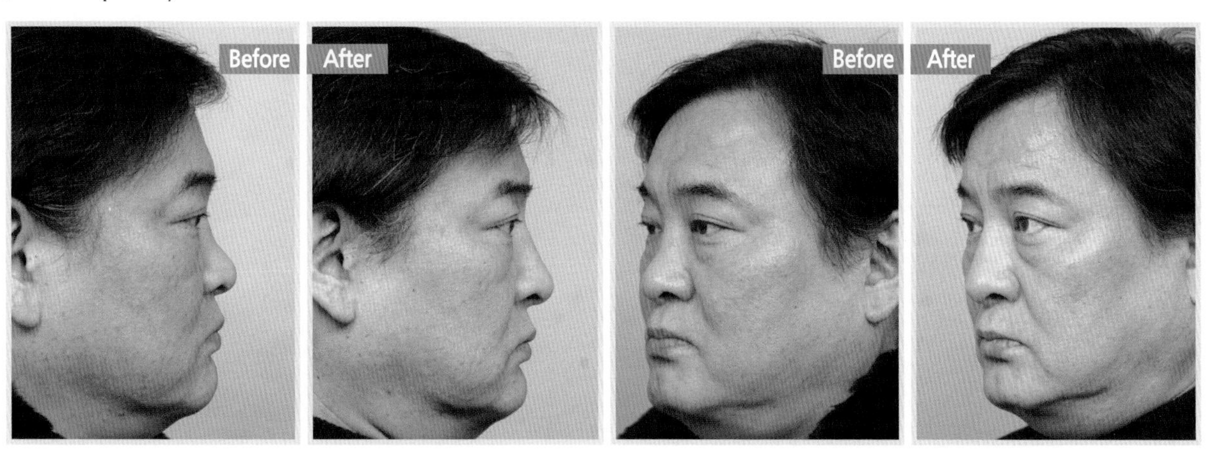

Lateral and Oblique: Saddle nose deformty was corrected. Tip definition was improved.

Case 2

A 25-year-old male visited for a deviated nose and bulbous tip.

Analysis
Frontal: Deviated nose, bulbous tip, wide alar base, thick skin
Basal: Poor tip projection, short columella
Lateral and Oblique: Saddle nose, low tip height, poor tip definition

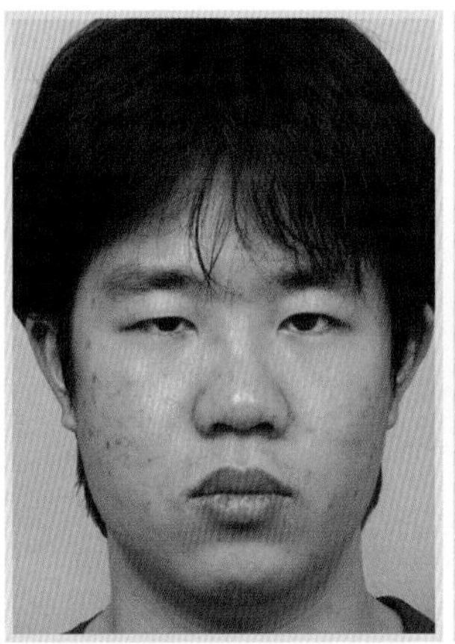 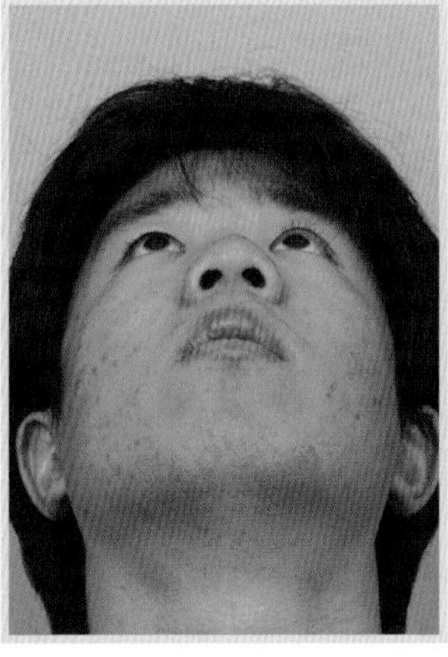 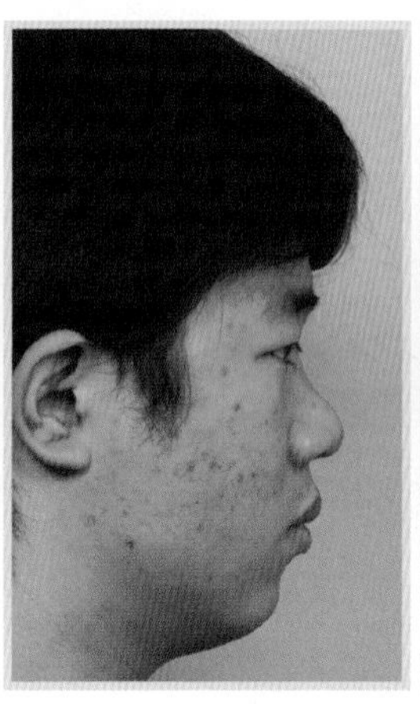 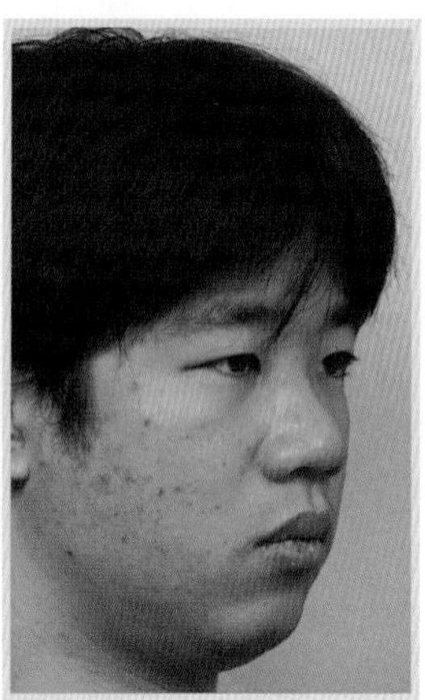

Operative Procedures

Open rhinoplasty approach
Septal mucoperichondrial flap elevation and harvest of septal cartilage
Caudal septum cutting and suture technique
Costal cartilage harvest
Medial and lateral osteotomies
Spreader grafting using costal cartilage (bilateral)
Caudal septal extension grafting using costal cartilage (bilateral)
Columellar strut application using septal cartilage
Multilayer tip grafting using costal cartilage
Dorsal augmentation using costal cartilage
Alar base resection (bilateral)

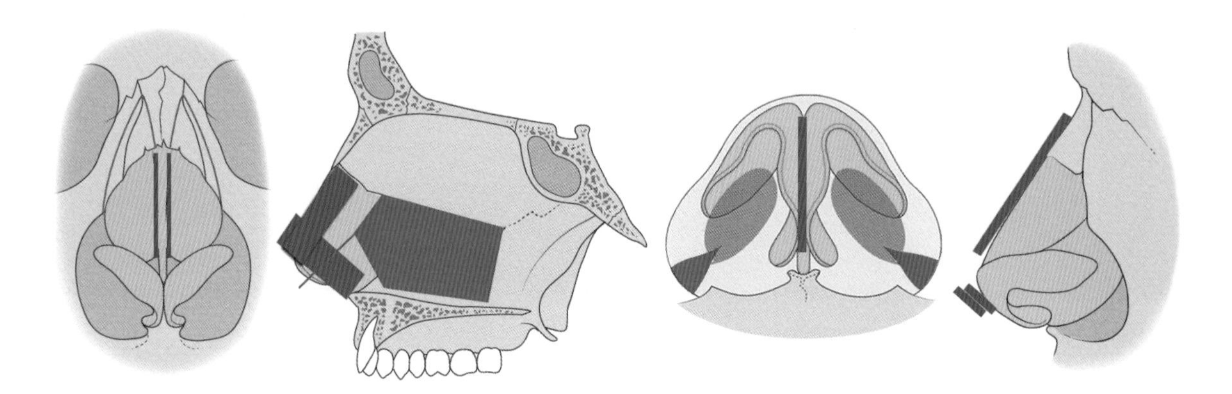

Postoperative Changes

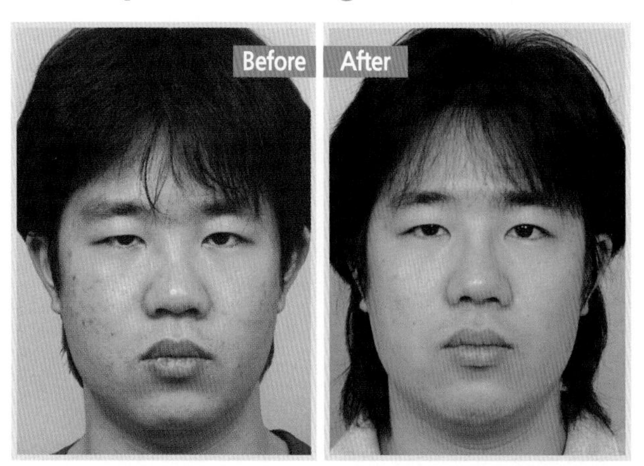

Frontal: Deviated nose was corrected. Dorsal height was augmented. Tip definition was improved.

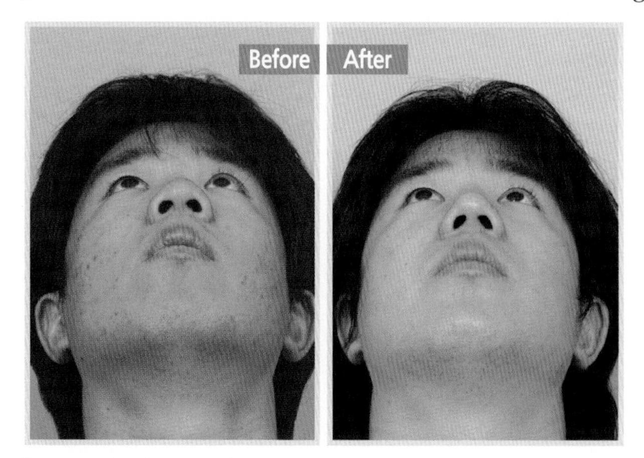

Basal: Elevated tip projection was achieved. Tip definition was improved. Alar base width was reduced.

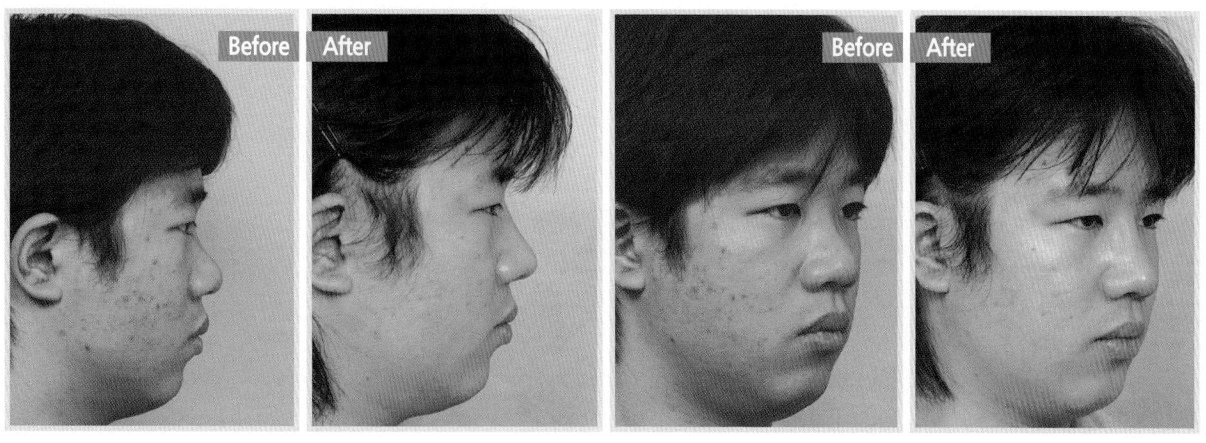

Lateral and Oblique: Saddle nose deformty was corrected. Tip projection was elevated. Tip definition was improved.

Case 3

A 46-year-old female visited for a saddle nose deformity acquired after septoplasty.

Analysis

Frontal: Flat nose, wide dorsum
Basal: Low tip height, mild nostril asymmetry
Oblique: Saddle nose, poor tip projection

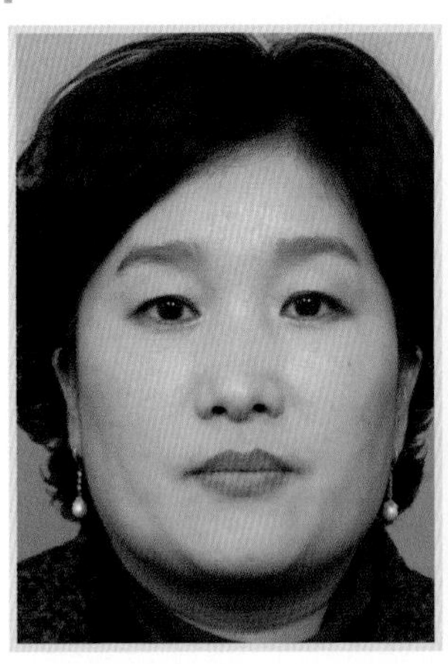
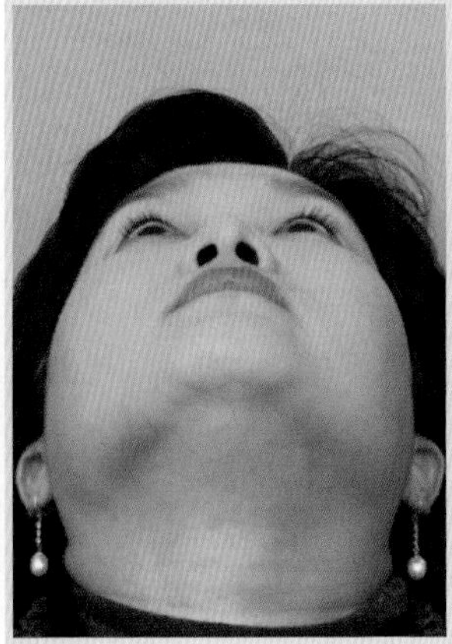
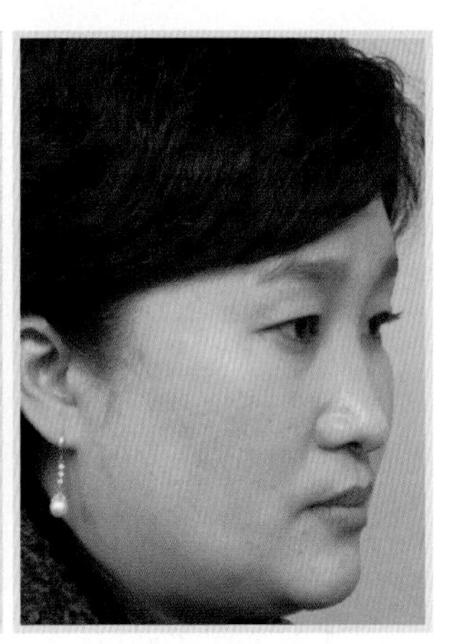

Operative Procedures

Open rhinoplasty approach
Costal cartilage harvest
Medial and lateral osteotomies
Caudal batten grafting using costal cartilage (bilateral)
Spreader grafting using costal cartilage (bilateral)
Columellar strut application
Shield grafting using costal cartilage
Dorsal augmentation with laminated costal cartilage covered with perichondrium

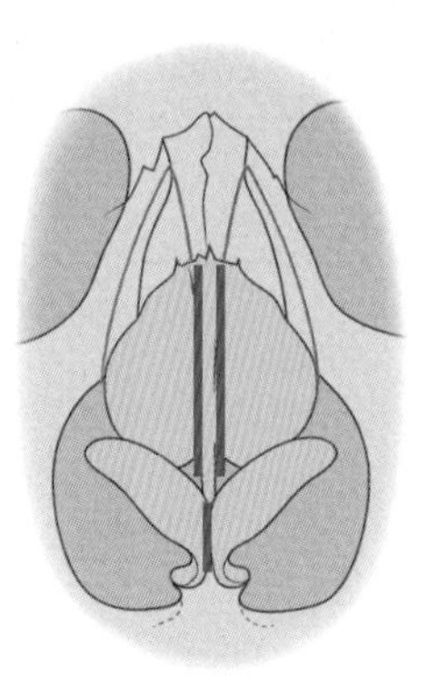
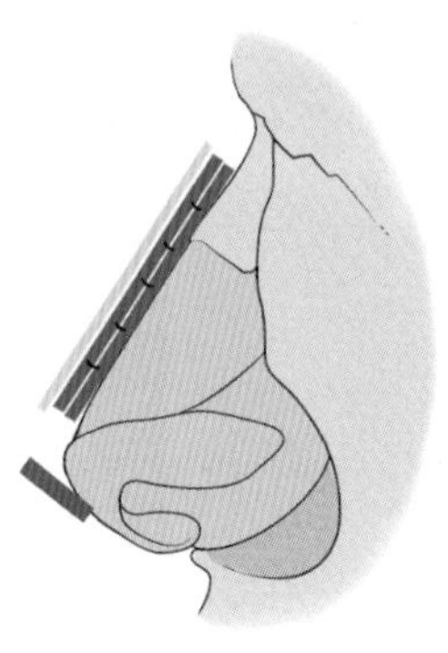
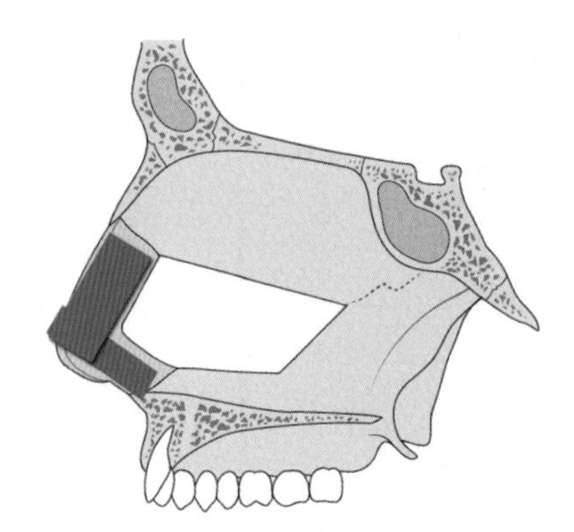

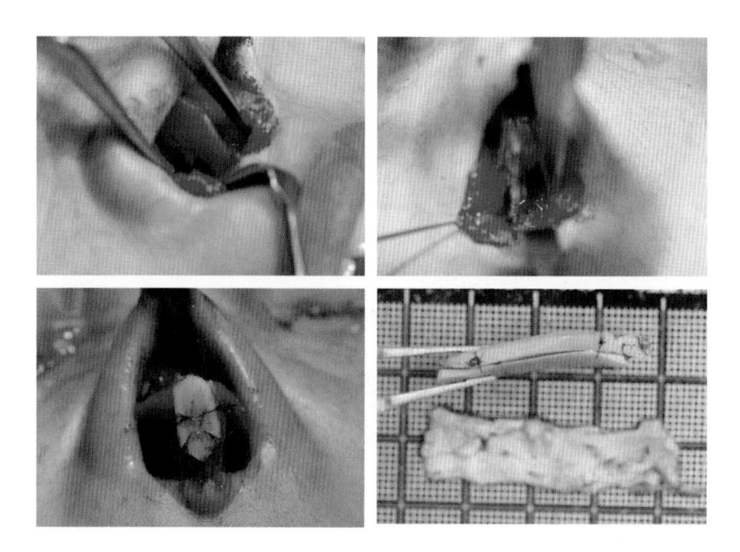

Postoperative Changes

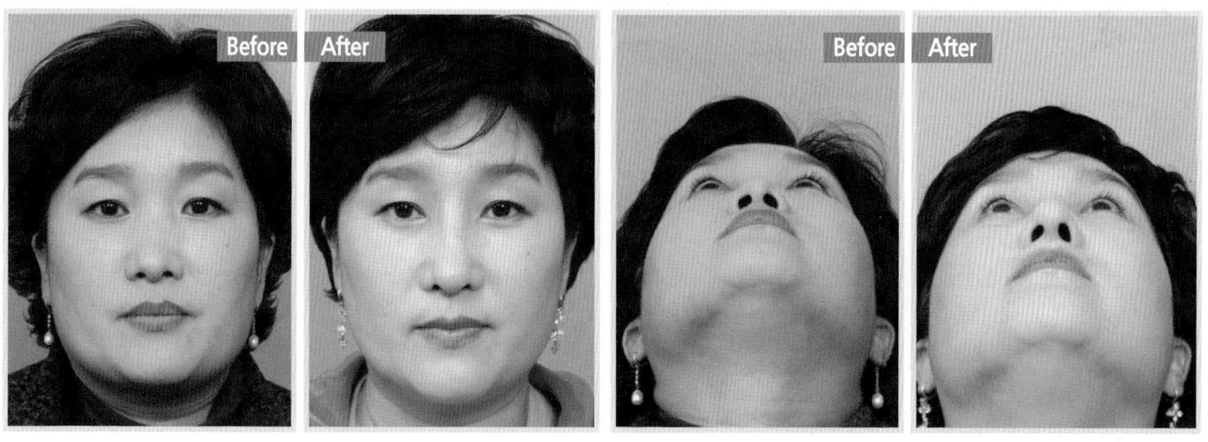

Frontal: Proper dorsal aesthetic lines were created following dorsal augmentation.

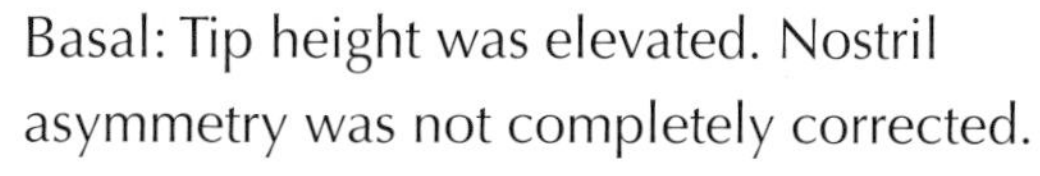

Basal: Tip height was elevated. Nostril asymmetry was not completely corrected.

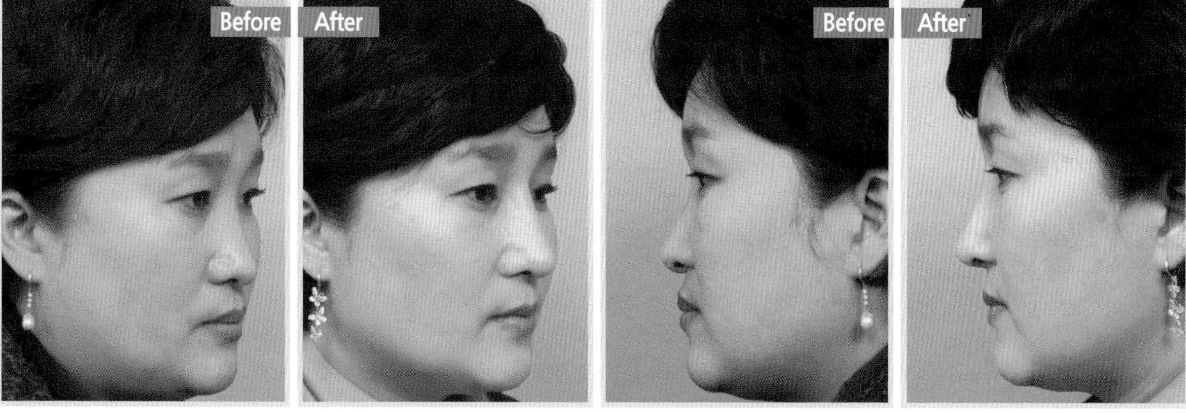

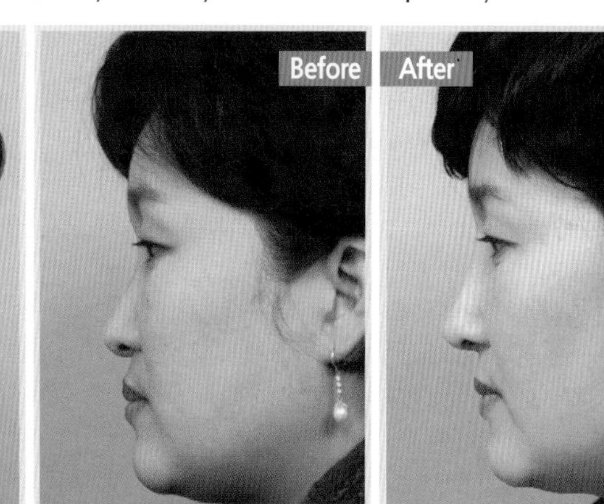

Lateral and Oblique: Natural looking dorsal line was gained through dorsal and tip augmentation. Slight concavity of nasal dorsal line remained.

Dermofat

Jun Mo Kim

I. Dermofat in Rhinoplasty

Among the various types of autologous tissue used in rhinoplasty, soft tissues and hard tissues differ greatly in their characteristics. Soft tissues include fat, dermofat, and fascia, while hard tissues include bone and cartilage. The proper use of soft tissue entails implanting it in the soft tissue of the nose which include smoothening of the nasal dorsum, correcting a focal depression, giving volume, or for camouflage purposes. Bone and cartilage would be best used to reconstruct the nasal skeletal framework.

Dermofat is easy to harvest thus has a low donor site morbidity, is resistant to infection, and is flexible enough to be made into various shapes easily. Free fat graft is also easy to harvest, is abundant, and is easy to inject. However, depending on the area of the nose, it has a volume reduction rate of 0-80% and a high rate of infection. It has higher survival rates in the radix and supratip areas, and significantly lower survival rates in the rhinion and nasal tip areas. Fascia has a relatively lower rate of absorption, thus it is easy to predict and control the surgical outcome. However, it is hard to harvest and comes in small amounts.

II. Donor Sites of Dermofat

In order to increase the success rate of dermofat grafting, choosing the proper donor site is critically important. The site should have a thick dermal layer, compact fat tissue composition, and should not induce visible postoperative scars. Dermofat can be harvested around the sacral area, buttock creases, groin, and scar-adjacent areas; successful harvest results from the posterior auricular area have also been published. Predictions that the dermis has a high survival rate among the components of dermofat graft call for harvesting from the body parts with a thick dermis. Comparing thickness of dermis from various areas shows that the sacral area has the thickest dermis. The thickness of dermis at the different harvesting sites of dermofat is listed in *Table 1*. The most commonly used donor site is also the sacral area, because of its low absorption rate due to its thick dermis, and low scar visibility. The author consider this area the ideal donor site because of its thick dermis and dense fat.

Table 1 Thickness of dermis in different donor sites(μm)

	Groin	Abdomen	Lateral gluteal area	Gluteal fold	Sacrum
Epidermis	57.3 ± 22.9	52.4 ± 9.9	59.9 ± 11.2	52.6 ± 16.0	86.1 ± 7.8
Dermis	681.0 ± 223.7	913.3 ± 271.7	1,018.7 ± 305.6	1,107.0 ± 272.6	1,510.7 ± 201.7
Total	738.3 ± 244.5	965.7 ± 271.1	1,078.6 ± 316.9	1,159.6 ± 270.8	1,596.9 ± 197.9

Adapted from Hwang K et al. Ann Plast Surg. 2001

III. Surgical Technique of Dermofat Grafting

The principles of dermofat grafting are the following: Selection of the donor site is of paramount importance. Careful handling of the graft and wide dissection of the recipient site is also important. Furthermore, the graft should be implanted promptly to the recipient site and properly sutured, with overcorrection necessary to some degree.

When harvesting dermofat from the sacral area, the patient is positioned face down, and the site sterilized with betadine. Keeping the midline at the sacral area, a 6.5×1.0 cm spindle-shape incision 2 cm above the coccyx is designed, and infiltrated with local anesthesia. After excising the designed dermofat, the epidermal layer is removed, trying to preserve as much fat layer as possible with the dermis *(Figure 1)*. The harvest site is then closed.

After harvesting the dermofat, the patient is positioned supine and prepped for rhinoplasty. From this point on, the rhinoplasty using dermofat is conducted as a typical rhinoplasty. One thing to keep in mind is that the nasal skin soft tissue envelope should be dissected wide enough to prevent the dermofat graft from receiving too much pressure. High absorption rates should also be considered in using this graft material. The cephalic part of the graft material should reach up to the desired location and the caudal part to the skin of the nasal tip or alar cartilage. Before inserting into the nasal dorsum, trim the graft appropriately and make sure to insert a dermofat graft containing sufficient amount of fat, matching the patient's desired nasal height.

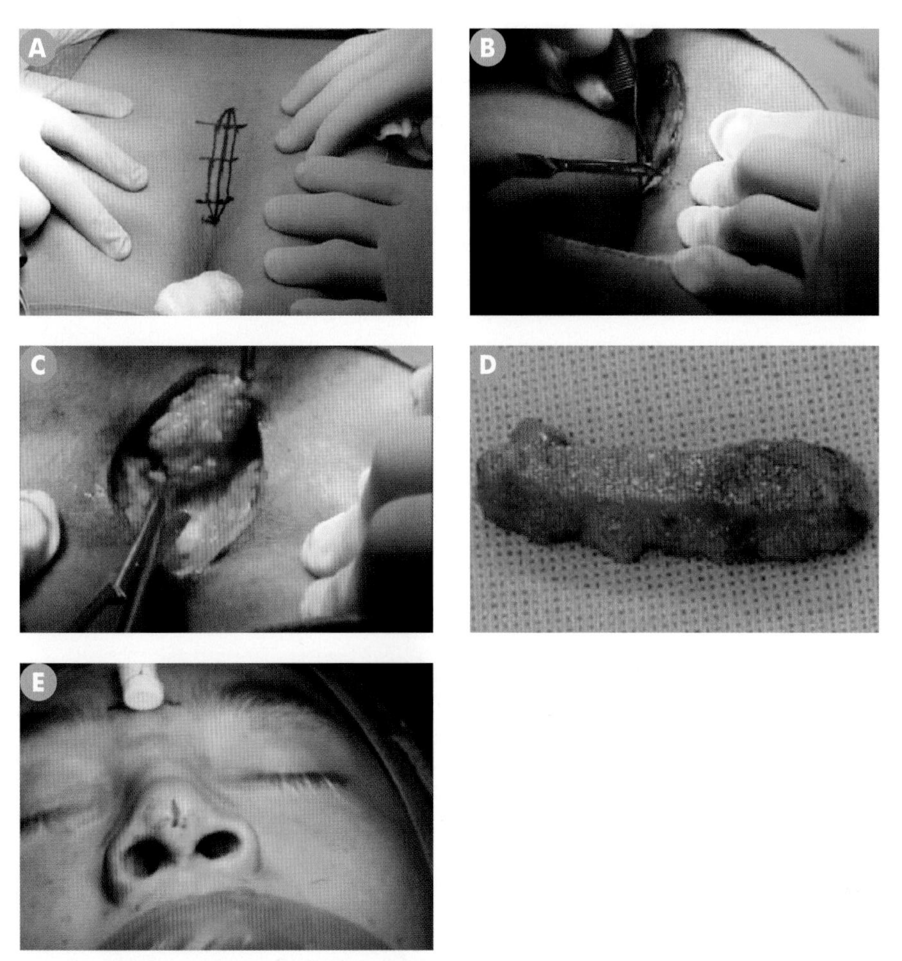

Figure 1 Designing the skin incision at the sacral area for dermofat harvest (A), removal of the epidermal layer before removal of the dermofat graft (B), harvesting dermofat with abundant fatty layer attached to the dermis (C), harvested dermofat is kept in saline-soaked gauze (D), and dermofat graft is implanted at the dorsum and externally sutured at the radix (E).

IV. Results of Dermofat Grafting

Some literature have reported superb results of dorsal augmentation using dermofat graft. However, many surgeons still raise doubts regarding its post-implantation absorption rates. According to one study, there is about a 50% loss of weight and volume of dermofat grafts from its initial state a year after implantation. This explains the necessity of overcorrection of approximately 20%, taking into account the average rate of absorption (20-30%: between 50% absorption of fat and 15-20% absorption of dermis). On the other hand, other reports claim that the postoperative absorption is lower than expected. A five-year follow-up of micrognathia correction using dermofat revealed that the graft remained unchanged in size and shape. A one and half-year follow-up study of 38 dermofat graft rhinoplasty cases showed that, in most cases, no evident change in size or shape could be observed. The degree of absorption appears to depend on patient's skin condition, smoking, alcohol consumption, difficulty of surgery, time required for surgery, and occurrence of hematoma or edema *(Figures 2, 3)*. Considering all these factors, dermofat seems to be a superb implant material obtainable from soft tissue, since it has lower absorption rates than fat graft and can be harvested in larger quantities than fascia implant. The author usually increase the dorsal height by 2-3 mm with augmentation using dermofat.

The author prefers to use dermofat when:

- ☑ The patient strongly prefers autologous tissue
- ☑ The skin is in bad condition due to multiple revisions
- ☑ The nasal bridge requires smoothening after osteotomy or humpectomy
- ☑ Alloplastic implants cannot be used due to thin nasal dorsal skin

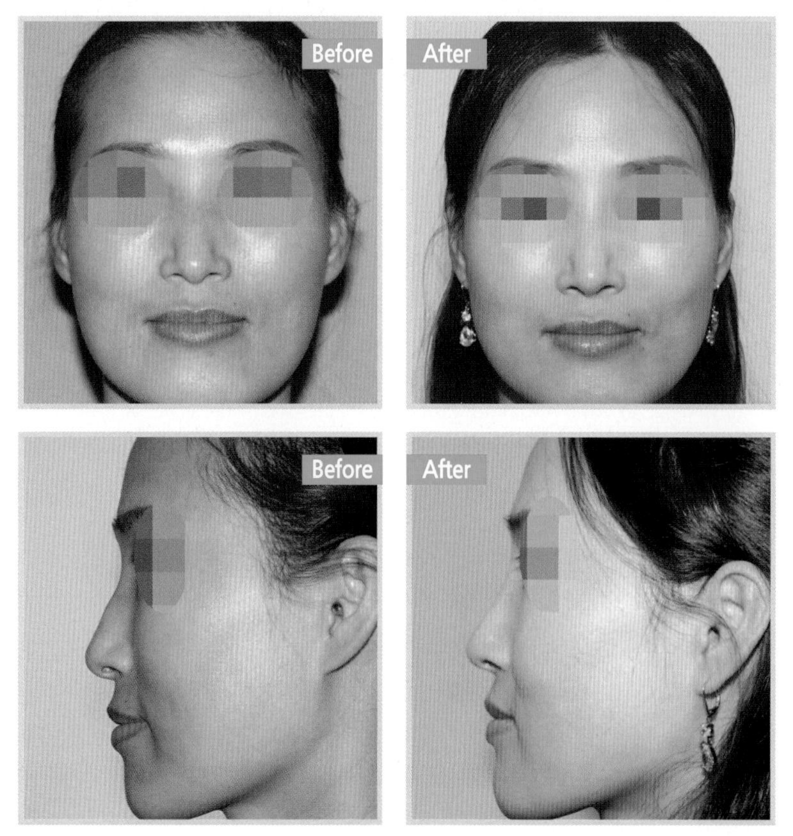

Figure 2 7-month postoperative result of dorsal augmentation using dermofat.

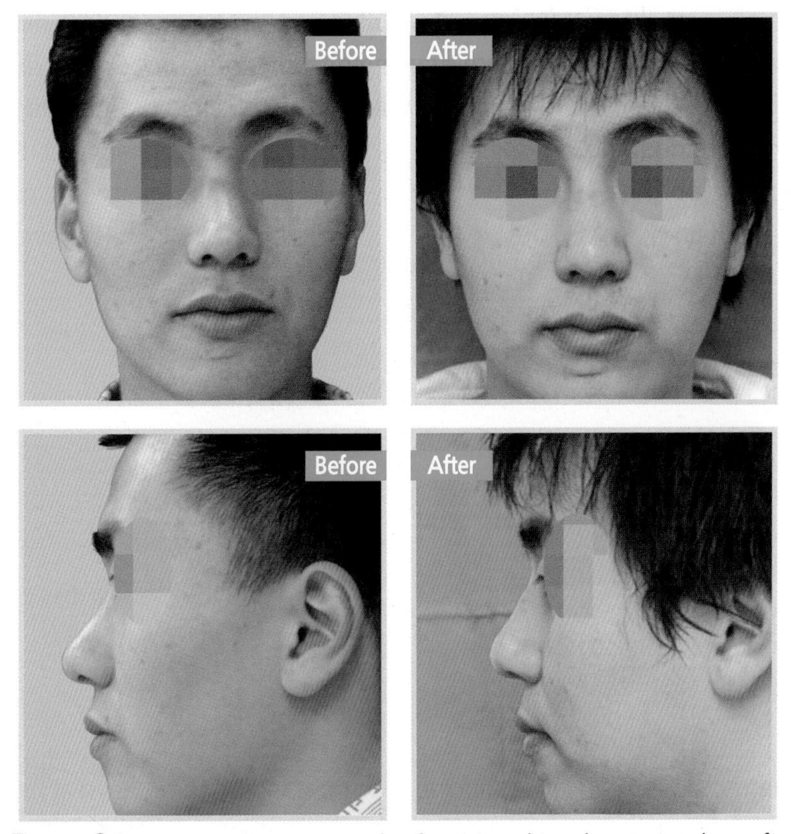

Figure 3 2-year postoperative result of revision rhinoplasty using dermofat

V. Complications of Dermofat Grafting

Complications include hematoma, seroma, inflammation, and infection. Such complications happen rarely and can be prevented through the use of antibiotics, meticulous hemostasis, and early drainage. Late complications include cyst formation due to skin appendages (residual subcutaneous glands from the implant's dermis, or hair follicles) included in the graft. Excessive absorption of graft or overcorrection of the dorsum is another aesthetic complication commonly expected in the use of dermofat grafts *(Figure 4)*.

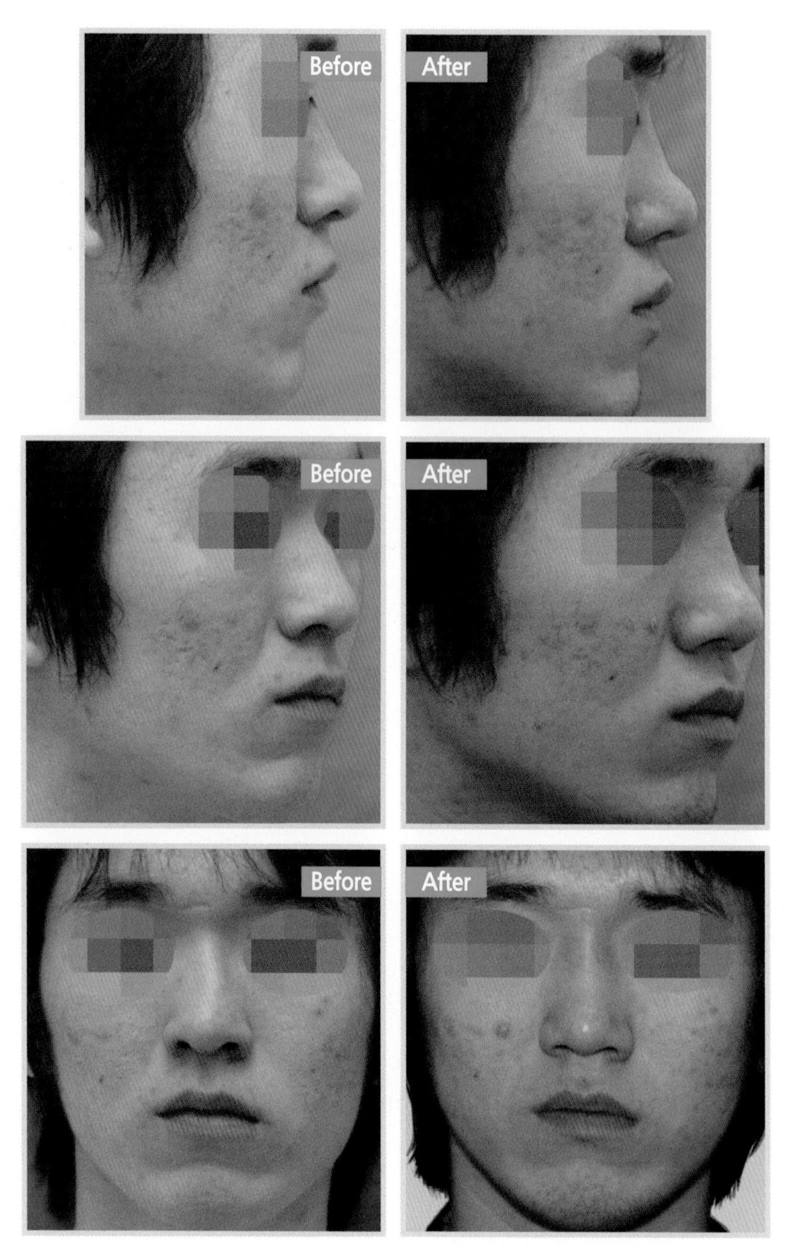

Figure 4 A patient showing loss of dorsal height due to absorption of the dermofat 2 months after rhinoplasty.

VI. Conclusion

Few will disagree that autologous tissue is preferable in rhinoplasty. However, dermofat is not without problems as with other autologous material. Dermofat makes it easy to create a natural curvature of the nose, and is relatively resistant to infection. But like other biological materials, its absorption rates are hard to predict. Overall, it has more benefits than fat or fascia among the types of autologous soft tissue. However, its learning curve and donor site morbidity should be considered seriously by the rhinoplasty surgeon.

References

1. Na DS, Jung SW, Kook KS, Lee YH. Augmentation rhinoplasty with dermofat graft and fat injection. J Korean Soc Plast Reconstr Surg 2011; 38: 53-62.
2. Erdogan B, Tuncel AT, Adanali G, Deren O, Ayhan M. Augmentation rhinoplasty with dermal graft and review of the literature. Plast Reconstr Surg 2003; 111: 2060-8.
3. Hwang K, Kim DJ, Lee IJ. An anatomic comparison of the skin of five donor sites for dermal fat graft. Ann Plast Surg 2001; 46: 327-31.
4. Kim JM, Seo MS, Seo BS, Kim SH. A case of revision augmentation rhinoplasty with dermofatgraft : 2 years follow-up result. J Rhinol 2006; 13: 132-5.
5. Kim YK. Augmentation rhinoplasty using dermofat graft. J Korean Soc Aesthetic Plast Surg 1999; 5: 33-8.
6. Park CH. Rhinoplasty using postauricular dermofat graft. J Rhinol 2005; 12: 46-9.
7. Romo T, Kwak ES. Nasal grafts and implants in revision rhinoplasty. Facial Plast Surg Clin North Am 2006; 14: 373-87.

Chapter 16 Fascia

Yong Ju Jang · Ian Loh

Autologous fascia is an appropriate graft material for use in rhinoplasty to increase the volume of the nasal soft tissue. This graft is helpful in filling volume but has no rigidity, so is unsuitable for structural grafting. Fascia is especially beneficial in that it creates a smooth dorsal contour, free of problems like graft visibility and dorsal irregularities that can arise after dorsal augmentation using cartilage. Another advantage is its considerably low risk of infection and delayed inflammation compared to alloplastic implants. Fascia is known to be absorbed steadily into the body, being substituted with the individual's own fibrous tissue.

I. Autologous Fascia

1. Temporalis Fascia

Though fascia can be obtained from various parts of the body, deep temporalis fascia, located above the ear, is the most commonly harvested one. Superficial temporalis fascia is too thin to be of good use. Temporalis fascia can be obtained in sizes of up to 5×5 cm through a 3-cm incision above the auricle *(Figure 1)*.

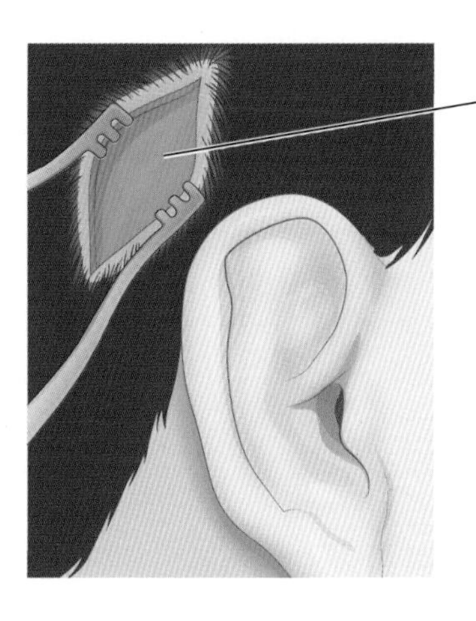

Figure 1 Temporalis fascia can be obtained in sizes of up to 5×5 cm through a 3-cm incision above the auricle.

2. Pectoralis Fascia and External Oblique Fascia

If costal cartilage harvesting is necessary during rhinoplasty, fascia can be obtained from the external oblique abdominal or pectoralis minor (areas exposed during costal cartilage harvesting) musele for various purposes. This fascia however, is hard to acquire in large amounts *(Figure 2)*.

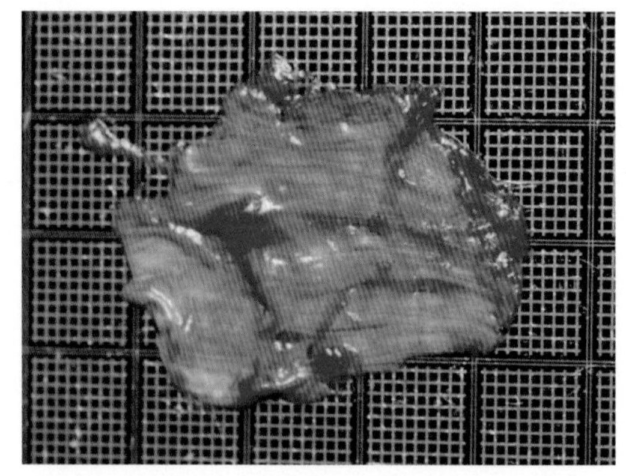

Figure 2 Chest muscle fascia obtained during costal cartilage harvesting.

3. Fascia Lata

1) Characteristics

Fascia lata is a good tissue useful in rhinoplasty. When compared to autologous deep temporalis fascia, fascia lata is much thicker, and when compared to temporoparietal fascia, a much larger volume of graft material can be obtained. The softness of fascia lata makes it suitable for radix or dorsal augmentation, and can also be used as an onlay camouflage graft or as a soft tissue augmentation graft for skin or dermis irregularities. Autologous fascia lata drapes well over the dorsum of the Asian nose, giving a softer, more rounded augmentation that is suited for Orientals. However, fascia lata is harvested in a separate location distant from the surgical area, cannot be used for structural grafting, and is inappropriate for cases that require a substantial degree of augmentation. Freshly harvested fascia also has a high water content and undergoes significant resorprtion immediately following grafting; which stabilizes in 6 weeks (does not result in more than 30% loss in augmentation). Augmentation requires the fascia be folded on itself, and when this is repeated too many times, the lack of rigidity results in the graft being unable to maintain its position and shape over the dorsum of the nose. Wrapping the fascia around a thinner cartilage core can overcome this problem, while maximizing the use of harvested autologous cartilage *(Table 1)*.

Table 1 Indications for Using Autologous Fascia Lata Grafts

Radix augmentation
Dorsal augmentation
Onlay camouflage graft
Softening contours of cartilage grafts
Soft tissue replacement/augmentation
Fascial envelope for diced cartilage graft

2) Relevant Anatomy in the Harvest of Fascia Lata

The fascia lata lies deep to the subcutaneous layer and encloses the entire musculature of the thigh. It is thickest over the lateral portion of the thigh where it condenses to form the iliotibial band (ITB). The ITB contributes to leg extension and maintaining hyper-extension of the knee when standing.

The fascia lata is of a good thickness over the anterior thigh but thins over the medial thigh.

The posterior border of the ITB is connected deeply to the lateral intermuscular septum. The fascia lata splits to ensheath the tensor fascia lata superior-laterally. This muscle is continuous inferiorly with the ITB. The intermediate cutaneous nerve of the thigh pierces the fascia lata on its anterior surface approximately 7.5 cm below the level of the inguinal ligament to supply the skin of the anterior thigh. The anterior branch of the lateral cutaneous nerve of the thigh travels in the fascia lata and pierces the fascia lata approximately 10 cm below the level of the anterior superior iliac spine (ASIS) to supply the skin over the anterior and lateral thigh. The supero-medial fascia lata is pierced by the great saphenous vein. The fascia lata also forms a condensation just above the knee which contributes to knee stability.

3) Harvest Method

(1) Surface Marking

The knee and hips are flexed and the hip is internally rotated. This accentuates the lateral intermuscular septum which is marked out. A 4 cm width of ITB anterior to the intermuscular septum is marked out to be preserved. The superior limit of the harvest is 17 cm distal to the ASIS. This avoids harvesting over the tensor fascia lata muscle. Harvesting at this level also avoids injuring the cutaneous nerves supplying the thigh. The fascia lata 10 cm proximal to the femoral condyle marks the inferior limit of harvest. This preserves the distal fascia lata around the knee which contributes to its stability. Using these landmarks, the area to be harvested is marked out. Harvest is avoided over the medial thigh as the fascia in this area is thin and there is increased risk of injury to the great saphenous vein and its tributaries *(Figure 3)*.

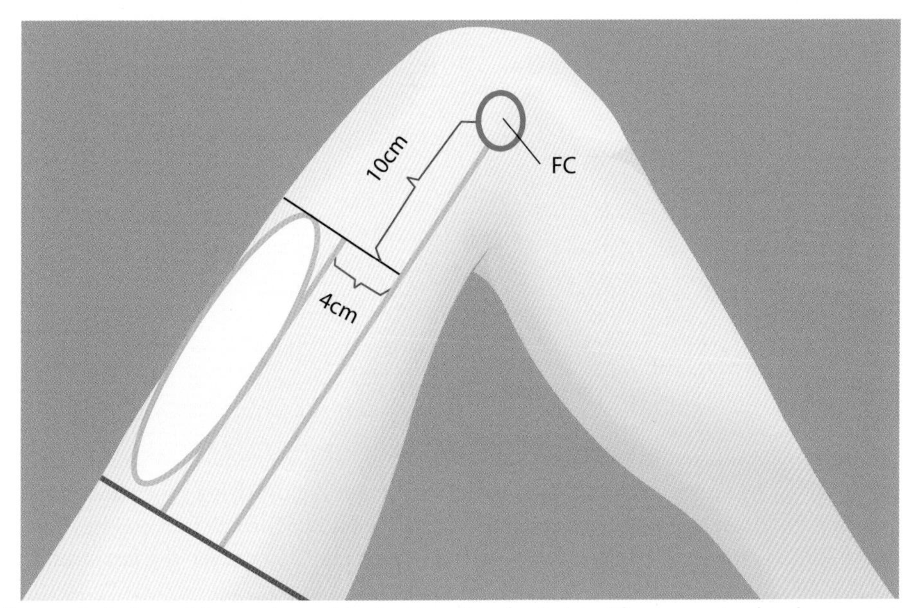

Figure 3 Green circle: lateral femoral condyle. Red bracket: fascia lata 10 cm proximal to knee not to be harvested. Purple line: horizontal line 17 cm distal to anterior superior iliac spine. Yellow oval: harvest site for fascia lata. Blue bracket (lined on sides with yellow lines): Iliotibial band.

(2) Harvest Method

Subcutaneous infiltration using tumescent solution is used 30 minutes prior to harvest. A superior 2 cm incision is made and deepened until the glistening white fascial layer is encountered. The subcutaneous tissue superficial to the fascial layer is separated from the fascia lata; a 5-10 cm horizontal incision is made through the fascia lata exposing the underlying muscles; next, the underlying muscles deep to the fascial layer are separated from the fascia lata. Dissection planes above and below the fascia are extended as distally as possible using blunt dissection once the correct planes are identified. The author uses a long blunt tipped Boies elevator for this purpose. The free edge of the cut fascia is grasped with an artery forceps and long parallel cuts are made perpendicular to the horizontal incision in the fascia lata. These are performed using a shearing action with long Metzenbaum scissors slightly opened at the tip. The artery forceps is now pushed forward in the subcutaneous plane until no further distal excursion is possible. The tip of the artery forceps is tented against the skin and a small stab incision is made over the site of tenting. A fine artery forc eps is used to dissect down onto the tented artery forceps tip. A second artery forceps is used to grasp the fascia lata, delivering the graft out of the stab incision like a piece of tissue from a tissue box *(Figure 4)*. When no further delivery of the graft is possible, it is transected at its root, flush against the skin. A large graft can be harvested using these small incisions *(Figure 5)*. The wound is flushed and closed in layers. The subcutaneous and deep dermal layers are closed using multiple PDS sutures and the skin carefully apposed using 5-0 nylon sutures. A pressure dressing is applied and compression stockings are issued to the patient after surgery.

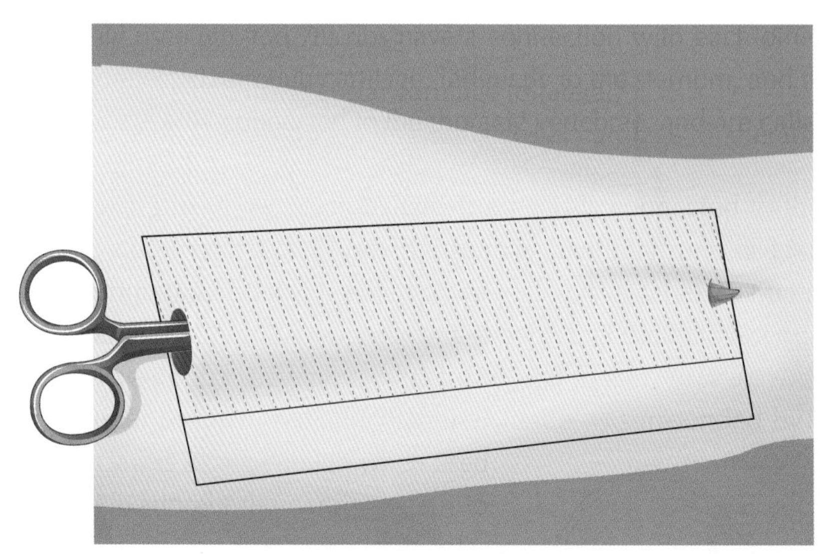

Figure 4 A 2 cm proximal incision is used to free the fascia lata from the overlying subcutaneous tissue and underlying musculature. Parallel long cuts have been made along the fascia. The cut free end has been grasped and passed under the skin distally, where a smaller stab incision has been made to deliver the fascia externally.

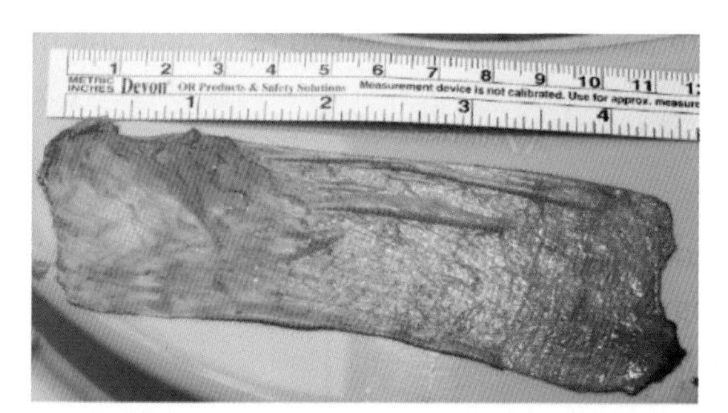

Figure 5 Harvested fascia. This is a modestly sized harvest measuring 12×4 cm, but much larger harvests are possible using small incisions as outlined earlier.

4) Postoperative Care

Some shrinkage and resorption of the graft is expected in the first 6 weeks. Thereafter, further resorption tends to be minimal. Postoperative pain tends to be minimal, with immediate ambulation possible in most patients. A small number of patients may develop cutaneous nerve neuralgia especially if the harvest is made too high. With compression dressing, hematomas and seromas are seldom seen. The need for deep tension sutures must be emphasized when closing the superior incision. The skin over the thigh moves readily on ambulation and broad scars can form if this is not done. With good wound closure, the superior incision heals well and remains well hidden, even when wearing shorts. The lower stab incision heals inconspicuously and becomes undetectable.

5) Complications

The following complications may occur:

- Muscle herniation
- Scar-related complications
- Neuralgia
- Weakness of knee extension
- Hemorrhage and seroma formation
- Infection
- Delayed ambulation

Muscle herniation, if it occurs, manifests immediately after the operation. This is mild and invariably resolves after 3 months. The use of compression stockings may shorten this process.

II. Homologous Fascia (Processed Fascia)

Autologous fascia requires additional surgery for harvest, thus entailing further complications, and has the disadvantage of having a limited amount for harvest. Such characteristics make its use somewhat limited. To overcome these shortcomings, the homologous fascia graft was developed *(Figure 6)*. Processed fascia as an implant material has the advantage of reducing harvest-induced donor site morbidity. Fascia obtained from a cadaver goes through many tissue processing methods to remove immune reactions and infection risks. Fascia processing follows normal processing methods used for homologous tissue; putting tissue collected from a cadaver donor that passed initial medical tests and that has no viral diseases, go through processes such as delipidization, osmotic treatment, oxidative treatment, solvent dehydration, and gamma irradiation. Though processing methods differ slightly for each company, there are no major differences. Another advantage of processed fascia is that it is easier to handle than autologous fascia harvested during surgery. Disadvantages of processed fascia are its possibly inadequate supply and high prices.

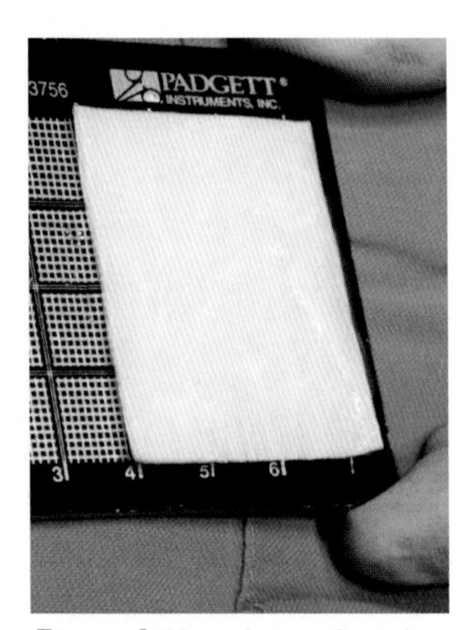

Figure 6 Homologous fascia lata.

III. Biological Characteristics of Fascia

The most critical point of concern when using fascia in rhinoplasty is the unpredictability of surgical results, due to postoperative absorption of the implant. The mechanisms of fascia resorption used as graft material during rhinoplasty include:

- Host-versus-graft reaction
- Graft infection

- ☑ Inward growth of surrounding connective tissue
- ☑ Volume reduction due to surrounding tissue's pressure

A number of studies have been published regarding, the resorption of implanted fascia. Baker, et al. have reported ample preservation of autologous temporalis fascia one year after rhinoplasty, while other animal experiments have shown that inserting temporalis fascia, harvested from a human, inside an athymic rat exhibits no signs of absorption even after time. On the contrary, Guerrerosantos, et al. have reported that about 10% of rhinoplasty patients for whom fascia grafts were used exhibit partial resorption of the graft, with frequency increasing with each additional/secondary surgery. Miller, et al. reported 20% decrease of overall volume due to condensing fibrous tissue 4-6 weeks after surgery, recommending slight overcorrection in light of these results. In the authors' research on autologous fascia and Tutoplast®-processed fascia lata, animal testing exhibits similar reactions for both autologous and homologous fascia (minor thickness reduction and histological reactions), thus indicating the fascia's suitability as implant material for rhinoplasty. However, based on the authors' clinical experience, morphological and aesthetic changes due to resorption should always be considered thoroughly when using fascia for rhinoplasty.

IV. Applications of Dorsal Augmentation Using Fascia

The authors use fascia for the following cases:

- ☑ Correction of minor contour irregularity
- ☑ Cosmetic augmentation in patients with very thin skin
- ☑ When dorsal augmentation is required as revision surgery for alloplastic implant complications
- ☑ Multiply revised noses that exhibits severe contraction
- ☑ When primary reconstruction of the nasal dorsum is required to treat active infection from prior surgery that used an alloplastic implant

V. How to Use Fascia

A number of techniques are available when using fascia on the nasal dorsum. The following methods can be used for both autologous and processed fascia.

1. Using Fascia Only

This method stacks multiple layers of fascia together for dorsal augmentation. Most cases make use of thick fascia lata. The authors prefer an open approach when using fascia for the dorsum. Antibiotics are administered before surgery, and after opening the processed fascia, is immerse in saline mixed with antibiotics for five minutes. The fascia is then cut into long pieces of 0.8×3-4 cm, suitable for the dorsum size. When cutting fascia, cutting it parallel to the fibers' directions is helpful in prevention of bending or curving in the long run. Three to four layers are stacked and the margins beveled carefully to prevent visibility in radix area. If a hematoma collects in the dorsum after surgery, the risk of infection becomes higher, thus applying pressure to the dorsum to let blood out is required. Taping and an external splint is then applied. Using fascia alone has a higher resorption rate compared to the combined use with cartilage *(Figure 7)*.

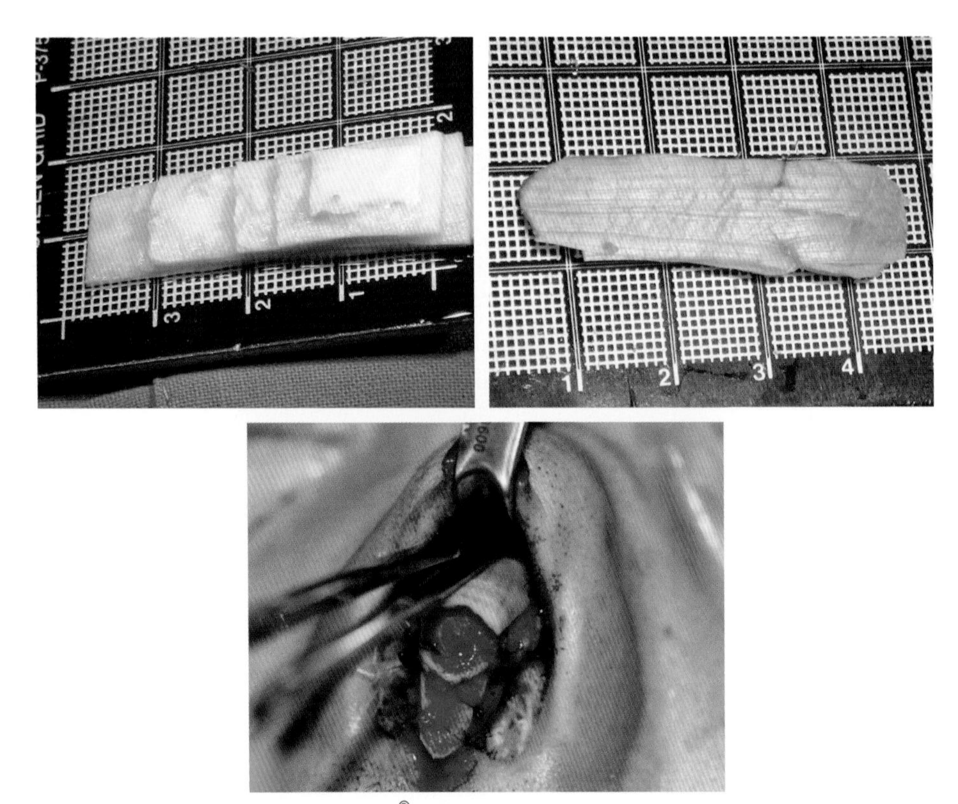

Figure 7 Designing Tutoplast® processed fascia lata for dorsal augmentation.

2. Overlapping Fascia with Cartilage

When the surgeon wants a greater degree of dorsal augmentation using fascia, one can place crushed septal cartilage or diced conchal cartilage between the fascia and nasal dorsum *(Figure 8)*. Diced cartilage or crushed cartilage can be inserted in the supratip cartilaginous dorsum or the entire dorsum. If crushed too much, cartilage resorption rate increases. Therefore, the surgeon should crush the cartilage lightly and gently, just enough to remove its original shape. Fascia covering the crushed or diced cartilages can soften the irregularity created by the cartilage, thus creating a better looking, smooth dorsum. This method has less postoperative volume reduction of the nasal dorsum compared to using fascia alone.

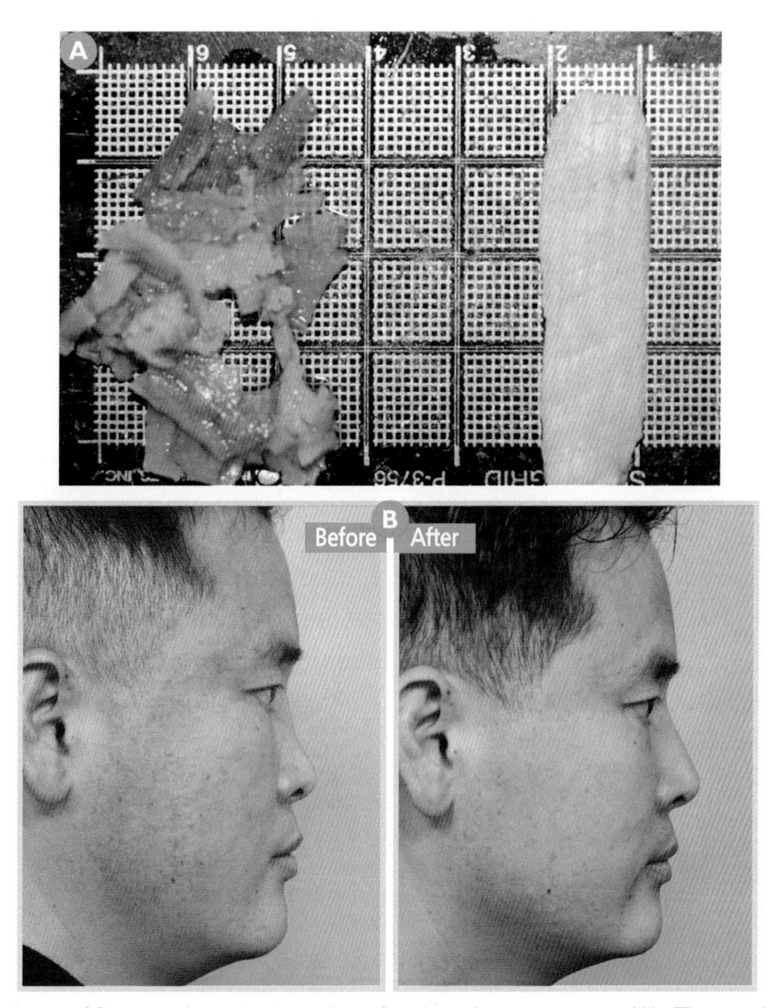

Figure 8 Combined use of fascia and crushed cartilage for dorsal augmentation (A). The crushed cartilage should be placed under the fascia. Patient showing good improvement of dorsal contour after use of fascia and cartilage (B).

3. Fascia-Wrapped Diced Cartilage

This method involves dicing conchal or septal cartilage and wrapping with fascia to be implanted in the dorsum. Conchal cartilage is most suitable as the inner contents *(Figure 9)*. Especially, if the perichondrium of the conchal cartilage is preserved, the cartilage pieces will not scatter after dicing, thus simplifying its use. Fascia-wrapped diced cartilage can be made to cover the entire nasal dorsum, and reducing its size to half makes it appropriate for insertion in cartilaginous dorsum. This method is easy to use, has relatively low visible surface irregularity, and low possibility of distortion. Its high resistance to infection makes it suitable for use in revision rhinoplasty.

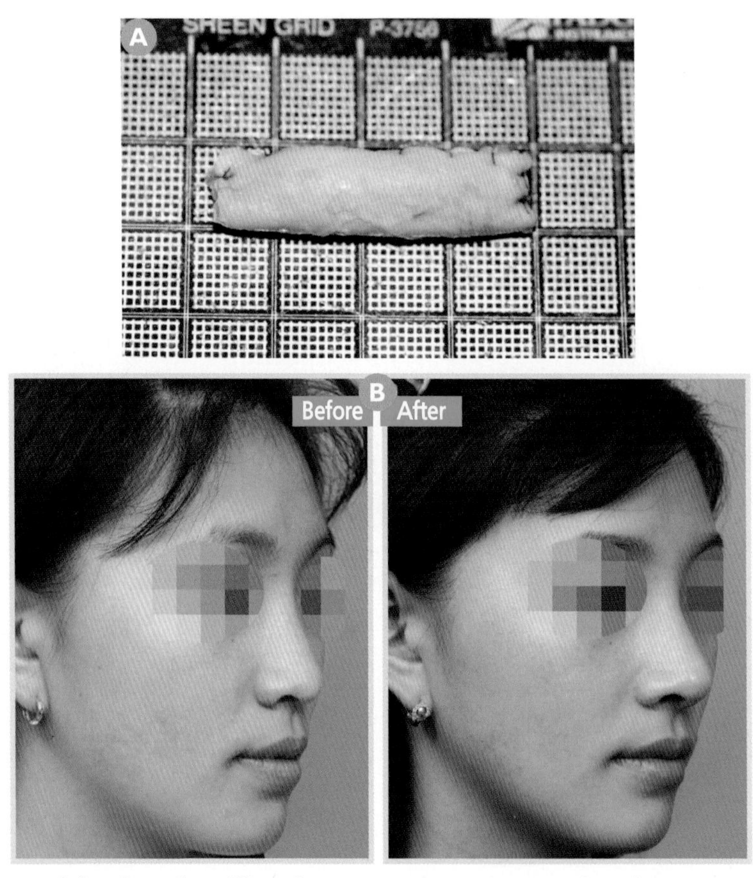

Figure 9 Fascia-wrapped diced cartilage (A) and a patient who underwent dorsal augmentation using fascia wrapped diced cartilage (B).

4. Sandwich Graft

This is a technique of wrapping the cartilage designed as a dorsal graft with fascia, and inserting it into the dorsum *(Figure 10)*. In this method, the cartilage graft is not crushed or diced; it designed as a graft for one-piece dorsal augmentation. This method prevents the edges of the cartilage graft from showing through the dorsum, thus is useful for creating a smooth nasal dorsum contour. This is advantageous in preventing dorsal implant visibility in the long run for patients with thin skin. Furthermore, this method helps keep the dorsal cartilage graft move less and stay stable after surgery. Inserting this graft is relatively easy even for surgeries using the endonasal approach, however, cartilage can still become visible when the fascia is absorbed.

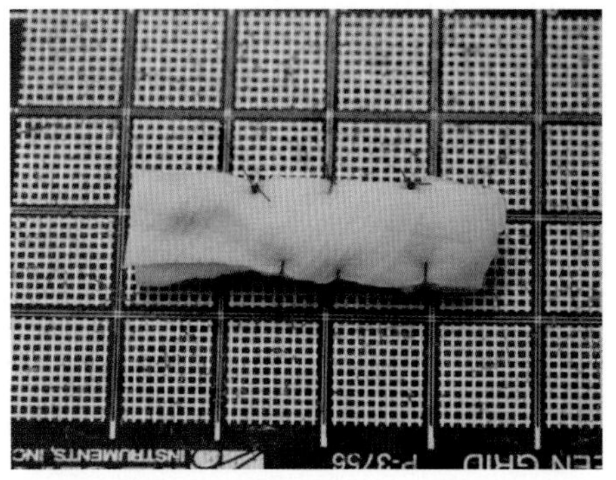

Figure 10 Sandwich graft: septal cartilage wrapped with fascia.

VI. Fascia Use in Tip Surgery

The following uses are possible in nasal tip surgery. The most common use is covering the cartilage tip grafting, and camouflaging overly sharp tip graft edges. This method can buy time in preventing initial tip graft visibility for patients with thin skin. This method is done by using one or two layers of fascia to wrap the tip graft *(Figure 11)*.

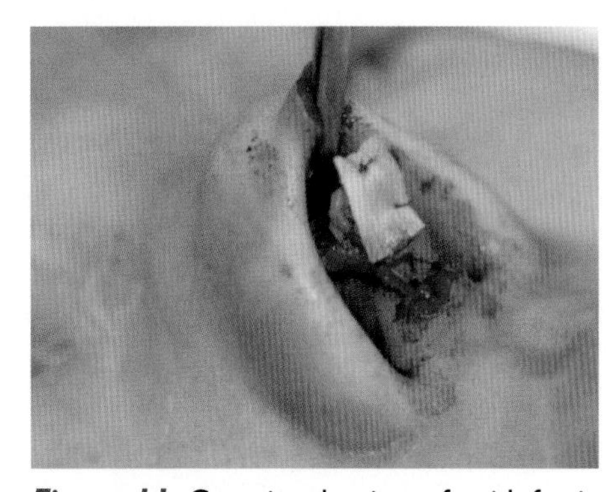

Figure 11 Covering the tip graft with fascia to prevent graft visibility.

Another method is to cut the fascia into little squares or rectangular blocks and close the transcolumellar incision first, and then insert the designed fascia as an onlay graft of the tip. This method is used when there is not enough cartilage remaining for use during surgery, or the projection of the nasal tip seems a little inadequate after closing the incision. Fascia inserted into the tip is usually made in sizes within 1 cm^3 *(Figure 12)*. In one study which followed up 82 such patients for over two years revealed that about 30% exhibited undesirable aesthetic results as the nasal tip became wider. However, there were no complications like infection, graft migration, or extrusion. Therefore, this method can create a smooth tip contour when used selectively for patients with thin skin; however, it is difficult to expect major projection, and tip definition may be compromised.

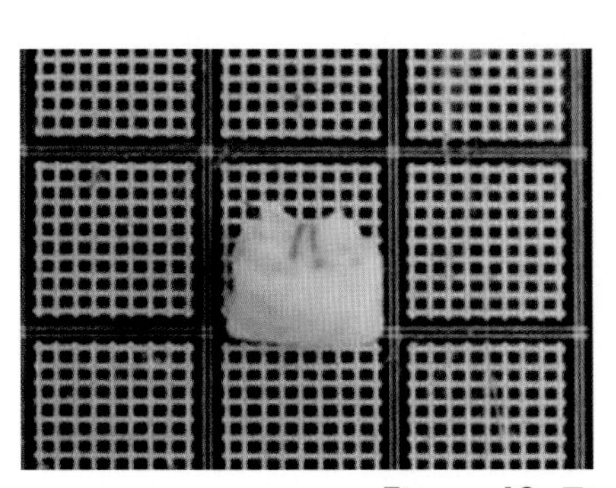

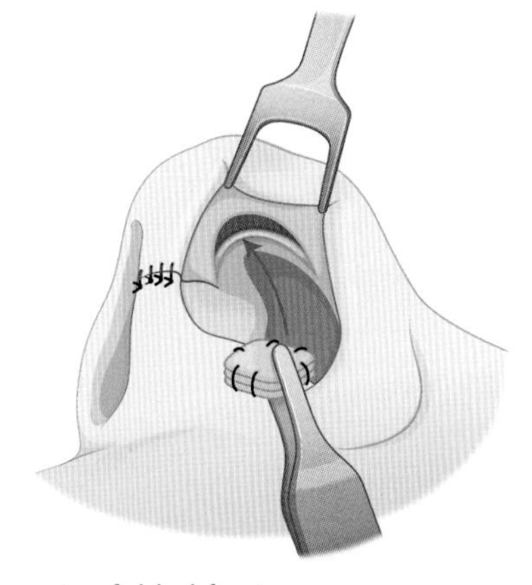

Figure 12 Tip onlay grafting using folded fascia.

VII. Complications

1. Resorption

This is the biggest shortcoming of fascia. Both using fascia alone and using it with cartilage can have the same issues. Based on the authors' experience, resorption rates differ among each individual and the quality of fascia. Some patients can preserve beautiful dorsal lines for years, while other patients exhibit symptoms such as irregularity or loss of dorsal height due to resorption of the graft *(Figure 13)*. Contraction of the dorsal skin resulting in an upturned nose appearance can happen in the long run *(Figure 14)*. Slight overcorrection using thick fascia may not provide the best immediate aesthetic results, but provides better results in the long term. According to the authors' experience, about 10% of patients demonstrated dissatisfaction due to postoperative resorption.

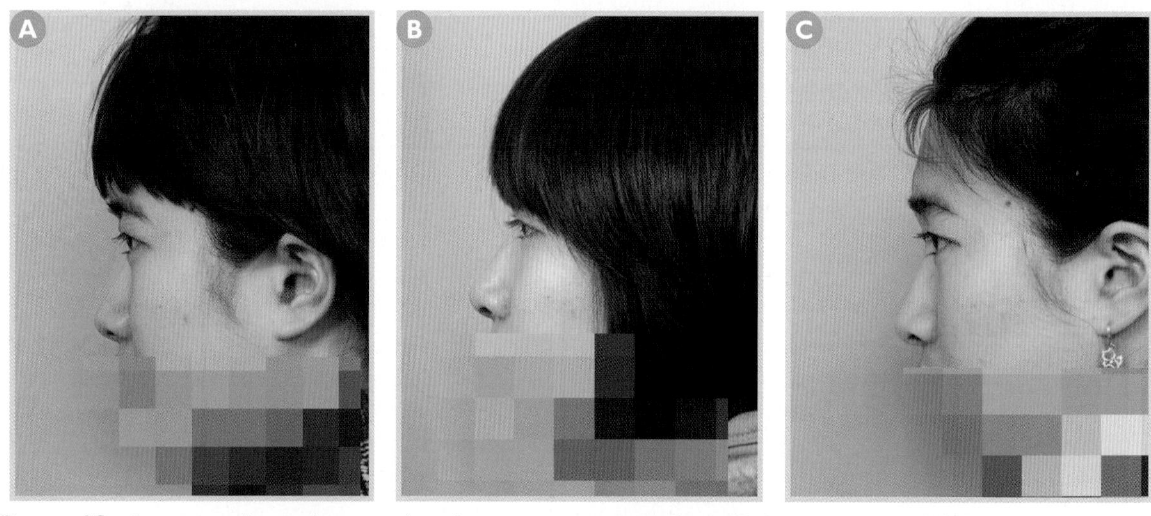

Figure 13 A patient who underwent dorsal augmentation using fascia. Before operation (A), 3 months after operation (B), and 18 months after operation (C), showing a considerably lowered dorsum.

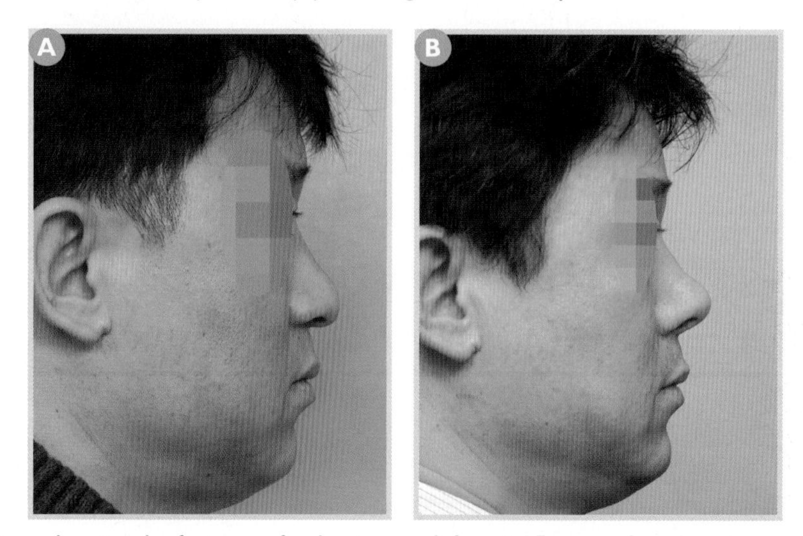

Figure 14 A patient showing the features of a short nose deformity 5 years after dorsal augmentation using processed fascia. Before surgery (A) and after surgery (B).

2. Infection

This complication occurs mostly within two weeks after surgery, and often accompanies hematoma or seroma accumulation in the nasal dorsum. To prevent infections, make sure there is no collection of blood or any tissue fluid by sufficiently pressing the nasal dorsum as the surgery ends. When there is an infection, prompt removal the implanted fascia can fix the problem. Once the fascia bonds with tissue, delayed infection becomes highly unlikely.

3. Deviation

When using fascia for the entire dorsum, the dorsal implant may bend unevenly, or if with cartilage may tilt to one side. External manual compression can correct minor deviations, but severe deviations require revision surgery.

References

1. Anthony PS, Steven AM, Rubina C. Biophysical and microscopic analysis of homologous dermal and fascial materials for facial aesthetic and reconstructive uses. Arch Facial Plast Surg 2002; 4: 164-71.
2. Baker TM, Courtiss EH. Temporalis fascia grafts in open secondary rhinoplasty. Plast Reconstr Surg 1994; 93: 802-10.
3. Daniel RK, Calvert JW. Diced cartilage grafts in rhinoplasty surgery. Plast Reconstr Surg 2004; 113: 2156-71.
4. Daniel RK. Grafts. In: Rhinoplasty: An atlas of surgical techniques. Springer-Verlag, 2002; 267-9.
5. Erkan T, Ozcan C, Binnaz HO, Volkan A. Comparison of alloderm, fat, fascia, cartilage, and dermal grafts in rabbits. Arch Facial Plast Surg 2008; 10: 187-93.
6. Guerrerosantos J. Temporoparietal free fascia grafts in rhinoplasty. Plast Reconstr Surg 1984; 74: 465-74.
7. Issing W, Anari S. Sandwich technique in nasal dorsal augmentation. Eur Arch Otorhinolaryngol 2011; 268: 83-6.
8. Jang YJ, Song HM, Yoon YJ, Sykes JM. Combined use of crushed cartilage and processed fascia lata for dorsal augmentation in rhinoplasty for Asians. Laryngoscope 2009; 119; 1088-92.
9. Jang YJ, Kim JH. Use of tutoplast-processed fascia lata as an onlay graft material for tip surgery in rhinoplasty. Otolaryngol Head Neck Surg 2011: 144; 528-32.
10. Jang YJ, Wang JH, Sinha V, Song HM, Lee BJ. Tutoplast processed fascia lata for dorsal augmentation in rhinoplasty. Otolaryngol Head Neck Surg 2007; 137: 88-92.
11. Karaatin MV, Orhan KS, Demirel T. Fascia lata graft for nasal dorsal contouring in rhinoplasty. J Plast Reconstr Aesthet Surg 2009; 62: 1255-60.
12. Miller TA. Temporalis fascia grafts for facial and nasal contour augmentation. Plast Reconstr Surg 1988; 81: 524-33.
13. Yu MS, Park HS, Lee HJ, Jang YJ. Histomorphological changes of tutoplast-processed fascia lata grafts in a rabbit rhinoplasty model. Otolaryngol Head Neck Surg 2012; 147: 239-44.

A 27-year-old female visited for a flat nasal dorsum with deviation. She suffered nasal trauma about 15 years ago.

Analysis

Frontal: Flat nose, poor brow-tip aesthetic line
Basal: Low tip projection
Oblique: Low dorsal height, poor tip projection

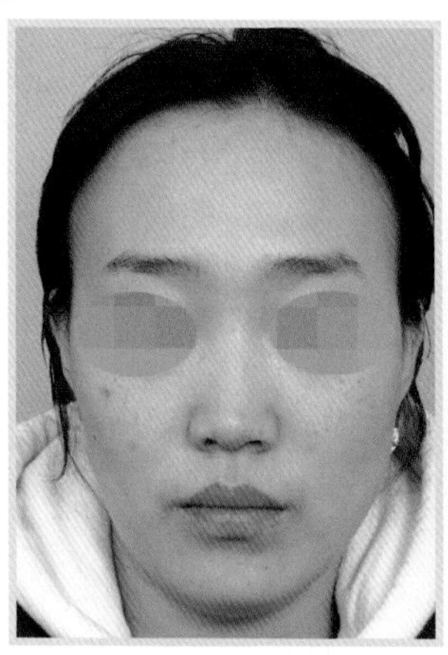
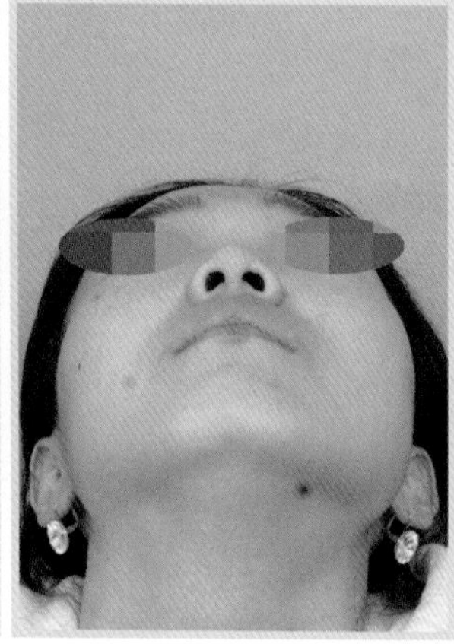
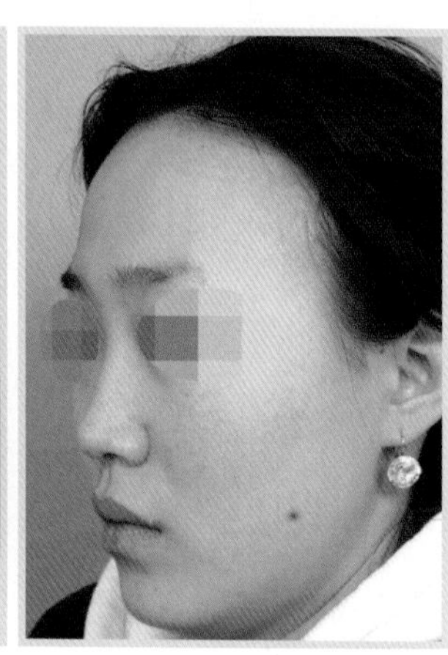

Operative Procedures

Open rhinoplasty approach
Harvesting of septal and conchal cartilage
Caudal septal extension grafting using septal cartilage (bilateral)
Multilayer tip grafting using conchal cartilage
Dorsal augmentation using crushed cartilage and fascia lata

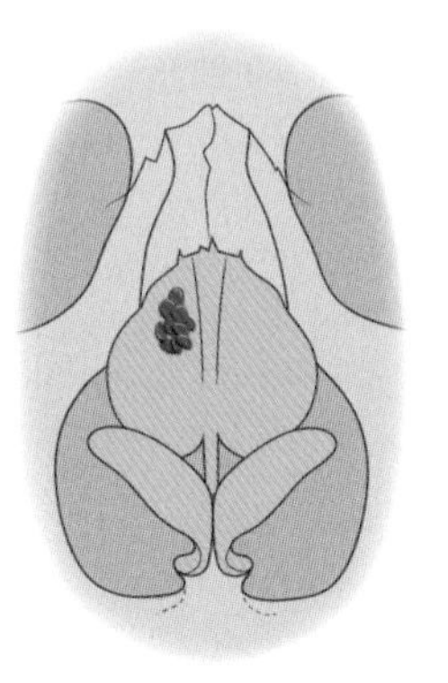
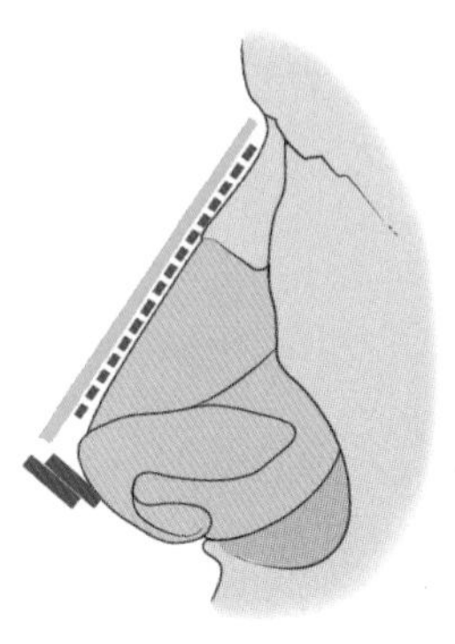
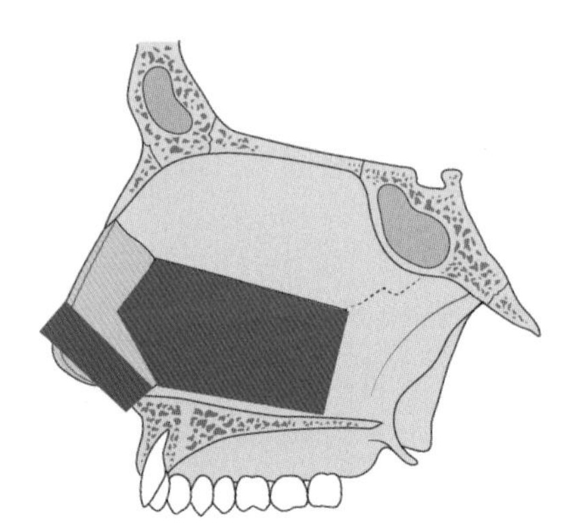

Postoperative Changes

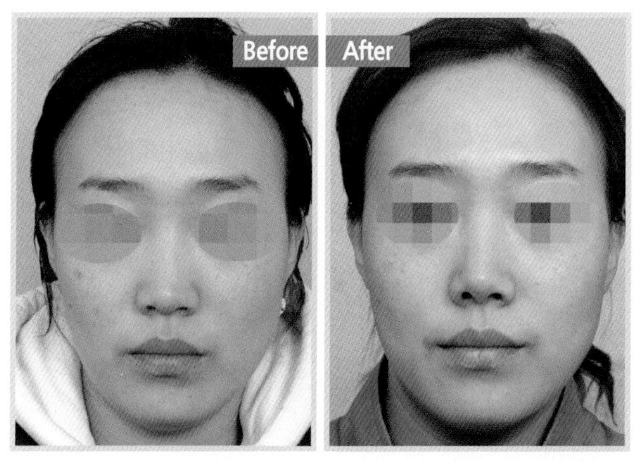

Frontal: Proper dorsal aesthetic lines were achieved after dorsal augmentation.

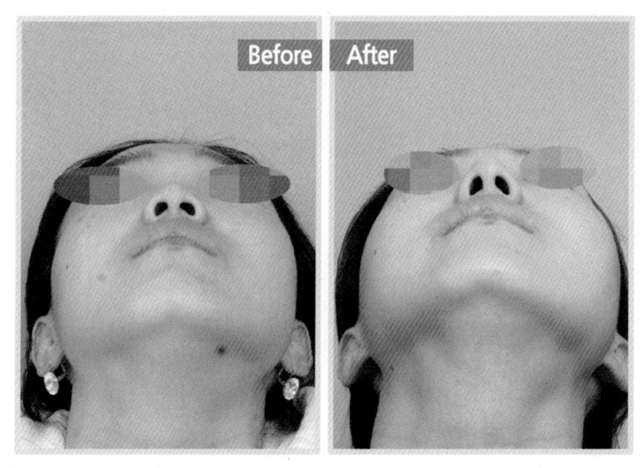

Basal: Tip projection was improved.

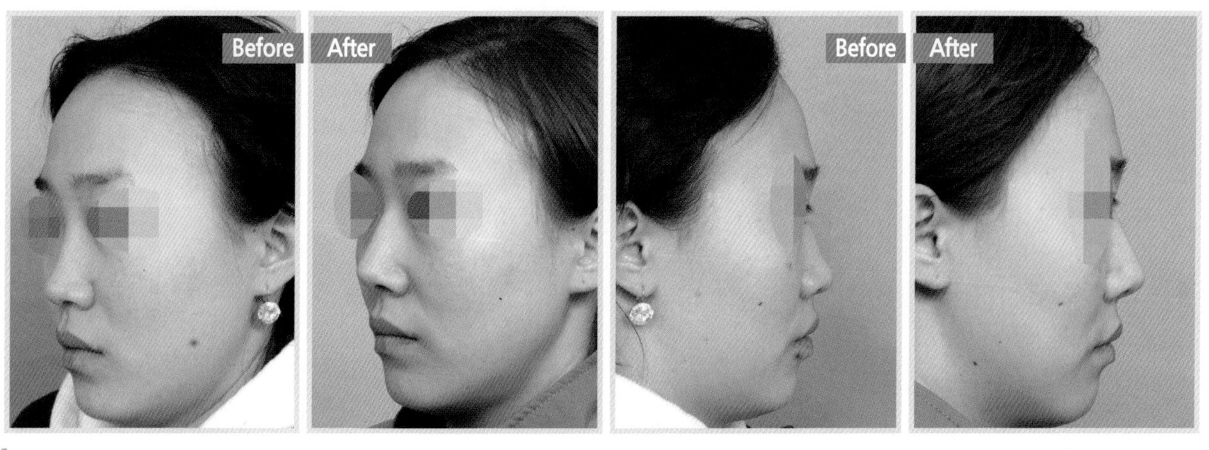

Lateral and Oblique: Dorsal height elevation and tip projection were achieved. Nasofrontal angle was narrowed.

Case 2

A 51-year-old female visited for a dorsal hump and deviated nose acquired after a nasal bone fracture.

Analysis
Frontal: Slightly depressed left nasal dorsum with mild dorsal deviation
Basal: Asymmetry of domal heights of the nasal tip
Lateral and Oblique: Slight dorsal convexity

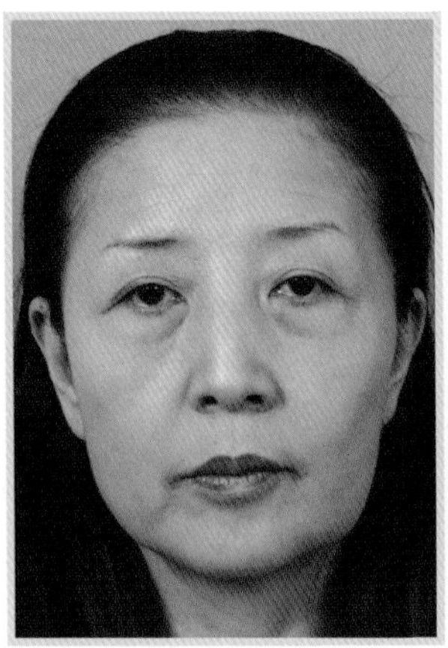
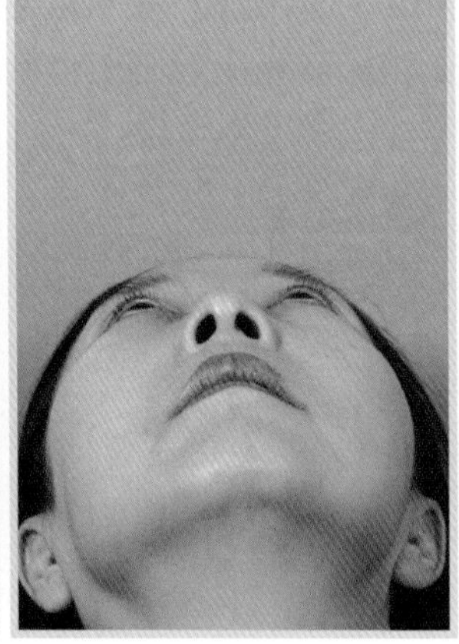
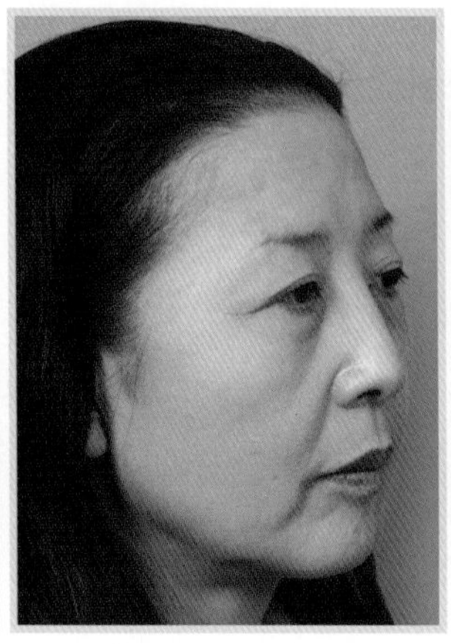
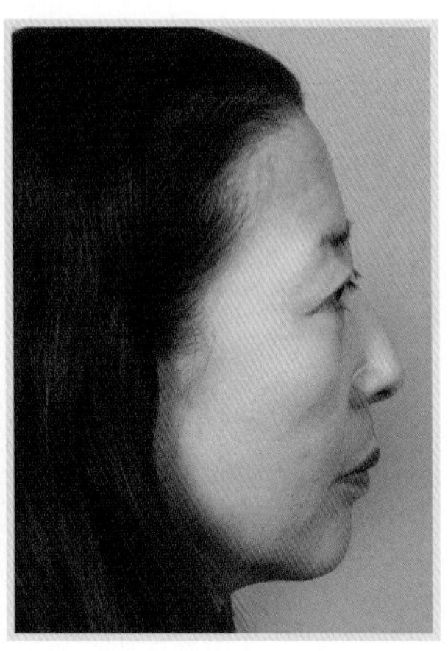

Operative Procedures

Open rhinoplasty approach
Medial, lateral, and percutaneous root osteotomies
Hump rasping
Caudal septal extension grafting using septal cartilage (bilateral)
Columellar strut application
Tip onlay grafting using folded processed fascia lata
Dorsal augmentation using processed fascia lata

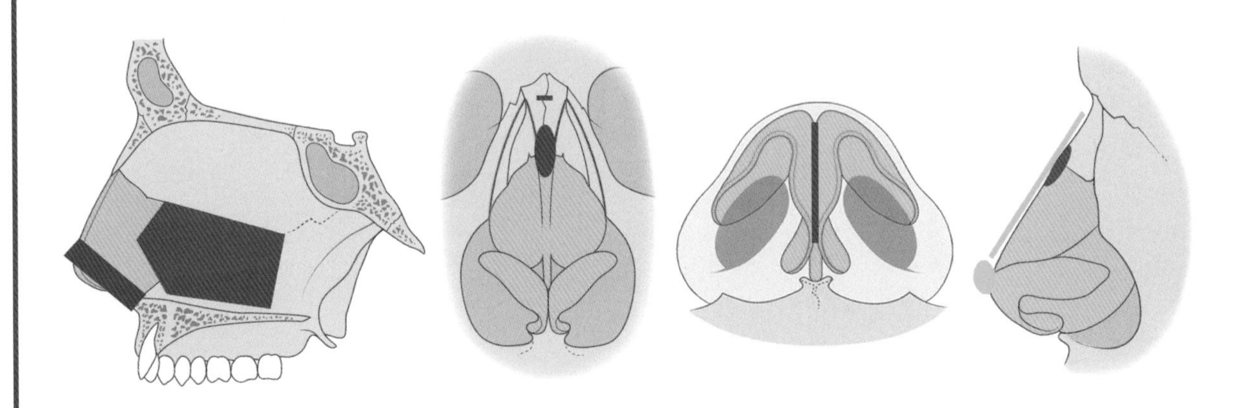

Postoperative Changes

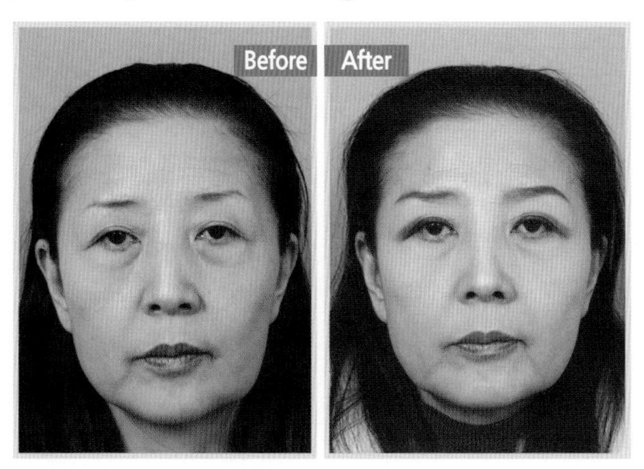

Frontal: Nasal deviation was corrected.

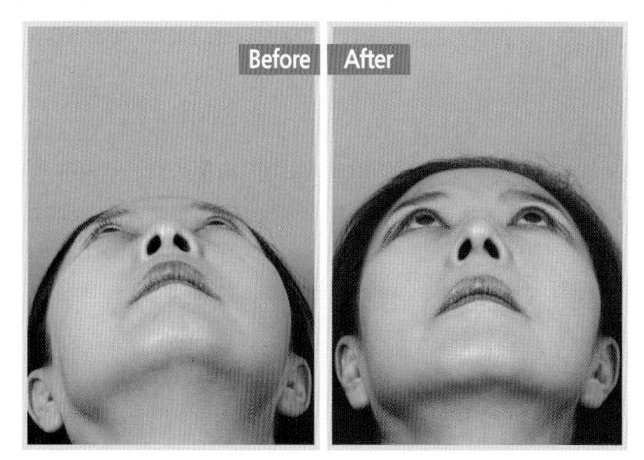

Basal: Domal heights were restored. Tip lobule was lengthened.

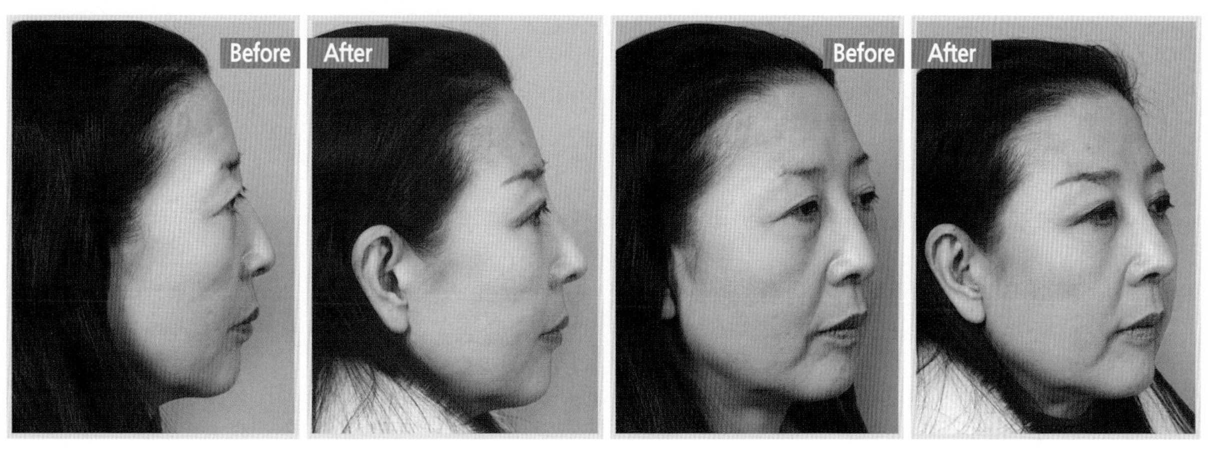

Lateral and Oblique: Tip projection was improved. Dorsal convexity was corrected through hump reduction.

AlloDerm

Myeong Sang Yu

I. Characteristics and Structure of AlloDerm

Various materials are used in rhinoplasty to create the desired nasal shapes. Although autologous tissue such as cartilage, bone, and fascia are ideal for rhinoplasty, they are sometimes difficult to obtain in sufficient amounts, and require additional procedures for harvesting which could damage the donor site. Such reasons have promoted the development of synthetic materials such as Silicone, Gore-Tex and Medpor, but none seem perfectly compatible with the human body just yet, prompting further research.

AlloDerm (LifeCell Corporation, Branchburg, NJ) is an acellular dermal matrix created by removing the epidermis from cadaveric skin, processing the dermis to remove the remaining epidermis and dermis cells that can have immune reactions, then freeze-drying it to preserve only its skeletal structure such as collagen fibers, elastin, and proteoglycans *(Figure 1)*. The 3-dimensional structure of the original dermis is not damaged, while basement membrane, elastin, and vascular channels are preserved. Therefore, the dermal skeletal structure, after implantation, meets an influx of fibroblasts and produces new blood vessels and nerve tissue, making integration and engraftment easy in addition to becoming homogeneous with the patient's own tissue.

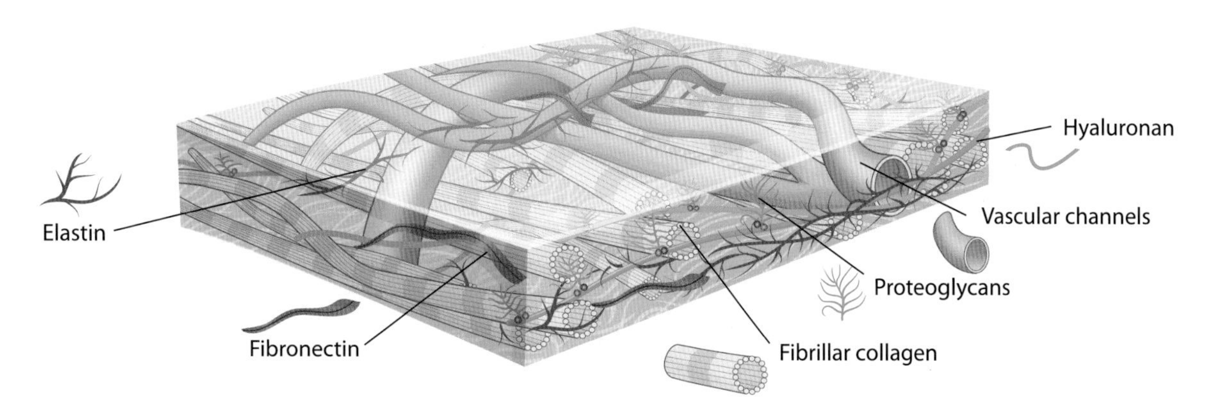

Figure 1 The 3-dimensional structure of AlloDerm.

II. Types of AlloDerm

AlloDerm can be classified into two types based on certain properties. The sheet type is stored freeze-dried as sheets of various sizes ranging from 1×2 cm to 16×20 cm and 0.33-3.3 mm thickness, and rehydrated for 30 minutes before use *(Figure 2A)*. Sheet type include: Graft AlloDerm (usually used in areas with skin loss due to burns, external injury, or other accidents), Hernia AlloDerm (used for abdominoplasty and reinforcing or reconstruction of areas with abdominal fascia loss), and Breast AlloDerm (used as a substitute for inner lining in breast reconstruction using breast implants or tissue expander). The second type is powder type, made by micronization of acellular dermal tissue and which is used as an injection filler after combining with a diluting agent *(Figure 2B)*. It can be used for injection laryngoplasty or correction of soft tissue loss.

Rhinoplasty usually involves sheet type AlloDerm, and is either cut into appropriate sizes after meeting thickness requirements or stacked together to increase thickness. Powder type AlloDerm, like any other filler, is used by injecting the needed amounts into the nasal dorsum or tip.

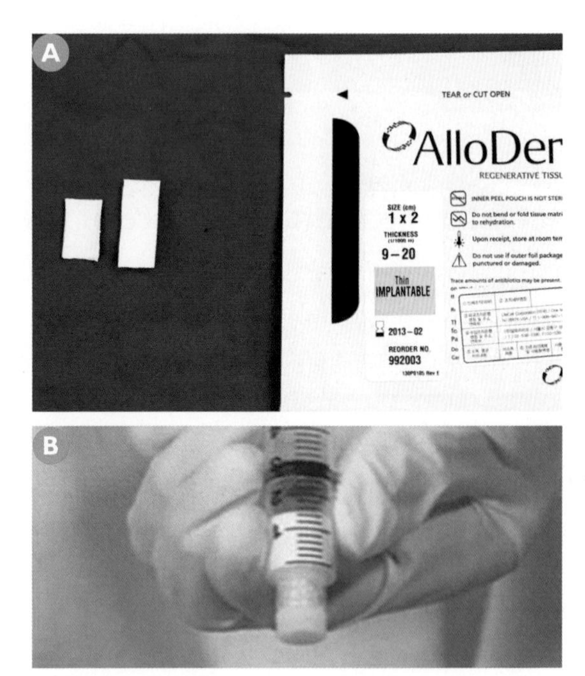

Figure 2 Types of AlloDerm; sheet type (A) and powder type (B).

III. Advantages and Disadvantages of AlloDerm in Rhinoplasty

1. Advantages

Since AlloDerm is manufactured and distributed as square sheets, it is relatively easier to design it accordingly for surgery. Furthermore, its various sizes and thicknesses makes adjustment of thickness required for augmentation easier. Its high elasticity and expansibility enable easier manipulation during surgery and makes it effective for evening out irregular surfaces on the dorsum or tip. Furthermore, since it has a soft texture and low rigidity, it can give an aesthetically natural texture to patients with grafts showing through the the tip or dorsum due to thin skin. Because its color resembles natural skin tones, it does not show through skin and can make up for the shortcomings of silicone or Gore-Tex by being used together to cover their surfaces. Its sheet form, with appropriate thickness and elasticity, makes it possible to place it stably inside desired locations on the nasal dorsum. Most of all, as homologous material collected from other people's bodies, immune-reaction inducing factors have been removed and revasculization and remodeling happen swiftly after implantation, reducing risks of postoperative infection and rejection.

2. Disadvantages

The biggest limitation of AlloDerm is the possibility of partial absorption as time progresses after surgery, all the more made unpredictable due to varied absorption rates among patients. When used for dorsal augmentation, it has been known that 20-30% of implanted AlloDerm is absorbed within a year after implantation. AlloDerm is more expensive than silicone or Gore-Tex, and moreover it bonds actively with surrounding tissues over time, becoming difficult to remove in cases that require revision. Furthermore, its low rigidity provides little structural support, making its contour clearly visible on an uneven nasal dorsum and has limited thickness possible for augmentation compared to silicone or Gore-Tex.

IV. Carving and Inserting AlloDerm

Sheet type AlloDerm ranges in thickness from 0.3 mm to 3.3 mm. Therefore, one must use a sheet with the same thickness as desired augmentation levels or stack multiple layers for higher degrees of augmentation. When stacking, rather than folding one layer multiple times to adjust thickness, cut the implant into same sizes and stack increase thickness to reduce postoperative absorption and prevent graft movement. Furthermore, when stacking, use Nylon or PDS to suture both ends to prevent separation, then use iris scissors to trim the edges. It is then inserted in the nasion and supratip, according to the shape of nasal dorsum.

AlloDerm can be inserted using either an open approach or a closed approach. First of all, when elevating the skin flap, create a precise pocket in the precise location like with other grafts. With the open approach, direct vision allows the graft to be stitched to the surrounding tissue and suspended even if the pocket is large *(Figure 3)*. Since inserting and fixation of AlloDerm can be difficult with the closed approach, it is important to place the edge of the graft in the precise location of the proximal part—the radix—during insertion. Insertion in a precise pocket does not require additional suture-fixation, but when creating a pocket exactly fitting the graft is difficult,

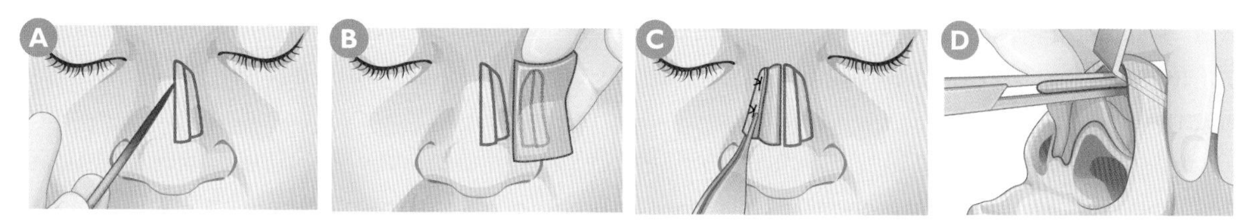

Figure 3 Open approach technique. The area to be augmented was carefully outlined with methylene blue or a marking pen (A). Placing the graft onto the marked area leaves a tattoo on the graft itself and the graft is cut to size (B). The graft was folded onto itself and stabilized with 5-0 PDS sutures (C). Wide sufficient dissection of the pocket is performed through an open approach, and then the AlloDerm graft is inserted under direct vision (D).

one can consider suture-fixation of the graft to the radix skin. The sutures are removed a week later *(Figure 4).*

AlloDerm's low rigidity makes it susceptible to crumpling around the edge, thus high attention is required. One must conduct tactile checks on the nasal dorsum after implantation to detect any folds/wrinkles. If nasal dorsum is uneven, the contour could show directly through the skin, thus it is important to straighten the nasal dorsum before surgery to get a smooth nasal dorsum after surgery. When it is difficult to undergo this process, partially insert additional AlloDerm pieces to achieve the desired nasal dorsal contour.

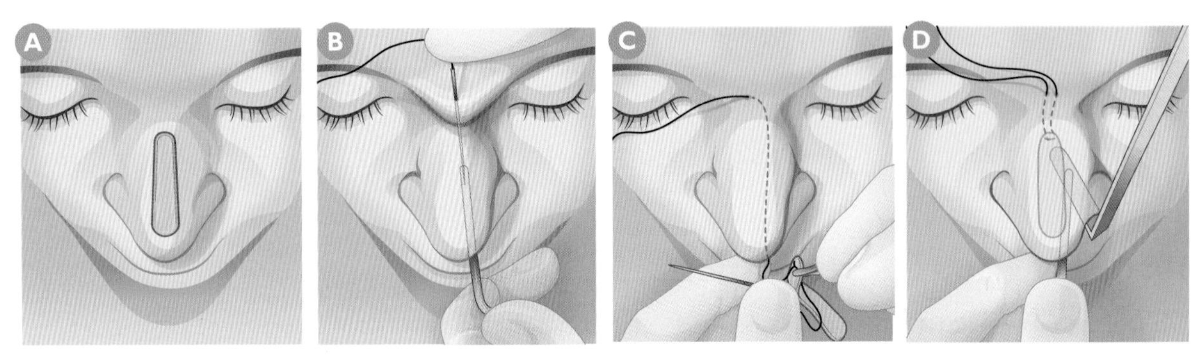

Figure 4 Closed approach technique. Preoperative markings with methylene blue of the area to be augmented and the graft is cut to size (A). A dissection of the exact-sized pocket is then undertaken through a closed approach, then a needle is inserted through the skin into the hollow cylinder of a metal suction tip (B). The very edge of the proximal portion of the AlloDerm graft is pierced with the needle (C). The needle is advanced out through the skin area immediately adjacent to the initial needle puncture entry site in the radix. And then AlloDerm graft is gently pulled into its recipient site pocket (D).

V. Precautions for AlloDerm Usage for Dorsal Augmentation

When using AlloDerm for dorsal augmentation, one must keep in mind the possibility and unpredictability of absorption of implanted AlloDerm. According to various reports, though there have been no cases of complete absorption, about half of the patients exhibited partial absorption over time. Generally, 20-30% is absorbed on the nasal dorsum and 10-15% is absorbed on the nasal tip, with most absorption taking place in the first year after surgery. Additional absorption rarely occurs after the first year. Stacking multiple layers does not increase absorption. The tendency to be absorbed is higher when used on the bony dorsum, in revision cases with thin skin, and patients with vascular diseases such as nasal telangiectasia. Therefore, if the patient's skin is thin or if used for augmentation of the bony dorsum, one must take extra care. When using AlloDerm for dorsal augmentation, always keep in mind overcorrection of 20-30% taking into account the rate of absorption. Since it is hard to judge the exact height of nasal dorsum during surgery due to edema, determine the degree of augmentation and thickness of AlloDerm before surgery.

Another point to consider is AlloDerm's tendency to bond with surrounding tissue and the ensuing difficulty in graft removal after one month. In rare cases, a seroma can occur after surgery, but it can easily be treated by aspiration or pressure taping. Other cases may exhibit edema lasting for months, but most are reported to have recovered within four months.

Though AlloDerm is easy to use and has many merits as a dorsal graft, it cannot be called the ideal dorsal graft due to its unpredictability in absorption, high prices, and limited augmentation levels. Therefore, when there are multiple options, discuss its characteristics fully with the patient before usage.

VI. Various Uses of AlloDerm in Rhinoplasty

1. Using with other Materials for Dorsal Augmentation

1) Silicone or Gore-Tex

Though AlloDerm can be used alone for dorsal augmentation, its various shortcomings (low rigidity, high absorption rates, and limited height increase) call for simultaneous use of other materials. Despite their many advantages, silicone and Gore-Tex, commonly used in Asian patients, can exhibit graft visibility in patients with thin skin due to their high rigidity or seem unnatural due to their hard texture. Furthermore, since silicone makes it impossible for surrounding tissue to bond with the graft, graft movement may occur. In such cases, using AlloDerm on top of silicone can prevent silicone or Gore-Tex from showing, creating a natural dorsal line. In addition, AlloDerm also bonds easily with the surrounding tissue, helping the graft stay stable at the desired position *(Figure 5)*.

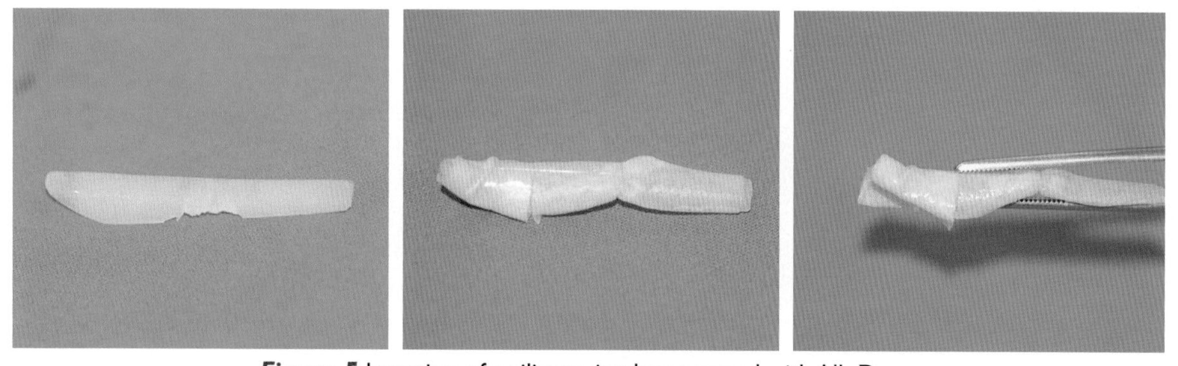

Figure 5 Insertion of a silicone implant covered with AlloDerm.

2) Diced Cartilage Grafts

Diced cartilage is appropriate for volume augmentation due to its high biological compatibility and low infection and extrusion rates compared to alloplastic implant materials. Diced cartilage wrapped in autologous fascia or Surgicel® has been commonly used in dorsal augmentation to prevent movement of cartilage and dorsal irregularity from cartilage fragments. However, recent studies have revealed the possibility of Surgicel® inducing inflammation in the surrounding tissue to facilitate absorption. Autologous fascia too has the problems of requiring additional surgical time and injury to the donor site. To make up for these problems, using AlloDerm instead of Surgicel® or fascia to wrap diced cartilage has been introduced *(Figure 6)*.

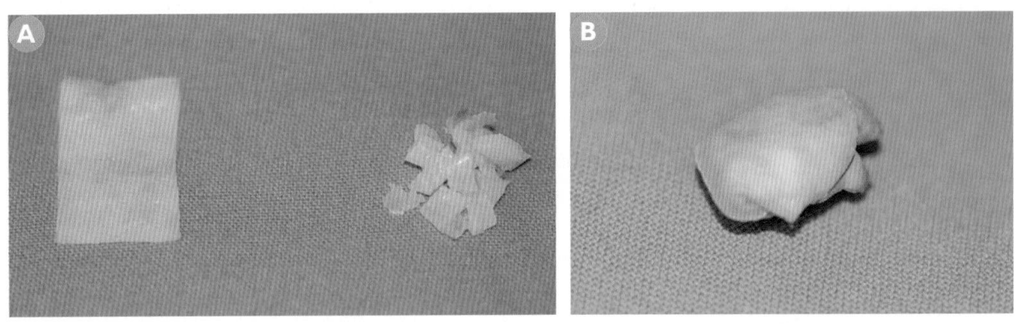

Figure 6 AlloDerm and diced cartilage (A). Diced cartilage wrapped in AlloDerm for use in tip augmentation (B).

2. Nasal Tip Surgery

The rigidity of AlloDerm is weaker than even that of sheet-type Gore-Tex, making it inadequate for structural support and susceptible to absorption at the tip, just like on the dorsum. Using AlloDerm creates a seemingly natural and high nasal tip right after surgery, but it can be absorbed over time to become lower and somewhat bulbous. Therefore, using AlloDerm alone for tip surgery is not recommended. If possible, it is best to use autologous cartilage for the nasal tip, and using AlloDerm on top of cartilage grafts can help prevent graft visibility in patients with thin skin *(Figure 7)*.

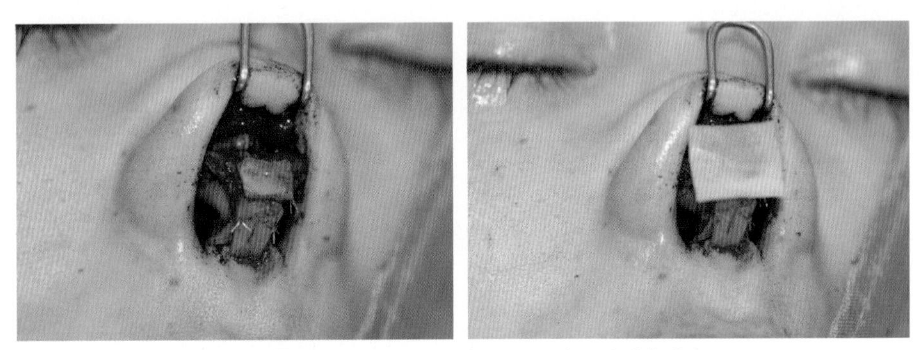

Figure 7 Cartilage tip graft covered with AlloDerm.

3. Correcting Dorsal Irregularities

Trauma on the nose or complicated prior rhinoplasties can make the nasal skin thinner or leave scars, causing cartilaginous or bony structures below the skin to feel irregular or protrude visibly. Crushed cartilage or autologous fascia can be used to camouflage these effects, but autologous fascia is associated with donor site morbidity. Since AlloDerm comes in various thicknesses, has high elasticity, and is strong against infection or foreign body reactions, it can be used effectively to correct various forms of dorsal irregularities *(Figure 8)*.

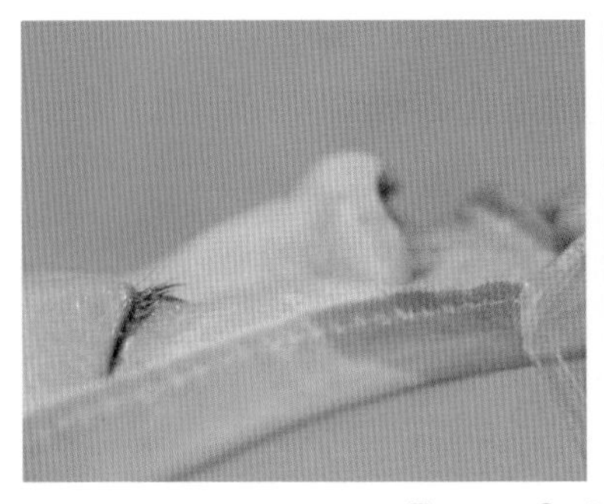
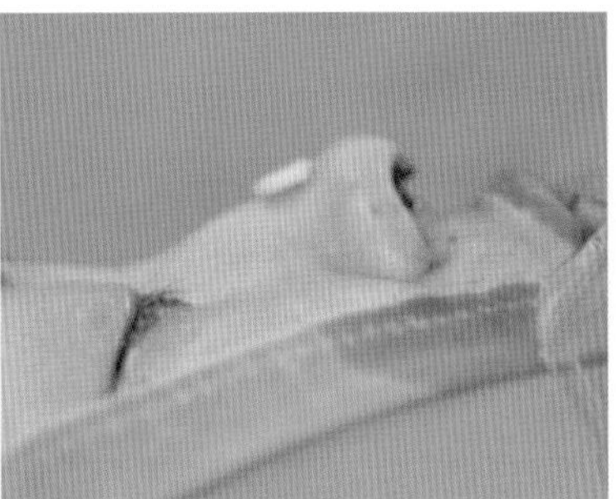
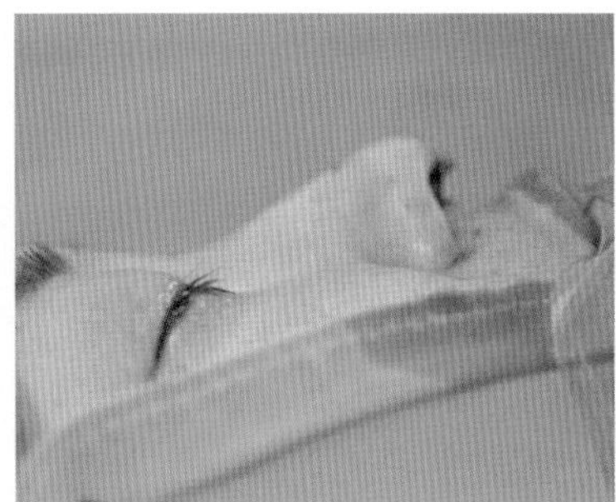

Figure 8 Correction of supratip irregularity using AlloDerm.

4. Revision Rhinoplasty

Patients who want or need secondary rhinoplasty sometimes exhibit graft visibility or their implant can be felt from the outside. Furthermore, the dorsal skin can become thinner or bond with nasal bone to leave rough outlines on the nasal dorsum as a complication of the initial surgery. Oftentimes, some patients have a limitation in acquiring autologous tissue due to depletion or usage from the first surgery. Homologous implants like AlloDerm can be useful for such patients. And since AlloDerm has a thin and natural texture and can be modified into various shapes, it can be used effectively for patients with thin skin or these who require camouflage of the dorsum or tip irregularity.

References

1. Gryskiewicz JM, Rohrich RJ, Reagan BJ. The use of AlloDerm for the correction of nasal contour deformities. Plast Reconstr Surg. 2001;107:561–570.
2. Gryskiewicz JM. Waste not, want not: The use of AlloDerm in secondary rhinoplasty. Plast Reconstr Surg. 2005;116:1999–2004.
3. Hong YT, Park SH, Kim SY. Histologic changes and photographic analysis of AlloDerm at tip plasty of the nose. Arch Aesthetic Plast Surg. 2006;12:140-144.
4. Jackson IT, Yavuzer R. AlloDerm for dorsal nasal irregularities. Plast Reconstr Surg. 2001;107:553–558.
5. Jang YJ, Park CH. Practical septorhinoplasty. Koonja Publishing Inc. 2007.
6. Kridel RW, Foda H, Lunde KC. Septal perforation repair with acellular human dermal allograft. Arch Otolaryngol Head Neck Surg. 1998;124:73–78.2
7. Life Cell co.Ltd. homepage. http://www.alloderm.co.kr/alloderm.html.3.
8. Sajjadian A, Naghshineh N, Rubinstein R. Current status of grafts and implants in rhinoplasty: Part II. Homologous grafts and allogenic implants. Plast Reconstr Surg. 2010 ;125(3):99e-109e.
9. Livesey SA, Herndon DN, Hollyoak MA, et al. Transplanted acellular allograft dermal matrix: Potential as a template for the reconstruction of viable dermis. Transplantation 1995; 60:1–9.
10. Tobin HA, Karas ND. Lip augmentation using an alloderm graft. J Oral Maxillofac Surg. 1998;56:722–727.

Silicone

In Sang Kim · Yong Ju Jang

Silicone was the first material to be used in facial plastic surgery, and is a broadly used artificial implant material. A silicone implant has a smooth surface, is easy to design, and brings excellent aesthetic results, thus is the most commonly used implant material in Asia.

Rhinoplasty using silicone is common in Asian countries, but not so much in the Western hemisphere. The reason for this phenomenon is that Asians have thicker skin tissue than Caucasians, thus have lower risks of complications like implant extrusion. Normally, silicone implantation conducted by an experienced surgeon is likely to have few complications. However, when surgeons with insufficient understanding of, and experience with silicone conduct rhinoplasty using silicone implants, many problems could arise— not because of the inherent demerits of silicone but because of the surgeon's misjudgments or technical errors. Minimizing such errors can prevent various problems.

I. Characteristics of Asian Rhinoplasty

Augmentation rhinoplasty is one of the most common aesthetic plastic surgeries in Asia. Therefore, patients have high aesthetic expectations, while also expecting fast recovery, prompt return to everyday life, and reasonable prices. Typical anatomical characteristics of the Asian nose call for long and big grafts to increase the size of the nose, but autologous cartilage, excluding costal cartilage, come in limited amounts, and surgery using costal cartilage requires a lengthy operation time, prolonged healing period, and high surgical fees. Furthermore, the fact that costal cartilage harvest will leave a scar in the chest gives patients an additional psychological burden. Moreover, costal cartilage presents issues such as warping and absorption, is too hard, and is relatively more difficult to carve. On the contrary, silicone has no warping, can be used in various sizes, is easy to carve, and has a smooth surface, possessing more, in purely aesthetic terms, advantages than autologous cartilage.

II. Physical and Chemical Characteristics of Silicone

Silicone refers to all organic compounds made from the chemical element Silicon (Si). Silicone has been commercially available since the 1940s, and Silastic® is a trademark of the company Dow Corning. Silicon Dioxide (SiO_2), also known as silica, is a mineral present in quartz and sand that is used to manufacture glass. Medical grade silicone is usually in the structure of dimethylsiloxane, composed of silicon, oxygen, and two methyl groups. Physical characteristics of silicone vary according to the degree of polymerization, length of chain structure, level of cross-linking between chains, and type of material added for cross-linking. These factors allow forms ranging from having lower viscosity than water to being very hard. Short chains take liquid or oil form, thus are used as lubricants or sealants, while long (5000-9000 units) and repeatedly cross-linked chains are used in various medical fields such as silicone rubber. Silicone rubber used for medical implants can be produced with various levels of hardness, and is normally marketed in the medical field as soft, medium, or firm types. Various chemicals are added in the synthesis of silicone for cross-linking, impurity control, and surface coating purposes, and while silicone itself is inert in the body and not toxic, impurities or added chemicals may create toxicity. Therefore, medical grade silicone has a higher production cost from following different processes and using physically harmless catalysts. Various organizations such as Good Manufacturing Practices (GMPs) of the U.S. FDA, U.S. Pharmacopeia (USP), and International Organization for Standardization (ISO) provide standards for medical implants, and the USP's Class VI is normally considered the minimum requirement for medical implants. This standard requires confirmation, by animal testing, of safety of over 5 years from intramuscular insertion. Standards of companies like Dow Corning are also used as production criteria. Medical grade silicone from Dow Corning is required to pass skin reaction, cell culture, and toxicity tests, and requires further observation (microscopic and naked eye) of intramuscular and subcutaneous insertion for 90 days by animal testing. Dow Corning's biomedical grade silicone requires additional testing for hemolysis, cytotoxicity, and cell mutation on top of the aforementioned criteria.

III. Characteristics and Advantages of Silicone

Silicone has the following advantages:

- ☑ Excellent biocompatibility
- ☑ Stable to heat and withstands a wide range of temperature (-60-260℃)
- ☑ Cannot be dissolved by enzymes
- ☑ High elasticity, flexibility, and form restoration
- ☑ Has no holes on the surface and is hydrophobic
- ☑ Has a sleek and smooth surface, and can be carved very precisely
- ☑ Has various levels of hardness
- ☑ Easy to remove when problems occur
- ☑ Less costly

IV. Designing and Insertion of the Silicone Implant

In order to design a silicone implant, the surgeon should have in mind the desired shape of the nose after surgery, and accordingly decide the shape and thickness of each region of the implant, and determine how to harmonize the relationship between the nasal dorsum and tip depending on the method of tip surgery. Furthermore, the surgeon must consider the implant's length, width, angle in the radix area, and shape of cross-sections of each area.

For proper carving of the silicone implant, not only the external shape of the nose, but also each patient's anatomical characteristics of the bony and cartilaginous part should be well understood by the surgeon. Radiological examination such as cephalogram or nasal bone view taken before surgery provides the required information *(Figure 1)*.

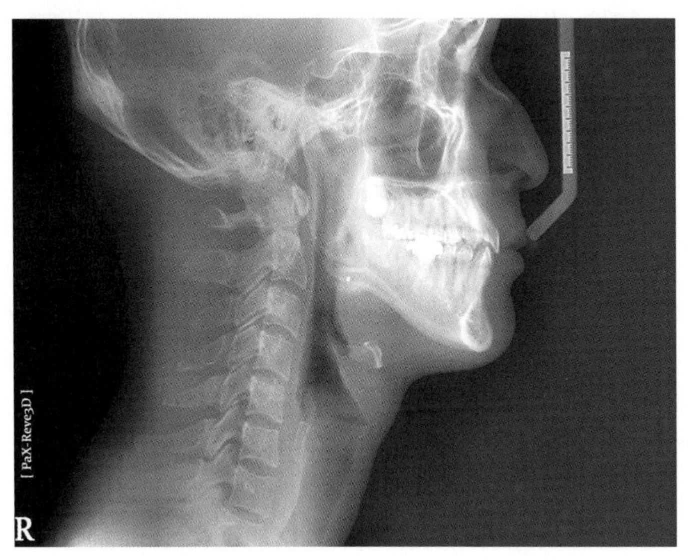

Figure 1 Cephalogram taken before surgery.

Radiological examination can reveal the degree of anterior projection of the nasal bone, shape of nasofrontal angle, and the soft tissue thickness at the different nasal regions. In cases of revision rhinoplasty, the shape and thickness of the inserted implant can be known beforehand by radiologic examination. It is also possible to make a plaster model of the patient's nose or use a three-dimensional surface scan to preoperatively design the implant. Radiological examination therefore can help with general surgical planning, but since it cannot accurately show internal anatomical structures (skin and soft tissue thickness of each region, bony structure or convexity, etc.) of the nose, precise carving based only on a plain radiograph is difficult and further modification is required during surgery.

Rather than using prefabricated and uniformly shaped implants, it is sometimes better to use custom implants for each patient. Silicone implants can be carved during surgery by using a #15 surgical blade, surgical scissors, carving knives, or sterilized razors. It is also possible to shape the implant before surgery using a milling machine and then sterilize the implant before usage. There are various implant designs *(Figure 2)*, and the general precautions in designing the implant are described below.

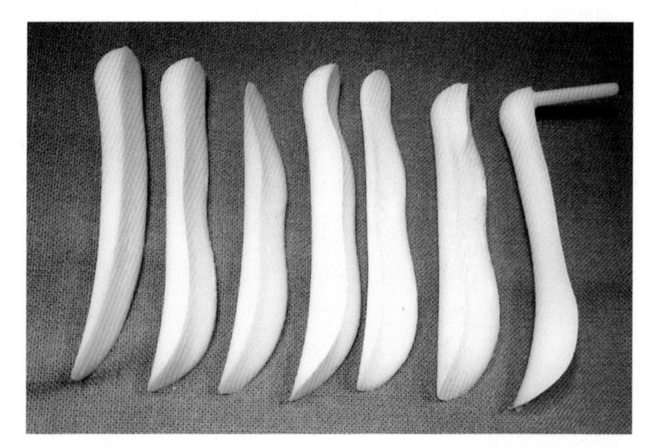

Figure 2 Different types of silicone implants

In the radix, precisely locate the thickest part of the implant's proximal area, or depending on the anatomical variation, the upper end of the implant in the deepest part of the nasofrontal angle. In the area where the nose connects to the forehead, keep the implant's margin from being too long and taper the margin smoothly. Especially for patients who have a wide nasofrontal angle and exhibit a gentle transition, be careful not to raise the glabella too high, and shape the cephalic end of the implant very thinly, so that the radix shows a gentle curve.

The nasal starting point (nasion) should be formed at somewhere between the mid-pupillary line and double eyelid line based on the patient's desired nasal height and initial shape. But it is usually acceptable to adjust the level of nasion to be formed around the level of upper eyelashes *(Figure 3)*.

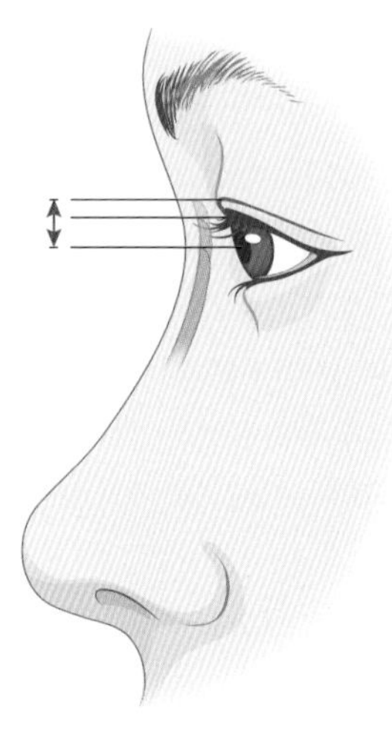

Figure 3 The nasal starting point. It should be formed at somewhere between the mid-pupillary line and double eyelid line based on the patient's desired nasal height and initial shape.

When modifying the shape of the implant, most cases require the implant's thickness to decrease and become concave around the rhinion, because the nasal bone protrudes the most in that area. If the convexity of the rhinion area is not that prominent and nasal tip is relatively well projected, a substantial modification of the implant around the rhinion might not be necessary. The nasal skeleton, composed of the nasal bone and cartilage, is low in the nasion, protrudes the most in rhinion area, and becomes lower again at the anterior septal angle. Therefore, the implant's shape must become thinner in rhinion and slightly thicker as it approaches the anterior septal angle, with the level of thickness depending on the anatomy of the individual patient *(Figure 4)*.

The lower part of nasal dorsum, the part that carries through to the alar cartilage and dome of the tip, from the anterior septal angle area, is an area that requires great care in order to create a smooth, ideal line from the dorsum to the tip without any gaps. Implant design of this area differs depending on each different tip surgery technique *(Figure 5)*.

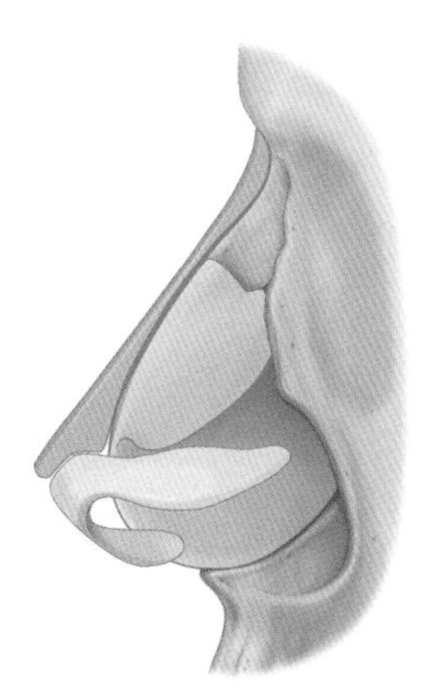

Figure 4 The implant's shape must become thinner in rhinion and slightly thicker as it approaches the anterior septal angle.

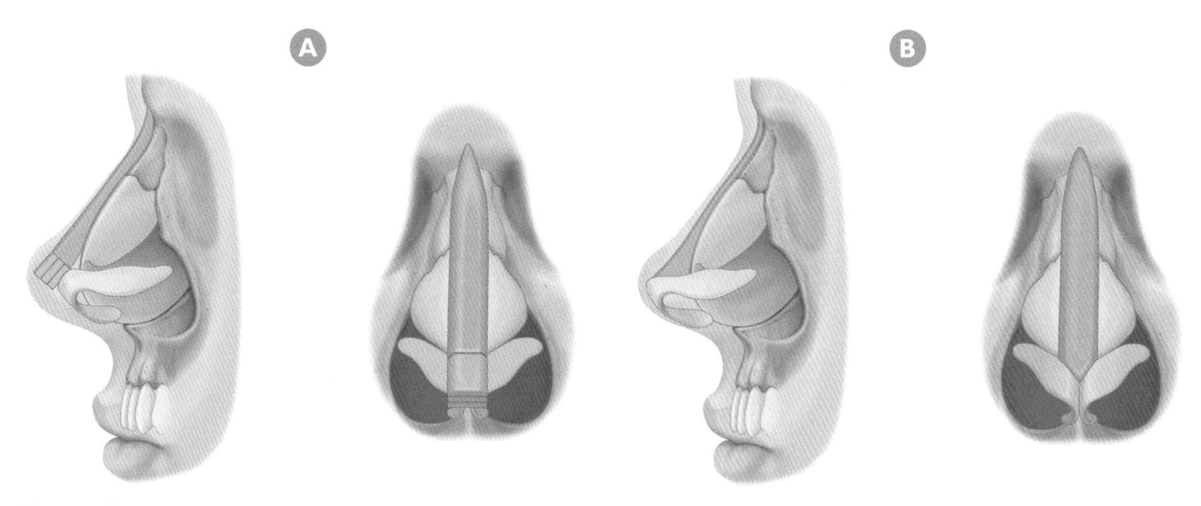

Figure 5 Implant design of the lower part differs depending on the tip surgery technique. Implant design for tip onlay graft (A) and for without tip grafting (B).

Following these general precautions could still create differences between the expected shape of the nose—influenced by the thickness or elasticity of patient's skin soft tissue envelope and tip support strength—and actual external shape. Therefore, in an open rhinoplasty approach, the surgeon must repeat the maneuver of covering the implant with the skin soft tissue envelope by temporary closure, and adjust the thickness of implant before final closure of the transcolumellar incision. The shape of the implant varies greatly according to patient's nasal anatomy or the surgeon's preferences, and while each situation might require appropriate modification, the generally recommended conformations are the following:

1. Caudal End of the Implant Reaching the Cephalic Divergence of the Alar Cartilages

This type of implant is used when there is considerable difference in height between the anterior septal angle and the alar cartilages, or when a septal extension graft has been used for anterior projection of alar cartilage. The caudal end of the implant is located in the space between anterior septal angle and alar cartilage, creating a smooth transition between the nasal dorsum and the nasal tip. The caudal end of the implant is carved in a sharp, angulated shape to fit the cephalic divergence of the alar cartilages, and is fixed to the surrounding cartilage tissue using sutures *(Figure 6)*.

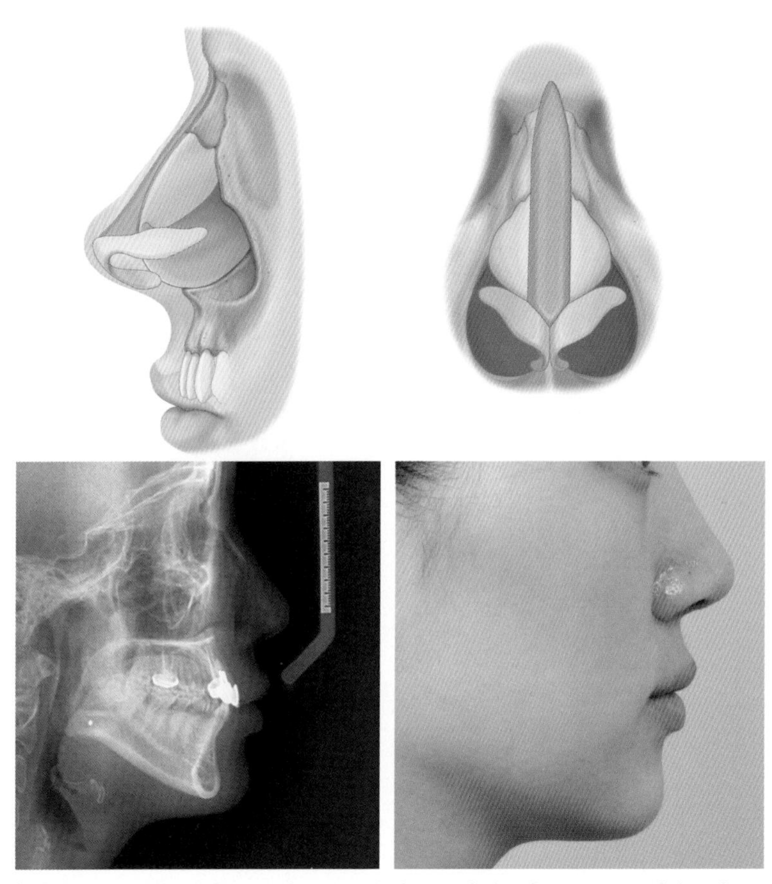

Figure 6 Silicone implant designed to reach the cephalic divergence of the alar cartilages.

The main advantage of this type is that it is easy to create a smooth transition from the nasal dorsum to the nasal tip by adjusting the thickness of the caudal end of the implant depending on the degree of projection of the nasal tip. However, this fact also means that it is difficult to make the nasal dorsum high when there is insufficient tip projection. Furthermore, if tip projection is inadequate or if nasal tip deprojection occurs over time, the prominence of the implant's end could be visible and the connection between nasal dorsum and tip could slightly depress, thus giving the nose an unnatural dorsal line. A slightly modified form of giving the implant's end a slight angle, starting from anterior septal angle area, and thinning it gradually can be used to surface the implant's tip above the alar cartilage. This method is helpful in rhinoplasty that raises nasal dorsum without tip plasty *(Figure 7)*.

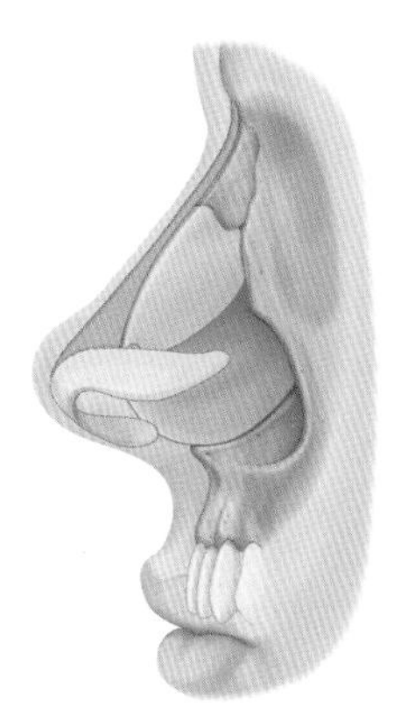

Figure 7 Silicone implant designed to be placed over the domal portion of the alar cartilages at its distal end.

2. Caudal End of the Implant Connecting Directly to the Tip Onlay Graft

This type connects the implant's caudal end directly to the tip onlay graft without any gaps, and the implant's end differs in thickness according to the height of the onlay tip graft and number of layers. This type is especially helpful when using a tip onlay graft as the main method of tip projection, as it gives a smooth transition between nasal dorsum and tip, free of gaps. This method lets the surgeon easily customize the thickness of the caudal end of the implant depending on the overall height of the tip onlay graft *(Figure 8)*.

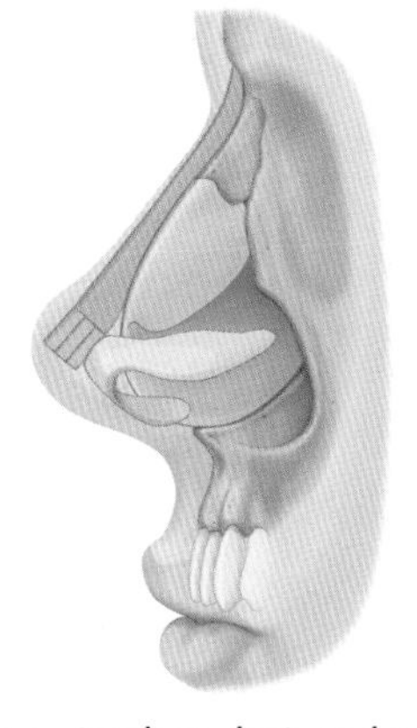

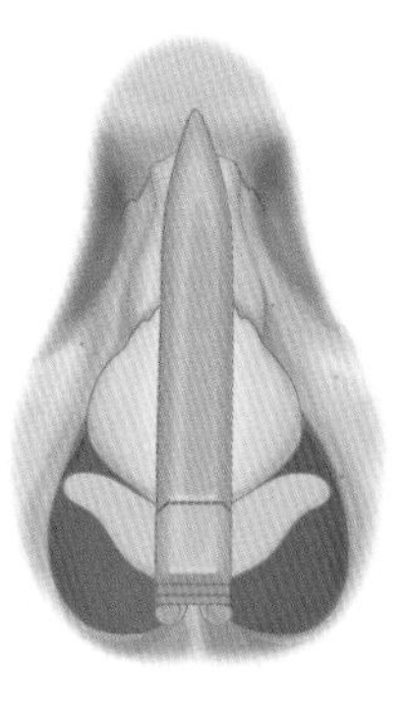

Figure 8 Silicone implant designed to come in direct contact with a tip onlay graft.

This type may keep the implant afloat in the nasal dorsum in the anterior septal angle area, and while theoretically this phenomenon may pose problems in that the potential dead space could increase the possibility of postoperative infections or implant movement, serious problems do not arise due to the formation of the fibrous tissue around the implant filling up the dead space over time.

Stacking tip onlay grafts to improve tip projection has side effects such as too much lengthening of the infratip lobule and creating an unnatural nasal tip shape, so the surgeon must precisely modify the height and shape of the onlay graft to get a more natural-looking tip shape. In an open rhinoplasty setting, trimming the implant into the precise length in which its caudal end meets exactly with the onlay graft without disconnection, temporarily inserting the implant to measure the length that puts it in the desired location, then cuting off the caudal end overlapping with the length covered by the onlay graft can be done later.

A simpler type would be to make the implant reach the caudal end of nasal tip and place one or two layers of autologous cartilage in the form of an onlay or shield graft over the caudal or upper part of the caudal end of the silicone implant *(Figure 9)*.

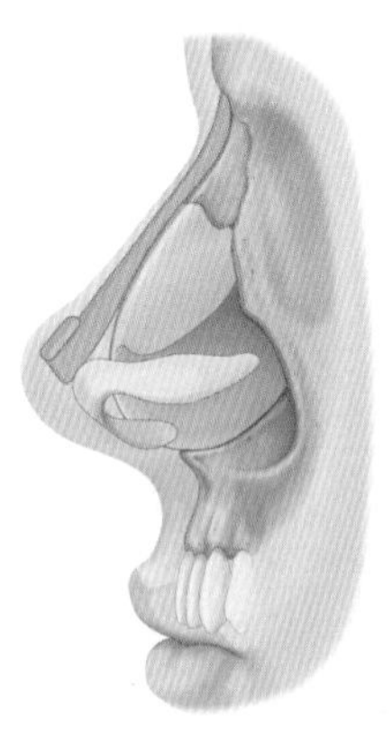

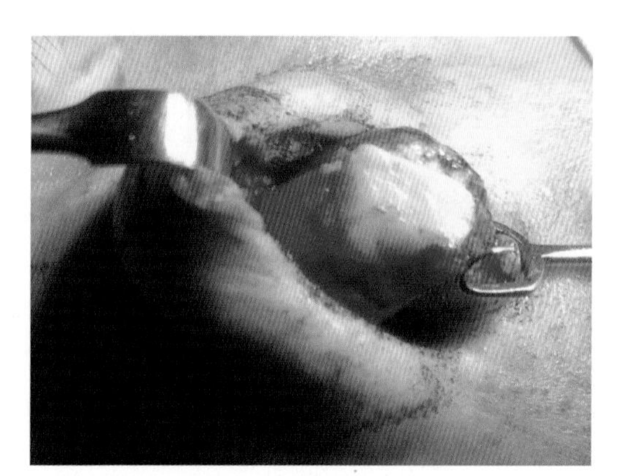

Figure 9 Silicone implant with tip onlay graft on the top of the caudal end. This can create an over-rotated looking nose.

This method utilizes the thickness of the implant's caudal end to adjust the height of nasal tip, and uses autologous cartilage as a supplement to reduce risks of damaging the nasal tip skin due to direct contact with the implant. However, the autologous cartilage used over the silicone is likely to cause visible tip graft contour, and the thick silicone makes the infratip lobule too big for the tip to look natural. Furthermore, although the tip height increases, its proportional length remains the same, thus giving the nose an over-rotated look.

3. L-Shaped Silicone

This type is used to raise both the nasal tip and dorsum using silicone. When using the L-shape implant, if the surgeon gives the tip too much tension in hopes of achieving a tent-pole effect, the skin of the nasal tip could become too thin in the long term. Therefore, many cases involves using autologous cartilage over the implant's bending area, and the silicone that is placed in the tip can be replaced with a softer silicone. Furthermore, to avoid excessive tension on the skin, implants with a slightly shorter vertical segment are also used *(Figure 10)*.

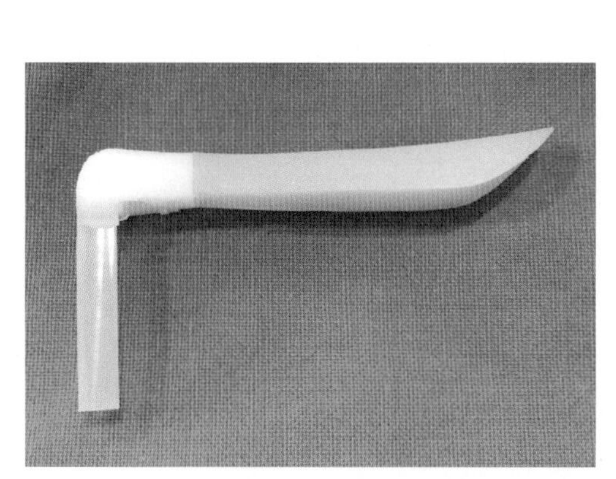
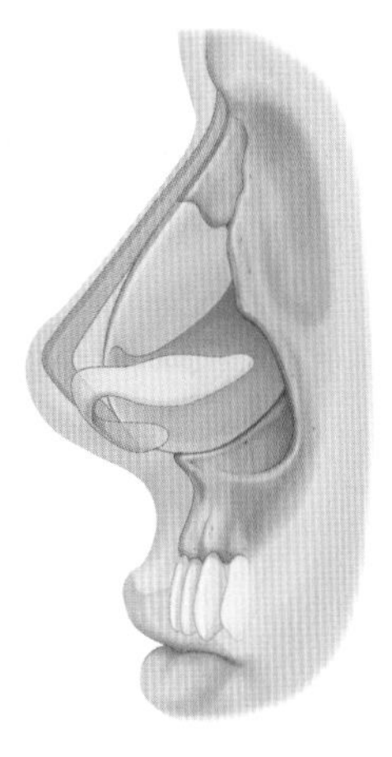

Figure 10 L-shaped silicone.

This type is advantageous in that it improves the dorsum and tip shape relatively swiftly and at once without any transcolumellar incision, and it could provide very satisfactory results in properly selected patients. However, this method is inadequate to make the nose look longer, thus giving an over-rotated look, and is inappropriate for patients with short noses or with cephalic rotation of the nasal tip. Another limitation is the thick and unnatural shape of infratip lobule it creates *(Figure 11)*.

Additionally, the vertical segment of L-shape implant could result in columellar asymmetry by

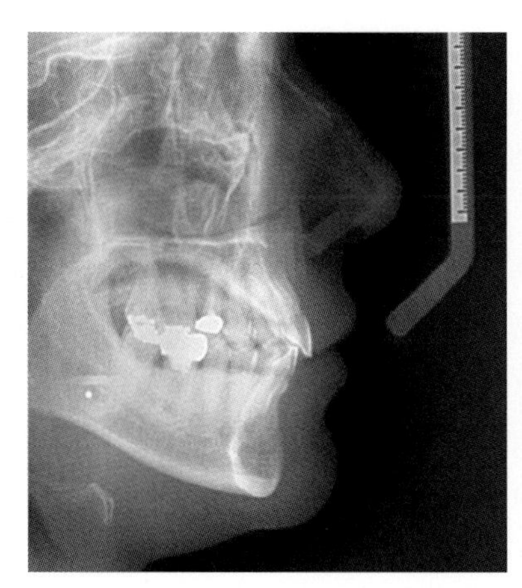
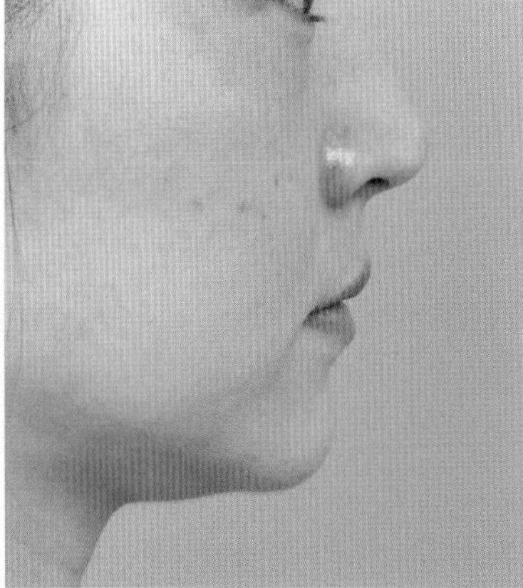

Figure 11 A patient showing unnatural-looking infratip lobule due to L-shaped silicone implant.

inducing damage or deformation of the lower lateral cartilages, and forming fibrous capsules and scar tissue around the implant. This deformity is notably difficult to correct. In the long term, a rocking phenomenon or see-saw phenomenon could gradually decrease the tip height, creating a very unnatural look after surgery *(Figure 12)*.

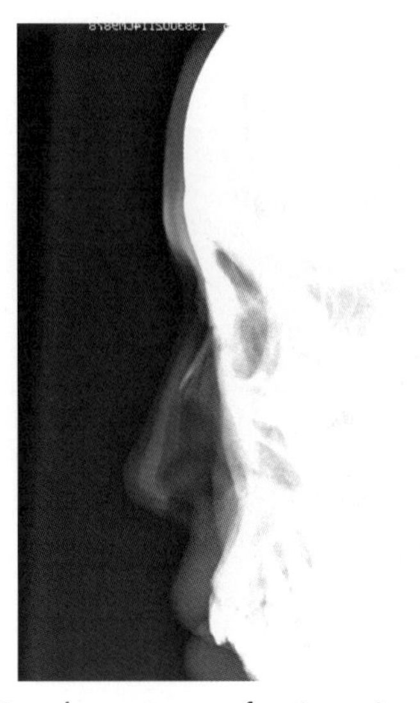

Figure 12 Rocking phenomenon after insertion of L-shaped silicone.

V. Complications

Although silicone is chemically inert, this fact does not necessarily mean inertness in the body. In the past, silicone gel injections were sometimes used for augmentation. Silicone gel is used for injections, and is composed of 20-60 μm particles. Particles of this size can be engulfed by macrophage, resulting in death of the macrophage and causing granulomatous inflammation. Furthermore, gel particles could spread to the lymph nodes, brain, kidney, liver, and lungs. If leaked through the injection area, it forms masses surrounded by granulomas or capsules, becoming palpable through the skin. However, these problems are not present in solid silicone rubber, thus solid implants are relatively much safer.

Negative perception to silicone implants for rhinoplasty is prevalent in the Western part of the world due to common complications of silicone implants. Ham, et al. (1983) reported a complication rate of 20.8% in about 1500 silicone implant rhinoplasty patients. On the contrary, Shirakabe, et al. (1985) reported only a 0.48% complication rate from 2500 such patients. This discrepancy demonstrates how complication rates differ greatly based on the surgeon's technique and experience. Generally reported complication rates are: 2-4% for extrusion, 4% for infection, and 3% for displacement. One study reported a 6.5% rate of implant removal. Interestingly enough, compared to various reports published in the 60s and 70s, recent studies show much lower rates of complications from silicone implants. These changes are thought to be due to improvements in implant design, conservative surgical techniques, surgeons having more experience, and use of softer silicone. Many surgeons in Asia perceive complication rates of silicone implant as acceptable, in part due to more experience with rhinoplasty using silicone implants compared to Western surgeons. Complications from silicone implants are largely divided into those caused by inherent traits of silicone itself and those from the surgeon's technical and judgmental errors. In order to enjoy successful surgical results, it is essential to minimize the unavoidable problems from inherent physical characteristics of this material, and to try every effort to reduce technical and judgmental errors.

1. Problems Caused by Inherent Physical Characteristics

1) Capsule Formation

Silicone has no holes on its smooth surface, so the surrounding tissue cannot penetrate the implant. Therefore, silicone is situated within a secluded space wrapped by a fibrous capsule *(Figure 13)*. In cases where complications such as contraction do not occur, the fibrous capsule prevents the implant from bonding with skin, prevents skin damage, and somewhat maintains thickness of the skin and soft tissue. The capsule can also fill the potential dead space created by the implant which is not in direct contact with the nasal dorsum. Thus, during revision, certain situations require incisions on or partial removal of the outer capsule to stretch the skin sufficiently. However, it is best to limit removal of the outer capsule (that is in direct contact with the skin) to prevent thinning of the skin and irregularities of the nasal dorsum caused by over-removal *(Figure 14)*.

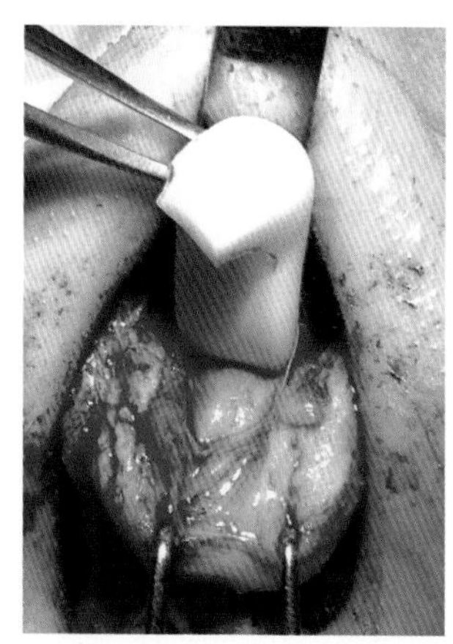

Figure 13 Silicone implant surrounded by capsule formation.

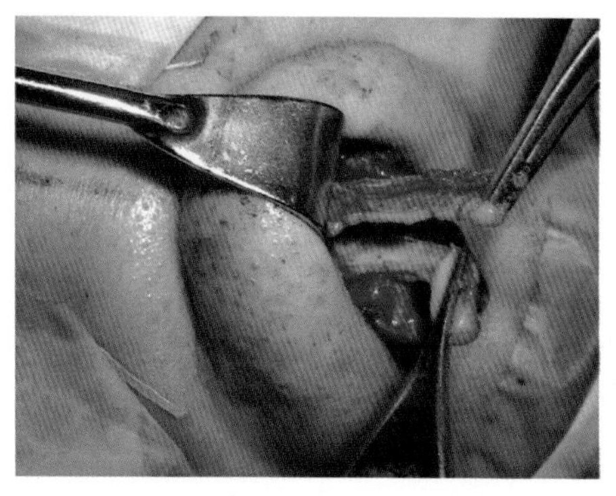

Figure 14 Intraoperative photo of outer capsule and inner capsule.

On the other hand, the fibrous capsule has a potential side effect of making the area susceptible to infection by preventing antibiotics from effectively penetrating the area around the implant, and by letting the silicone implant create a dead space within the capsule as it moves around inside.

In certain situations, the capsule causes severe complications, most notably contraction. In severe cases of contraction, a contracted nose could arise, and the implant could become deformed due to contraction of the asymmetric capsule. Formation of an excessively thick and wide capsule and contraction is known to be caused largely by bacterial infection, with individual immunologic status and excessive tissue damage known as additional factors.

To prevent over-production of capsule and its ensuing complications, the surgeon must take care not to let inflammation or infection occur during, or after the surgery, while minimizing tissue damage and hemorrhage during the operation. Reports say that irrigants containing antibiotics can reduce capsular contraction, and that prescribing anti leukotriene agents such as Zafirlukast can decrease capsule formation. Additionally, some claim that conducting allergic tests on silicone before surgery can also be beneficial.

2) Physical Stimulation and Damage

Over time, an implant can cause complications such as stimulating the skin making it thinner, damaging the skin and its appendages, causing skin contraction, and telangiectasias. The slight, yet repetitive damage caused by the solid implant can harm the mucous membranes creating chronic recurrrent inflammation, or small defect to induce bacterial infections from the nasal cavity. To minimize such physical damage from silicone implants, the implant should be designed to attach to the nasal dorsum and have close to zero movement, while having appropriate length and width to fit in the area it will occupy. Additionally, using a softer material for implantation can help reduce physical stimulation.

3) Calcification

When removing implanted silicone from the nasal dorsum after a long period of time, the surgeon may come across partial calcification of the silicone *(Figure 15)*. There are many theories speculating on the mechanisms of surface calcification in silicone implants: saturation of calcium ions due to the negative charge on the surface of silicone, discharge of intracellular calcium ions due to tissue damage, or scar tissue formation on the periosteum, or muscle tissue damage due to continuous friction. Calcified implants form a harder and rougher surface, increasing stimulation to the overlying skin, and letting the irregular surface show through the skin. Calcification has a tendency to become worse as time progresses. Efforts should be made to reduce mechanical stimulation and damage to the surrounding tissue since calcification is also related to such factors.

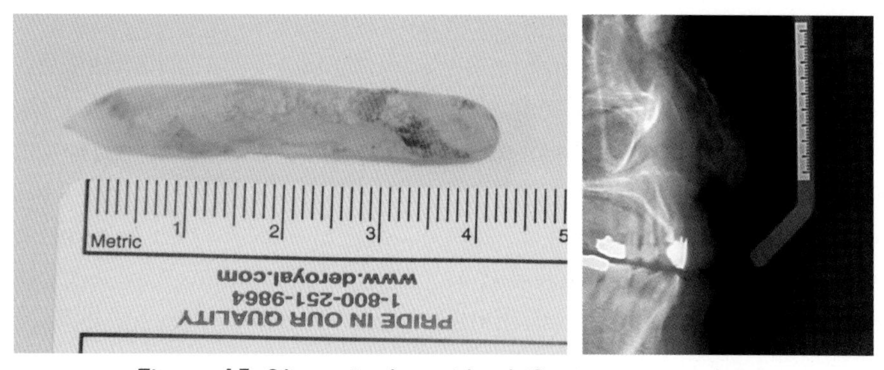

Figure 15 Silicone implant with calcification on its surface.

4) Immune Responses

There is debate regarding whether silicone causes autoimmune responses, and although it is uncertain for now, there have been reports of anti-silicone antibodies and induction of nonpecific autoimmune response against silicone. There is also a theory that patients with underlying diseases or high susceptibility to autoimmune diseases show autoimmune responses to silicone more frequently. What is clear is that silicone creates inflammatory fibrosis in the surrounding tissue, regardless of systemic or hematological immune function.

2. Other common complications

1) Extrusion

Extrusion rates of silicone implant varies from 0.48-50%, probably due to the differences in surgical technique, shape of implant, and the surgeon's level of expertise. In putting too much tension on the nasal tip skin with the intention of giving a tent-pole effect through the implant, especially in the L-shaped silicone that has a long columellar segment, the risk of both skin damage in the nasal tip and implant extrusion increases. Even with other types of silicone, if the implant reaches nasal tip or is too long, the nasal tip skin thins over time, and as a result there is the risk of implant extrusion *(Figure 16)*. The implant can also extrude into the nasal cavity through the mucous membrane due to inadequate fixation of the implant, mucous membrane damage from implant movement, or inflammation. Such implant extrusions can be easily prevented by appropriate trimming of implant length or tip surgery using autologous cartilage.

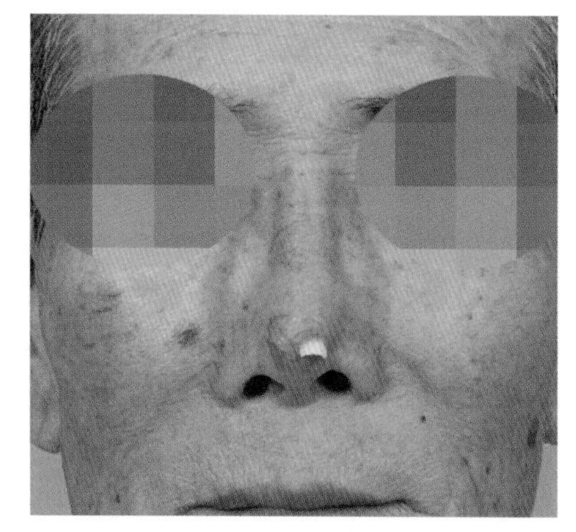

Figure 16 A patient showing extruded silicone implant through the nasal tip skin.

2) Implant Displacement, Movement

Implant deviation is a very common complication *(Figure 17)*. To prevent displacement of the implant, the implant should preferably be placed below the periosteum of the nasal bone, but since the periosteum is attached firmly to the bone and is easily torn, it is difficult to place the implant perfectly underneath the periosteum. Thus, it is actually common for implant to be inserted above the torn periosteum, but partial covering of implant can be expected during the healing process of periosteum. If it is inserted too superficially, the implant will move and show. Since silicone implants have a higher risk of movement compared to materials such as Gore-Tex (a material that is soft and porous on the surface), it is important to use a splint for precise fixation right after surgery, and to maintain it for about a week. It is also important to design the implant according to the patient's anatomical characteristics. For example, in cases of asymmetric nasal bones or a deviated nose, carving the bottom side of implant asymmetrically (thickness or width) to conform the slopped nasal bone can be helpful.

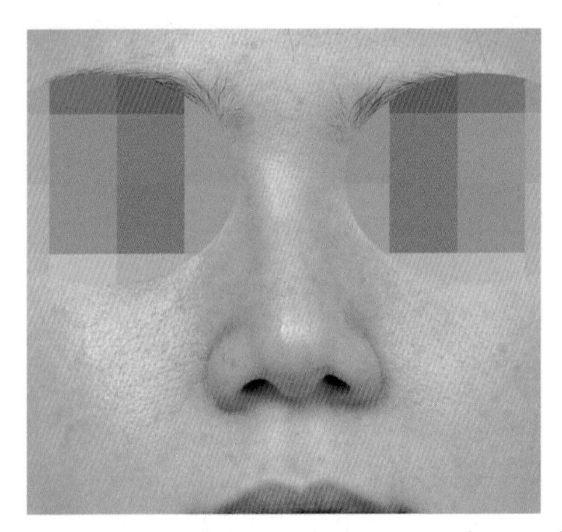

Figure 17 A patient having deviated silicone implant on her dorsum.

The radix in particular is prone to induce much more movement and malposition of implants. And since this area differs greatly for each patient, it is better to examine the patient's anatomical characteristics carefully before surgery. There is also a large difference between the radices of males and females. For female patients, the radix often has a smooth/gentle curve, thus requiring the implant to be carved with a gradual thinning towards the cephalic end, free of square ends. On the contrary, for male patients, the radix is much more prominent and shows a sharper nasofrontal angle, thus the implant should be designed accordingly. Furthermore, in the glabella, it is important to keep the cephalic end of the implant from overly extending into the forehead and to keep the implant margin from looking prominent.

Creating a pocket of the appropriate size is also important. The risk of implant displacement is higher if the space to be implanted with is too large. The same applies for spaces that are too small where the implant is placed unstably, becoming deviated, and moves. Implant deviation due to an asymmetric pocket creation is more common in rhinoplasty using an endonasal approach than in those using an open approach. The implant pocket is created by setting the median line as the center, and dissecting adequately (to be only a little larger than the implant) and symmetrically. In order to prevent implant displacement, making several holes in the implant or making cuts on its edge to prevent its movement may be helpful. However, some claim that it may not be helpful for short-term fixation immediately after surgery when implant movement is high, or that it may cause delayed hematoma due to hemorrhaging from implant movement triggered by the irregularly formed fibrous capsule around the implant.

Anatomically, the nasal dorsum is most protruded at the rhinion. If this anatomical convexity does not match well with the undersurface of the implant, it can move like a rocking chair. Even with implants that seem to match well with the glabella right after surgery, the implant can rise in the glabella and the implant of nasal tip area can be pushed downwards, and be buried deep within tissue due to skin tension with tip support decreasing over time. This phenomenon is called a rocking phenomenon or a see-saw phenomenon *(Figure 12)*.

If there is constant movement of the implant, chronic skin irritation and chronic inflammation can occur. It can also cause thinning of skin and resorption of nasal bone below the implant due to physical/mechanical irritation. Pressure from postoperative hematoma can displace the implant, and the space created by the hematoma provides room for implant movement that can cause displacement. In the long term, the implant can also become deviated due to capsule contraction.

For patients with facial asymmetry, the implant can look deviated according to the angle of perception, despite successful placement of implant; furthermore, if the nasal dorsum becomes higher following dorsal augmentation, the preexisting facial asymmetry could be perceived more easily. Therefore, sufficient explanation about this possibility should be given to the patient before surgery. However, since facial asymmetry can be considered quite common when taking into account slight asymmetry, it is not that special a case, and in such situations the implant should be inserted to create a nasal dorsum looking as straight as possible. Rather than setting the implant in the middle of the glabella, aligning it vertically with the center of nasal tip gives a straighter look.

3) Infection

Alloplastic implants are susceptible to infection, and when infected, exhibits typical signs such as erythema, swelling, and purulent secretions *(Figure 18)*. However, temporary erythema and swelling in the form of subclinical infections can occur recurrently. Subclinical infections are thought to occur when the number of bacteria is low, or if bacteria lie on the surface of silicone in the form of biofilm *(Figure 19)*.

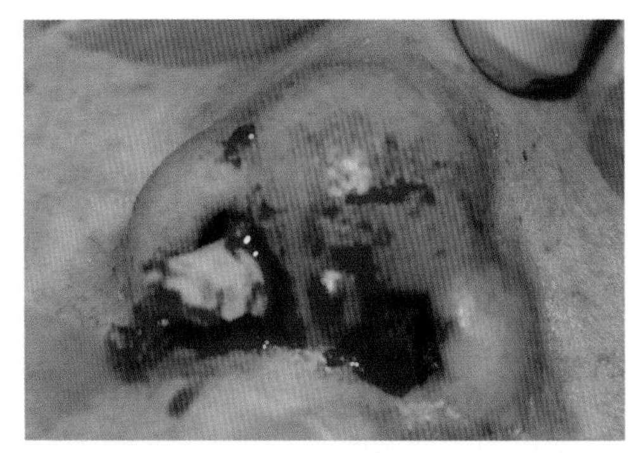

Figure 18 Intraoperative photo of silicone removal extruded through the nasal cavity.

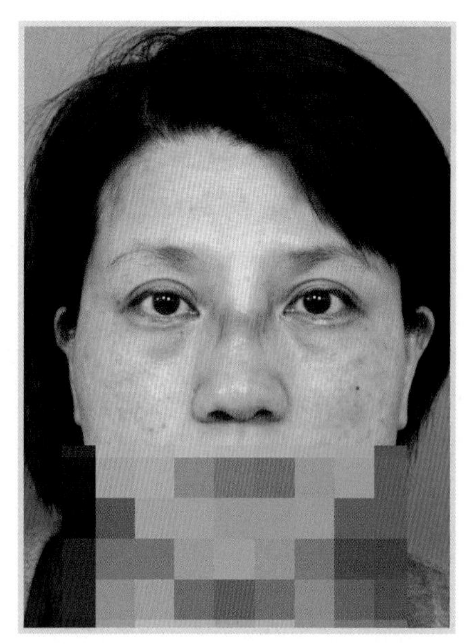

Figure 19 Silicone-induced subclinical infection manifesting as recurrent erythema on the nasal dorsum.

Thorough sterilization of the surgical field is necessary for reducing infection, especially in the nasal vestibule and the nasal cavity. Inserting gauze soaked in antiseptic solution further inside of the nasal cavity to separate the already sterilized nasal inlet area from the inner space during surgery is also helpful. It is also better to isolate the area around the mouth from the surgical field using a mask or sterilized gauze. During surgery, it is important to prevent the breakage of natural barriers such as a mucous membrane injury. A lengthy surgical time that can increase the risk of infections should be avoided. Though osteotomy is not contraindicated during augmentation using silicone implants, in cases that involve a significant modification of the normal anatomical structure like osteotomies, infection should be a chief concern. An implant that was carved during surgery should be immersed in sterilizing solution before implantation, and it is helpful to sterilize the surgical field again, or to change surgical gloves before handling or inserting the implant.

4) Using Overly Hard Silicone

A hard implant causes minute and repetitive damage to the skin or nasal mucosa, has a higher risk of inducing skin changes, chronic inflammation, or infection. Thus, choosing a softer type of silicone can be helpful. Soft silicone had good elasticity and form restoration, but can become slightly curved following insertion due to pressure from the soft tissue of nasal dorsum, thus it is relatively more difficult to create the desired nasal shape.

5) Aesthetically Improper Implant Designs

Improper aesthetic designs include: too narrow or too wide, too long or too short, too square or

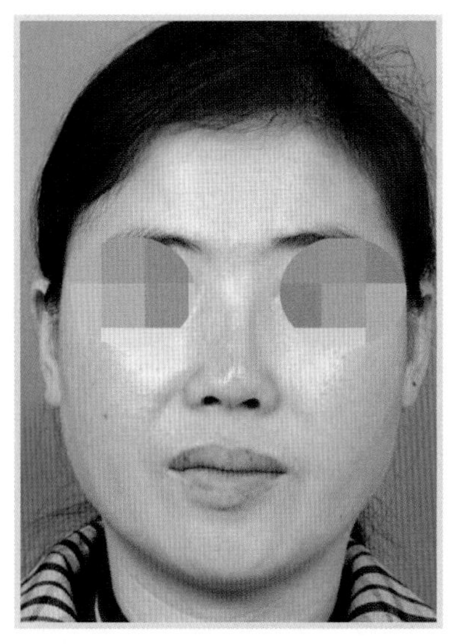

Figure 20 A patient showing undesirable aesthetic effect by a narrow and deviated dorsal implant.

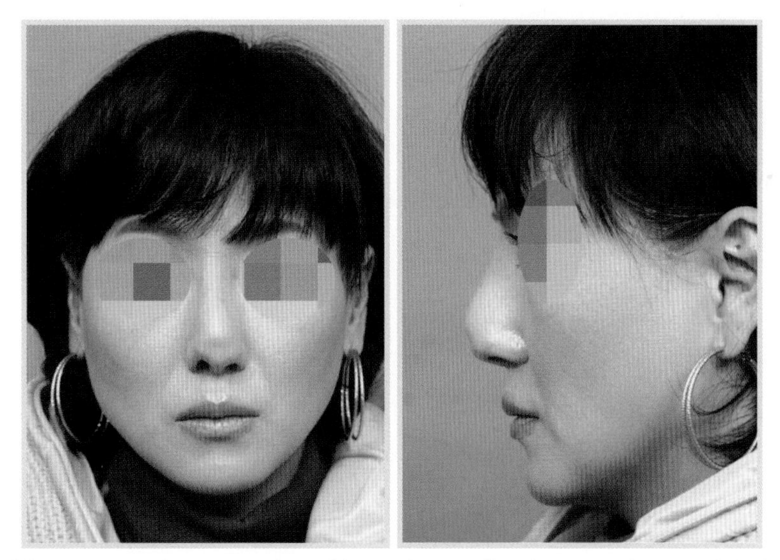

Figure 21 A patient showing undesirable aesthetic effect by a too short and thick implant.

prominent edges, too thin or too thick, rough edges or surfaces, and incompatible with patient's desired aesthetic goal *(Figures 20, 21).*

One of the most common mistakes is the implant being too thick in the radix, creating an obtuse nasofrontal angle and giving a strong/prominent, unnatural, and artificial look. This point should be considered especially for patients with a high radix and gentle slope.

If the implant is too thick or wide, or has an inadequately tapered margin, the implant's outline can become visible through the skin as if there is a stick under the nasal skin. An overly narrow implant also makes the implant visible and appears unnatural. The width of the implant should normally be 7-8 mm, but can be varied to a 6-10 mm range depending on the patient's wishes.

For patients with a convex dorsum, rather than trying to conceal the hump with implant pieces, the surgeon should reduce the hump as smoothly as possible to the maximum point allowed, while keeping an open roof to a minimum. Then the surgeon makes the nasal dorsum appear smooth by making the implant thinner in the hump region to accommodate for the remaining protrusion. Anatomically, the rhinion is the most protruded area in the nasal dorsum, so it is better to make the middle section of implant concave or moderately thinner even if there is no prominent hump. For some cases, it is also helpful to reduce the projection of nasal bone by gentle rasping. If there is a hump with a low radix and tip, raise the radix and tip first, then design the implant accordingly.

VI. Conclusion

Dorsal augmentation using silicone is an essential part of Asian rhinoplasty, and can bring about excellent aesthetic outcomes with relative ease. Though there are disadvantages due to the inherent characteristics of the implant such as the risk of infection, most complications are caused by the surgeon's judgmental or technical errors, and such errors can be minimized through learning and experience. Therefore, a rhinoplasty surgeon must fully understand, and be able to handle silicone implants. In order to obtain the best results using silicone implants, meticulous surgical planning and aesthetically appropriate implant design is crucial, along with mastery of the various tip surgery techniques.

References

1. Ahn J, Honrado C, Horn C. Combined silicone and cartilage implants: augmentation rhinoplasty in Asian patients. Arch Facial Plast Surg 2004; 6: 120-3.
2. Berghaus A, Stelter K. Alloplastic materials in rhinoplasty. Curr Opin Otolaryngol Head Neck Surg 2006; 14: 270-7.
3. Hong JP, Yoon JY, Choi JW. Are polytetrafluoroethylene (Gore-Tex) implants an alternative material for nasal dorsal augmentation in Asians?. J Craniofac Surg 2010; 21: 1750-4.
4. Jang YJ, Moon BJ. State of the art in augmentation rhinoplasty: implant or graft?. Curr Opin Otolaryngol Head Neck Surg 2012; 20: 280-6.
5. Lam SM, Kim YK. Augmentation rhinoplasty of the Asian nose with the"bird" silicone implant. Ann Plast Surg 2003; 51: 249-56.
6. Lee MR, Unger JG, Rohrich RJ. Management of the nasal dorsum in rhinoplasty: a systematic review of the literature regarding technique, outcomes, and complications. Plast Reconstr Surg 2011; 128: 538e-50e.
7. Peled ZM, Warren AG, Johnston P, Yaremchuk MJ. The use of alloplastic materials in rhinoplasty surgery: a meta-analysis. Plast Reconstr Surg 2008; 121: 85e-92e.
8. Sajjadian A, Naghshineh N, Rubinstein R. Current status of grafts and implants in rhinoplasty: Part II. Homologous grafts and allogenic implants. Plast Reconstr Surg 2010; 125: 99e-109e.
9. Tham C, Lai YL, Weng CJ, Chen YR. Silicone augmentation rhinoplasty in an Oriental population. Ann Plast Surg 2005; 54: 1-5.
10. Wang TD. Multicenter evaluation of subcutaneous augmentation material implants. Arch Facial Plast Surg 2003; 5: 153-4.
11. Wang JH, Lee BJ, Jang YJ. Use of silicone sheets for dorsal augmentation in rhinoplasty for Asian noses. Acta Otolaryngol Suppl 2007; 558: 115-20.
12. Zeng Y, Wu W, Yu H, Yang J, Chen G. Silicone implant in augmentation rhinoplasty. Ann Plast Surg 2002; 49: 495-9.

Case 1

A 23-year-old female visited for a flat nose deformity.

Analysis

Frontal: Flat nose, wide bony dorsum
Basal: Wide alar base, broad tip
Lateral: Underprojected tip

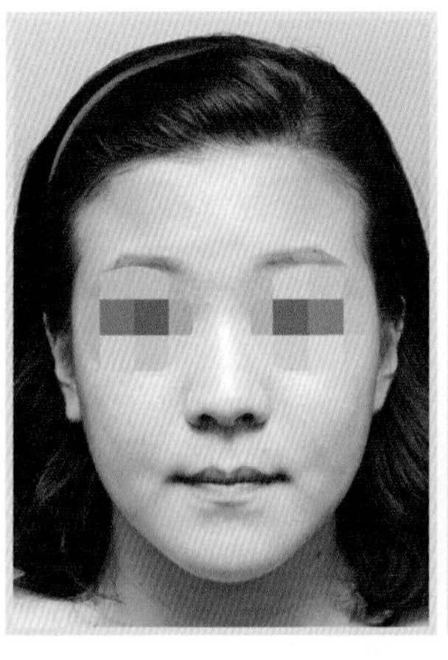
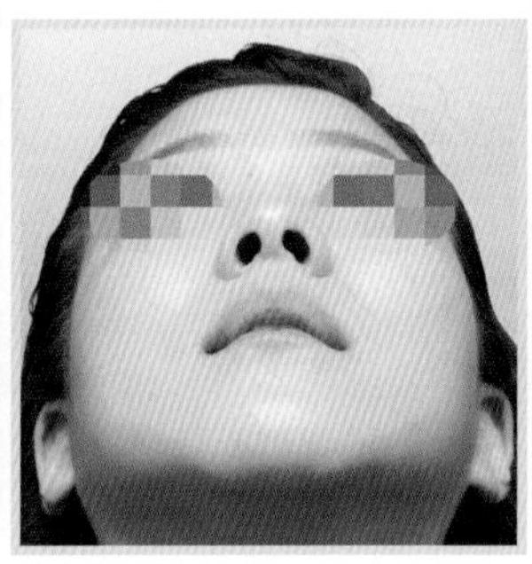
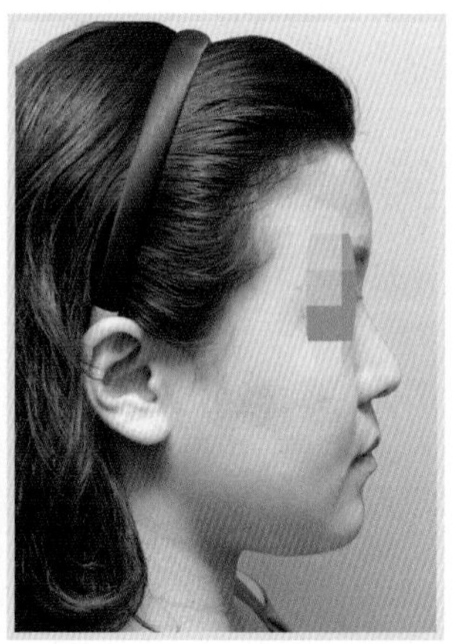

Operative Procedures

Open rhinoplasty approach
Conchal cartilage harvest
Septal cartilage harvest
Medial and percutaneous lateral osteotomies
Septal extension grafting (anterior extension type)
Stacked onlay tip grafting using conchal cartilage
Rim grafting (bilateral) fixed to tip graft
Shield grafting
Dorsal augmentation using silicone
Alar base resection (bilateral)

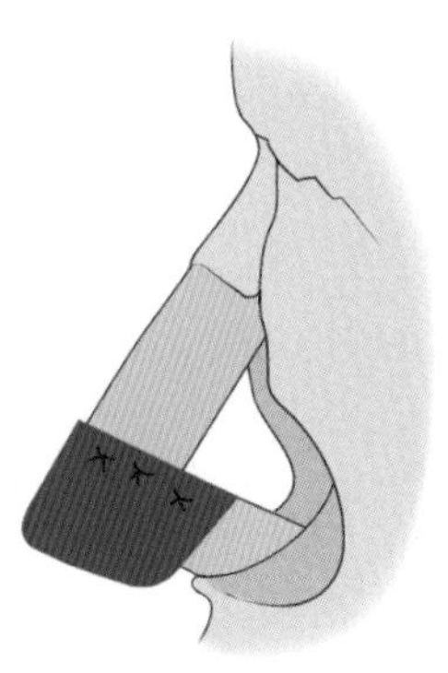
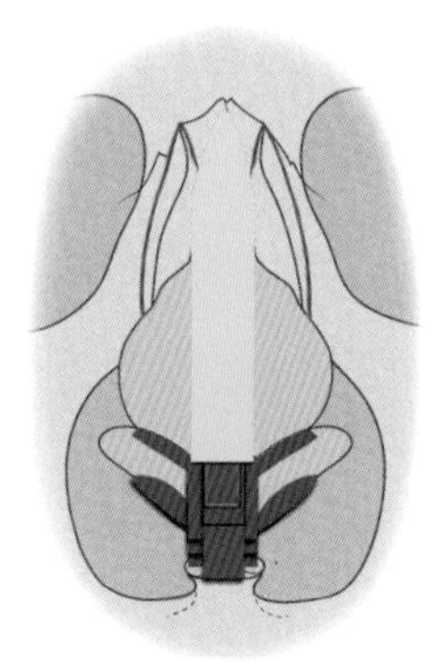
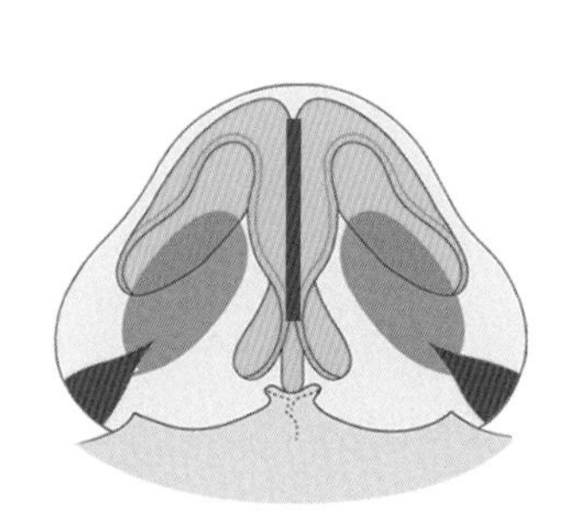
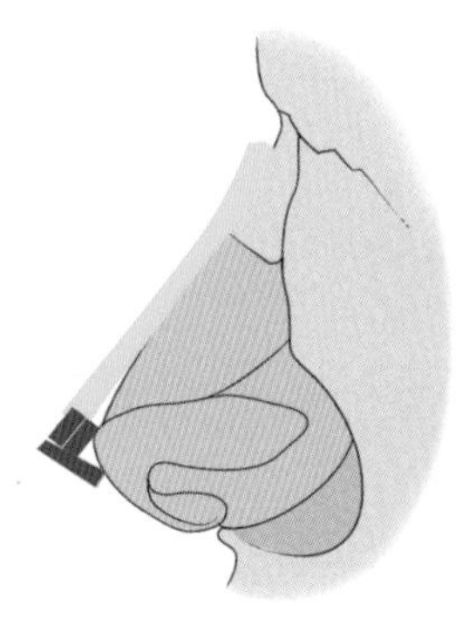

Postoperative Changes

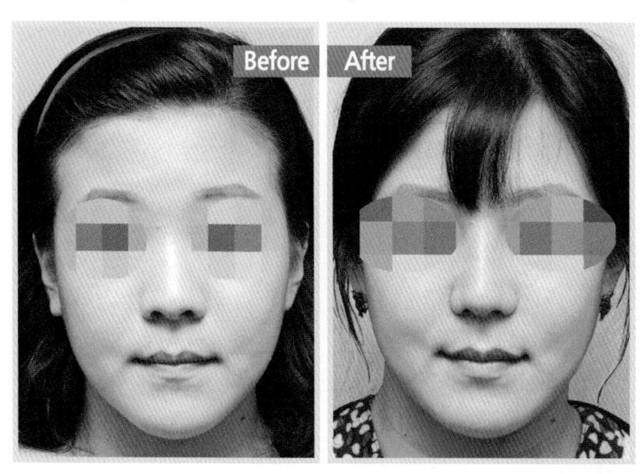

Frontal: Dorsal contour was improved. Dorsal width and alar base width were reduced. Nostril show was decreased by the rim graft shield graft and alar base resection.

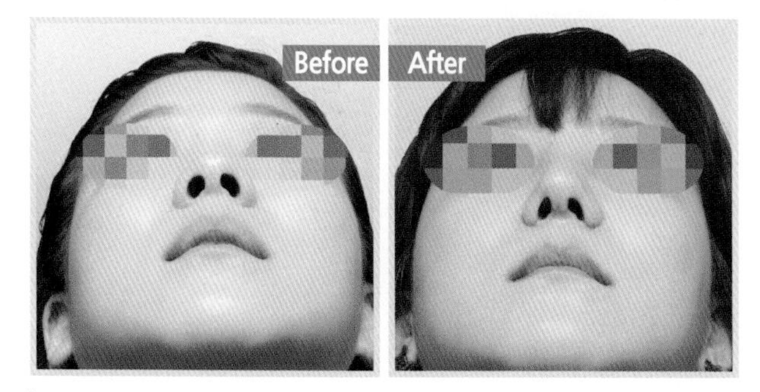

Basal: Tip projection was increased. Tip definition was improved. Alar base width was reduced.

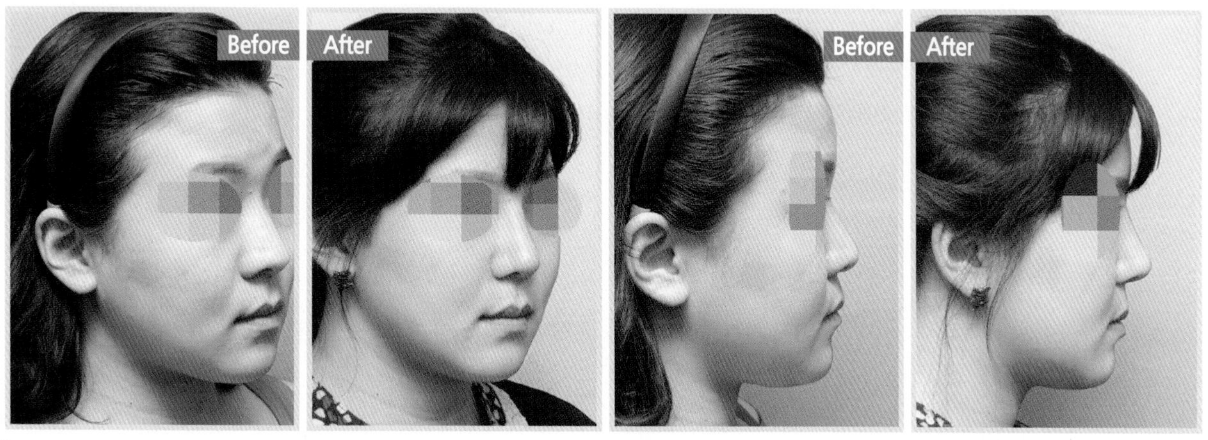

Lateral and Oblique: Dorsal height was augmented. Tip definition and projection were improved. Balanced facial profile was achieved through an improvement of dorsal aesthetic lines.

Case 2

A 22-year-old female visited for a hump nose deformity.

Analysis Frontal: Narrow midvault, mildly deviated nose (C-shaped)
Basal: Underprojected, pointed tip with nostril asymmetry associated with facial asymmetry
Lateral: hump nose

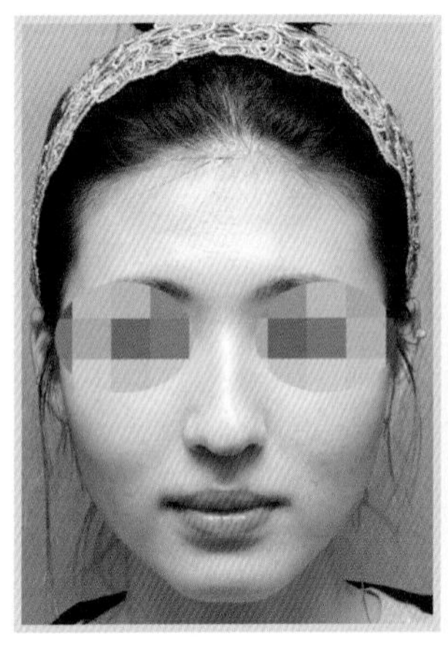
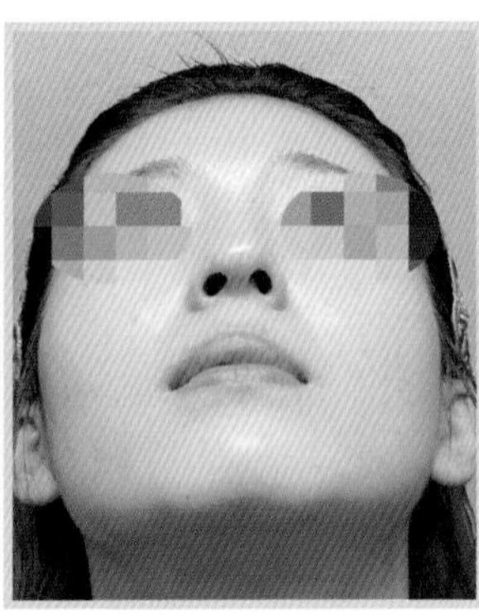
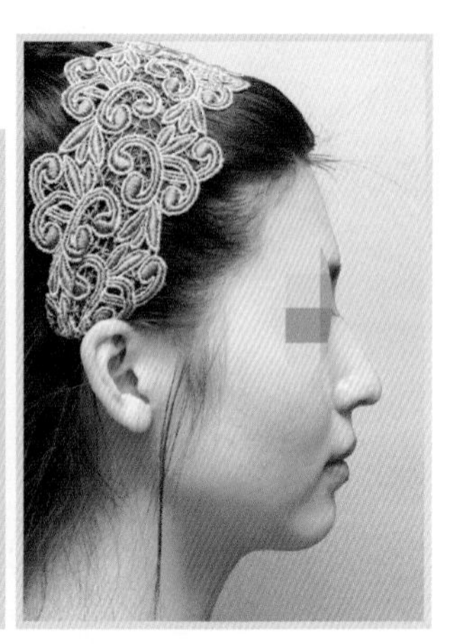

Operative Procedures

Open rhinoplasty approach
Conchal cartilage harvest
Septal cartilage harvest, septoplasty, turbinoplasty
Hump resection
Spreader grafting (left)
Septal extension grafting (anterior extension type)
Stacked onlay tip grafting using conchal cartilage
Rim grafting (bilateral) fixed to tip graft
Dorsal augmentation using silicone

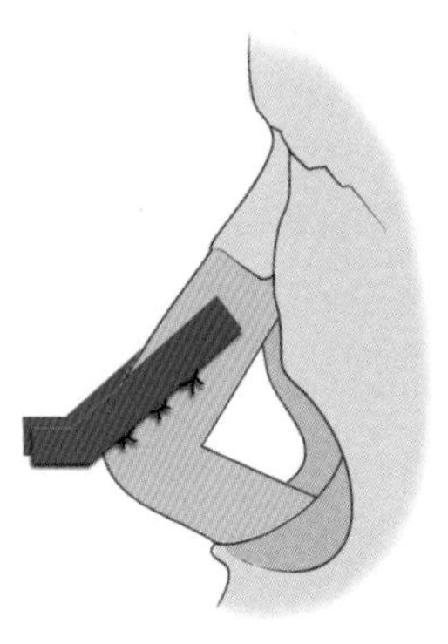
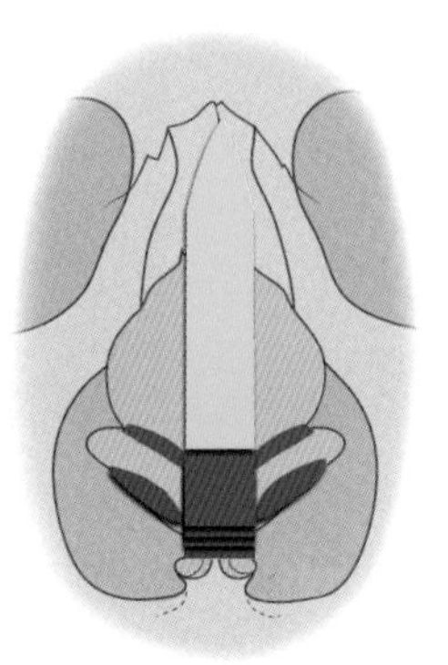
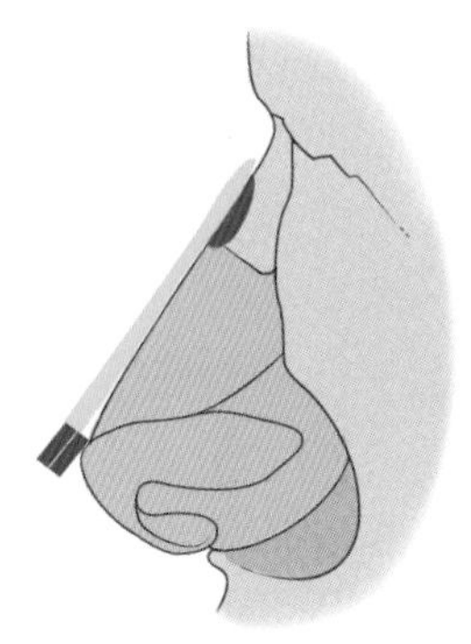

Postoperative Changes

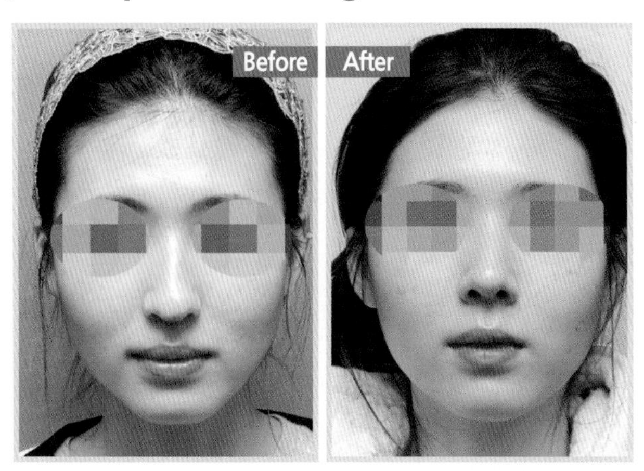

Frontal: Dorsal contour was improved. Midvault widening was obtained. C-shaped deviation was improved. Linear deviation remained due to the facial asymmetry. Tip definition, tip projection, and rotation were improved.

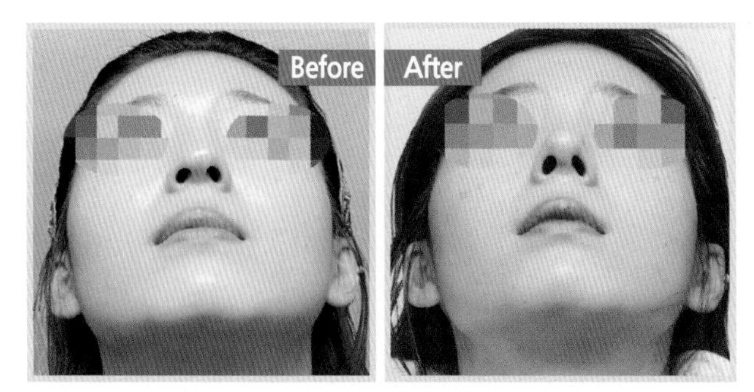

Basal: Tip projection and definition were improved. Nostril asymmetry was remained.

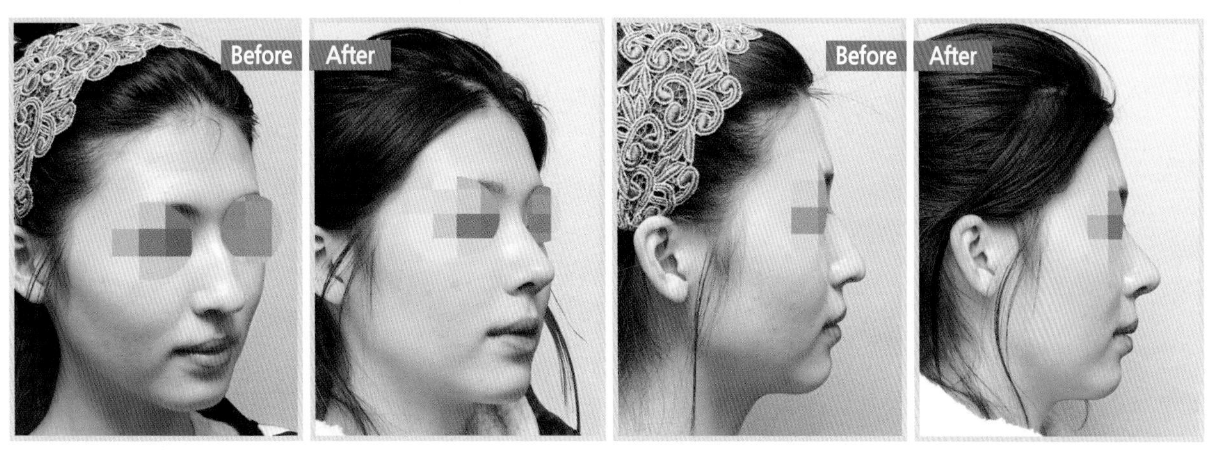

Lateral and Oblique: Profile was improved after hump removal. Tip projection and rotation were increased. Dorsal height of distal third was improved through dorsal augmentation. Supratip depression was corrected by tip projection and rotation. Proximal dorsal height showed no change.

Gore-Tex

Yong Gi Jung · Yong Ju Jang

I. History of Gore-Tex Usage

Expanded polytetrafluoroethylene (e-PTFE) is a synthetic material first created in 1969 that has a unique porous structure which gives it great waterproof properties without preventing air from passing through. It first received recognition as a substitute material for human tissue in 1972 after being used in cardiovascular surgery. Since then, it has become a common substitute for human tissue in various fields including cardiovascular surgery, urologic surgery, repair of hernias, and pediatric surgeries. Despite the millions of cases using e-PTFE in the human body, there has been no report of carcinogenesis, thus testifying on its safety.

Neel, et al. conducted animal testing in 1983 to assess the suitability of e-PTFE for facial plastic surgery, and published excellent results to opening e-TPFE usage in aesthetic surgery. In augmentation rhinoplasty, Rosthein and Jacobs were the first to publish cases using e-PTFE (1989). It has become a widely used material since the US Food and Drug Administration's (FDA) approval of its usage for facial plastic surgery and rhinoplasty in 1993.

II. Physical Properties

e-TPFE is a polymer created from a double bond between two carbon atoms that each have bonded with two fluorine atoms, and is expressed as (–CF2=CF2-)n. This polymer is pressure-molded with dyes under extreme pressure, creating a microporous structure of PTFE polymers (composed of PTFE nodules connected to PTFE microfibril). The resulting e-PTFE compound cannot be chemically degraded due to the strong bonds between carbon and fluorine, and is biologically inert. Such fluorine-carbon bonds cannot be broken by any biological enzyme, thus maintaining a high level of physical stability once inserted in the human body. Furthermore, the negatively charged fluorine acts as a barrier to lower the surface energy of the polymer, making it unlikely to bond with surrounding material. This electrical negativity of e-PTFE also keeps blood from penetrating and prevents blood clots.

The hydrophobic nature of e-TPFE grafts attracts proteins such as albumin, immunoglobulin G, fibrinogen, fibronectin, and proteoglycans to its surface once implanted. Such proteins aid fibroblast attachment with the implant which is beneficial for the structural support of the implant. An e-TPFE polymer has innumerable micropores, with each pore about 10-30 μm in size, with an average of 22μm *(Figure 1).*

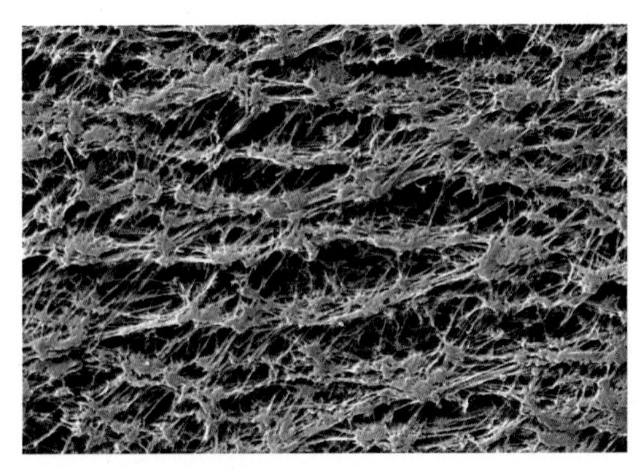

Figure 1 Expanded polytetrafluoroethylene (ePTFE). Scanning electron micrograph of Gore-Tex showing numerous micropores.

In general, bacteria can penetrate through most spaces larger than 1 μm in diameter, making the pores within e-PTFE susceptible to penetration and settlement of bacteria within the implant. In contrast, macrophages that play a crucial role in the body's defense system can only pass through spaces over 50 μm due to their much larger size. Theoretically, e-PTFE has a structure vulnerable to infection, since bacteria can pass but macrophages cannot. However, in clean surgeries such as primary rhinoplasty that often has environments with low bacterial concentration, micropores of such sizes are known to have no direct causal relationship with infection. On the other hand, in a contaminated surgical field with high bacterial concentration, the very porous e-PTFE can be susceptible to infection. Considering these facts, it is best not to use e-PTFE in areas with prior infection or contaminated surgical fields, and to immediately remove the implant if infection occurs.

The porous structure of e-PTFE also affects the interaction between the implant and the surrounding tissue. Fibroblasts and many other cells can penetrate through its micropores, and connective tissue such as fibrous tissue, collagen, and capillary vessels can grow into the implant over time. Such bonding keeps the graft firmly fixed to the surrounding tissue after being inserted into the nasal dorsum, preventing issues that could arise from implant movement and from interaction with surrounding tissue (such as excessive formation of capsules as with silicone implants).

Ideal conditions of alloplastic dorsal implants are the following:

- ☑ Biocompatibility

- ☑ No absorption or reduction of volume over time
- ☑ Easy to handle and carve
- ☑ No risk of inflammation or spreading disease
- ☑ Not too hard in order for it to naturally match with the patient's soft tissue

Based on many clinical trials, it can be said that e-TPFE has the ideal physical properties that meet most of the above conditions. It is not too hard like silicone (the most commonly used material in Asian rhinoplasty), thus is not as uncomfortable when inserted into the nasal dorsum, cannot be easily palpated through the skin, and can be carved and stacked into desired shapes and sizes due to the relative ease in handling. Furthermore, since light cannot pass through (unlike silicone), the nasal dorsum does not seem transparent under a strong light after surgery, thus looking more natural. However, although its distinctive porous structure gives the nose an initial softness, it can also make the graft become thinner over time. Reports state that the most widely used type of e-PTFE, Gore-Tex (W.L., Gore & Associated Flagstaff, AZ) sheets, have exhibited an average thickness decrease of 29% over time, with reduction rates positively correlated with original implant thickness. Therefore, dorsal augmentation using Gore-Tex sheets should take this factor into account before deciding on the height of implant. On the other hand, there are new e-PTFE products that do not decrease in thickness after insertion. PureForm 3D® (Surgiform Technology, Ltd., Lugoff, SC) and SFAM® (Surgiform Facial Augmentation Material) sheets are composed of 100% e-PTFE like Gore-Tex, but have a denser structure, thus can maintain their original thicknesses in the postoperative period.

III. Types of e-PTFE

As already mentioned, until recently, the most widely used e-PTFE product for dorsal augmentation was the Gore Subcutaneous Augmentation Material (SAM). However, further supply has come to a halt following Gore & Associate's decision to stop producing SAM as material for facial plastic surgery. Another type of e-PTFE material from Gore & Associates that can replace the Gore SAM is the Gore soft tissue patch. This material was developed to replace the membranous tissue loss in cardiac surgeries, hernia repairs, or urologic surgeries, and comes in thin sheets that can be cut and overlapped into implants of desired heights, making it suitable for use an the nasal dorsum. However, it is soft, thus is difficult to handle and can decrease in thickness after insertion. Furthermore, since it is thin, the surgeon must go through stacking procedure if he/she hopes to raise the height of dorsum significantly *(Figure 2)*.

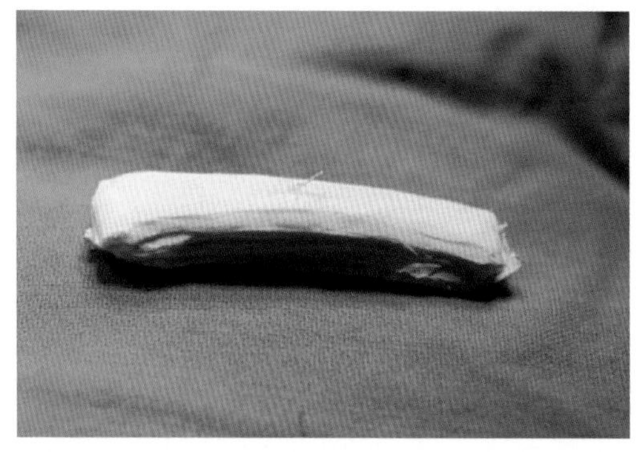

Figure 2 Stacked e-PTFE sheets prepared for dorsal augmentation

Recently, e-TPFE material other than Gore SAM have been developed and used. Surgiform is a facial plastic surgery material composed of 100% e-PTFE that is becoming more popular. Surgiform comes in two types: Pureform 3D implant *(Figure 3A)* is a prefabricated implant ready to be inserted into the nasal dorsum like silicone, and SFAM sheet and block *(Figure 3B)* that requires carving by surgeons like the original Gore SAM. Surgiform is produced harder than the original Gore-Tex; it has a denser structure that makes it easier to handle and carve. SFAM sheets come in sizes of 1-3 mm of which the surgeon can choose from based on need.

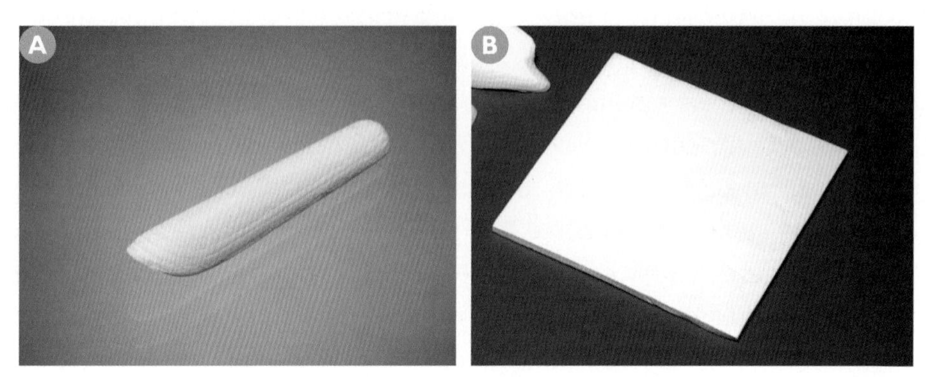

Figure 3 Surgiform 3D implant (A) and sheet (B).

IV. How to Use in Surgery

In rhinoplasty, it is best to shape the e-PTFE implant after procedures on other areas like nasal tip and septum have been finished, and aesthetic relations between tip and dorsum have been considered. Precautions for handling e-PTFE are the following:

- ☑ Put on a new pair of surgical gloves with the powder completely removed.
- ☑ Surgical tools used to shape the implant such as scissors, knife, and caliper should also be new, free of contamination by blood or secretions (no hands technique).
- ☑ Put implant inside a syringe mixed with antibiotics or povidone-iodine solution and induce permeation of the solution into the pores by exerting negative pressure *(Figure 4)*, or immerse in povidone-iodine solution before surgery.
- ☑ Unpack the e-PTFE right before implantation to minimize implant's exposure to the outside environment.

As already mentioned, e-PTFE has a structure with micropores of 10-30 μm in size that makes it vulnerable to penetration from bacteria of 5-10 μm in size. The above precautions can minimize the implant from coming into contact with contaminants before insertion. When using prefabricated implants like PureForm 3D implants, it is important to trim it well to ensure adequate attachment of implant's undersurface to the anatomical components of the nasal dorsum such as the upper lateral cartilages, septal cartilage, and nasal bone. If this is not done, there will be dead space between the implant and nasal skeleton, from which fluid collection and implant migration could occur. This dead space may also increase the frequency of infections after surgery and keeps the implant from staying fixed.

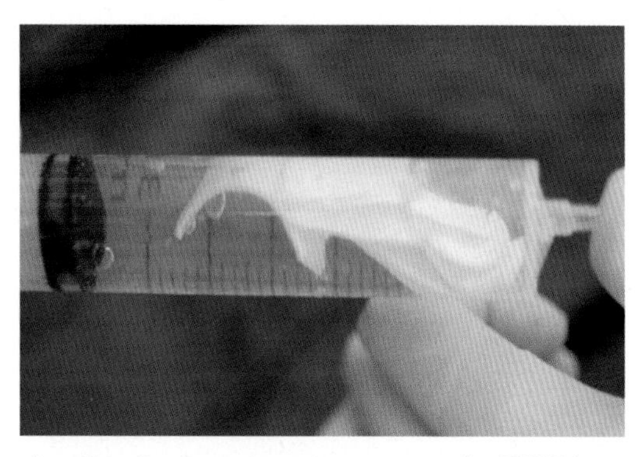

Figure 4 Inducing permeation of antibiotics into the micropores of e-PTFE by exerting negative pressure on the syringe containing antibiotic solution.

Though prefabricated implants are commonly used, more commonly used is the sheet type e-TPFE implant. This type of implant is highly flexible in its usage in that the surgeon can modify its shape freely, based on need. However, they should be able to perform very delicate carving in order to get a good surgical outcome. Although the desired shape of the implant after carving may vary according to nasal length and shape. The implant is normally designed to have 7-10 mm width and 3.5-5 cm length *(Figure 5)*.

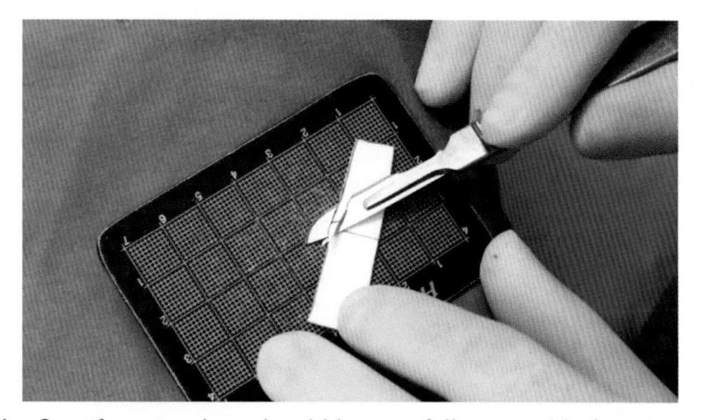

Figure 5 The margin of the Surgiform implant should be carefully carved before insertion into the nasal dorsum.

Since the thickness of commonly used e-PTFE is usually 1-2 mm, multiple sheets should be stacked to get considerable increase in dorsal heights. The convenient part about using the sheet implant is that augmentation levels can be adjusted for each different region easily, even for patients with a focal prominence or depression in dorsal height. If the surgeon conducts partial augmentations in regions such as the radix and nasal dorsum, using multiple layers for such regions can achieve getting desired dorsal line *(Figure 6)*. This material is especially useful for radix augmentation in hump-nose patients or focal augmentation in the cartilaginous dorsum for slight saddle-nose patients. It is easy to create the desired shape of the dorsal line by adjusting the degree of augmentation at the different areas of the nasal dorsum (differential augmentation).

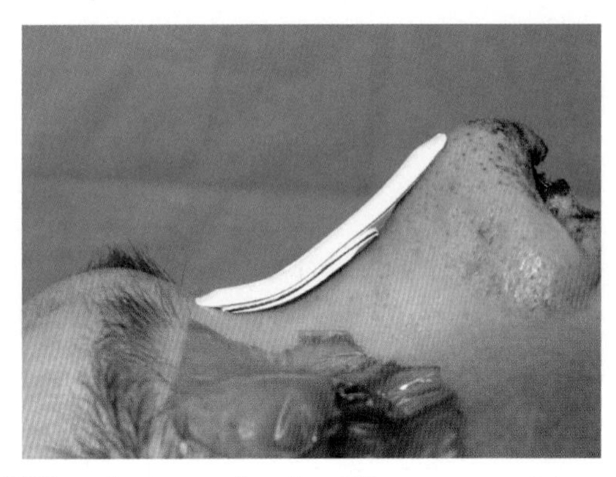

Figure 6 Different layers of e-PTFE can be inserted at the different parts of the nasal dorsum in order to meet the desired aesthetic goal.

One thing to keep in mind is that when using multiple layers of e-PTFE, the upper sheet should be carved narrower than the lower sheets to create a natural-looking nasal shape. Therefore, when designing a thick augmentation material of over 4-6 mm height, design the bottom sheet wide enough to make the whole cross-section a trapezoid shape. After stacking to the appropriate height, the sheets should be suture-fixated using 4-0 PDS, 5-0 PDS, or nylon. Before trimming the margins with a #10 blade following stacking, the process becomes easier if the middle part is sutured with number 4-0 PDS *(Figure 7)*. The process should be done on a hard, flat surface. When using Surgiform SFAM sheet, a strengthened form of e-PTFE, good beveling of the sheet's margins is essential, especially for sheets of over 2 mm thickness. If not beveled enough, the implant's margins can be felt through the skin after surgery. This beveling can be done easily with a #10 blade *(Figure 5)*.

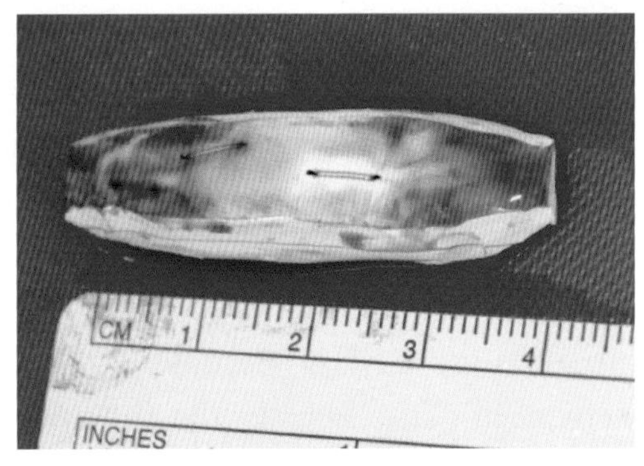

Figure 7 When the e-PTFE implants are stacked, suture fixation at the mid portion can ease beveling of the margin and insertion into the nasal dorsum.

When the desired shape is achieved, keep the implant immersed in a povidone-iodine solution for over 5 minutes, and wash with clean saline right before insertion. Even when using a single layer of Gore-Tex of Surgiform, margin beveling should be conducted before inserting the implant.

V. Inserting the Implant

As important as the precise carving of the implant is in obtaining the ideal nasal shape after surgery, is the preparation of nasal dorsum receiving the implant in achieving good surgical results and preventing postoperative complications. The most basic and important principle is to elevate the sub-SMAS (superficial muscular aponeurotic system) plane flap correctly. Damage to the skin-soft tissue envelope following improper flap elevation can hinder blood supply, increasing vulnerability to infection and mechanical trauma. It is important to know that in the nasal bone area, postoperative implant movement can be prevented by placing the implant in the subperiosteal plane. Extra care should be taken in dissecting the exact subperiosteal plane. When using prefabricated implants like the PureForm 3D, making the nasal dorsum flat by reducing any dorsal convexity increases stability of implant and reduces dead space. In contrast, when using a smooth and easily bent sheet type implant, since differential augmentation is possible, keeping the nasal dorsum's natural curves can ensure a more natural surgical outcome. Any bleeding should be checked and controlled carefully during surgery because a hematoma after surgery increases the risk of infection and implant migration. When using alloplastic implant materials like e-PTFE, it is best not to use gauze or cotton pads in the nasal dorsum for hemostasis. Using such materials might leave tiny pieces of fiber in the surgical field, which could act as a nidus for infection or inflammation after surgery. If the use of gauze or cotton is inevitable, it is advisable to thoroughly irrigate the surgical field with saline to eliminate any trace of foreign materials.

When using the e-PTFE sheet, especially when stacking multiple layers, it is better to make a pocket slightly wider than the size required when using silicone, because a narrow pocket could fold or wrinkle the implant's margins during insertion. After preparing the nasal dorsum fully, copious irrigation of the pocket for removal of tissue debris, bone dust, and possible pathogens right before implant insertion helps reduce infection and inflammation. Saline alone, saline with antibiotics, and diluted betadine povidone-iodine can all be used as irrigating solutions, and no studies have proven which solution is the best. Leftover e-PTFE should not be reused if possible, and if inevitable, divide it before carving and sterilize it in a different package, minimizing exposure to air. Various forceps can be used during insertion depending on the surgeon's preferences, and the bayonet type forceps is very convenient. If the pocket for the implant is narrow or precise, or if insertion in the radix is intended, use of a guide suture using Nylon or PDS can be helpful. When performing rhinoplasty via an open approach, inserting the implant right at the midline is not a difficult procedure, but the midline placement of the implant may be more difficult through an endonasal rhinoplasty approach, thus the surgeon should pay more attention to ensure the proper placement of the implant precisely in the middle.

VI. Prevention and Treatment of Complications

One most crucial thing to keep in mind when using alloplastic materials like e-PTFE is preventing postoperative infections. In general, infection rates are reported to be 2-3% for primary surgery, and 4-5% for revision rhinoplasty. However, the surgeon can reduce the risk of infection by adhering to various principles of infection prevention. Especially when e-PTFE was used in the nasal dorsum, infection or inflammation could occur months, even years after surgery, requiring implant removal. It has yet to be determined whether these delayed inflammations are a form of primary infection or a form of secondary infection caused by an initial immune function-related inflammation. The authors lean towards the latter theory. Although delayed inflammation can be treated easily if detected early, if untreated, this could cause irreversible damage to the skin covering. Therefore, it is important that symptoms and signs of delayed inflammation are explained thoroughly to patients who underwent rhinoplasty with e-PTFE. These patients should be advised to visit the hospital immediately if erythema, swelling, or tenderness occurs in the nasal dorsum *(Figure 8)*.

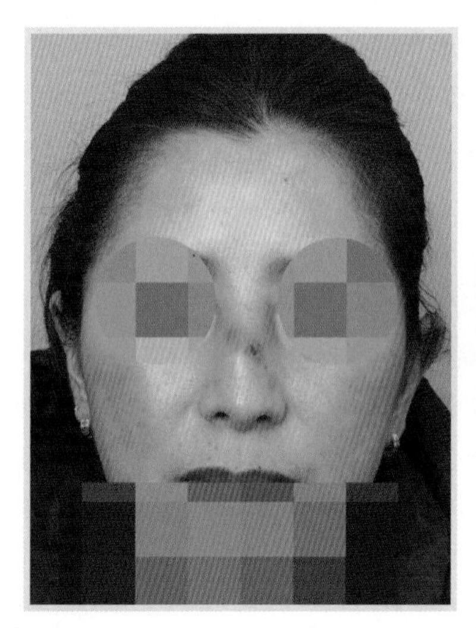
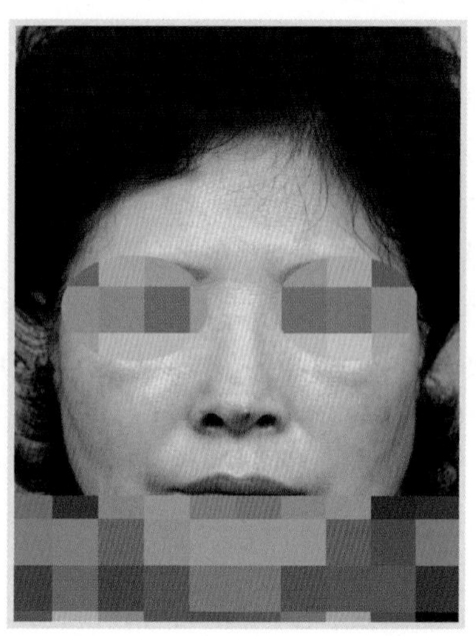

Figure 8 Delayed inflammation after use of Gore-Tex at the nasal dorsum and the nasal tip.

As mentioned previously, e-PTFE has a porous structure, and thus must be kept unpacked as little time as possible before insertion. If the underlying nasal mucosa is damaged while conducting medial or other osteotomy, cephalic trimming on the lower lateral cartilage, or creating a pocket for a spreader graft by separating the upper lateral cartilage from the septal cartilage, there is a possibility of inducing a communication route between the nasal dorsal pocket for implant insertion and the nasal cavity, increasing the risk of ascending infection. Thus, mucosal damage calls for heightened caution during these procedures.

Since ascending infections could occur through the incision site, it is important to maintain enough distance between the implant and the incision line, and to close the incision meticulously. However, if the distance between the implant tip and the domal portion of the nasal tip becomes large for trying to maintain a space between the implant and incision, complications such as a supratip depression could occur. In order to avoid this problem, the surgeon can either bevel the caudal end of the Gore-Tex implant precisely, or insert crushed cartilage or diced cartilage in the gap between the implant and the tip graft *(Figure 9)*.

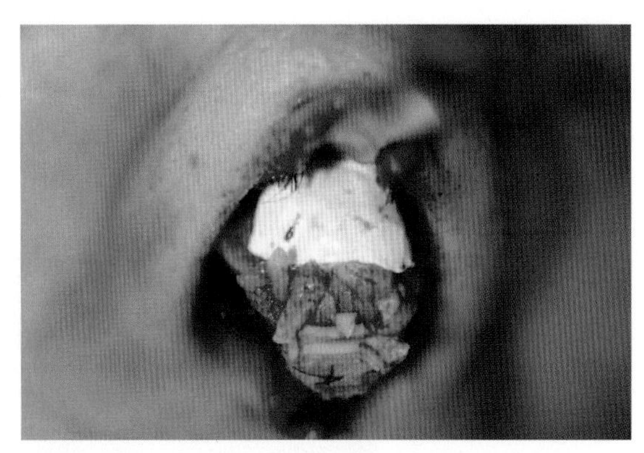

Figure 9 A gap between the caudal end of the Gore-Tex implant and tip graft can be filled with diced cartilage to prevent a supratip depression or discontinuity.

Infections could manifest in various forms after surgery. Intermittent erythema or pain can initially be managed by antibiotics and anti-inflammatory agents. However, if the inflammation progresses into a purulent lesion, the implant must be removed immediately. Since e-PTFE implants often exhibit tissue integration without forming capsules in the surrounding tissue, their removal is much more difficult than removing silicone implants. However, if inflammation is present, the implant has already separated from the tissue, making removal easier. If inflammation is not present, removal can be made easier by injecting enough local anesthetic agent between the implant and surrounding tissue before surgery. Surgiform, which has a denser structure than Gore-SAM, exhibits median traits of both silicone and Gore-SAM, neither forming capsules nor bonding excessively with surrounding tissue. Thus, it is relatively easy to remove. Other common complications are implant displacement, deviation, and bending. These complications are due to the gradual displacement of implant during healing, or technical errors like imprecise insertion of the implant into the nasal dorsum *(Figure 10)*.

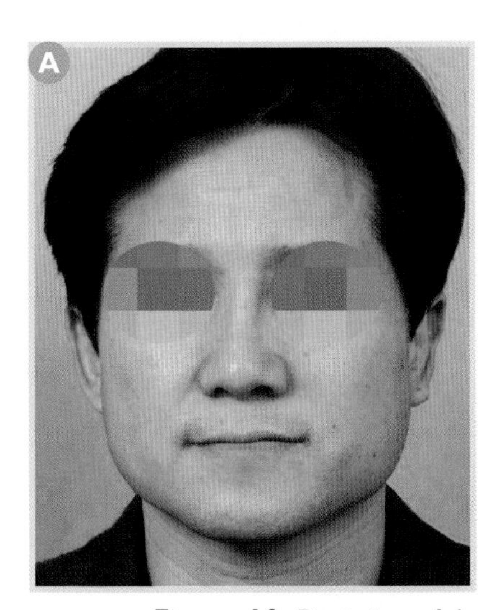

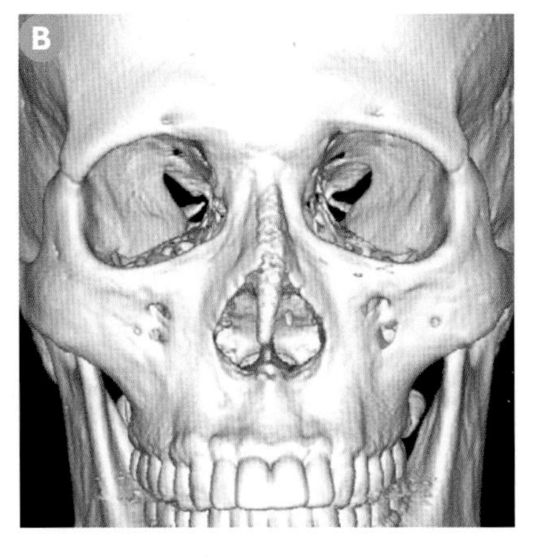

Figure 10 Deviation of dorsally-implanted e-PTFE implant.

Inserting sheet type e-PTFE without care can bend the implant's margins; therefore, the surgeon must pay attention not to make the margin wrinkled or bent. Using e-PTFE in the nasal tip is a very dangerous practice, and the authors experienced a number of patients who manifested delayed infection caused by e-PTFE placed in the nasal tip *(Figure11)*.

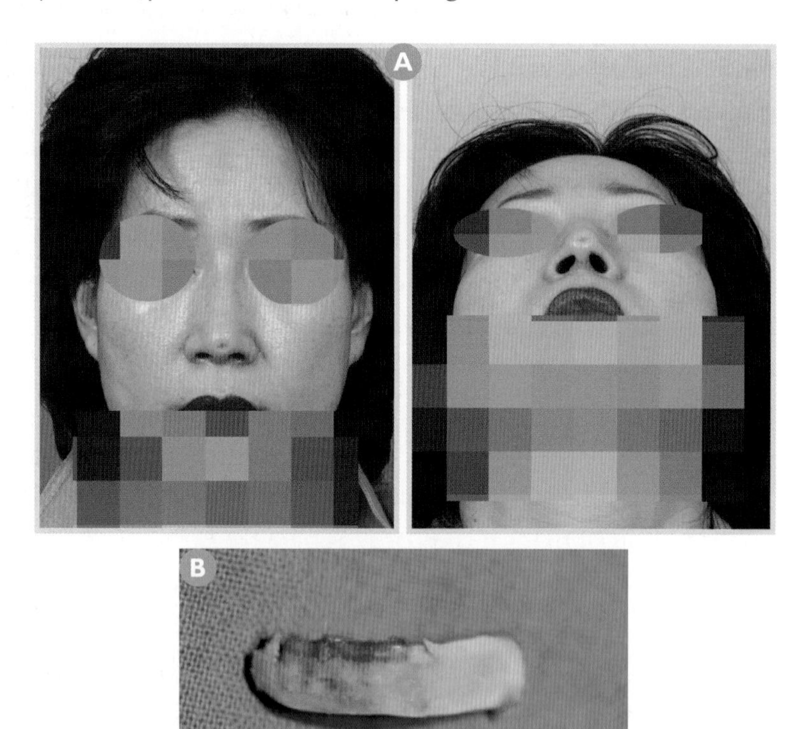

Figure 11 Delayed inflammation at the tip area due to an e-PTFE implant used as a columellar strut.

References

1. Conrad K, Gillman G. A 6-year experience with the use of expanded polytetrafluoroethylene in rhinoplasty. Plast Reconstr Surg 1998; 101: 1675-8.
2. Hanel KC, McCabe C, Abbott WM. Current PTFE grafts: a biomechanical, scanning electron, and light microscopic evaluation. Ann Surg 1982; 195: 456-63.
3. Ham J, Miller PJ. Expanded polytetrafluoroethylene implants in rhinoplasty: literature review, operative techniques, and outcome. Facial Plast Surg 2003; 19: 331-9.
4. Inanli S, Sari M, Baylancicek S. The use of expanded polytetrafluoroethylene (Gore-Tex) in rhinoplasty. Aesthet Plast Surg 2007; 31: 345-8.
5. Jung YG, Kim HY, Dhong HJ. Ultrasonographic monitoring of implant thickness after augmentation rhinoplasty with expanded polytetrafluoroethylene. Am J Rhinol Allergy 2009; 23: 105-10.
6. Jung YG, Kim KH, Dhong HJ. Ultrasonographic monitoring of new expanded polytetrafluoroethylene implant thickness after augmentation rhinoplasty. Am J Rhinol Allergy 2012; 26: 137-41.
7. Merritt K, Shafer JW, Brown SA. Implant site infection rates with porous and dense materials. J Biomed Mater Res 1979; 13: 101-8.
8. Neel HB, 3rd. Implants of Gore-Tex. Arch Otolaryngol 1983; 109: 427-33.
9. Schoenrock LD, Chernoff WG. Subcutaneous implantation of Gore-Tex for facial reconstruction. Otolaryngol Clin North Am 1995; 28: 325-40.
10. Singh S, Baker JL, Jr. Use of expanded polytetrafluoroethylene in aesthetic surgery of the face. Clin Plast Surg 2000; 27: 579-93.
11. Serin GM, Polat S, Aksoy E, Baylançiçek S, Inanli S. Importance of placing Gore-Tex in the subperiosteal plane for augmentation rhinoplasty. J Craniofac Surg 2012; 23: e359-61.
12. Tang L, Eaton JW. Inflammatory responses to biomaterials. Am J Clin Pathol 1995; 103: 466-71.
13. Wang TD.Gore-Tex nasal augmentation: a 26-year perspective. Arch Facial Plast Surg 2011; 13: 129-30.
14. Zhang X, Peng Q, Xu Y. Methods for carving expanded polytetrafluoroethylene prostheses in augmentation rhinoplasty and their impact on nose shape. Plast Reconstr Surg 2012; 130: 906-8.

Case 1

A 47-year-old female visited for a flat nose deformity.

Analysis

Very low dorsum
Wide dorsum
Wide alar base
Severely underprojected tip
Nostril asymmetry
Endoscopy: Septal deviation

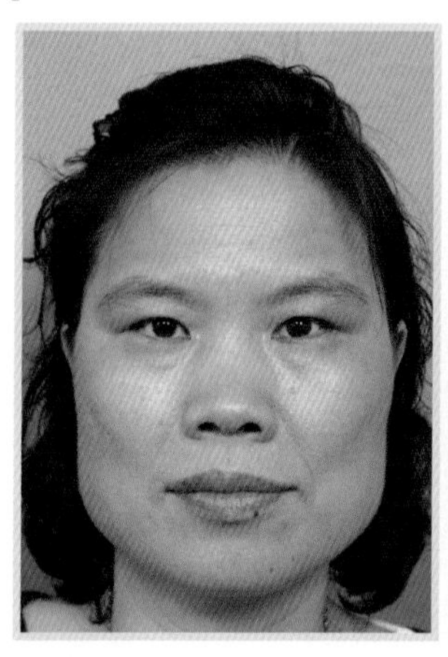
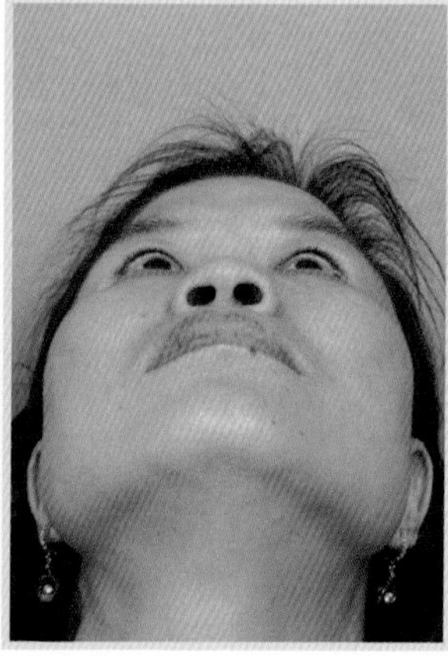
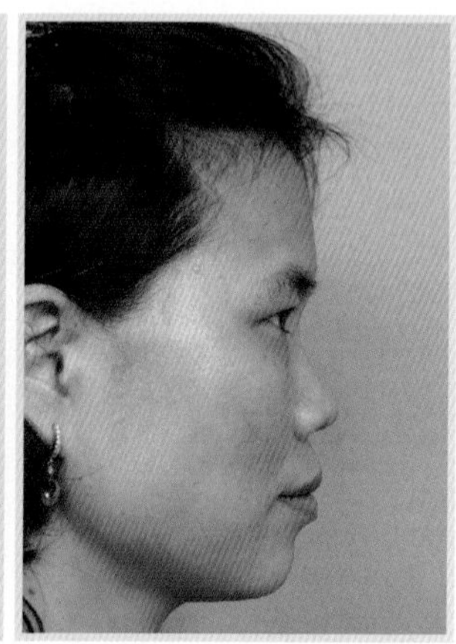

Operative Procedures

Open rhinoplasty approach
Septoplasty and harvesting of septal cartilage and bone
Caudal septal extension grafting
Transdomal and interdomal suturing of the alar cartilages
Multilayer tip grafting with cartilage backstop graft using conchal cartilage
Dorsal augmentation using Gore-Tex
Tip graft camouflaging using homologous pericardium
Alar base resection (bilateral)

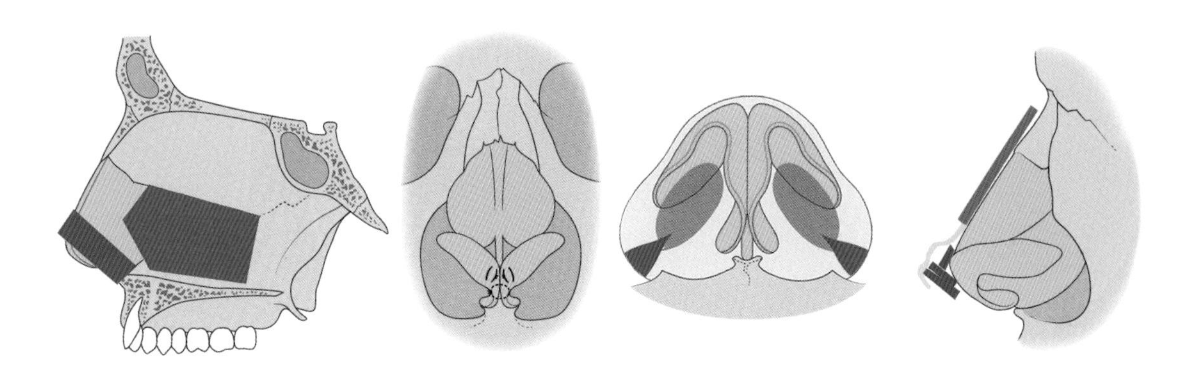

Postoperative Changes

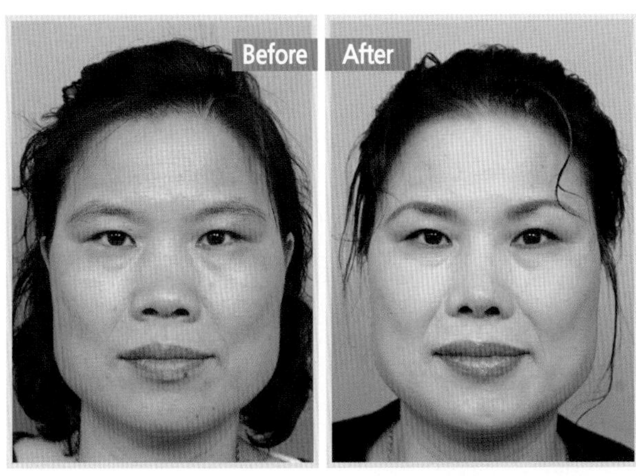

Frontal: Dorsal contour was improved. Alar base width was reduced.

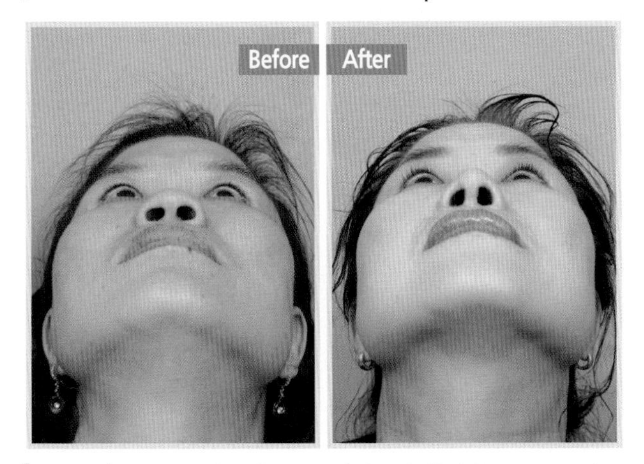

Basal: Tip projection and tip definition were improved. Alar base width was reduced. Nostril asymmetry was aggravated.

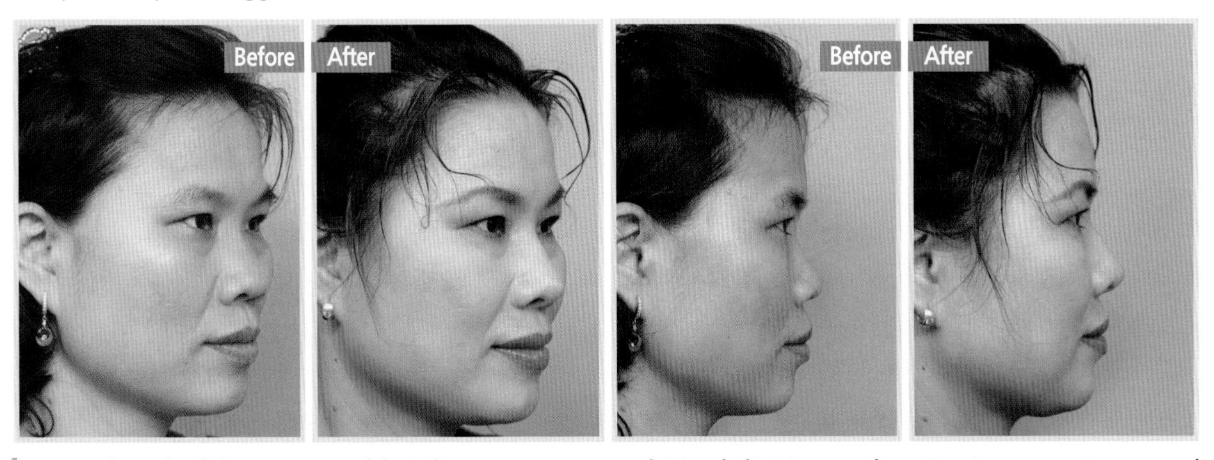

Lateral and Oblique: Dorsal height was augmented. Tip definition and projection were improved.

Case 2

A 25-year-old female visited for her flat and short nose deformity.

Analysis

Frontal: Very low dorsal height
Basal: Wide ala
Lateral and Oblique: Underprojected tip
Endoscopy: Septal deviation

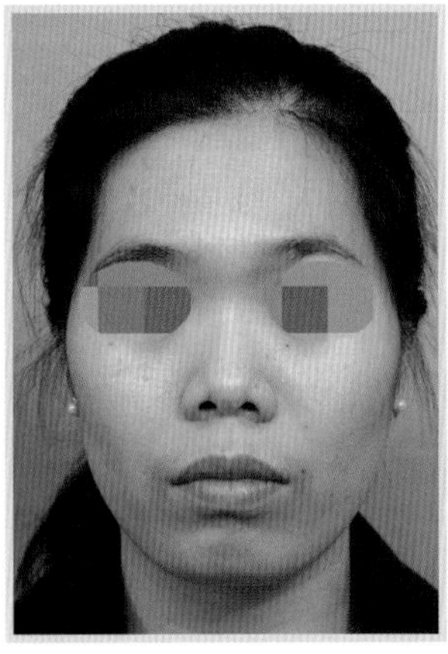
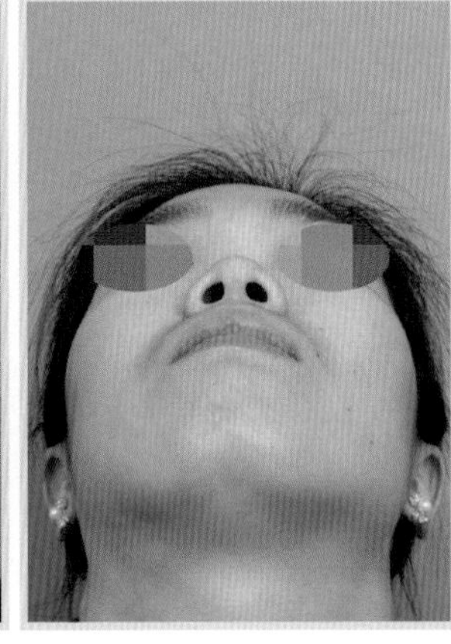
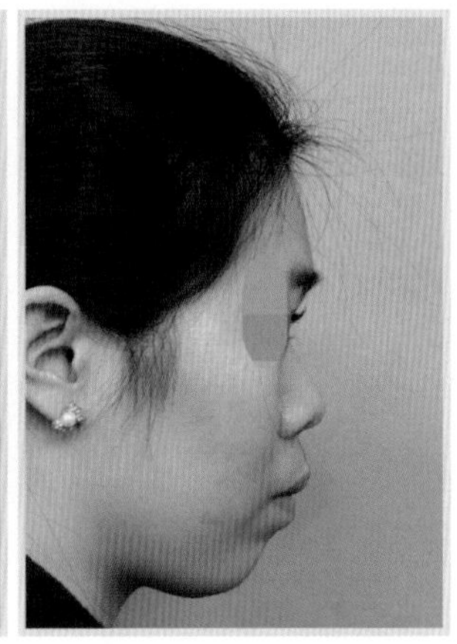

Operative Procedures

Open rhinoplasty approach
Septoplasty and harvesting of septal cartilage and bone
Caudal septal extension grafting using septal cartilage (left)
Multilayer tip grafting using conchal cartilage
Dorsal augmentation using processed fascia lata and Gore-Tex
Alar base resection (bilateral)

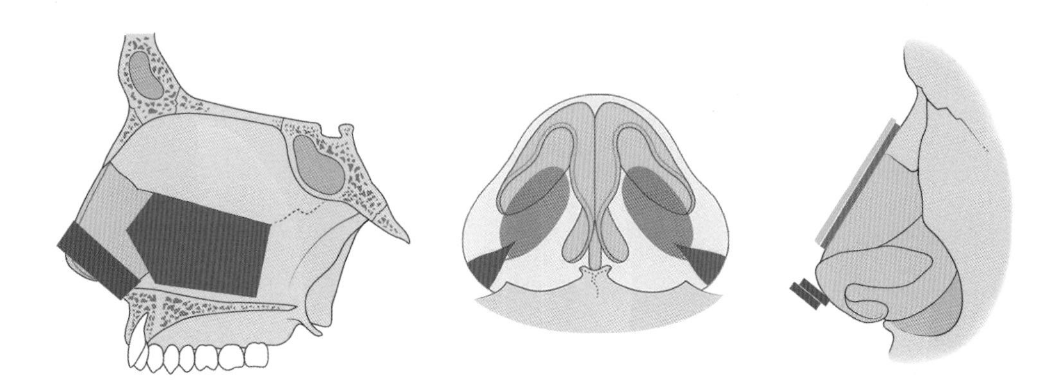

Postoperative Changes

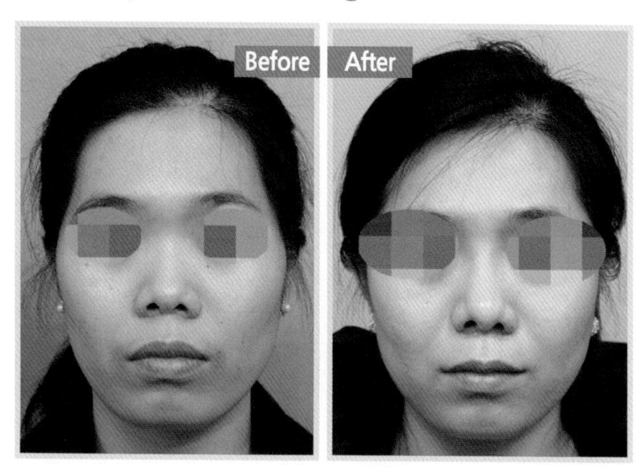

Frontal: Dorsal aesthetic lines were improved through dorsal augmentation and tip surgery.

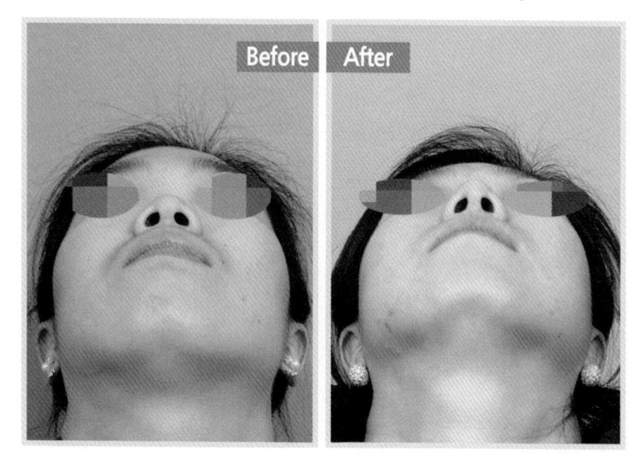

Basal: Tip projection was improved. Alar base width was reduced.

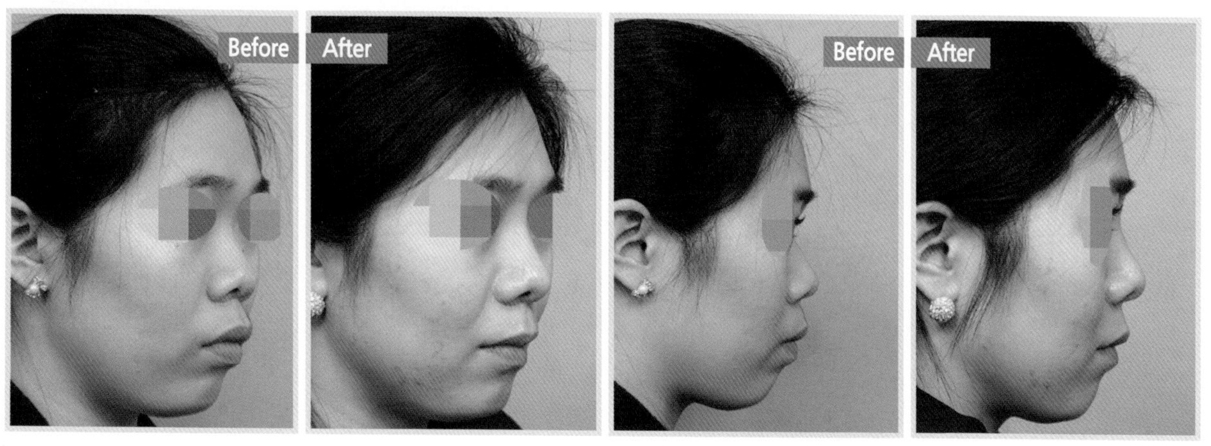

Lateral and Oblique: Dorsal height was augmented. Tip projection was improved. Tip was rotated caudally.

Medpor

Jin-Young Min · Yong Ju Jang

I. Medpor Implants

Medpor (Porex Surgical, IVC College Park, GA), a biocompatible material composed of porous high-density polyethylene (PHDPE), is commonly used and has been proven to be a reliable implant material. Medpor has been used clinically for skull base reconstruction, orbital wall reconstruction, external ear reconstruction, and facial reconstruction since the 1980s. This is also being used more and more frequently in rhinoplasty, particularly as ever finer and more delicate special implants become available for the bridge of the nose, the middle third, the septum, and as replacements for the alar cartilages. Medpor is a high-density polyethylene with a structure of interconnected pores ranging 125-250 μm in size. Its hardness is similar to cancellous bone, yet it is quite flexible. Polyethylene composes 54% of its volume, and pores compose the rest. The pores provide space for blood vessels and fibrous tissue to grow inward and for collagen to embed, thus ensuring proper bonding with the implant site with high integration and stability *(Figure 1)*. This process of tissue ingrowth has been reported to occur within four weeks of insertion. Additionally, the proliferation of surrounding blood vessels prevents or minimizes implant infection.

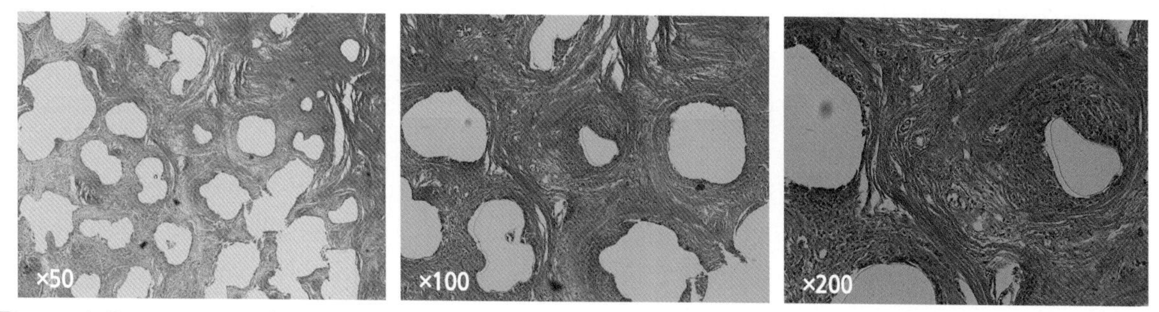

Figure 1 Cross-section of the Medpor implant removed from the nose. Note extensive fibrovascular ingrowth into the implant pores.

The advantages of Medpor are:

- Foreign body reactions are rare: nonantigenic and nonallergenic.
- When heated, the material can be punctured with a needle or cut, and can be molded to in the desired sizes and shapes, then cools back into a firm structure. Medpor sheets can easily be cut with surgical scissors.
- The implant can be prefabricated in various shapes such as sheet type, block type, dorsal type, dorsal tip type, L-type, batten type, and saddle type.
- Its porous nature permits ingrowth of connective and vascular tissue, increasing mechanical stability of the implant and lowering the risk of implant migration and infection.
- Implant resorption is minimal and its biomechanical properties provide durability for a long time.

The disadvantages of Medpor are:

- It has an increased incidence of implant extrusion compared with autologous grafts.
- Implant removal is relatively difficult in cases of revision surgery.
- The stiffness of Medpor makes patients feel uncomfortable.

II. Patient Selection for Medpor Implants in Rhinoplasty

The use of Medpor implants can be considered for patients when autogenous materials are unavailable or insufficient for multiple grafts. However, patients who have received multiple revisions or have a history of external injuries have a higher risk of extrusion due to the compromised circulation and altered wound healing process. Furthermore, heavy smokers and patients who take drugs such as corticosteroids or chemotherapeutic drugs may represent impaired wound healing process, therefore requiring additional caution prior to using Medpor implants.

III. Application of Medpor Implants in Rhinoplasty

Unlike Gore-Tex, Medpor can be used not only for dorsal augmentation but also for structural grafting, since it possesses flexibility, firmness, and the ability to fuse well with the surrounding tissues. Furthermore, Medpor can be useful when revision rhinoplasty is needed to correct functional problems and unsatisfactory aesthetic results. Many reports have been published regarding the effectiveness of using Medpor not only for dorsal augmentation but also for other purposes including columellar struts, septal extension grafts, and spreader grafts *(Figure 2)*. Especially in columellar strut procedures for Asians, Medpor is considered as a useful substitute for autologous cartilage due to its relatively low complication rate and capability of achieving significant tip projection and tip rotation. However, risks of implant extrusion and secondary infection should always be kept in mind.

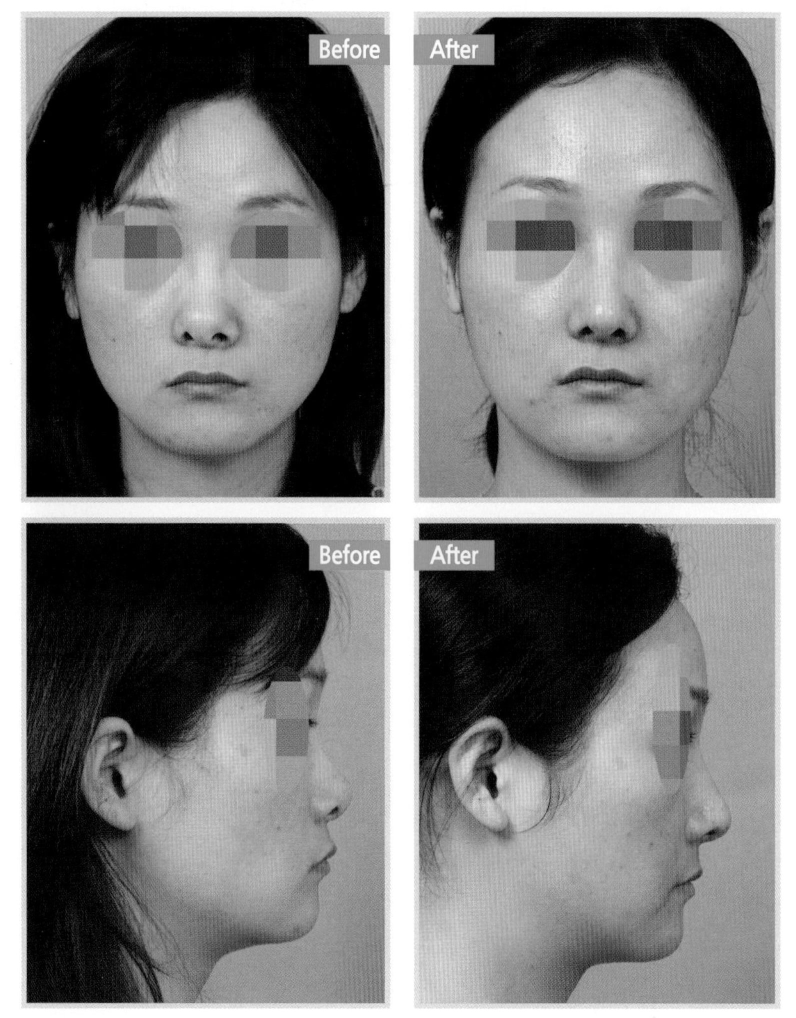

Figure 2 Preoperative and postoperative views of a patient who underwent dorsal augmentation using a Medpor implant.

IV. Surgical Technique of Rhinoplasty Using Medpor Implants

1. Use of Antibiotics Before and After Surgery

Perioperative intravenous antibiotics covering streptococcus and staphylococcus organisms are recommended. After surgery, it is better to use oral antibiotics for one week to prevent bacterial colonization around the implant.

2. Handling Medpor Implant

In all rhinoplasties in which Medpor is used, the surgeon should sterilize the surgical field meticulously. Before insertion, the implant should be soaked in antibiotic or sterilizing solution and rinsed well before actual insertion. The surgeon should try to minimize the time between unpacking the Medpor to its insertion into the nose. To prevent contamination of implant, powdered gloves should not be used. Additionally, it would be helpful to keep the implant from touching the surgical cloths or towels on the operative field to prevent contamination with microfiber *(Figure 3)*.

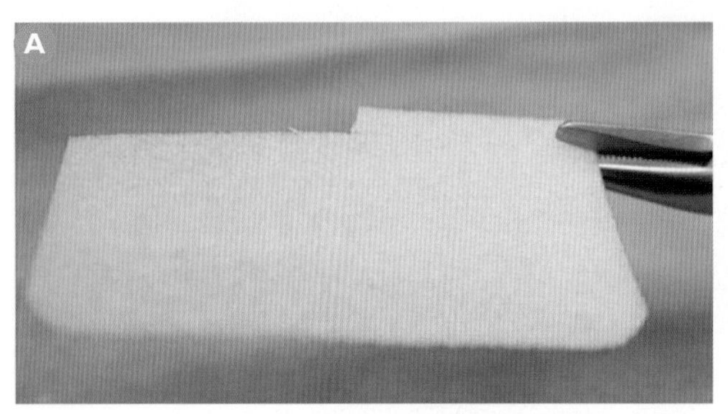

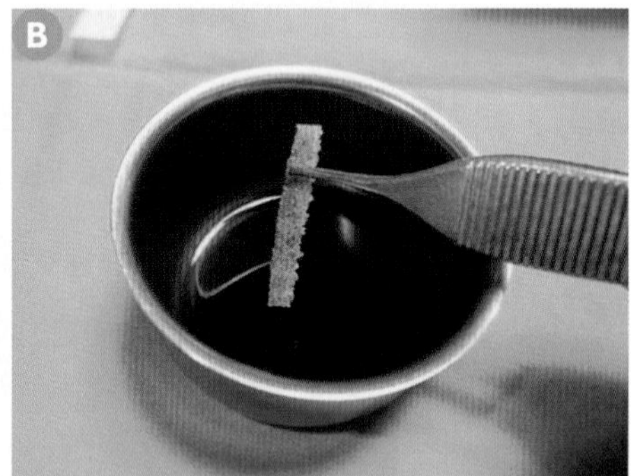

Figure 3 Preparation of the Medpor implant before its placement. The surgeon should keep the implant from touching surgical cloths or towels in the operative field to prevent microfiber contamination (A) and the implant should be soaked in antibiotic or sterilizing solution prior to its use (B).

3. Dissection of Operation Field and Wound Closure

A pocket should be created approximately 10% larger than the implant itself. An external rhinoplasty approach is useful since it provides the wide exposure that allows direct visualization for dissection and pocket creation. Regardless of implant type, elevation of the proper layer of soft tissue flap is essential. The nasal superficial musculoaponeurotic system (SMAS) layer should be well preserved, and the dissection should be conducted beneath SMAS to preserve the nasal blood supply. Dissection beneath the SMAS layer preserves the normal circulation to the nasal skin-soft tissue envelope, and thus decreases the risk of skin breakdown and implant extrusion. Placing the Medpor implant close to the incision line, which increases the risk of wound breakdown, infection, and extrusion, should be avoided. Covering the surface of the implant with autologous tissue such as fascia or cartilage can be helpful to prevent implant extrusion through the skin or nasal mucosa. In addition, a meticulous closure of the incisions is beneficial for minimizing bacterial contamination and prevention of complications.

V. Complications

The common complications are infection and implant extrusion. Both complication rates with Medpor implants in rhinoplasty are reported to be 2.7-7.4% *(Figure 4)*. Although it is generally thought that removal of Medpor from the nasal tissue may be difficult due to extensive vascular ingrowth and strong adhesions between the implant and soft tissue, sometimes it is relatively not so difficult to remove the implant from the surrounding tissue. In some cases, the surgeon can opt to preserve a remnant of the Medpor implant rather than completely removing it. This results in less injury to the surrounding tissue. In addition, removal of the Medpor implant from the extrusion area, carving the implant into a smaller size and inserting it again does not cause major problems *(Figure 5)*.

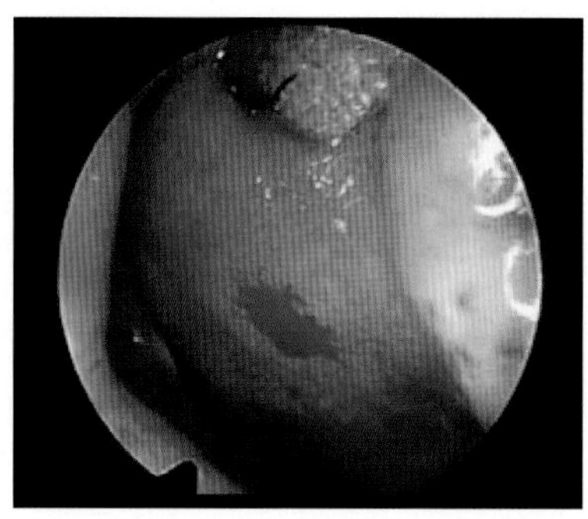

Figure 4 Endoscopic photo of a patient showing persistent discharge due to the exposed Medpor implant through a defect in the septal mucosa.

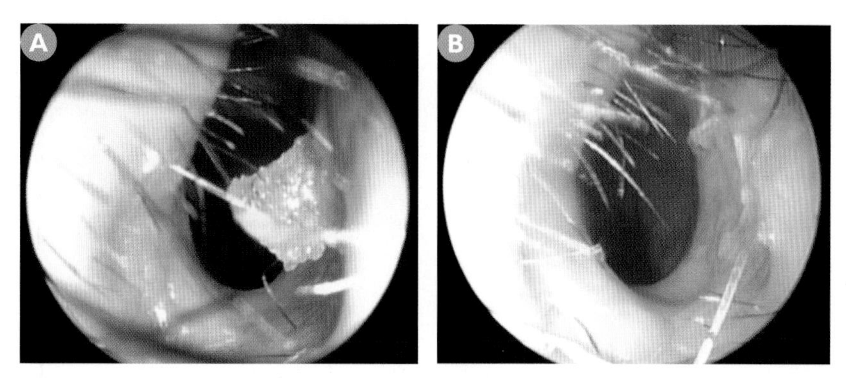

Figure 5 Extrusion of a Medpor implant. Visible Medpor implant in the nasal cavity (A) and postoperative view after removal of extruded Medpor implant (B).

References

1. Berghaus A, Mulchand G, Handrock M. Porous polyethylene and proplast: their behavior in a bony implant bed. Arch Otorhinolaryngol 1984; 240: 115-23.
2. Berghausand A, Stelter K. Alloplastic materials in rhinoplasty. Curr Opin Otolaryngol Head Neck Surg 2006; 14: 270-77.
3. Kim YH, Kim BJ, Jang TY. Use of porous high-density polyethylene (Medpor) for spreader or extended septal graft in rhinoplasty: aesthetics, functional outcomes, and long-term complications. Ann Plast Surg 2011; 67: 464-8.
4. Ozturk S, Sengezer M. Coskunand U, Zor F. An unusual complication of a Medpor implant in nasal reconstruction: a case report. Aesthet Plast Surg 2002; 26: 419-22.
5. Ozdemir R, Kocer U, Tiftikcioglu YO. Axial pattern composite prefabrication of high-density porous polyethylene: experimental and clinical research. Plast Reconstr Surg 2005; 115: 183-96.
6. Skouras A, Skouras G, Karypidisand D, Asimakopoulou FA. The use of Medpor alloplastic material in rhinoplasty: experience and outcomes. J Plast Reconstr Aesthet Surg 2012; 65: 35-42.
7. Wellisz T. Clinical experience with the Medpor porous polyethylene implant. Aesthet Plast Surg 1993; 17: 339-44.2

Injectable Fillers

Hyoung Jin Moon

Rhinoplasty is one of the most commonly performed operations in the field of cosmetic surgery. Rhinoplasty is performed more frequently among Asians due to the low nasal bridge and flat tip. However, standard rhinoplasty procedures using implants and autologous grafts require longer recovery time, are expensive, and have many complications related to synthetic implants, because of which many patients hesitate to have the surgery. Moreover, it requires a considerable amount of training to become a competent rhinoplasty surgeon who can create good results. Due to these reasons, doctors and patients seek a procedure that is less invasive, simpler, has fewer complications, has a quick recovery, and is inexpensive. Rhinoplasty using fillers is the procedure that meets such demands *(Figure 1)*.

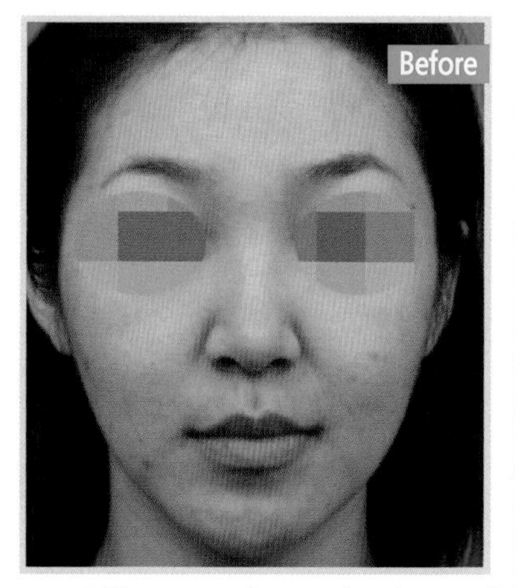

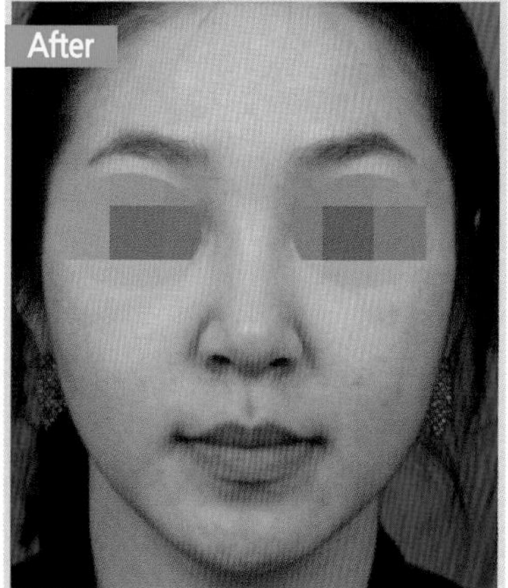

Figure 1 Proper use of fillers can change the shape of the nose simply and safely as demonstrated in the cases.

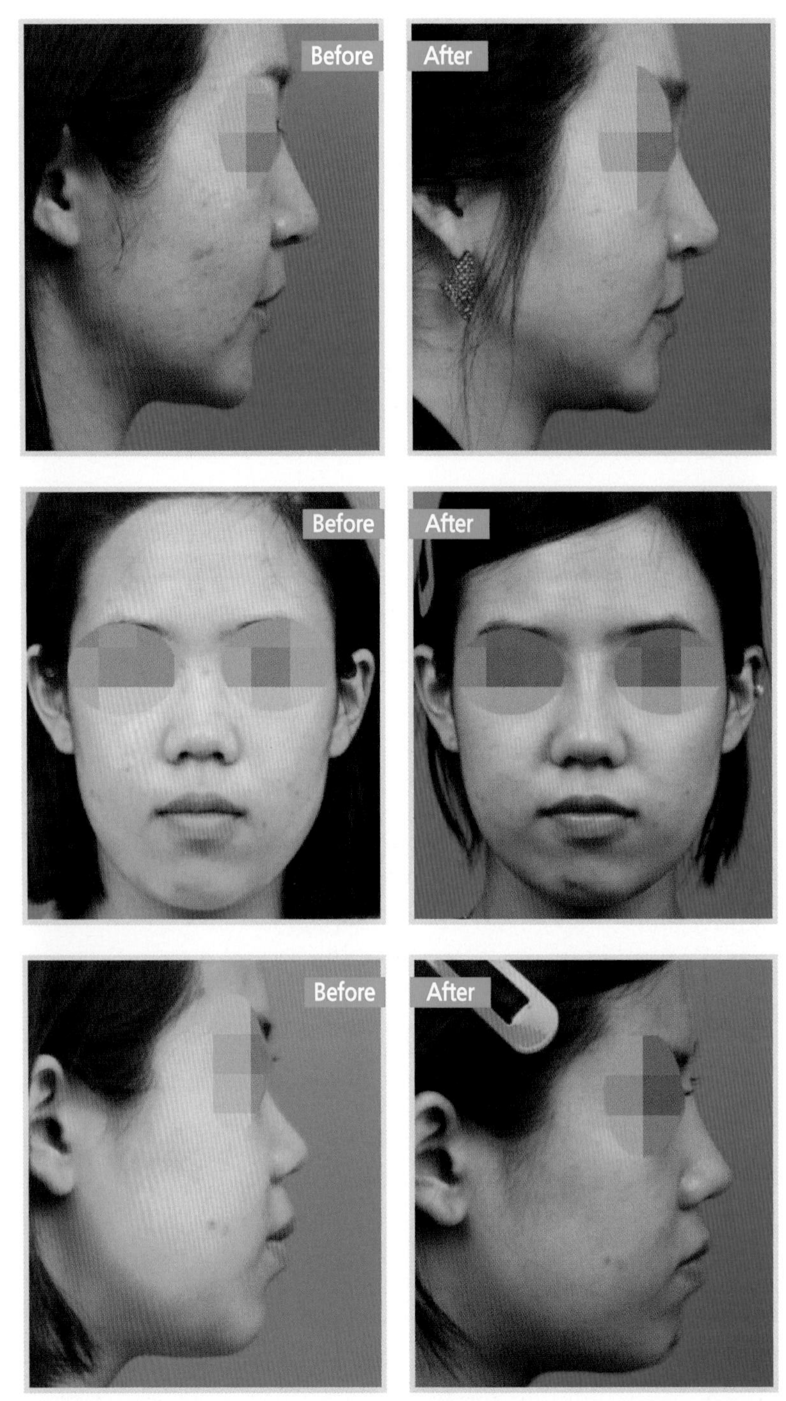

Figure 1 (continued) Proper use of fillers can change the shape of the nose simply and safely as demonstrated in the cases.

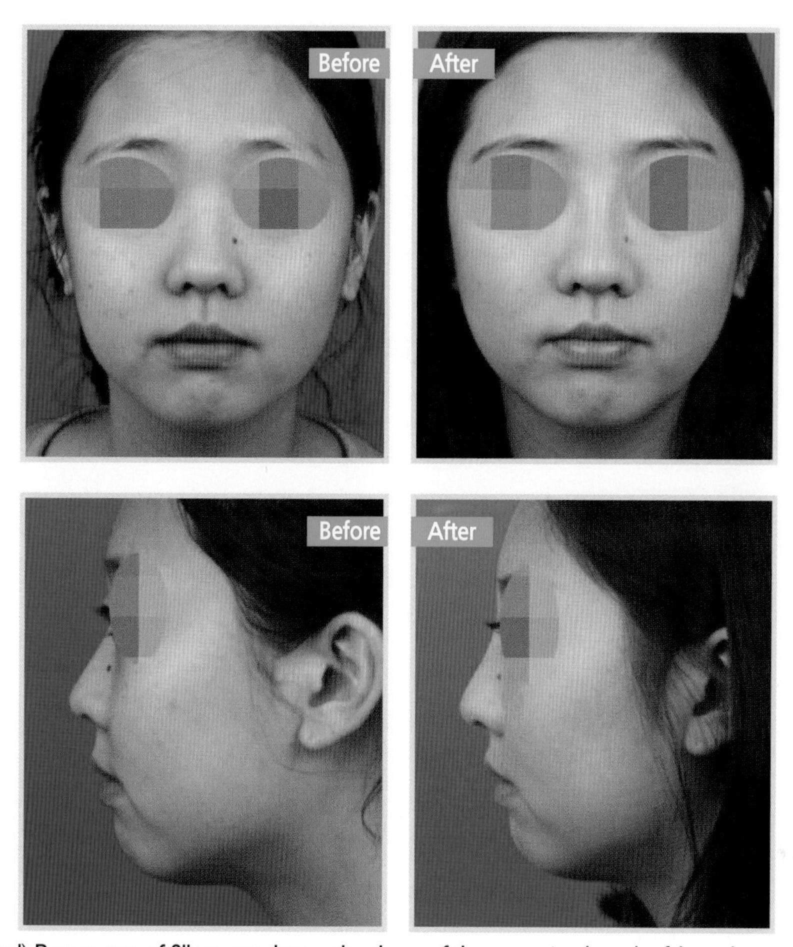

Figure 1 (continued) Proper use of fillers can change the shape of the nose simply and safely as demonstrated in the cases.

I. Types of Fillers

Fillers, by definition, refers to all substances that can increase volume by injection. Most well-known types of fillers include hyaluronic acid, collagen, paraffin, and liquid silicone. Fillers are generally categorized by its components, but occasionally they are also classified by the duration of their effects, such as temporary fillers with longevity of less than 2 years and semi-permanent fillers with 2 to 5 years. Fillers with effects lasting for over 5 years after injection are referred to as permanent fillers. Moreover, fillers can also be divided into volumizer fillers and stimulator fillers according to their mechanism of action. Fillers in which the injected substances form volume by themselves such as collagen and hyaluronic acid are referred to as volumizer fillers. Fillers in which the main components stimulate fibroblasts and synthesize collagen or cause an inflammatory reaction, resulting in the deposition of fibrous tissue thereby increasing volume, are referred to as stimulator fillers *(Table 1)*. Most types of fillers introduced in Korea thus far are relatively safe. However, severe side effects are reported in some filler products, such as granuloma formation or inflammation due to tissue reaction. Therefore, it is necessary to select the correct filler by thoroughly examining the characteristics of each product. An appropriate filler does not have untoward tissue reaction and is safe, easy to use, with long-lasting effects, no migration within the tissues, and no allergic reactions.

Table I Different types of fillers

Kind	Longevity	Chemical component	Representative commercially available products	Action
Temporary filler	6-9 months (12 months when combined with BoTox®)	Hyaluronic acid	Restylene®, Juvederm®, Belotero®	Volumizer
	1-2 years	Calcium hydroxyapatite	Radiesse®	Volumizer (collagen rebuilder)
Semi-permanent filler	2-4 years	Poly -L-Lactic Acid	Sculptra®	Stimulator
	2-4 years	Blood	Selphyl®	Stimulator
Permanent filler	5-10 years	Polymethylmethacrylate	Artesense®	Stimulator
	> 5years	Liquid silicone	SilSkin®	Volumizer
	> 5years	Polyacrylamide gel	Aquamid®	Volumizer

II. Anatomy for Filler Rhinoplasty

Filler rhinoplasty can be successfully performed only if the nasal anatomy is thoroughly understood, and its characteristics comprehended. It is a procedure that sculpts the nasal shape by injecting materials in the space between the skin and nasal skeleton composed of cartilage and bones. A solid nasal skeleton forms the support for the injected filler, maintaining the shape properly after the procedure, producing an aesthetically satisfactory result. Therefore, if the nasal skeleton is deformed or weak, it is difficult to obtain satisfactory postoperative results. The surgical outcome of filler rhinoplasty generally reflects not only the individual capabilities of the surgeon but also the difference in the anatomical structures of the patients, as well as the surgeon's awareness of such individual variations. All aspects must be considered, including thickness and quality of the skin and soft issues, as well as size, shape, and strength of structures such as bones or cartilage.

1. Nasal Soft Tissues

The nasal skin is an important factor to be considered before performing filler rhinoplasty. Patients with thick oily skin suffer from more severe edema after the procedure compared to patients with thin skin. Moreover, there is a disadvantage that it is difficult to form a solid three-dimensional shape. However, an advantage is that slight irregularities or asymmetry that may occur after the procedure is shown relatively less than on patients with thin skin. In general, Asians have thicker skin, more subcutaneous tissues, and more oily skin than Caucasians. The skin-soft tissue envelope of the nasal dorsum is thick near the nasion and thinnest near the rhinion. The part between the skin and bones or cartilage consists of four layers: the superficial fatty layer, fibromuscular layer, deep fatty layer, and periosteum or perichondrium. Major blood vessels or nerves distributed on the external nose passes through the superficial musculoaponeurotic system (SMAS) layer or the fatty layer. Thus, to minimize vascular injuries or nerve damage, it is most ideal to inject fillers in the superficial fatty layer located between the SMAS layer and the dermis. Moreover, the superficial fatty layer is relatively wide and has rough and loose tissues compared to other areas, which has the advantage of increasing volume easily by injecting fillers *(Figure 2)*.

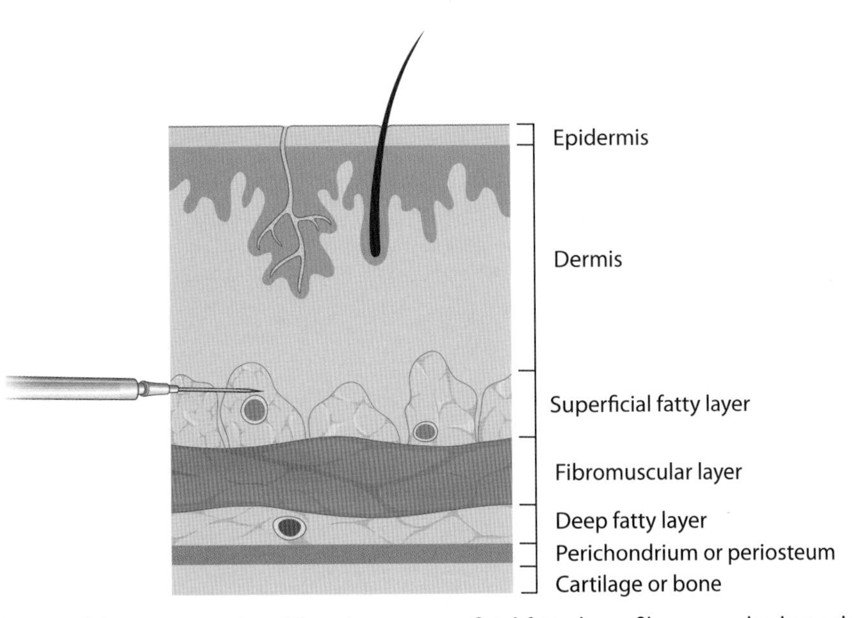

Figure 2 Soft tissues of the nose consist of four layers: superficial fatty layer, fibromuscular layer, deep fatty layer, and periosteum or perichondrium. To minimize vascular injury or nerve damage, it is most ideal to inject fillers in the superficial fatty layer located between the SMAS and the dermis.

Among muscles distributed on the nose, the following are relevant in filler injection: the depressor septi nasi muscle starts from orbicularis oris and ends at the medial crura of the lower lateral cartilage. This muscle lowers the nasal tip when the person smiles or makes a facial expression. To suppress the action of this muscle prior to filler injection, botulinum toxin is injected to paralyze this muscle. If the procerus muscle located on glabella contracts strongly, the filler injected in the glabella may migrate, and thus it is also desirable to paralyze it in advance using botulinum toxin. The levator labii superioris alaeque nasi broadens the nasal width and lowers the nasal tip when smiling; in the patient whose nasal tip descends excessively or whose nose width broadens greatly, this muscle must also be paralyzed using botulinum toxin before injection of fillers *(Figure 3)*. The dilator naris muscle must be paralyzed in the patient whose nose width is excessively broad.

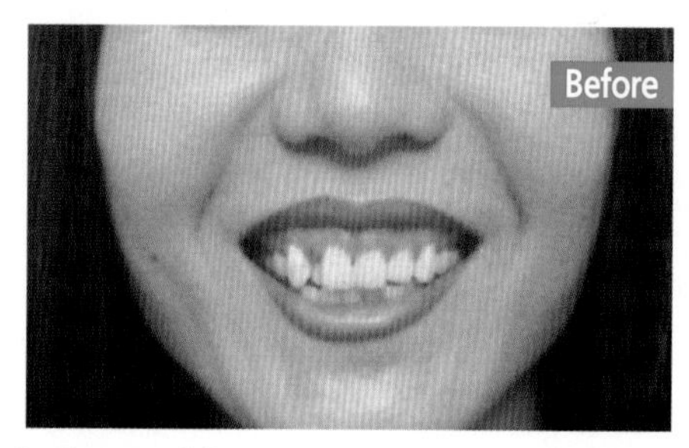

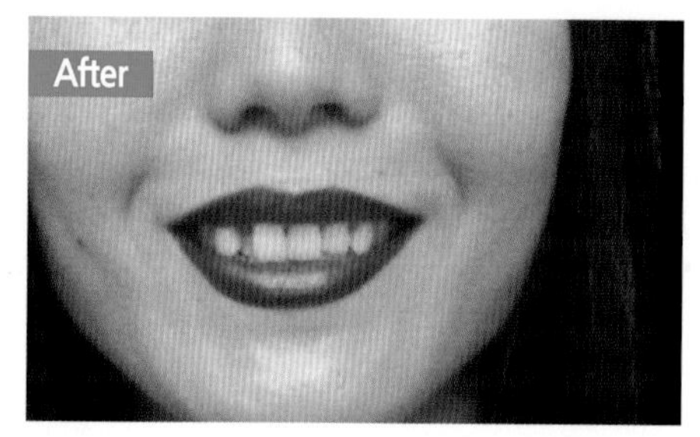

Figure 3 If the levator labii superioris alaeque nasi is paralyzed using botulinum toxin, it can correct nasal tip ptosis or alar widening appearing when one smiles. In addition, it can soften the too distinct upper part of nasolabial line.

2. Blood Supply of the External Nose

One of the main complications that may occur after filler injection is skin necrosis due to venous congestion and intra-arterial embolization. To prevent these complications, the surgeon must be familiar with the anatomy of the blood supply of external nose. The skin- soft tissue envelope of external nose receives blood from both the internal carotid artery through the ophthalmic artery and the external carotid artery through the facial artery. The ophthalmic artery supplies the upper part of the nose through the dorsal nasal artery and the external nasal branch of the anterior ethmoidal artery. The superior labial artery and angular artery that are branches of the facial artery mostly supplies on the lower part of the nose. They form the columellar artery and lateral nasal artery. The nasal tip receives blood through the lateral nasal artery from the above and the columellar artery from below *(Figure 4)*.

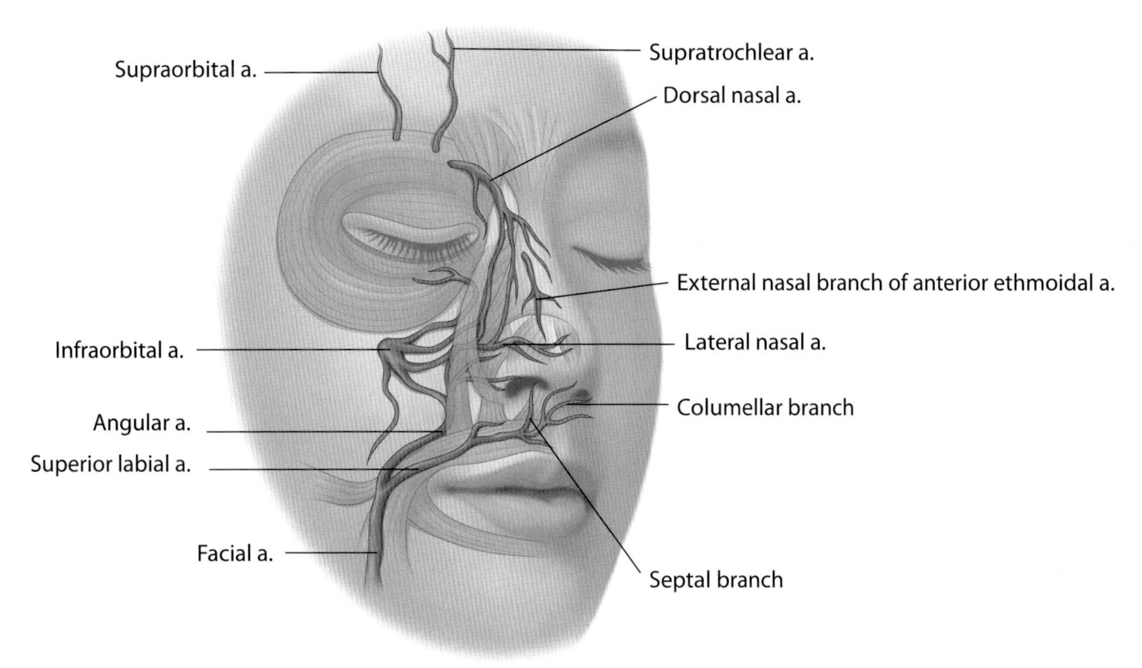

Figure 4 Arterial distribution of the external nose.

III. Selection of Patients

To carry out rhinoplasty effectively using fillers, it is necessary to distinguish patients whom we can expect good postoperative results from those who cannot. For patients whom we cannot expect good results, it is better to recommend standard surgical procedures. The patients that generally tend to show good results are those with:

- Minor humps
- Minor deviations
- High nasal tip and low nasal bridge
- Slight irregularity due to previous surgery

The patient groups that do not show good results are those with:

- Severe hump or deviation
- Upturned nose
- Bulbous nose
- Patients who underwent dorsal augmentation using implants
- Patients who received paraffin or liquid silicone injection previously

IV. Surgical Technique

Filler rhinoplasty can largely be divided into injection on the nasal dorsum and injection on the nasal tip. The nasal dorsum is supported by relatively rigid and fixed structures such as the nasal bone and upper lateral cartilages, and thus can easily be augmented with fillers. On the other hand, the nasal tip has a weak supporting structure especially in Asians, which makes it difficult to be projected or lengthened by filler injection alone. Filler rhinoplasty mostly use the linear threading technique in which the injection needle is inserted and partially retreated repeatedly while injecting the filler. A long 2.5-inch needle can be used to inject the filler in one skin puncture, or a short 0.5-inch needle can be used to inject the filler in several skin punctures. A cannula with a blunt edge is can also be occasionally used for the procedure, which is recommended for beginners due to the relatively low risk of complications such as intravascular injection, but the blunt canula makes it difficult to perform the procedure precisely. Another thing to be cautious about is injecting in the precise layer, as the diameter of the recommended needle and the injected layer varies according to the filler. If the filler is not injected in the appropriate surgical plane, a bump may occur or the filler absorption quickens. The most important thing in filler rhinoplasty is to perform the procedure properly so that the filler stays at the midline. The most frequent complaint after standard augmentation rhinoplasty is asymmetry. This also occurs in filler rhinoplasty. To minimize these complications, the surgeon must always mark the midline on the nasal bridge and perform the procedure on that midline. It is desirable to form a smooth and even dorsal contour by massaging the irregularly elevated area after injection. The area with excessive injection must be pushed down with pressure toward the base, and the area with insufficient filler must be given additional material. Slight edema occurs after the procedure, and thus re-injection must be performed only after two weeks. Special dressings or prescriptions for antibiotics are not necessary.

1. Nasal Dorsum

Anesthesia before filler injection can be performed adequately by applying local anesthetic cream for approximately 40 minutes prior to the injection. The effect is maximized by using plastic wrap on the cream. The surgeon marks the midline on the patient's dorsum after anesthesia. The midline must be marked accurately to prevent complications such as asymmetric injection or intravascular injection. Then the surgeon marks the point from which the augmentation will begin with the filler, finding the point that forms the ideal nasofrontal angle by pinching up the skin on glabella with fingers. For Asians, the line that connects the double eyelids on both sides is the point from which the nasal augmentation begins. Filler injection is performed by largely dividing the nose into four parts: the radix, rhinion, supratip, and tip. This is because the thickness or quality of subcutaneous tissue for each area as well as the strength of the supporting structure vary, and thus it is necessary to use different surgical methods for each area. After marking the four divided parts of the nose, the surgeon marks depressed areas that require filler on the left and the right of the midline *(Figure 5)*.

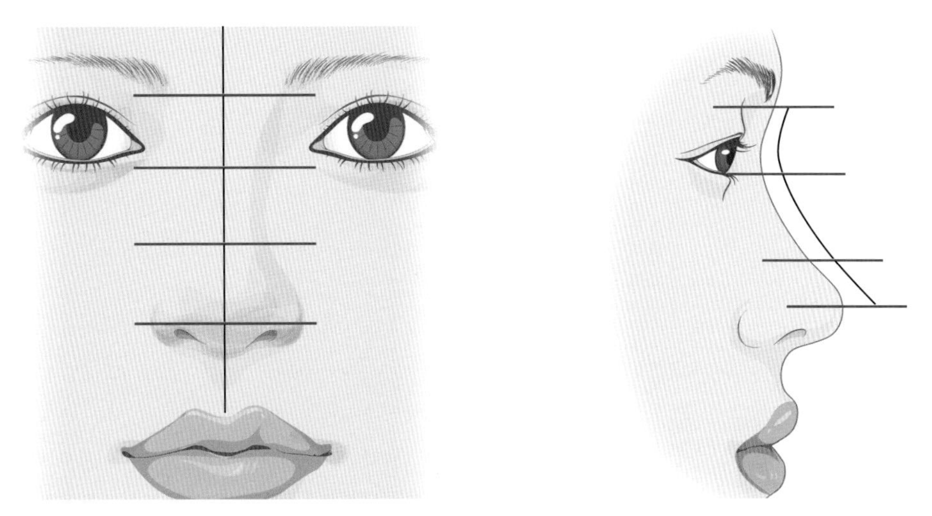

Figure 5 The surgeon marks the nasal midline on the patient's dorsum before injection. The midline must be marked accurately to prevent complications such as asymmetry or intravascular injection. Then the surgeon marks the point from which the augmentation will begin. For Asians, the line that connects the double eyelids on both sides is the point from which the nasal augmentation begins.

The radix and supratip areas have thick soft tissues. Moreover, the base consisting of cartilage and bone is little bit concave. Therefore, if filler is not injected sufficiently in these areas, the filler in the radix and supratip areas will be compressed by pressure of the soft tissues after some time, and may form a hump nose *(Figure 6)*.

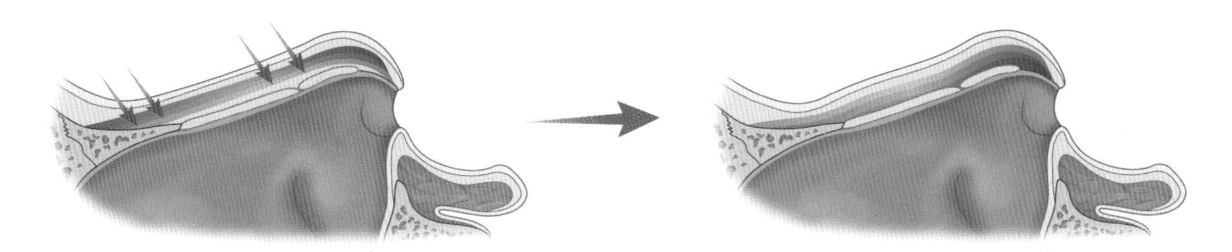

Figure 6 The radix and supratip areas have thick soft tissues. Moreover, the base consisting of cartilage and bone is a little concave. Therefore, if filler is not injected sufficiently in these areas, the filler in the radix and supratip areas will be compressed by the pressure of soft tissue after some time and may form a hump nose.

The filler is usually injected in the order of radix, rhinion, tip, and supratip area. The tip is injected before the supratip area because the supporting structure of the nasal tip is weak especially for Asians, and thus it is difficult to determine in advance how much the nasal tip can be projected by filler injection. If the supratip area is augmented before the tip, a polly beak deformity that makes the nasal tip seem droopy may occur if the nasal tip is not adequately augmented *(Figure 7)*.

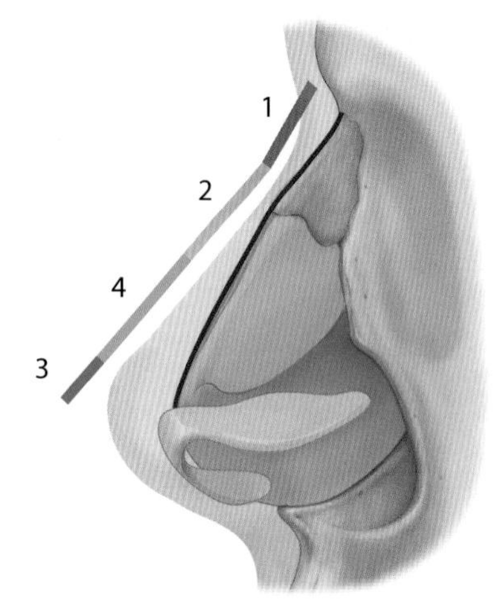

Figure 7 Filler is usually injected in the order of radix, rhinion, tip, and supratip area.

2. Nasal Tip

Using fillers, patients can receive tip augmentation simply at the outpatient clinic. Despite the disadvantages of short longevity compared to surgery and the limited capability of augmentation in terms of achievable height, injection rhinoplasty is preferred by patients with reluctance to standard rhinoplasty or those who want a shorter downtime after procedure. Areas that are injected for augmentation using fillers are the nasal spine area, intercolumellar space, dome area, and alar margin *(Figure 8)*. Filler injection in the nasal spine area has the effect of lifting the nasal tip by increasing nasal tip support, and if the nasolabial angle is acute, it can correct this as well. It is desirable to inject by holding the membranous septum with the fingers so that the filler, when injected on the nasal spine area, does not expand the membranous septum toward nasal cavity, but stay at the intended location. If the filler migrates inward, and expands the membranous septum, the patient may suffer from nasal obstruction. Thus, the surgeon must check whether the filler has migrated toward the nasal cavity even after injection, and if the filler has expanded the membranous septum, if so, it must be mobilized to the infero-medial direction by molding with fingers. In general, 0.5cc of filler is used in the nasal spine area. Filler injection in the intercolumellar space enhances the support of the nasal tip as the injected filler acts as a pillar. It can also correct columellar retraction to a certain degree. For this purpose, 0.2-0.3 cc of filler is used.

Filler injection at the apex of the tip, or domal area, is performed to project and shape the nasal tip by giving additional volume. The injected area varies according to the direction to which the domal area is to be augmented. Generally, 0.2 cc of filler is injected, and it is recommended to inject in the subcutaneous layer. When injecting fillers in the domal area, it is safe to inject at the center to reduce unexpected injuries of blood vessels as they are located on the sides of the tip defining point. Alar retraction, in which the edges of alar lobule are retracted, can also be corrected by filler injection. However, if a scar is formed due to previous surgery, injection is not recommended as it may cause complications such as skin necrosis or irregularity.

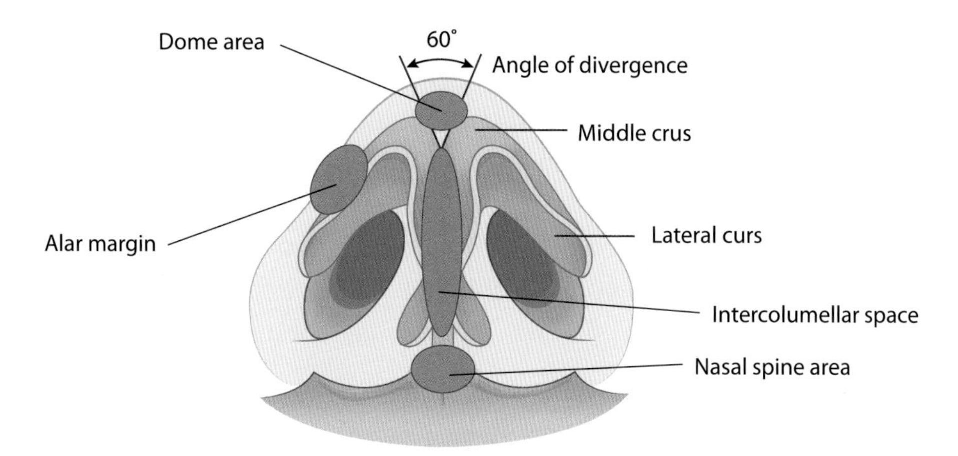

Figure 8 Areas that are mostly injected with fillers are the nasal spine area, intercolumellar space, dome area, and alar margin.

3. Surgery of the Paranasal Areaa

For better aesthetic outcomes of rhinoplasty, it is better to augment the paranasal area along with the nose. Areas that require the filler injection are the forehead, around the nose, and the chin. This is to create a better dorsal aesthetic line. In the past, alloplastic implants such as silicone and Gore-Tex were most commonly used for augmentation of the paranasal area, but recently fat injection is more commonly used. Fat injection however has unpredictable graft survival rate and may cause donor site morbidity. Thus, filler injection on the paranasal area is gradually becoming popular as a more non-invasive procedure. When performing filler injection at the paranasal area, fillers for the subcutaneous layer are more frequently used than fillers injected in the dermal layer. Injection of filler into the paranasal area is effective, simple, and has fewer side effects; however, the surgeon must explain to the patients that it may be gradually absorbed as time passes.

V. Complications

Surgery using fillers is relatively safe, but complications may occur as in other types of surgery. Fortunately, most complications can be prevented by choosing safe fillers and employing appropriate injection techniques. Typical postoperative complications include swelling, erythema, bruising, discoloration, lumps, irregularity, granuloma, and infection in rare cases. The most serious complication is skin necrosis due to impaired circulation.

1. Bruising

Bruising is one of the most frequently occurring complications after filler injection, and is caused by injured blood vessels by the needle. To reduce bruising, it is better to minimize puncturing the muscle layer whenever possible, and to inject under good illumination with the surgical lights on in order to prevent inadvertent injuries of blood vessels. The surgeon must make patients discontinue intake of blood thinners such as aspirin a week prior to the procedure. Placing an ice pack on the injected areas after the injection helps prevent bruising. Special injection needles or cannula are occasionally used to minimize injuries of blood vessels. If bleeding occurs after filler injection, the needle entrance area must be covered with gauze, and given pressure for a few minutes to prevent severe bruising. It is necessary to remind the patients that bruising is a temporary phenomenon and does not influence the ultimate surgical outcome. Moreover, the surgeon must explain that the bruises may darken for a few days and slowly disappear over 10 days.

2. Asymmetry

As in the typical rhinoplasty procedure, asymmetry is one of the common complications of filler rhinoplasty. To prevent asymmetry, the needle tip must be located precisely on the midline of the nose, and the direction of the needle's bevel must face the midline without slanting toward one side *(Figure 9)*. When injecting fillers to a patient with a deviated nose, it is better to inject filler in smaller, fractionated doses while observing the change in the overall shape.

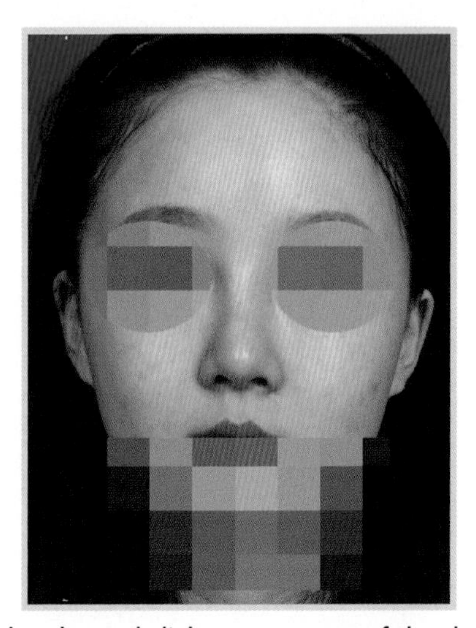

Figure 9 Patient who showed slight asymmetry of the dorsum after injection.

3. Visible Implant

If filler is injected too close to the skin surface, the injected area becomes bumpy or the filler may show through; thus, it is desirable to inject the filler in the appropriate surgical plane. If the skin surface becomes bumpy or the filler shows through because the filler is injected too superficially, the surgeon can massage the area and push the filler deeper, which solves the problem *(Figure 10)*.

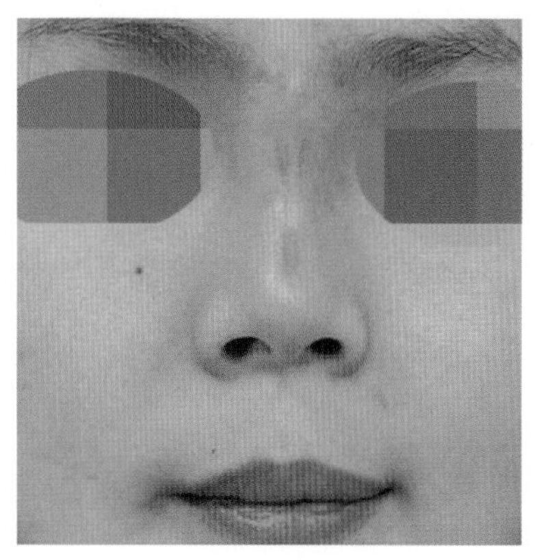

Figure 10 If the filler is injected too superficially (close to the skin surface), the injected area becomes bumpy or the filler may show through.

4. Hypersensitivity Reaction

Rarely, a hypersensitivity reaction to the chemical components of the filler may occur. Pain and erythema, accompanied by pruritus and fever are typical symptoms and signs. In most cases, the symptoms improve spontaneously. If the reactions are severe, they can be improved by warm compression and administration of systemic corticosteroids. If the erythema persists, it can be treated by a V-beam laser *(Figure 11)*.

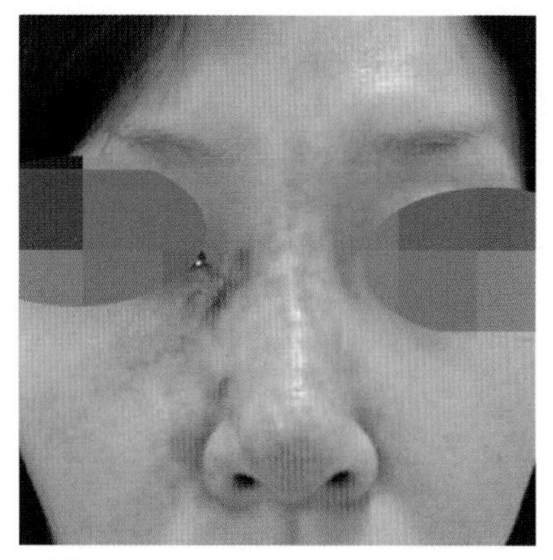

Figure 11 Hypersensitivity reaction to the filler.

5. Granulomas and Nodules

Occasionally, masses can form around the injected area after filler injection. These masses can be classified into granulomas and nodules. A granuloma is an immune response formed as the immune related cells such as lymphocytes gather to remove foreign substances. Granulomas have irregular shapes, and shows an excessive inflammatory reaction in the injected areas. To treat granulomas, one can locally inject costicosteroids or remove it surgically. Nodules are globular in shape and usually are solid in consistency. The injected filler itself can form a lump that makes a nodule without causing an inflammatory reaction. It must be removed surgically, or if the injected filler is hyaluronic acid, hyaluronidase needs to be injected.

6. Skin Necrosis

The most serious complication that may occur after rhinoplasty using injectable fillers is skin necrosis caused by deficient blood supply. Deficient blood supply may be due to intravascular or extravascular causes. Direct filler injection into an artery is an example of an intravascular cause. Deficient blood supply due to extravascular causes occurs when blood vessels are externally compressed due to excessive filler injection or pressure during filler injection, or when there is excessive edema and inflammatory reaction caused by components of the filler.

Symptoms and signs vary according to cause. Out of 52 patients referred to the author with skin necrosis after filler injection since 2006, 6 (11.5%) patients showed skin necrosis caused by direct filler injection into an artery, 43 (82.7%) had congested venous blood vessels, and 3 (5.8%) had skin necrosis probably due to vascular compression due to edema and an inflammatory reaction around the blood vessels *(Figure 12).*

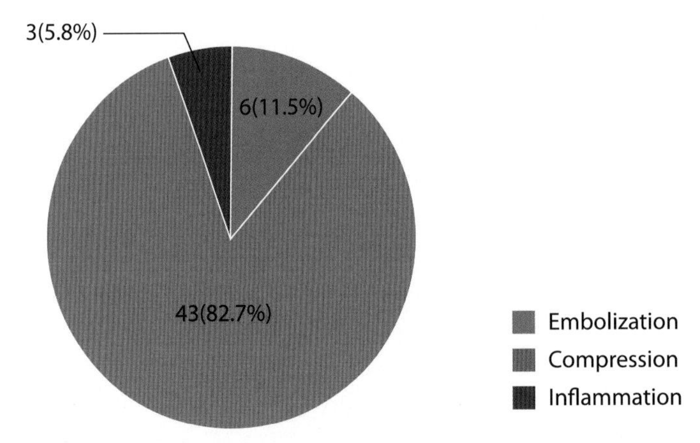

Figure 12 Out of 52 patients referred to the author due to skin necrosis after filler injection, 6 (11.5%) patients showed skinal necrosis caused by direct filler injection into arterial blood vessels, 43 (82.7%) had congested venous blood vessels, and 3 (5.8%) had skin damage due to edema and, an inflammatory reaction.

1) Intra-Arterial Embolization

(1) Pathogenesis

Arterial embolization after filler injection is mostly due to direct filler injection into the dorsal nasal artery when injecting filler into the nasal dorsum. The dorsal nasal artery is a blood vessel that runs longitudinally about 3 mm away from the nasal midline. This blood vessel is immobile and is fixed by surrounding tissues; thus, if the needle is inserted in parallel to the direction of the artery, the tip of the needle can be located inside of this artery. The dorsal nasal artery anastomoses with the ophthalmic artery, infratrochlear artery, and angular artery. Thus a skin lesion due to intra-arterial emoblization can manifest in a geographic pattern. Furthermore, it may be accompanied by ophthalmological symptoms as it is connected to ophthalmic artery *(Figure 13)*.

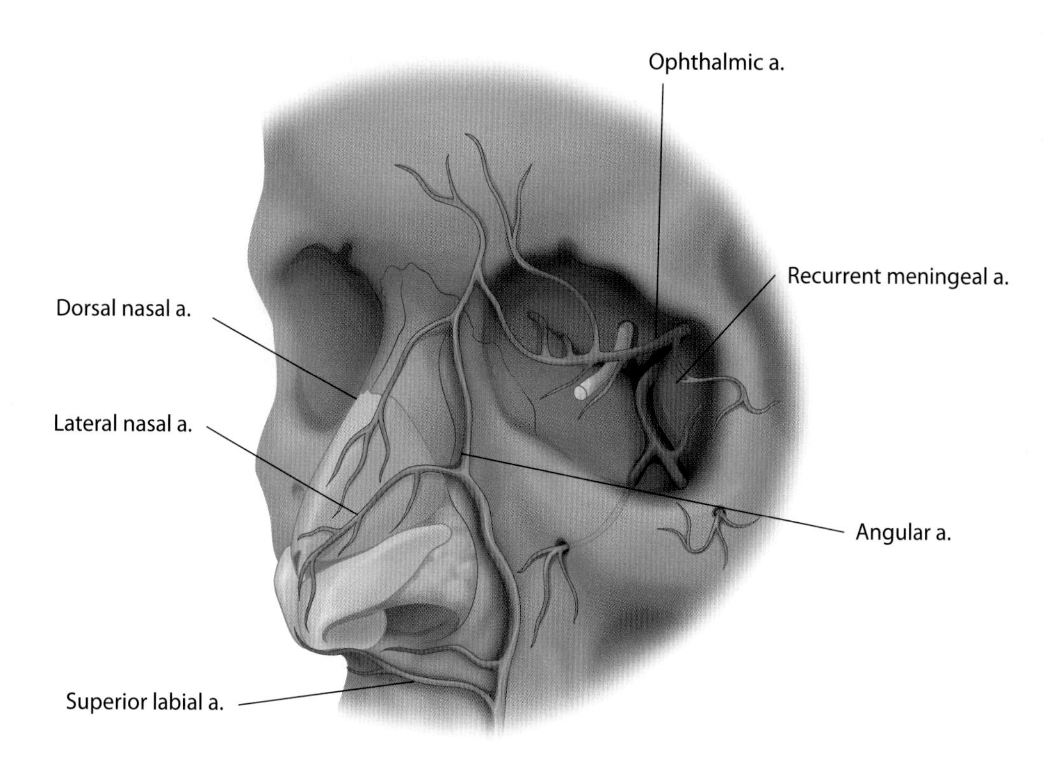

Figure 13 Embolization after filler injection is most commonly due to direct filler injection into the dorsal nasal artery. The dorsal nasal artery is a blood vessel that runs longitudinally about 3 mm away from the midline.

(2) Symptoms and Signs

The frequency of intra-arterial embolization is relatively low, but the clinical manifestations are extremely severe. If the filler is injected directly into an artery, patients suffer from intense pain, and some can feel as if something is spreading from the injected area. Ischemia occurs in the areas supplied by the blood vessels where filler embolization has occurred, turning the skin pale. The ischemic area will show edema within a few hours, and the area around ischemia will show congestion as a rebound phenomenon. After 24 hours, a number of ulcerative lesions accompanied by crusting and erythema occur, which aggravates as time passes and leads to tissue loss within a few days *(Figure 14)*.

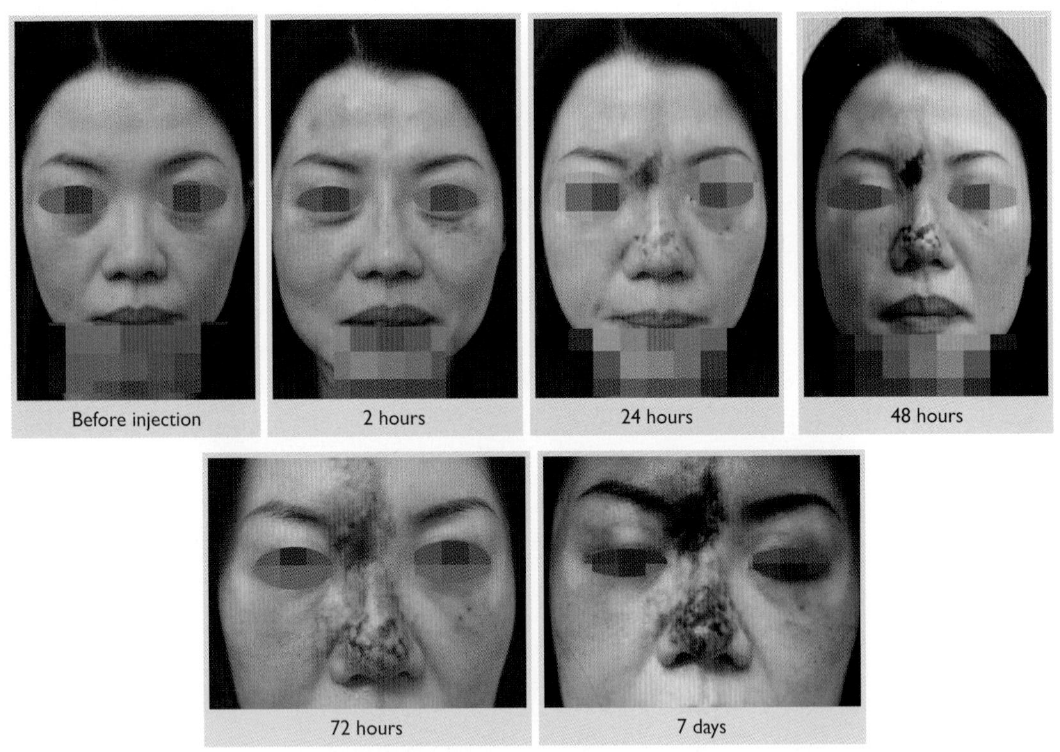

Figure 14 Serial photographs of a patient who experienced skin necrosis due to arterial embolization.

(3) Prevention

To avoid direct filler injection into the dorsal nasal artery, it is necessary to inject the filler by always positioning the needle at the center, as the dorsal nasal artery runs 3 mm away from the nasal midline. If the filler must be inevitably injected on the side of the nose for the correction of deviated nose, the surgeon must never move the needle parallel to the running direction of the blood vessel. If the needle is inserted from the nasal midline and directed laterally to the side for injection, bleeding may occur due to damaged blood vessels by forming a certain angle with the running direction; yet, it may prevent intravascular injection *(Figure 15)*.

(4) Treatment

If the patient feels severe pain during filler injection and the skin turns pale in a geographic distribution along the region in which the blood vessel runs, the surgeon must discontinue injection immediately and perform aspiration to withdraw as much filler as possible. If hyaluronic acid filler is injected, injection of hyaluronidase around the area is recommended. There is a report that injecting hyaluronidase around arterial blood vessels may cause some to penetrate the vascular endothelium, and enter the blood vessels. Low molecular heparin therapy reduces thrombus formation and embolization, but it is difficult to perform in the outpatient setting. It is important to supply sufficient oxygen to the area that shows ischemia. It is necessary to softly massage the area with a hot pack and apply 2% nitroglycerin paste to expand the blood vessels, and to start hyperbaric oxygen therapy if possible. The patient must be given appropriate antibiotics to prevent secondary infection. Intravenous injection of 10 μg of prostaglandin E1 once a day for five days may be helpful. If desquamation occurs and pustules form after one day, the surgeon must begin proper dressing. It may be necessary to perform wet dressing and administration of systemic antibiotics for faster wound healing.

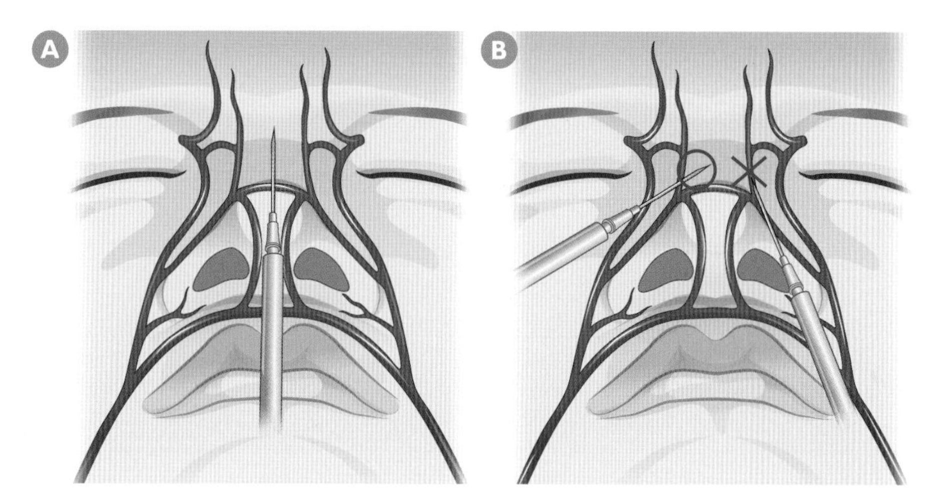

Figure 15 To avoid filler injection into the dorsal nasal artery, it is necessary to inject the filler by always positioning the needle point at the midline, as the dorsal nasal artery runs 3 mm away from the midline (A). If the filler must be injected on the side of the nose for correction of deviated nose, the surgeon must insert the needle on the midline and direct the needle point laterally along the side for injection to prevent intravascular injection (B).

2) Venous Congestion

(1) Pathogenesis

Skin necrosis due to deficient blood supply occurs more frequently due to blocked venous circulation by strong compressive force of excessively injected filler in the tissues, rather than direct injection into the veins.

(2) Symptoms and Signs

If venous vessels are externally compressed, arterial blood vessels that run along with them are also compressed in most cases, causing patients to feel severe pain around the injected areas immediately after injection, and turning the skin pale where the compressed arterial blood vessels supply blood. However, arterial circulation has a higher blood pressure and well-developed collaterals, and thus interruption in the arterial blood supply is a temporary phenomenon that improves quickly, normalizing the pale skin color and reducing pain. However, venous congestion can persist. If venous congestion continues, the patient will continue to feel dull pain, and the skin color around the impaired circulation darkens as time goes by, turning into dark purple after 24 hours, and later causing desquamation or pustule formation. Clinical signs of clear skin necrosis such as tissue loss and discharge are gradually shown within a few days, which recovers through the wound healing process *(Figure 16)*.

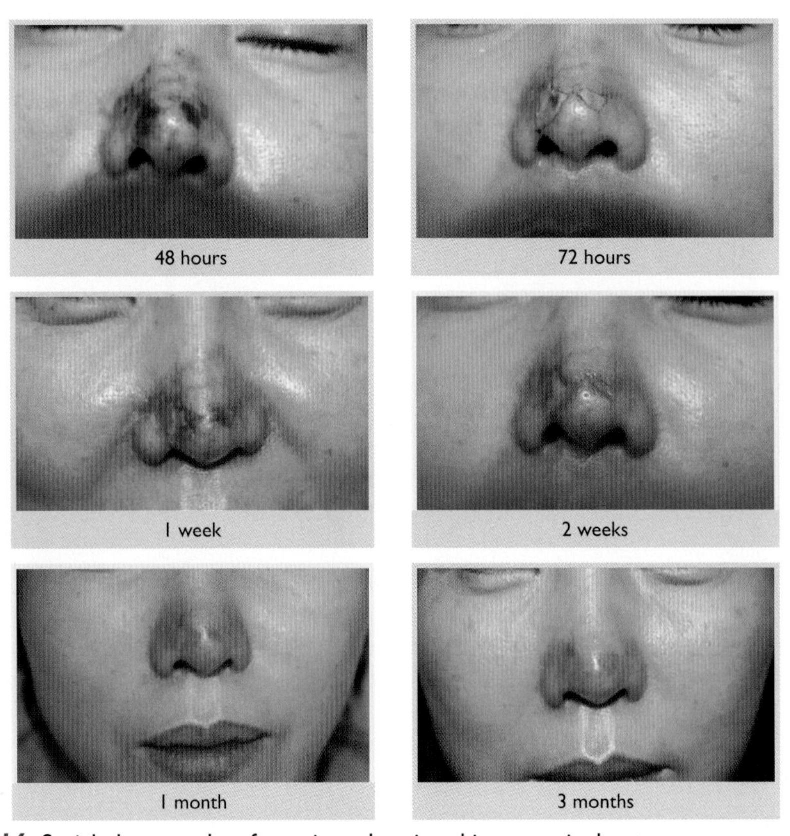

Figure 16 Serial photographs of a patient showing skin necrosis due to venous congestion.

(3) Danger Zone

Skin necrosis that occurs as a result of venous congestion after filler injection appears most commonly on the nasal tip area. Thus, injecting fillers on the nasal tip seems highly dangerous. However, in reality, impaired circulation actually occurs when the filler is injected near the cephalic area of the nasal tip, or the supratip area. The nasal tip area has broad subcutaneous area and is relatively soft. Moreover, as major blood vessels are located on the lateral aspect of the tip defining point, it is relatively safe to inject filler at the center part of the nasal tip. However, in the supratip area, blood vessels run right next to the dermis; thus, if the filler is injected in excessive amounts or with great pressure into the dermis or the subcutaneous area, the blood vessels are more likely to be compressed by the filler *(Figure 17)*. Moreover, the supratip area acts as a hub in which various arteries and veins run together while passing to and from the nasal tip. Therefore, if the blood vessels in this area are compressed and blocked, it may result in deficient circulation at the nasal tip.

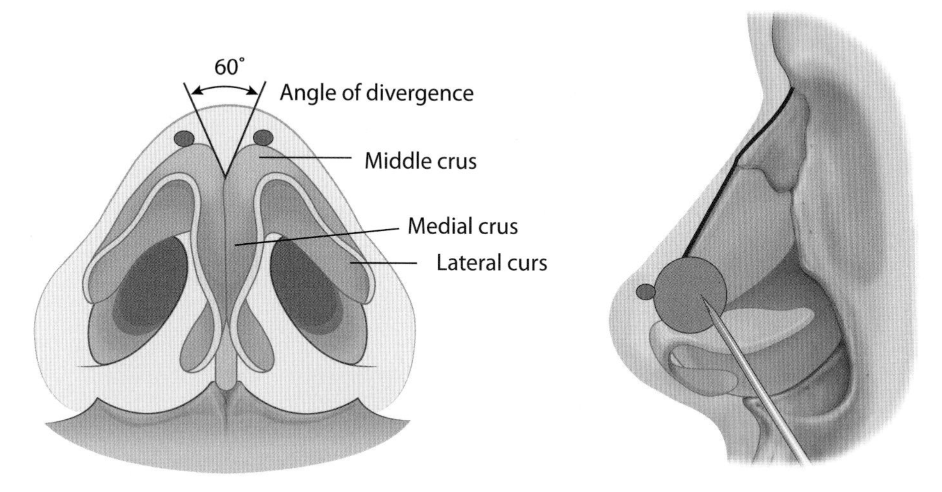

Figure 17 The danger zone for frequent occurrences of skin necrosis in filler injection is near the cephalic area from the nasal tip, or the supratip area.

(4) Prevention

As previously mentioned, if the filler is injected in excessive amounts or with too much pressure into the dermis or the subcutaneous plane of the supratip area, the injected filler can compress and block the blood vessels in the subdermal layer and cause skin necrosis. Therefore, it is recommended to inject the filler in the deepest layer possible above perichondrium, in small fractionated doses. When injecting filler in this area, the surgeon must carefully observe whether there is any change in skin color or pain.

(5) Treatment

If the nasal tip turns pale after injection and shows signs of vascular compression, the surgeon must discontinue injection immediately and adequately massage the nasal tip and the injected area with a hot pack. The surgeon must also make an opening on the injected area and remove the filler by squeezing it out from the surrounding area. If hyaluronic acid filler is used, the filler must be removed by injecting hyaluronidase. Some recommend hyaluronidase injection regardless of the kind of injected filler, because hyaluronidase loosens the tissues and reduces pressure exerted on blood vessels by the filler. The surgeon must then apply 2% nitroglycerin paste to expand blood vessels, and start hyperbaric oxygen chamber therapy if possible. The patient must be given appropriate antibiotics to prevent secondary infection. Use of prostaglandin E1 may be required. In most cases, unlike in arterial embolization, skin necrosis due to venous congestion can be treated without significant sequalae if appropriate measures are taken at an early stage. However, if not, the skin color turns dark purple after a day with skin necrosis. In that case, it is necessary to perform wet dressing and administration of antibiotics for faster wound healing.

3) Inflammatory Reactions and Edema

The protein components such as endotoxin contained in fillers may cause inflammatory reaction and edema, any may cause skin problems. Such complications occur most commonly when injecting fillers made of hyaluronic acid. The symptoms and signs appear few days after the injection in the form of erythematous edema, dermal hyperplasia, and pustule formation. These occur in the areas where the filler was injected, and they are improved easily by proper antibiotic treatment and dressing *(Figure 18)*.

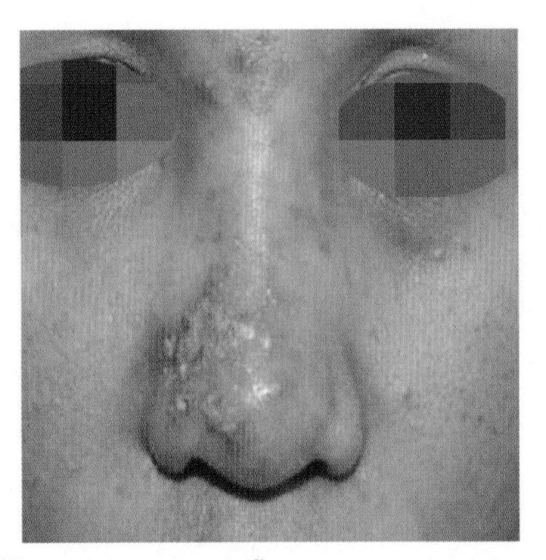

Figure 18 Endotoxin contained in fillers may cause inflammatory reactions and edema as shown in this patient.

References

1. Converse JM. The cartilaginous structures of the nose. Ann Otol Rhinol Laryngol 1955; 64: 220.
2. Daniel RK. The radix. In Daniel RK(eds): Rhinoplasty. Boston, Little, Brown, 1993, 151-168.
3. Gunter JP. Facial analysis for the rhinopalsty patient. Proceedings of the 14th Dallas Rhinoplasty Symposium; 1997 Feb 28- Mar 3, Dallas, USA. Southwestern, 1997, 45-55.
4. Gunter JP, Rohrich RJ. Augmentation rhinopalsty: Dorsal onlay grafting using shaped autogenous septal cartilage. Plast Reconstr Surg 1990; 86: 39-45.
5. Farkas LG, Kolar JC, Munro IR. Geography of the nose: A morphological study. Aesthetic Plast Surg 1986; 10: 191.
6. Gunter JP. Basic nasal tip surgery. Proceedings of the 14th Dallas Rhinoplasty Symposium. 1997 Feb 28- Mar 3, Dallas, USA. Southwestern, 101-15.
7. Lessard M, Daniel RK. Surgical anatomy of septorhinoplasty. Ann Otolaryngol Head Neck Surg 1985; 111: 25-9.
8. Letourneau A, Daniel RK. Superficial musculoaponeurotic system of the nose. Plast Reconstr Surg 1988; 82: 48-52.
9. Rohrich RJ, Gunter JP, Friedman RM. Nasal tip blood supply: An anatomic study validating the safety of the transcolumellar incision in rhinoplasty. Plast Reconstr Surg 1995; 95: 795-9
10. Sherris DA, Kern EB. Computer-assisted facial analysis. In Cummings CW, Fredrickson JM, Harker LA, et al(eds). Otolaryngology Head and Neck Surgery. 3rd ed. St. Louis: Mosby: 1998. p833-843
11. Straatsma BR, Straatsma CR. The anatomical relationship of the lateral nasal cartilage to the nasal bone and the cartilagenous nasal septum. Plast Reconstr Surg 1951; 8: 443-9.
12. Tardy Jr ME. Pratical surgical anatomy, In Rhinoplasty, Philadelphia, W.B. Saunders Co, 1997, 5-125.

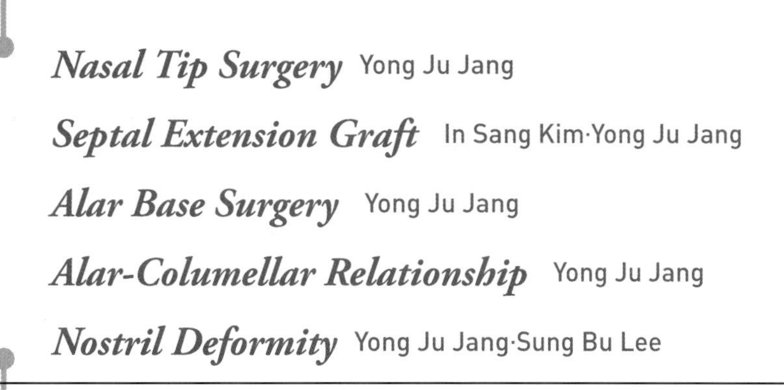

Section 05

The Lower Third

Nasal Tip Surgery

Yong Ju Jang

In rhinoplasty, tip surgery is either the primary objective or a major factor that plays a decisive role in determining the overall success of the surgery. A successful tip surgery becomes possible only when accurate diagnosis, adequate analysis, and precise execution of surgical techniques are in harmony. It is therefore important to have a thorough understanding of the anatomical characteristics of the lower lateral cartilages consisting of the nasal tip, the structures supporting the tip, and their mutual dynamics.

I. Anatomy

The lower lateral cartilage or alar cartilage is made up of the medial, middle (intermediate), and lateral crus *(Figure 1)*. The medial crus makes up the columella that acts as a supporting pillar of the nasal tip. In the columella, the two medial crura are firmly attached to each other by dense fibrous tissues, and covered with a subcutaneous fat-free skin. When the nasal base is viewed

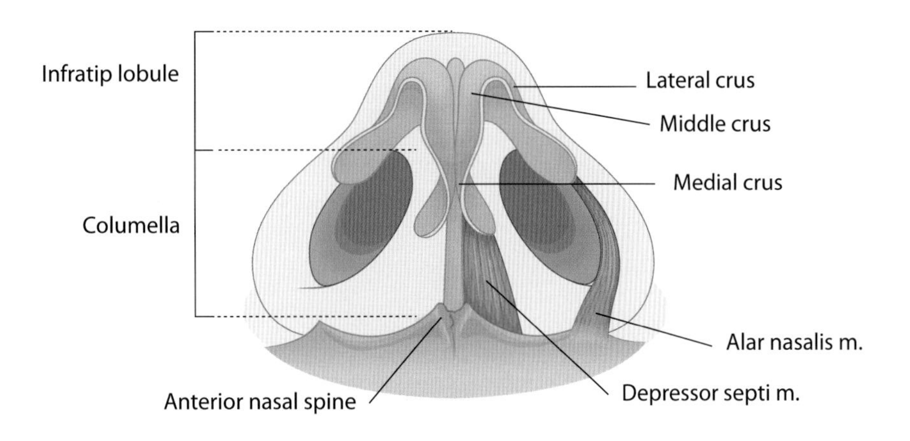

Figure 1 Anatomical components of the nasal tip.

laterally, the apex of the tip to the upper part of the nostril is called the infratip lobule, and the area below it is called the columella. The medial crus continues posteriorly to become the footplate and is connected to the caudal part of the nasal septum. The middle crus, a region with the greatest anatomical diversity, can be divided into the lobular segment and the domal segment *(Figure 2)*. However, during actual surgery, there are frequent occasions where the division and transition of each crus is indistinct and vague. The dome is the most prominent area of the lower lateral cartilage, and the dome on both sides is an important determinant of the shape of the nasal tip. There is an angle of divergence created by the middle crura, and is on average about 50-60˚ *(Figure 3)*. It is cosmetically unappealing if this angle is either overly narrow or excessively broad. The shape of the lower lateral cartilage among patients is quite diverse varying from those that are well-developed to those that are under-developed. It is difficult to perform a successful tip surgery on patients who are characterized by a gently curved lower lateral cartilage; round, fleshy and thick skin; a circular and gaping nostril; and a thick and broad infratip lobule. The lateral crus constitute most of the ala, and is tightly joined to the upper lateral cartilages by forming a scroll junction at its cephalic border *(Figure 4)*.

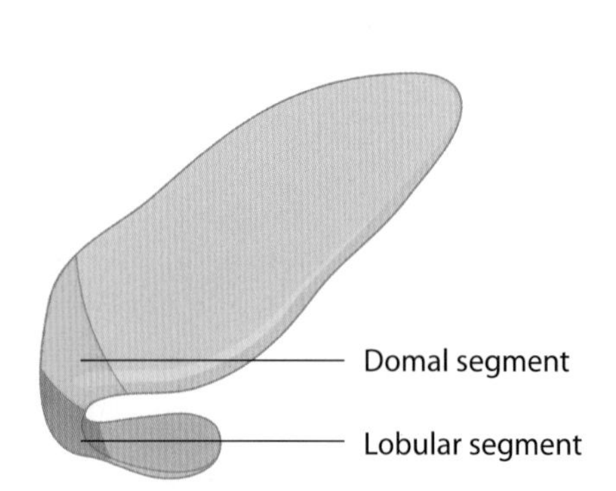

Figure 2 The middle crus is divided into the domal segment and lobular segment.

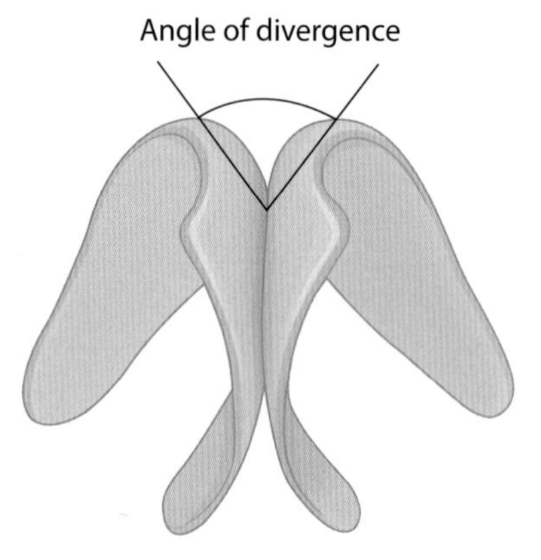

Figure 3 Normal angle of divergence is approximately 50-60˚.

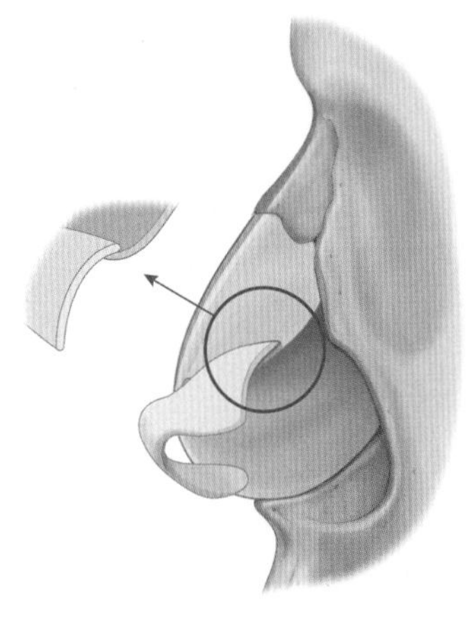

Figure 4 How the lower lateral cartilage is attached to the upper lateral cartilage.

The distance between the caudal margin of the lower lateral cartilage and the alar rim differs from location to location, and also varies greatly from person to person. Nevertheless, on average, the distance from the dome is about 6 mm, the distance from the mid-section of the lateral crus is about 5 mm, and the distance from the rear section of the lateral crus is about 13 mm. Therefore, when applying a marginal incision, the incision line should be made to follow the caudal margin of the lower lateral cartilage rather than the nostril margin. Note that the distance between the alar rim and the caudal margin of the cartilage may be greater among patients with an underdeveloped lower lateral cartilage. Unlike the upper lateral cartilage, the lower lateral cartilage is not directly supported by the septum and is only sustained by a number of soft tissues. The tip support mechanism, which can be sub-divided into the major tip support and minor tip support, is a point of emphasis in anatomical studies of the lower lateral cartilage and the nasal tip *(Figure 5)*. The elements of the major tip support include the shape and strength of the lower lateral cartilages, the junction of the medial crural footplates and the caudal septum, and the union between the lower lateral cartilage and upper lateral cartilage. The interdomal ligament, cartilaginous vault, and the membranous septum act as a minor tip support of the nasal tip.

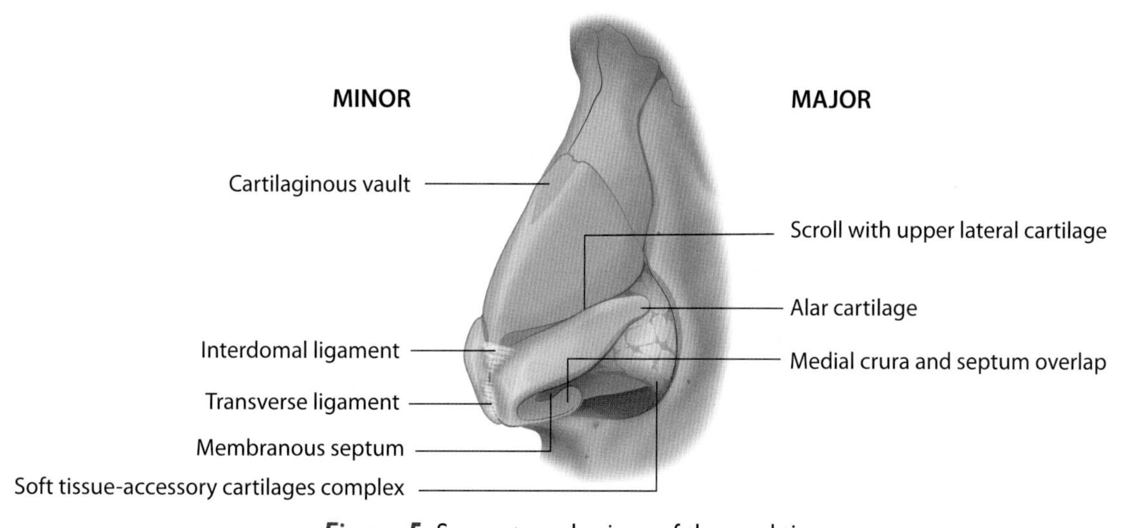

Figure 5 Support mechanisms of the nasal tip.

If the tip support is damaged during tip surgery, it can have short term and long-term effects on the shape of the tip. Thus, care must not only be taken to avoid such damage, but if a situation arises where such damage is encountered, efforts must be made to properly restore the support. Surgical techniques such as complete transfixion incision, intercartilaginous incision, cephalic resection, and division of the medial crus can compromise the tip support mechanism. In tip aesthetics of Asians, tip skin thickness has much more significant role in tip support. In the nasal tip with thin to moderate skin thickness, the contour of the underlying lower lateral cartilage can easily be expressed through the skin, and determines an ultimate tip shape; in extremely thick skinned individuals, the shape of the skin itself determines the overall shape of tip as the thick skin completely obscures the contour of the lower lateral cartilages. Therefore, in order to beautify the nasal tip of thick skinned patients, a tip grafting procedure using thick and angulated grafts can achieve the desired changes.

II. Aesthetic Analysis

To conduct a good tip surgery, an accurate analysis of the shape, width, definition, volume, rotation, position, projection, symmetry, and alar-columellar relationship of the tip is required. Such an analysis implies multi-directional observations from the front, side, oblique, and base.

1. Tip Defining Points

The tip defining points are made up of four anatomical markers which are the supratip break, the dome on either side of the lower lateral cartilage, and the infratip break (columellar breakpoint or columellar lobular junction). The frontal view displays the supratip and the infratip breaks positioned on a vertical line running down the center of the face. The dome of the lower lateral cartilages should be positioned at an identical distance from the nasal tip *(Figure 6)*. It is a point of emphasis that, when performing tip surgery, the tip defining points must be made to be definite if the shape of the tip is to look natural. To make each component of the tip defining points prominent, the skin must be thin and the cartilage well developed. However, for patients with thick skin, it may be more practical to adopt a surgical approach that disregard the concept of such tip defining points, seeking only to avoid making the tip overly round or overly sharp *(Figure 7)*.

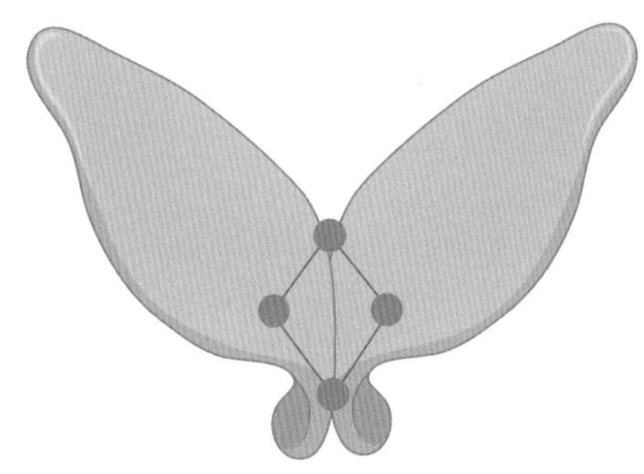

Figure 6 Tip defining points. This is formed by the four anatomical components: supratip break, dome of left and right lower lateral cartilages, and infratip break (columellar break point or columellar-lobular junction).

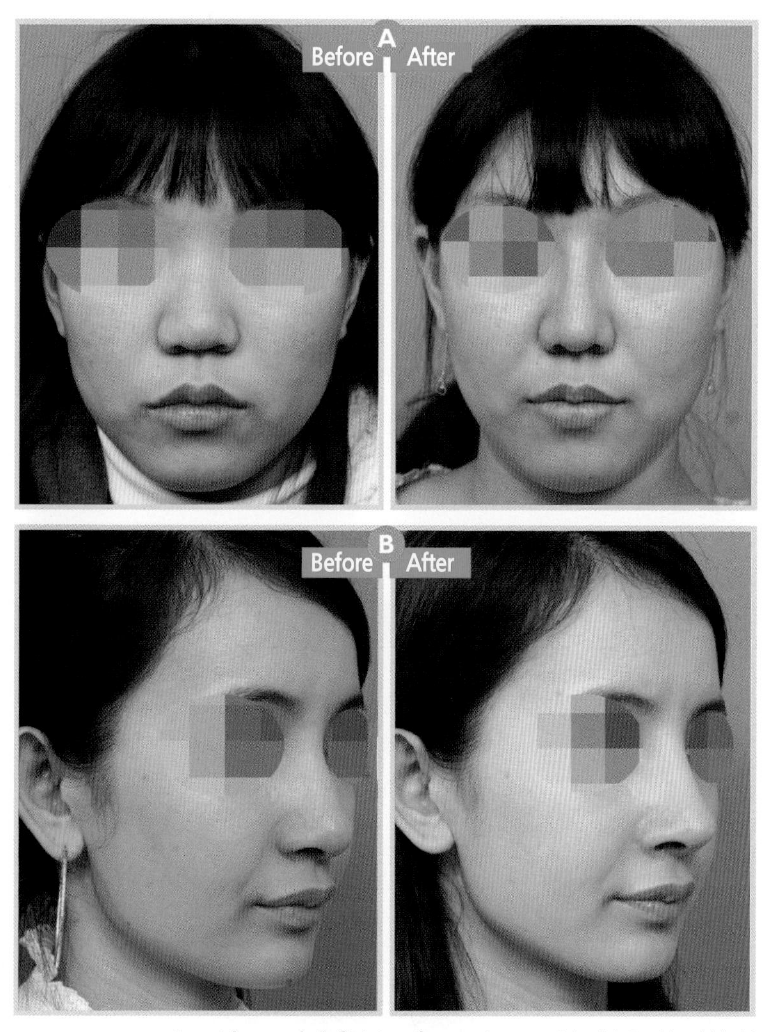

Figure 7 It is not easy to create a tip with good definition for patients with thick skin (A). However, it is easier to improve definition and projection for patients with relatively thin skin (B).

2. Profile Analysis

On the profile view, the tip position, rotation, and projection must be analyzed based on the anatomical landmarks such as radix, supratip break, infratip break, and alar crease, as well as the alar-columellar relationship. A suitable columellar-labial angle is 90-95° and the columellar-lobular angle must likewise exhibit a pleasing angle if the tip is to be determined cosmetically desirable *(Figure 8)*.

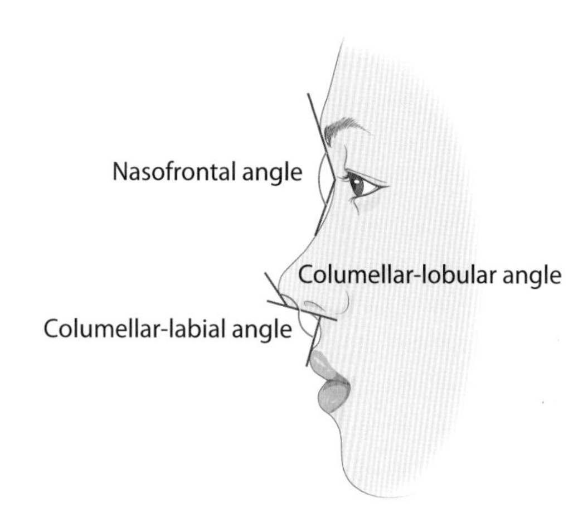

Figure 8 Aesthetic angles observed from the lateral view.

Most of the previous literature emphasize that the most ideal profile image possess the form of a double break, consisting of an infratip break and a supratip break. However, too much effort to create a supratip break may create the appearance of a supratip saddle, and an infratip break that is too prominent may make the nose look like an upturned short nose *(Figure 9)*. Moreover, patients with thick skin, the surgeon can never create distinct double break. In fact, Korean patients prefer a nose with a suitable dorsal height with natural transition to the tip rather than a nose with a clear supratip break and infratip break. It is therefore necessary to thoroughly understand this view in surgery. Analysis of patients' tip shape and actual anatomical characteristics shows that the tip shape varies according to the different shapes of lower lateral cartilages. When observed from the lateral view, a tip with good definition and projection shows antero-caudal projection of the lower lateral cartilages, showing a slight angulation in the domal region. With the skin covering, the tip will have a naturally projected shape *(Figure 10)*. However,

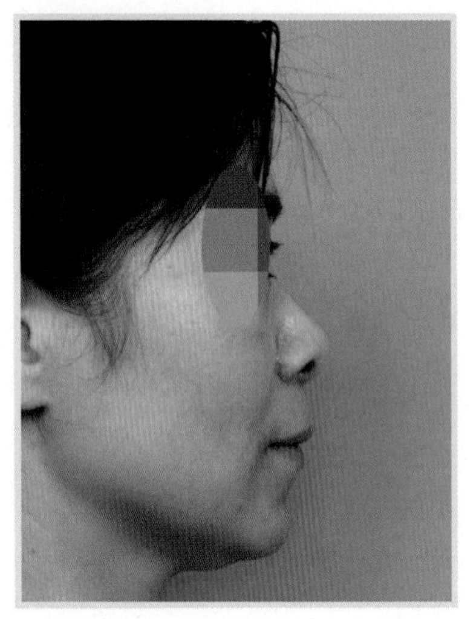

Figure 9 Profile of a patient with the appearance of a short nose due to a too distinct infratip break.

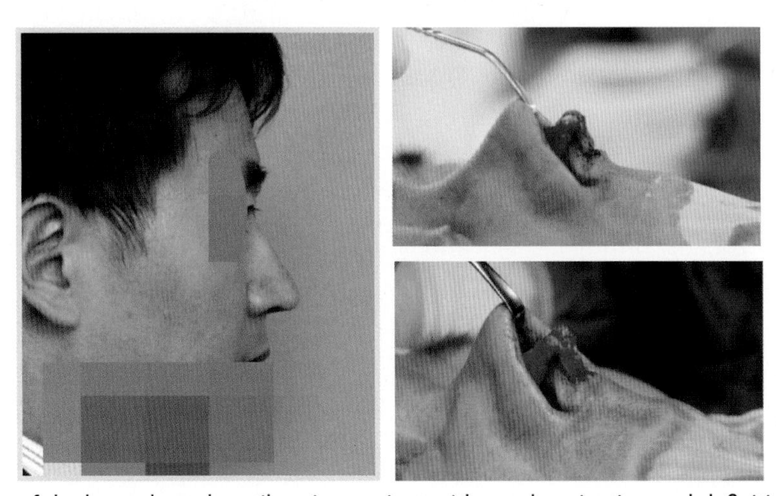

Figure 10 Shape of the lower lateral cartilage in a patient with good projection and definition of the nasal tip.

the intrinsic lower lateral cartilage shape in patients with an underprojected tip usually manifests as underprojected lower lateral cartilages with round contours rather than an appropriate antero-caudal projection *(Figure 11)*. If this patient has thick skin as well, the tip looks worse once covered by the thick skin. Therefore, the author's concept of tip surgery is for the tip structure to have antero-caudal projection to a certain degree, and show angulation in the domal region.

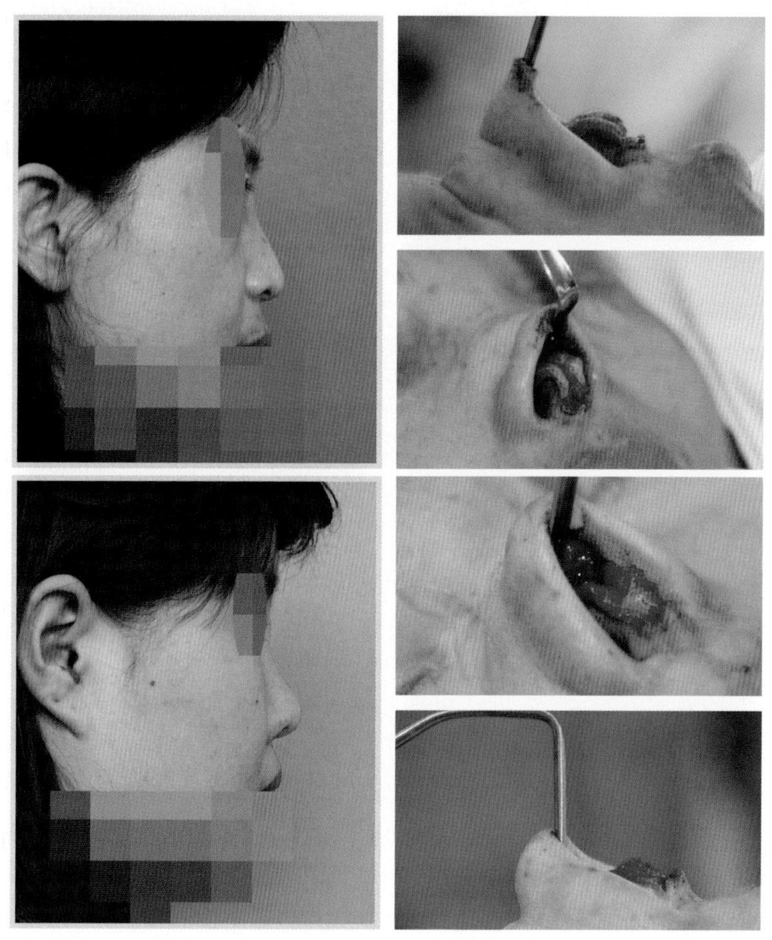

Figure 11 Patients with poor tip definition and projection. Most patients have roundly-contoured cartilage or thick skin.

3. Analysis from the Basal View

From the basal view, the overall triangular shape, the ratio between the infratip lobule and the nostril, as well as the shape of the nostril must be examined. When viewed from below, the nose is in the shape of an equilateral or an isosceles triangle, and the nostril takes on an egg like or tear-drop shape. The ideal ratio between the infratip lobule and the height of the nostril is 1:2, but among Koreans, a ratio closer to 1:1 can be seen frequently.

Nostril asymmetry is identified in the basal view. This asymmetry should be detected prior to surgery, and should be informed to the patient of its existence, as complete correction of this deformity is very difficult *(Figure 12)*.

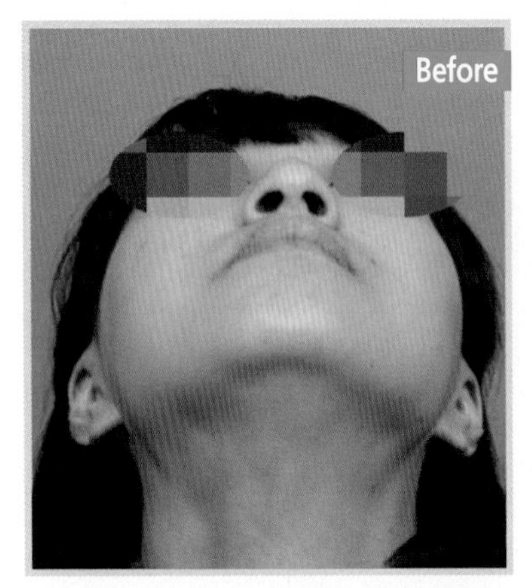

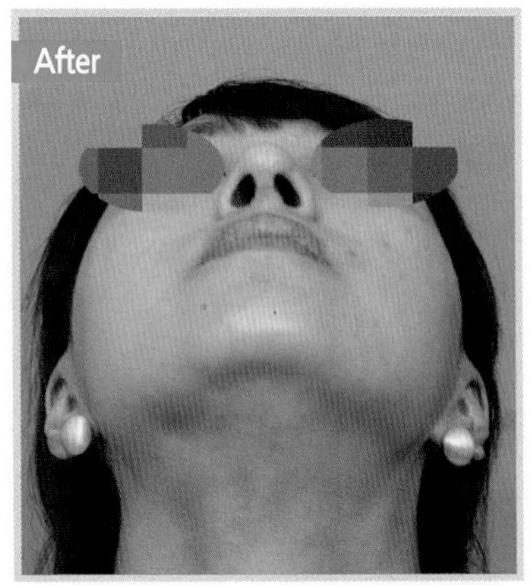

Figure 12 Basal photograph of a patient whose infratip lobule and nostril proportion improved after tip surgery, but the nostril asymmetry was not completely corrected

4. Analysis of the Morphological Characteristics of the Tip

When conducting a comprehensive aesthetic analysis of the tip, in addition to the perspectives discussed above, the analysis must be carried out with a clear understanding of the concepts of projection, rotation, definition, width, volume, and shape. The concept of definition relates to how angular the tip of the nose is, and how much of an impression is being conveyed that it is lean and protruding. Definition is determined by the extent of convexity in the dome as well as the level of the dome's prominence resulting from the interconnected level of concavity in the lateral crus. The thickness of the skin is a very important factor in determining the definition *(Figure 13)*. Width is an element that is determined by the interdomal distance and the thickness of the tip soft-tissue. In a frontal photograph, the width is represented by the distance between the two tip defining points. Projection represents the degree of the tip height. The tip projection is related to the shape of the lower lateral cartilages and the surrounding structures, for example, in accordance to the characteristics of the septum or the anterior nasal spine *(Figure 14)*. Rotation is a term used to express whether the tip is raised, or is droopy. Tip rotation is represented in terms of the tip angle and this also varies according to the intrinsic shape of the lower lateral cartilages and the shape of the surrounding structures *(Figure 15)*. The shape determining factors, in most cases, conform to the intrinsic shape of the lower lateral cartilages. In accordance to the shape of the lower lateral cartilages, particularly that of the lateral crus, various types of shapes such as broad nose, boxy nose, or pinched nose can be found. A cosmetically ideal nasal tip has a suitable outline, a height that accords well with the length of the nose, and maintains a proper angle when viewed laterally.

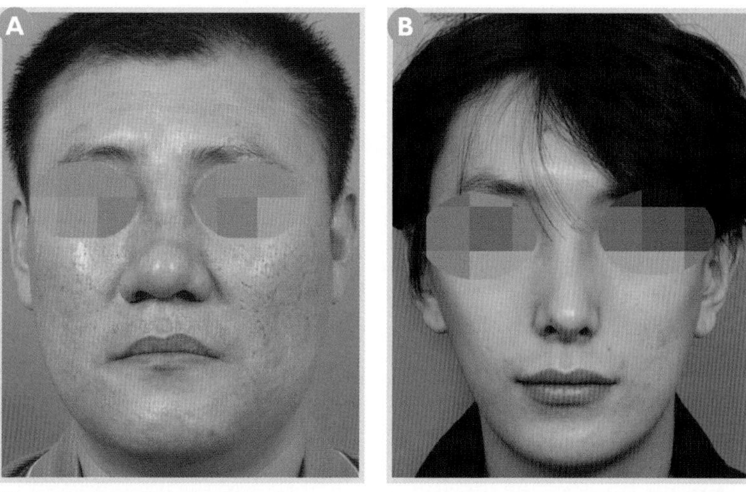

Figure 13 Patient with extremely poor tip definition (A) and relatively good definition (B)

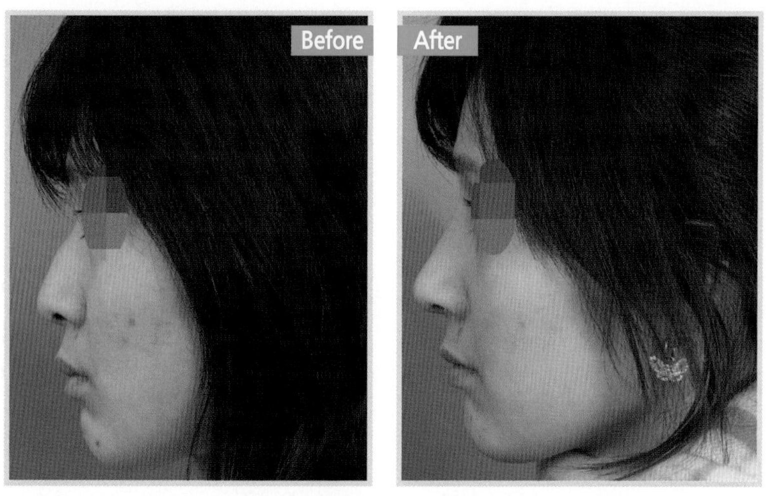

Figure 14 Example of a patient showing an increase of projection after tip surgery.

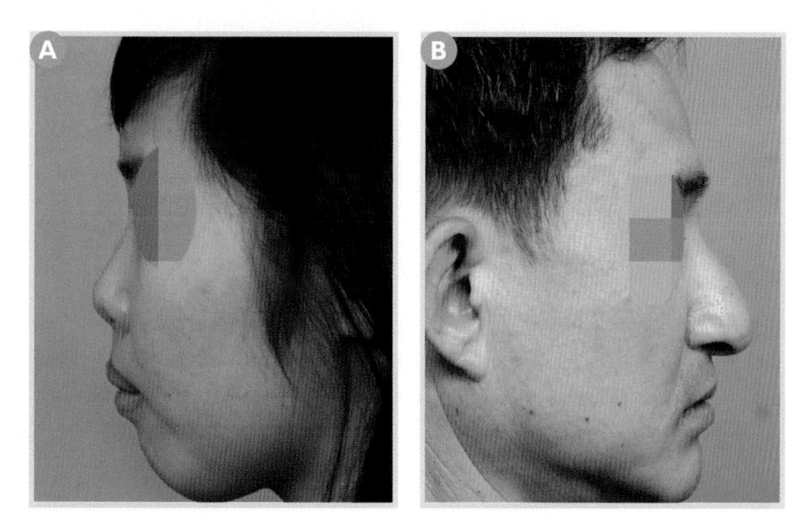

Figure 15 Example of two contrasting patients showing a great difference in tip rotation: cephalic rotation (A) and caudal rotation (B).

III. Surgical Approach

1. Endonasal Approach

In the endonasal approach, the following procedures can be done: cephalic resection through a nondelivery approach, cephalic resection through a delivery approach, transdomal suturing, interdomal suturing, and columellar strut insertion. This approach can also be used for the placement of the graft such as a shield graft or an onlay graft.

1) Nondelivery Approach

The nondelivery approach can be divided between the transcartilaginous approach *(Figure 16)* and the retrograde eversion approach *(Figure 17)*. The transcartilaginous approach is a method that involves applying an incision at the mid-section of the lower lateral cartilage, usually 4-6 mm from the caudal margin of the lateral crus. With this method, volume reduction of the lower lateral cartilages or other tip procedures are possible without any modification to the

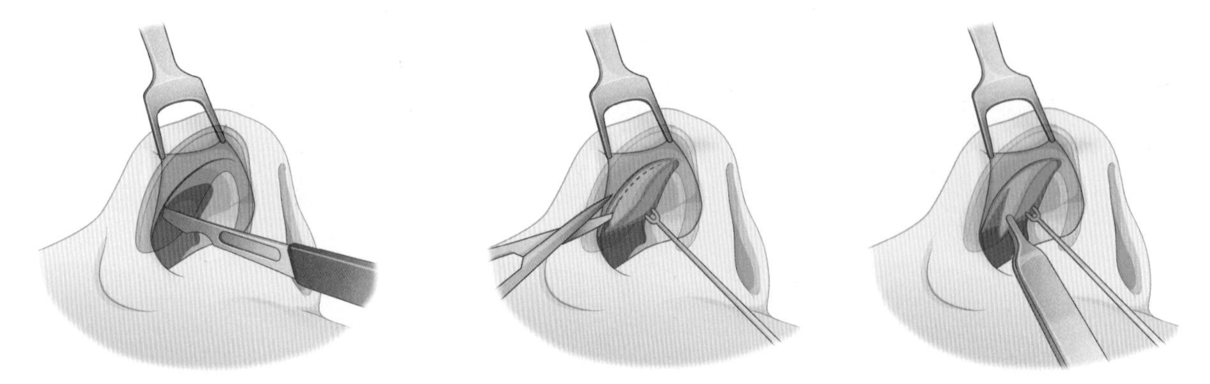

Figure 16 Transcartilaginous approach.

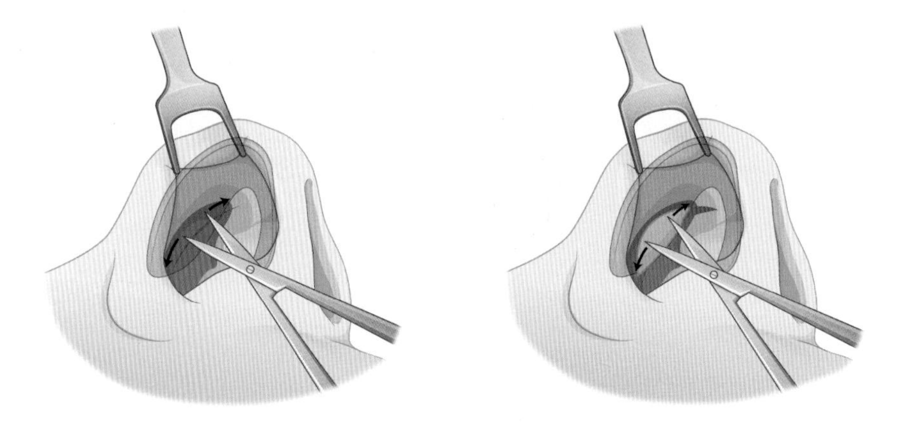

Figure 17 Retrograde eversion approach.

dome or nasal valve. An operation using the retrograde eversion approach involves, following an intercartilaginous incision, the retrograde undermining of the nasal vestibular skin from the rear to the front and exposing half of the cephalic area of the lateral crus *(Figure 17)*. This exposure is simple and causes little scar tissue, and the likelihood of postoperative distortion is low. However, the poor surgical field makes it difficult to maintain symmetry while performing the operation. Therefore, this method is used selectively in cases where there is only a minor deformity of the tip. However, the author does not believe this method to be practical for Asian patients because tip surgery cases that require a nondelivery approach to perform only a cephalic resection is quite rare among Asian patients.

2) Delivery Approach

The delivery approach is a form of operation that involves making an intercartilaginous incision, marginal incision, and septal incision followed by a dissection of the skin-soft tissue envelope. Next, the lower lateral cartilages are then drawn out in the form of a bipedicled chondrocutaneous flap. This approach can be chosen when the desired shape cannot be achieved simply with volume reduction of the lower lateral cartilage, so an additional manipulation of the caudal part of the lower lateral cartilage or the dome is required. The improved direct visualization of the lower lateral cartilages by the delivery approach makes it ideal when using various surgical techniques simultaneously. However, the drawback of this approach is that distortion of the nasal tip can result from the dissection, or postsurgical scarring, in addition to the irreversible damage of the lower lateral cartilages.

3) Extended Marginal Incision

If a marginal incision is sufficiently extended on both sides of the lateral crus and nasal floor, a good view of the nasal tip can be secured. Using this approach, a number of different suture techniques or grafting techniques can be performed more easily. This surgical technique is favored by many endonasal rhinoplasty surgeons as this allows greater maneuverability on the tip without performing an intercartilaginous incision *(Figure 18)*.

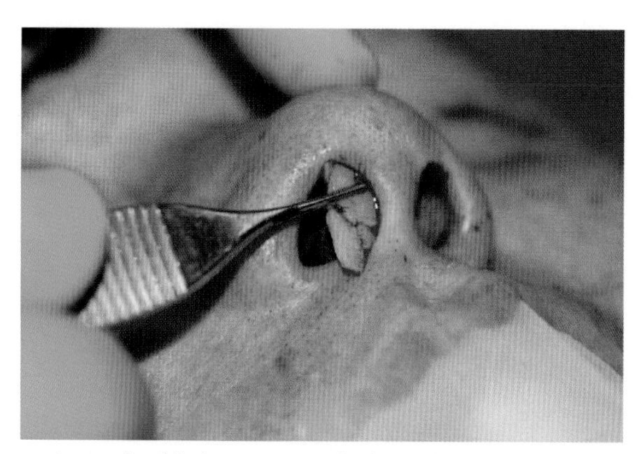

Figure 18 Inserting a double layer tip graft through an extended marginal incision

4) Limited Marginal Incision

A pocket can be formed by making a marginal incision in the caudal aspect of the middle crus and medial crus of lower lateral cartilages. Endonasal tip grafting can be performed by inserting cartilage in this pocket. A certain level of tip projection and rotation can be achieved by onlay tip grafting through this approach. Here, the graft insertion can be facilitated by making the pocket slightly bigger than the cartilage to be grafted. This limited marginal incision can also be used effectively in revision tip surgery to treat tip graft visibility or infection *(Figure 19)*.

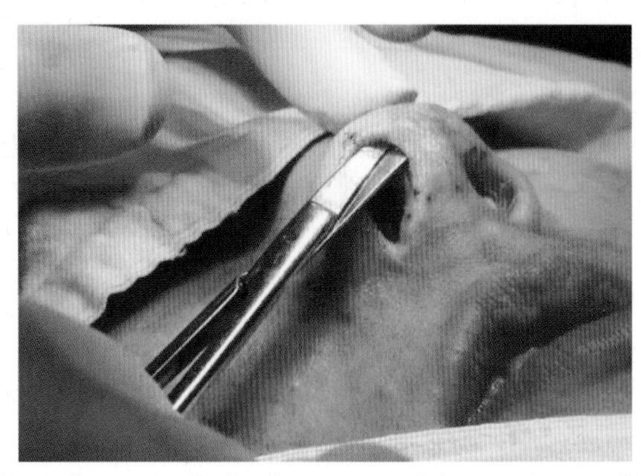

Figure 19 It is possible to effectively approach the dome area of the nasal tip with a limited marginal incision.

2. External Rhinoplasty Approach (Open Approach)

The external approach, which utilizes the marginal incision together with the transcolumellar incision, has several advantages. Primarily it is possible to observe the entire lower lateral cartilages. The use of this approach makes an accurate diagnosis possible and a suturing or grafting can be performed at a more accurate location. Also, the fact that the intercartilaginous incision is not being used lowers the risk of nasal valve obstruction, as well as making it possible to perform meticulous hemostasis. Other advantages are that it allows for the use of both hands and is useful for teaching purposes. However, disadvantages include: scarring in the transcolumellar incision, a risk of secondary inflammation, atrophy of the tip skin (resulting from dissection of the tip area), and prolonged operation time. In addition, as the surgery is performed while the skin is lifted up, there is a difficulty in accurately anticipating how the tip surgery technique will affect the final shape of the tip prior to closing the skin.

IV. Various Techniques of Tip surgery

The following section will describe the various techniques that can be used to bring morphological changes in the nasal tip. The techniques will be classified as follows and explained in this order.

1. Modification of Tip Soft Tissues

1) Defatting

In cases where the skin-soft tissue envelope of the nasal tip is too thick, it is almost impossible to create an ideal tip with distinct definition. Nevertheless, it is possible to make an effort for cosmetic improvement even in such patients. In the author's case, when the patient has an overly thick soft tissue at the tip, an external approach is used to expose the tip. During the process of dissecting the skin flap, rather than using the more common supraperichondrial dissection method, a method that elevates the flap with the yellowish fibro-fatty tissue left attached to the surface of the lower lateral cartilage is preferred. When the supraperichondrial dissection of the lower lateral cartilage is performed after the flap is elevated in this manner, the fibro-fatty tissue can be removed safely, and the tissue that is removed in this manner can be used as filler for other areas during surgery *(Figure 20)*. At times, the soft tissue attached to the elevated skin flap can be additionally removed. However, this procedure requires extreme caution as there is a risk that such additional procedure may cause irreversible damage to the skin. Most patients with a bulbous nose, which necessitates this technique, also have extremely poorly developed lower lateral cartilages. Therefore, the tip projection must be enhanced through transdomal sutures, interdomal sutures, a columellar strut, or onlay grafting. However, the author frequently solves the issue of tip bulbosity in thick-skinned patients with grafting using thick and angulated cartilage, not defatting. In this way, the preserved fibro-fatty tissue in the tip by not performing defatting, is much more beneficial by softening the angled edges of the graft, and is useful to prevent tip graft visibility that is likely to occur in the future.

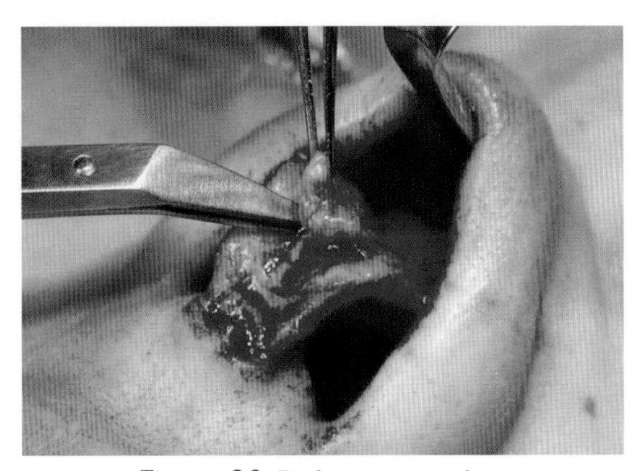

Figure 20 Defatting procedure.

2. Direct Modification of Lower Lateral Cartilage

1) Cartilage Excision, or Volume Reduction of the Lateral Crus

(1) Definition and Effects

Cartilage excision is also known as volume reduction. In this procedure, the method most commonly used by the author is cephalic resection (cephalic trim), which resects the cephalic area of the lateral crus.

(2) Classification

Two surgical techniques used in lower lateral cartilage excision are the complete strip and incomplete strip (interrupted strip) technique. The complete strip technniques maintains continuity of the lateral crus left after cephalic resection, preserving the width of lateral crus at 4-8 mm or 75% of the original volume. Leaving a little cartilage strip is enough if the patient's cartilage is strong, but a greater portion must be left if the cartilage is weak. If too much lower lateral cartilage is excised, the tip support will be damaged, which results in changes in the tip shape or nasal obstruction by valve collapse. The incomplete strip technique excises a part of the remaining lateral crus after cephalic resection, and suturing the segments together. This technique includes lateral crural overlay or medial crural overlay. Using this technique, a greater degree of cephalic rotation can be obtained if more lateral crus is excised, especially on the lateral side than the medial side *(Figure 21)*. Incomplete strip technique enables more cephalic rotation than the complete strip technique, but it is accompanied by loss of the nasal tip projection and has the disadvantage of not being able to easily and accurately predict the tip shape after healing.

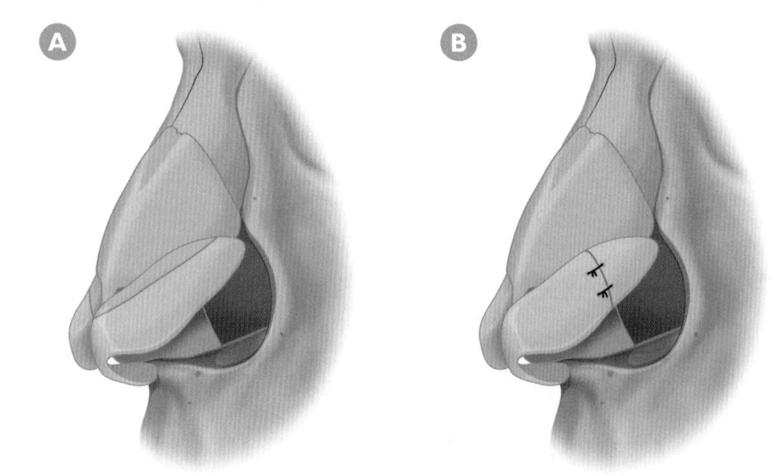

Figure 21 Cephalic resection of lateral crus (A) and lateral crural overlay technique (B), that is one of incomplete strip techniques.

(3) Indications and Surgical Technique of Cephalic Resection (Cephalic Trim)

This surgical procedure is the one of the most typical methods among the cartilage excision techniques. Performing this procedure will lead to the formation of fibrous tissue during the healing process. This will cause a contraction to occur resulting in the narrowing of the lateral crus area as well as a secondary cephalic rotation of the tip.

This method is performed to solve the following problems:

- ☑ Excess convexity of the ala due to too much convexity of the lateral crus
- ☑ Bulbous nasal tip due to bulky lower lateral cartilages
- ☑ Caudally rotated tip
- ☑ Excessive tip projection
- ☑ Lack of a triangular definition of the tip

Generally this technique is commonly performed on patients with well developed lower lateral cartilages. It should be applied with caution to those with poorly developed lower lateral cartilages. In the author's case, this technique is performed to improve the tip projection, rotation, and definition of patients with well developed lower lateral cartilages. In patients with a poor definition of the dome, a cephalic resection is first performed ahead of a transdomal suture *(Figure 22)*.

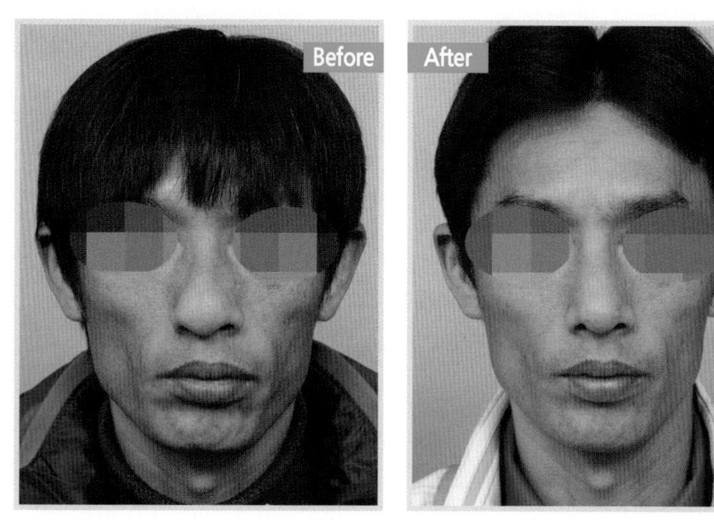

Figure 22 Example of a patient of which cephalic resection and tip graft procedure was performed for the purpose of volume reduction to correct tip bulbosity.

(4) Surgical Technique

Prior to performing cephalic resection, the area to be excised needs to be marked and then resection performed to ensure that the remaining cartilage strip on both sides are equal in shape and width. While performing this surgical procedure, care must be taken not to damage the mucosal lining the nasal cavity. Using a #15 blade, start the incision from the medial side to be excised, followed by dissection from the mucosa underneath. Then raise the area to be excised, and using a fine scissors, proceed to remove the cartilage in a lateral direction *(Figure 23)*.

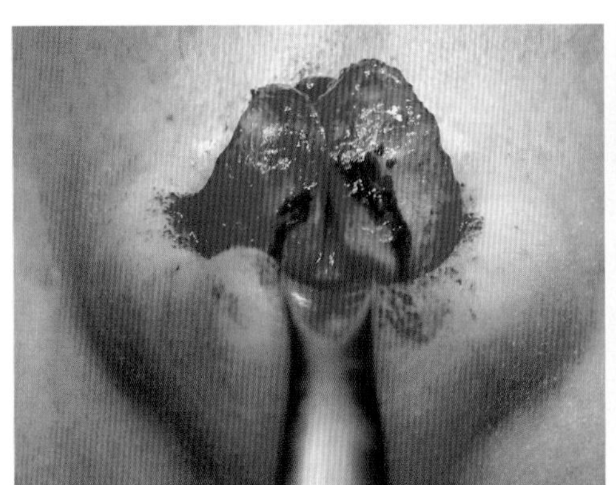
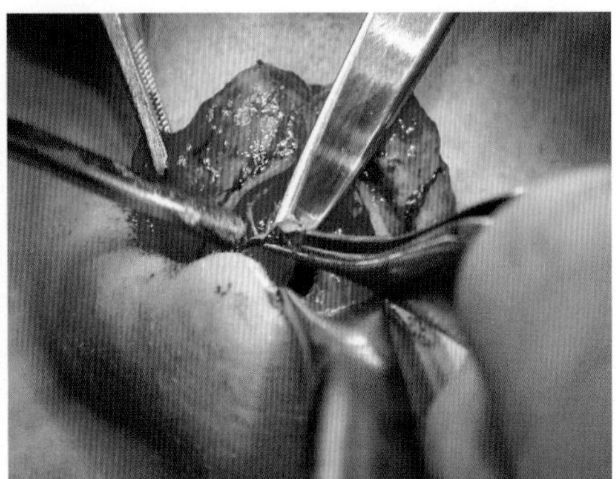

Figure 23 Intraoperative view of cephalic resection.

2) Medial Crural Overlay

This technique separates the medial crus from the underlying vestibular skin and incises it, overlapping it to desired amount to correct asymmetry or overprojection of the tip. This technique can be performed on only one side when there is asymmetry of the tip.

3) Lateral Crural Overlay

This technique involves dissecting off the lateral crus from the underlying vestibular skin, incising, and overlapping it *(Figure 24)*. This technique is effective in correcting tip asymmetry as well as a ptotic tip. Robust effect of cephalic rotation can be expected in patients with severe tip ptosis *(Figure 25)*.

4) Flip-Flop (Upside Down Repositioning) of the Lateral Crus

In rare occasions, the lateral crura are not symmetrical, with one side of the lateral crus convex and the other side concave, which can cause a deviated nose. When both sides of the lateral crus are extremely concave, this may result in alar concavity. One way to solve this problem is to excise the lateral crus from the dome area, and reconnect it after flipping it over *(Figures 26, 27)*. When applying this technique, the lateral crus must be freed from the underlying vestibular skin very carefully. The process can be facilitated by injecting topical anesthetic solution at the vestibular skin before dissection.

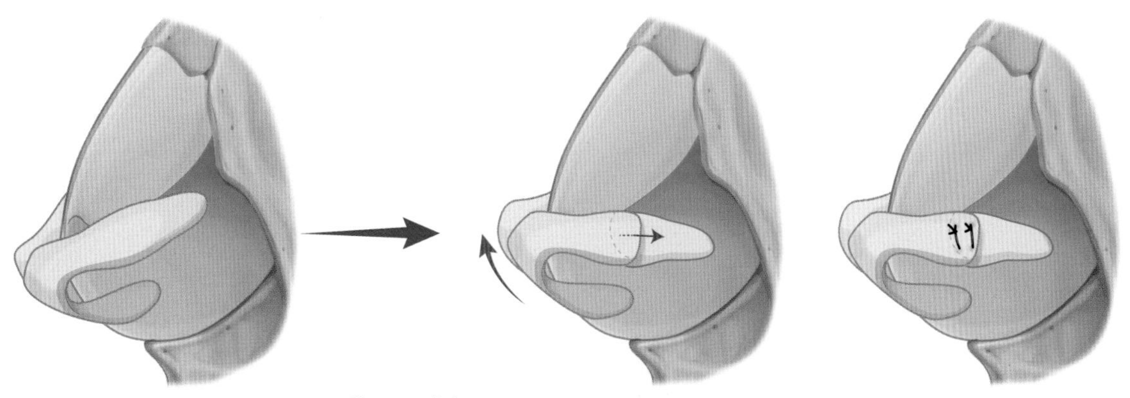

Figure 24 Lateral crural overlay technique.

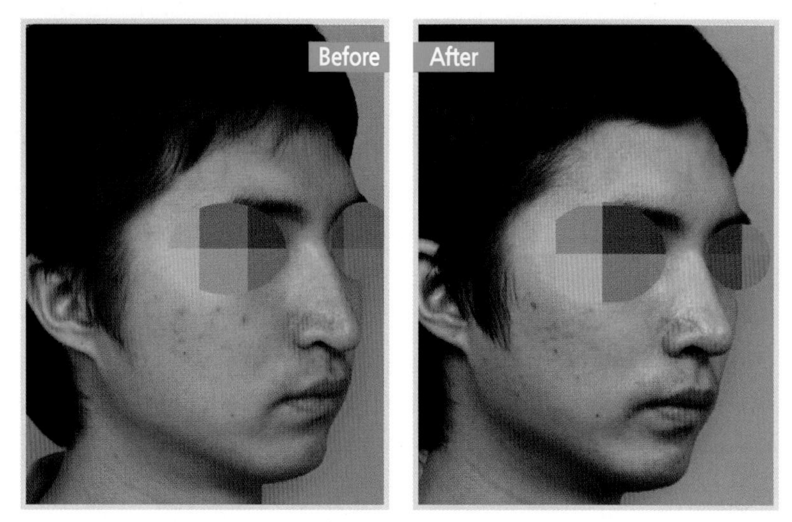

Figure 25 Example of a patient who experienced improvement of tip ptosis by applying lateral crural overlay technique.

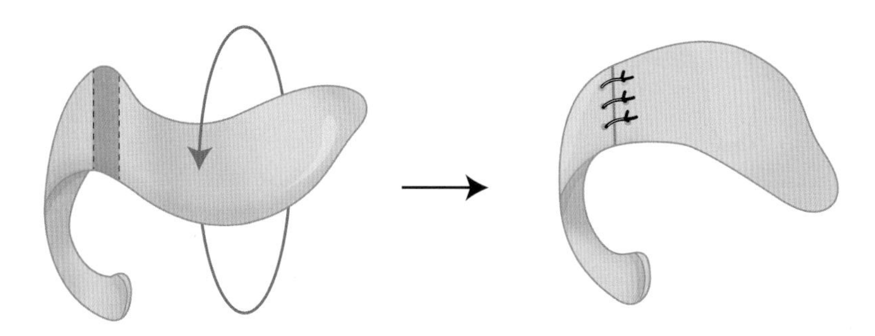

Figure 26 Flip flop (upside down repositioning) of lateral crus.

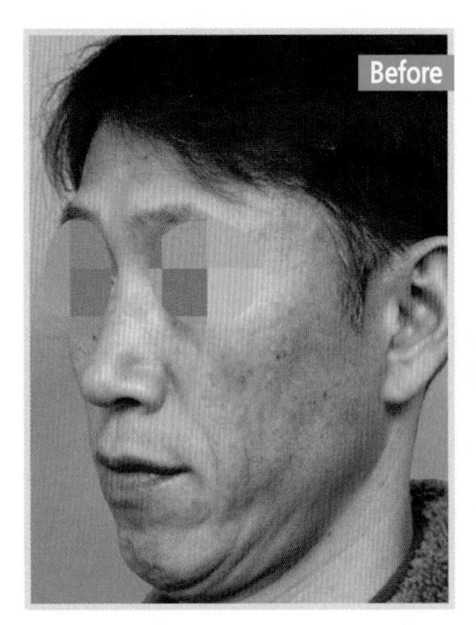

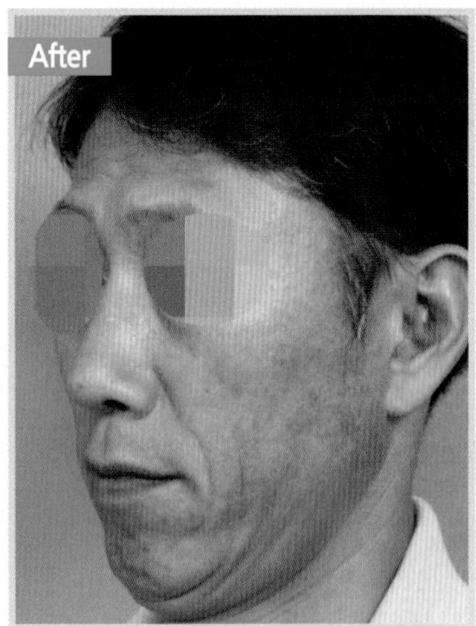

Figure 27 A patient whose supra alar concavity improved after surgery by applying the flip flop technique on left lateral crus.

3. Nasal Tip Suture Techniques

Suture techniques for the tip cartilage can be used effectively for narrowing the width of the tip or to increase tip projection. It is a particularly useful technique for cases where the lower lateral cartilage is relatively strong. Because the suture technique allows for the removal of the suture when the procedure does not produce the expected result, it is a flexible technique. The suture materials that can be used are the permanent nylon suture and semi-permanent PDS suture. It is easiest to perform the suture techniques via an external approach. To use the suture techniques in a closed approach, a delivery approach or extended marginal incision is needed. Common suture techniques that are in use today include the transdomal suture (dome creation suture), interdomal suture (dome equalization suture), and intercrural suture. Not all cases of tip surgery require all of the above listed suture techniques. Regardless of which suture technique is used, the objective is to create an anatomically ideal appearance. Moreover, it is not always possible to obtain the best results in the first attempt. The author mentioned in the introduction that it is aesthetically desirable to project the lower lateral cartilage complex in the antero-caudal direction, but it is not easy to create this change with only the suture techniques. In particular, in patients with poorly developed lower lateral cartilages or relatively thick skin, difficulties will be encountered.

1) Transdomal Suture (Dome Creation Suture, Dome Definition Suture)

(1) Effects and Indications

It is one of the most commonly used suture technique. In this method, the dome can be narrowed, elevated, and a slight concavity created at the lateral crus. When the transdomal suture performed on both sides of the dome is tied together, not only will the interdomal distance become narrower but a slight projection will also take place. If necessary, a suture with different width and shape can be performed on each side of the dome in order to balance the different shape of both sides. Unidomal suture technique can be performed to correct asymmetric projection and shape of both domes *(Figure 28)*.

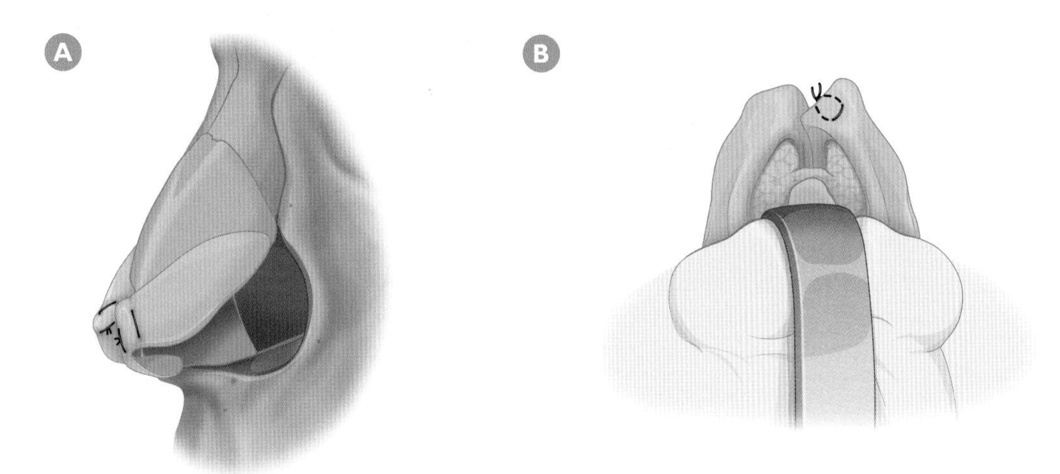

Figure 28 Bilateral transdomal suture (A), and unidome suture (B).

(2) Surgical Technique

Before suturing, the vestibular skin can be slightly dissected off after ballooning the soft tissues in the lower part of cartilage by injecting topical anesthetic agents *(Figures 29, 30)*. When making the transdomal suture, it is better to make the suture knot on the medial side than the lateral side. As suture material, 5-0 prolene, which is non-absorbable, and 5-0 PDS, which is an absorbable material that minimizes inflammation or extrusion can be used. If the transdomal suture is tied excessively tight, the dome will become too pointed. As a normal dome is round and free of acute angles, this should be avoided. To adequately improve the definition of the dome area as desired using a transdomal suture, an adequate amount of cephalic resection of the lower lateral cartilages should be performed prior to suturing. This is due to the fact that, if the lateral crus is

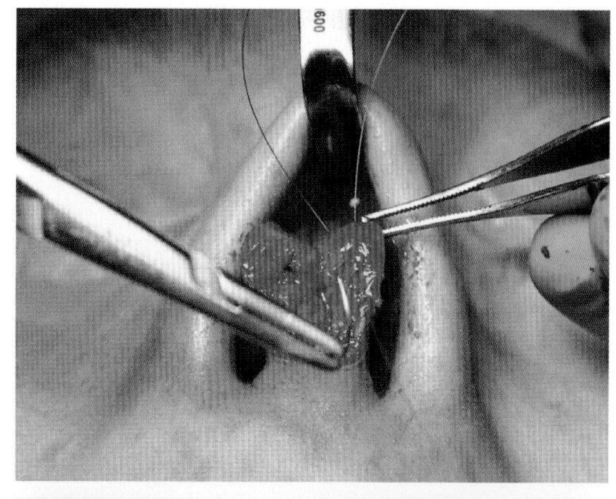

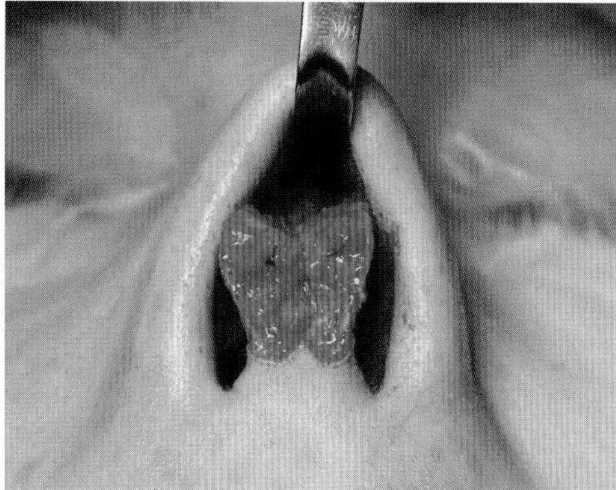

Figure 29 Intraoperative photo of transdomal suture using 5-0 PDS.

too broad and is not preceded by a cephalic resection, the width of the domal segment that is rendered convex will become too big leading to a cosmetically unsatisfactory shape.

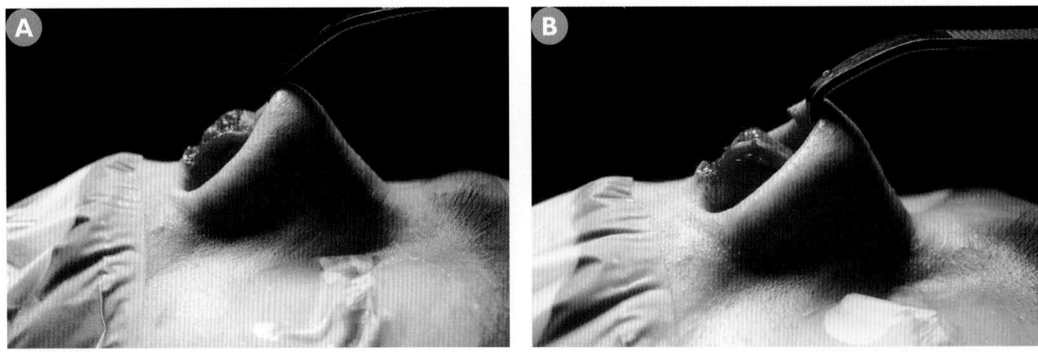

Figure 30 Increased tip angulation and projection after transdomal suture. Before surgery (A), and after surgery (B).

(3) Precautions

It is preferable that this surgical technique be done in cases of severe cartilage asymmetry, excessive rotation of the nasal tip, and in narrow lower lateral cartilages that easily bends. Among many Asian patients, the crural cartilage is very thin, and the midsection of the middle crus is indistinct so that the cartilage frequently gets overly folded by the suture. Thus, prior to surgery, the strength of the cartilage should be well examined in order to determine whether or not to perform this technique. Even when a flawless and symmetrical transdomal suture is performed, compared to the pre-suture state, the tip may become slightly rotated and distorted into an asymmetrical shape. If the suturing is performed with excessive tightness, it may result in over narrowing of the dome, abnormal interdomal angle, increase of lateral crural concavity, and rim retraction. If these problems occur, efforts must be taken to solve them by adding techniques such as interdomal suturing or intercrural suturing. If the author performs transdomal suturing, it is almost always accompanied by interdomal and intercrural suturing to make the tip shape ideal by solving the imbalance of both sides after transdomal suturing.

2) Lateral Crural Steal

If a great deal of tip projection is necessary, suturing with big bites of the cartilage is performed after dissecting the vestibular skin off from the bottom of the cartilage to make a much bigger part of cartilage folded. This lateral crural steal is a tip suture technique developed from the aforementioned transdomal suture. This technique is performed by suturing the lateral crus to the lobular segment of middle crus by horizontal mattress suture to increase the folded area. Accordingly, the medial crura become longer, while lateral crura become shorter *(Figure 31)*. This technique is effective in improving nasal tip projection and rotation.

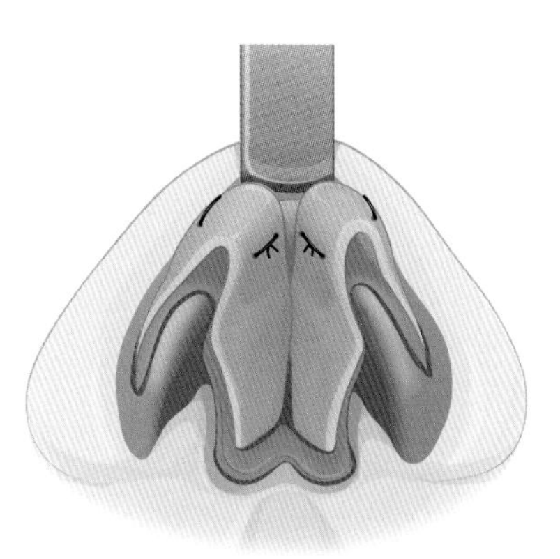

Figure 31 Increased tip projection using lateral crural steal technique.

3) Interdomal Suture (Dome Equalization Suture)

This technique also called a dome equalization suture, is mostly carried out after a transdomal suture. It is applied at the cephalic end of the middle crura right behind the dome using a 5-0 PDS or prolene, and it provides symmetry and stability to the lower lateral cartilages *(Figure 32)*.

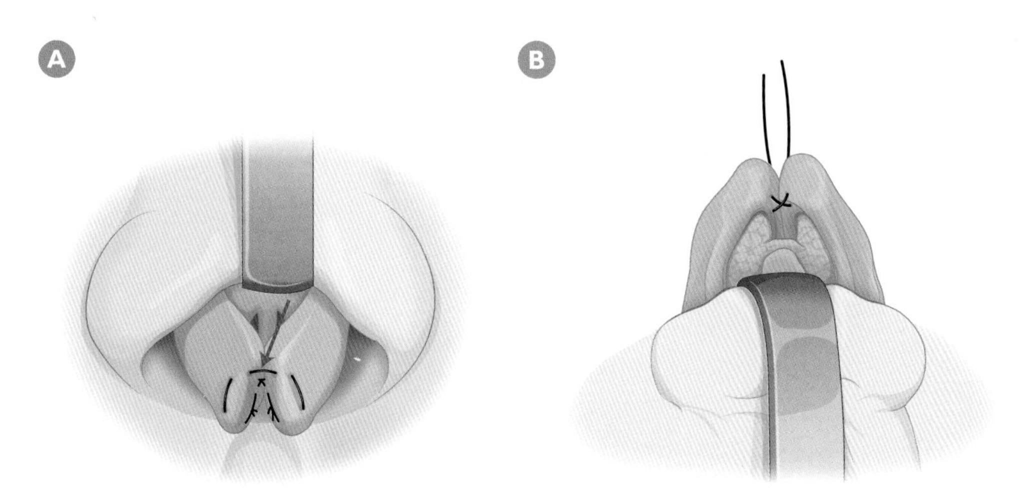

Figure 32 Interdomal suture with (A), or without (B) transdomal suture.

4) Intercrural Suture

This suture is positioned at the caudal side of the middle crura. As a result of this suture, the appearance of a divergent columella is improved and the width of the tip reduced. This suture also can bring about a slight improvement in the tip support and projection. If the intercrural suture is made too tight, the angle of divergence may be reduced excessively, leading to a slender columella, and causing the tip to have a very unnatural shape. When performing this procedure, make sure not to tie together the caudal margin of the cartilage, to control the tension, and to let the knot gets hidden within the caudal margin of the middle crura *(Figure 33)*.

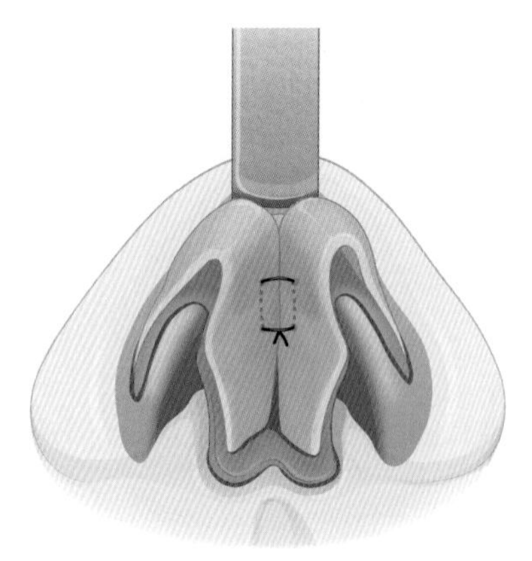

Figure 33 When performing intercrural suturing, the knot must be placed at the inner side of the middle crura.

5) Crural-Septal Suture (Septo-Columellar Suture)

A medial crura-septal suture that connects the medial crura and septum is a technique also referred to as projection control suture, which may cause nasal tip projection without causing deformation of the lobule. This is for anchoring the medial crus footplate to the caudal septum, and has the functions of improving tip rotation, changing the nasolabial angle, and strengthening the tip *(Figure 34)*.

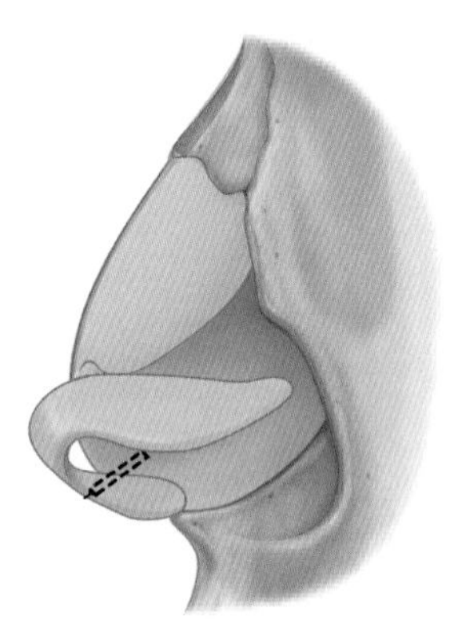

Figure 34 Nasal tip projection can be created by performing crural-septal suture.

The tongue-in-groove technique, which belongs to a type of crural-septal suturing, is done by suturing the caudal septal cartilage lying between the medial crura of both sides after pulling them backwards *(Figure 35)*. This technique can correct excessive columellar show, hanging columella, and ptotic tip. Using this technique, one can improve the nasal tip rotation and projection without direct modification on the cartilage of the tip lobule *(Figures 35, 36)*.

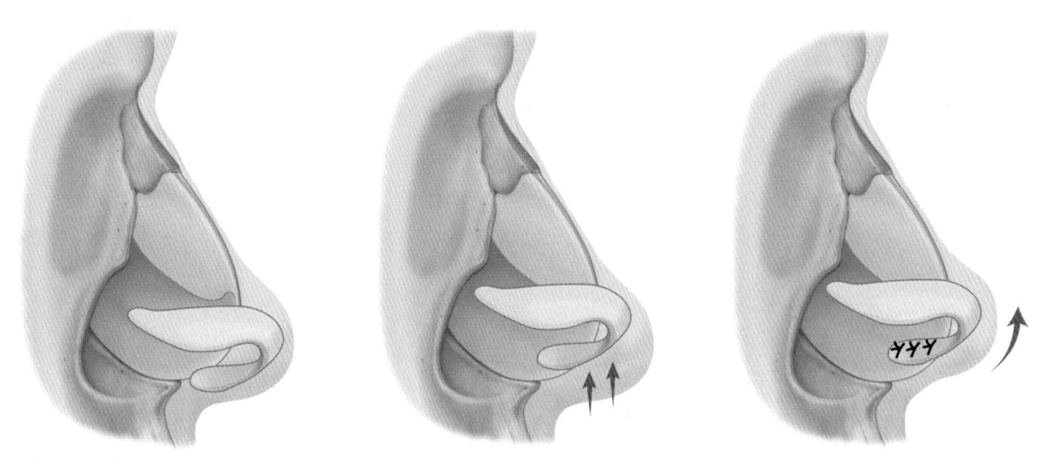

Figure 35 Nasal tip projection and rotation can be obtained using tongue-in-groove technique.

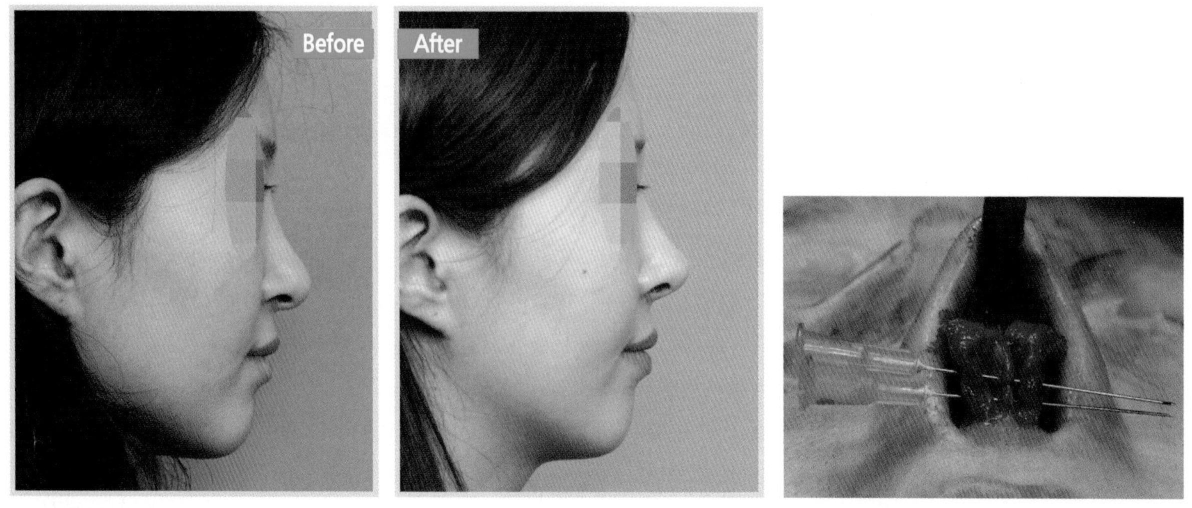

Figure 36 A patient whose hanging columella was corrected using tongue-in-groove technique and additional multilayer tip graft.

4. Cartilage Graft Technique

Tip grafting is an important technique that plays the most essential role in tip surgery of Asians, and can effectively improve tip projection and rotation, as well as definition.

1) The Concept of Tip Grafting

The nasal tip shape is determined by the interplay between the cartilaginous skeleton of the tip and the skin that covers it. Most importantly, the projection, direction, and strength of the lower lateral cartilages forms the nasal tip. The tip shape varies according to the shape of the lower lateral cartilages. When observed laterally, a tip with good definition and projection is, as mentioned in the introduction of tip surgery, shows antero-caudal projection of the lower lateral cartilages and slight angulation in the dome. In order to make under-projected and round-contoured lower lateral cartilages have antero-caudal projection, it is necessary to add shape and volume using cartilage grafting as if placing a sharp hill on an even mountaintop. This can be referred to as a "hill on the mountain", or adding the "second tip" on the existing tip *(Figure 37)*. The concept of creating a second tip is not needed in a subject who already has well-developed and well projected lower lateral cartilages.

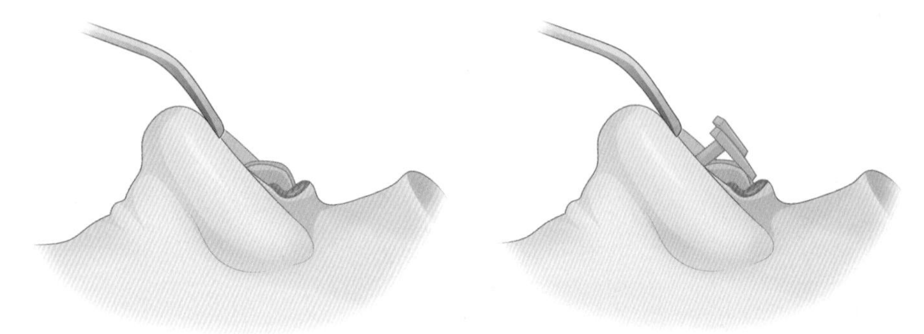

Figure 37 Concept of grafting that creates the second tip to create tip projection and improve definition.

2) Materials and Use of Graft

The most important thing to consider in selecting the materials for tip grafting is the quantity and quality of available cartilage and the thickness of skin. If a sharp stick is covered in a thin cloth as shown in the figure, the shape of the stick is revealed as it is *(Figure 38A)*. However, if an elastic and weak stick is covered with an extremely thick and heavy cloth, the stick will bent and the pole shape can't be reflected on the surface due to the thickness of the cloth *(Figure 38B)*. Therefore, to have a shape that is sharp to a certain degree, it is necessary to apply a strong and sharp pole on the inside *(Figure 38C)*. This analogy well describes the interaction between the skin and cartilage in determining the success of tip surgery. The stick indicates different qualities and shapes of cartilage, while the cloth indicates different skin types.

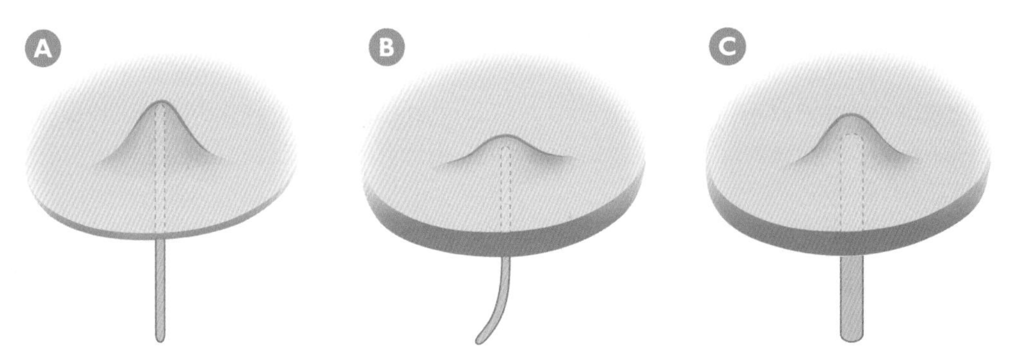

Figure 38 To produce the desired surgical result from patients with thick skin, it is necessary to build a tip graft with strong, thick, and angulated cartilage.

(1) Septal Cartilage *(Figure 39)*

Tip grafting can be performed easily if there is a sufficient amount of septal cartilage, but in many cases there is an insufficient amount available. Moreover, some patients, especially female patients in Korea, have extremely thin and weak cartilage that cannot bear the weight and tension of the skin covering the graft, thereby losing the shape designed by grafting. In particular, when tip surgery is performed using weak septal cartilage on patients with thick skin, the tip definition becomes rather worse after closing the skin, and the bulbosity increases. Furthermore, the thin septal cartilage graft is easily lacerated by suture material during the suture-fixation with the underlying lower lateral cartilages. However, if thick and rigid septal cartilage can be obtained, this is the most ideal tip grafting material as it can avoid additional morbidity to obtaining another cartilage elsewhere.

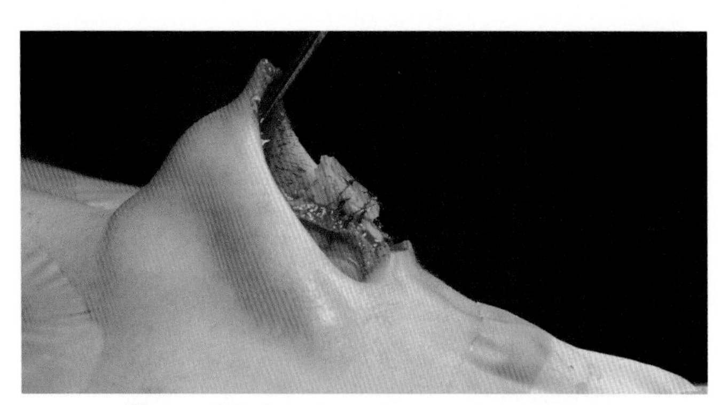

Figure 39 Septal cartilage used as tip graft.

(2) Conchal Cartilage

In using conchal cartilage in tip surgery, it is desirable to harvest it with perichondrium attached on both sides, or at least on one side of the cartilage. In this case, conchal cartilage can be used effectively for grafting as suture fixation with the lower lateral cartilage is easy, and the cartilage strength can be well maintained. As conchal cartilage has a natural curvature, it requires careful attention so that the direction of the curvature does not influence the surgical results. Utilizing the intrinsic curvature of the conchal cartilage effectively can contribute to getting an aesthetically desirable result. If the concave side of the conchal cartilage is positioned toward the caudal direction, improved tip definition, while avoiding cephalic bending at the same time, can be achieved in the patients with thick skin *(Figure 40)*.

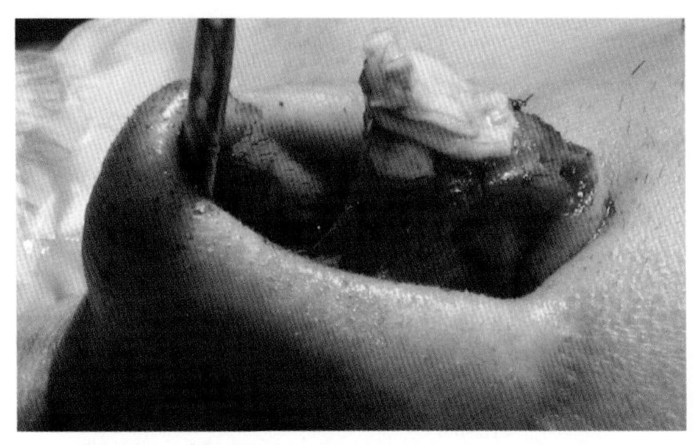

Figure 40 Tip graft using conchal cartilage.

(3) Costal Cartilage

This cartilage can also be used effectively in tip surgery *(Figure 41)*. If a patient with thick skin yet poorly developed tip cartilage wants a significant change in tip shape, the best way to satisfy this need is to perform tip grafting using costal cartilage. It is necessary to use relatively rigid cartilage for the change required as this shows externally through the thick skin; thus, septal cartilage or conchal cartilage cannot be used for this purpose *(Figure 42)*. However, a few difficulties can be encountered when using costal cartilage. As this cartilage is harder than other cartilages, suture fixation is slightly more difficult. It also requires more suture material than other cartilage. According to the author's experience, when large amounts of thick and hard costal cartilage are grafted on the tip, there is a risk that the core portion of these cartilages are not supplied well with blood, and thus tend to necrose, causing secondary infection.

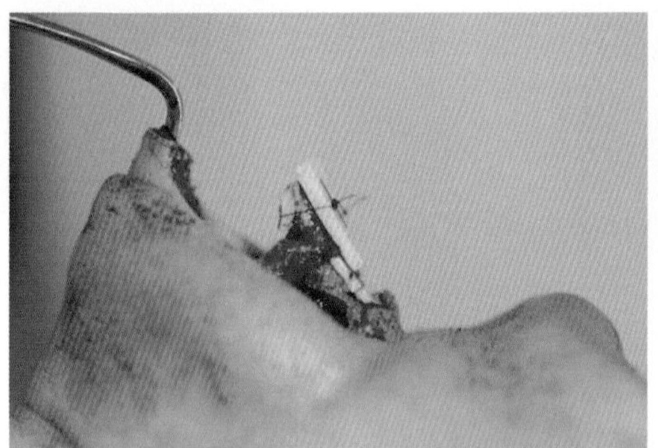
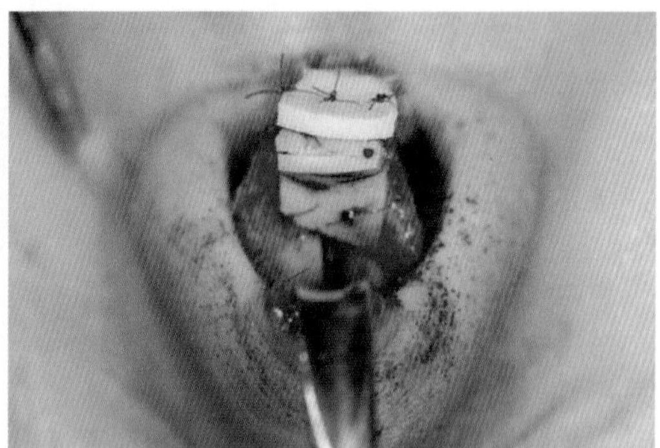

Figure 41 Tip graft using costal cartilage.

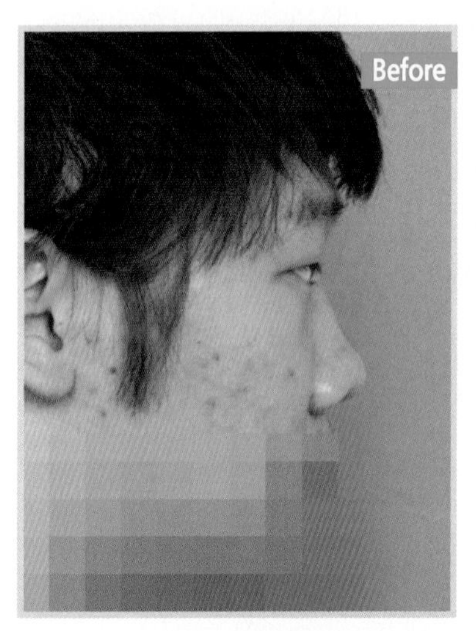

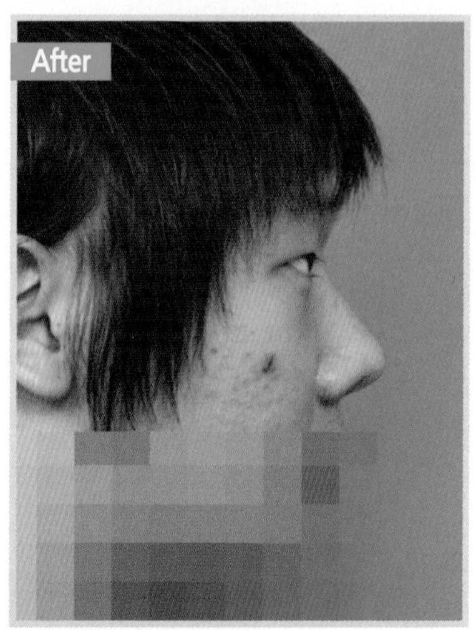

Figure 42 Tip grafting using costal cartilage is the most effective method if the desired effect is to create a big change in tip shape for patients with thick skin as shown in the example of the patient above.

3) Particulars of Tip Graft Technique

Various graft techniques described in the following section must be selected with a thoughtful consideration of quality and quantity of available cartilage as well as the patient's tip shape.

(1) Columellar Strut

A. Effects

This technique involves carving a long cartilage into a strut and positioning it between the middle crus and medial crus of both sides of the lower lateral cartilages *(Figure 43)*.

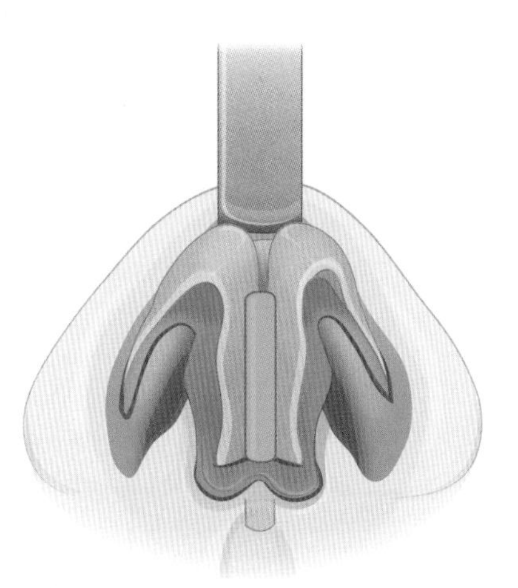

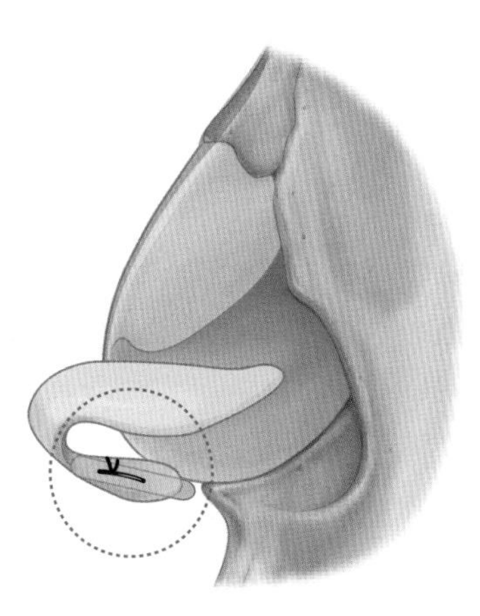

Figure 43 Columellar strut placed between the middle crus and medial crus of the lower lateral cartilages on both sides to act as a support.

Changes that can be made through this technique are as follows:

- Enhancement of the nasal tip support
- Moderate degree of tip projection
- Alteration of the nostril shape, improvement of symmetry
- Alteration of the columellar lobular angle

In tip surgery, columellar strut alone cannot bring about fundamental changes in the shape of the tip cartilage. So, this technique should be considered as a foundation work on which additional tip grafting such as shield graft and onlay graft can be placed in better stability.

B. Selecting the Cartilage for Use as Graft

The columellar strut is usually made of septal cartilage, but when a stronger graft is needed, costal cartilage can be used. When there are concerns over the use of costal cartilage, conchal cartilage can also be used. In such a case, to overcome the intrinsic curvature of the conchal cartilage, it is desirable to suture two pieces of conchal cartilages that are bent towards opposite direction into a straight two-fold graft before being used.

C. Classification

The columellar strut can produce a tip projection effect even when it does not get in direct contact with the maxillary spine. In such a case, it must be positioned 2-3 mm above the maxillary spine. This is called a floating type columellar strut. When necessary, a fixed type strut that is fixed to the nasal spine or maxilla can be fashioned.

D. Surgical Technique

To place a columellar strut, the soft tissue between the medial crura must be dissected in the direction of the nasal spine in order to create a pocket. The length of the strut must conform to the distance between the middle crus and the pocket created by dissecting downwards from the middle crus. However, it is difficult to talk about a uniform distance as the amount of cartilage obtainable and the length of the crus may vary from patient to patient. It is recommended that the width of the strut be over 3 mm in order for it to be well placed between the medial crus. At times, the strut itself may be curved and, in such a case, it can cause an asymmetry of the tip, so proper action to counter this situation must be taken before concluding the surgery. Suturing the strut is performed near the columellar breakpoint. The process involves beginning from one side of the vestibular mucosa, piercing the cartilage all the way to the mucosa at the opposite side of the strut and using a PDS suture in a mattress pattern. During this process, if the desired location is pierced with a 25 gauge needle for temporary fixation, the strut will be became immobile making the suturing that much easier.

E. Complications

A columellar strut may result in cephalic rotation of the tip or columellar deviation.

(2) Shield Graft (Infratip Lobular Graft)

A. Definition and Effects

This is a graft that is positioned onto the middle and medial crus of the lower lateral cartilages. The name shield graft is derived from the fact that it is shaped in the form of a shield *(Figure 44)*.

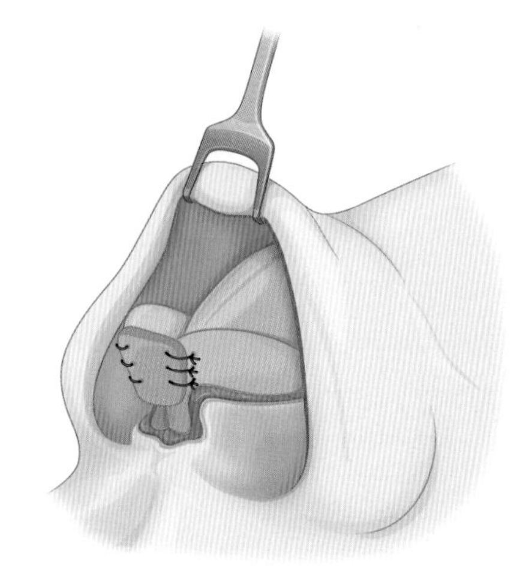

Figure 44 Typical form of shield graft.

The technique has the following effects:

- ☑ Increase in tip projection
- ☑ Improvement of tip definition
- ☑ Making the infratip lobule more distinct

This technique mostly has the effect of increasing tip projection by extending the length of the infratip lobular segment. If the length of the graft is long, in addition to the increase in tip projection, one can expect an increase in the overall length of the columella. Should the length of the graft be short and placed on the infratip lobule portion, there is a possibility that the graft will bend backwards, causing a cephalic rotation of the nasal tip. An important factor in selecting this technique is the shape of the tip cartilage. If the tip cartilage shows an adequate domal angulation, a single shield graft can produce the effect of increasing projection. However, patients with round-contoured tip cartilage and poor projection will experience an aggravation of the round contour of the tip when a shield graft is inserted, thereby not improving the tip definition.

B. Surgical Technique

While carving the graft, beveling of the periphery of the graft should be performed using a knife, or the cartilage should be crushed so that the graft margin does not become visible through the skin. This procedure is particularly necessary among those with thin skin. The graft must be shaped like a shield or a ginkgo leaf, and the top part must be broad so that both ends of the top side can indicate tip defining points. However, performing this technique may make the columellar lobular angle blunt and infratip lobule unnaturally long, and increase the risk of excessive rotation of the tip. The leading edge of this shield graft must be slightly higher than the height of the existing dome of the tip *(Figure 45)*.

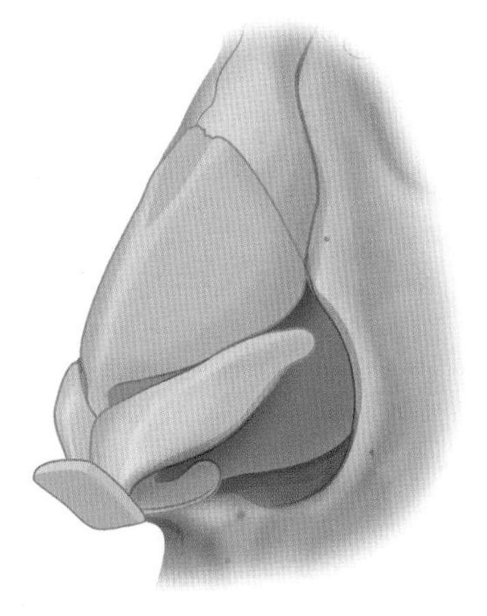
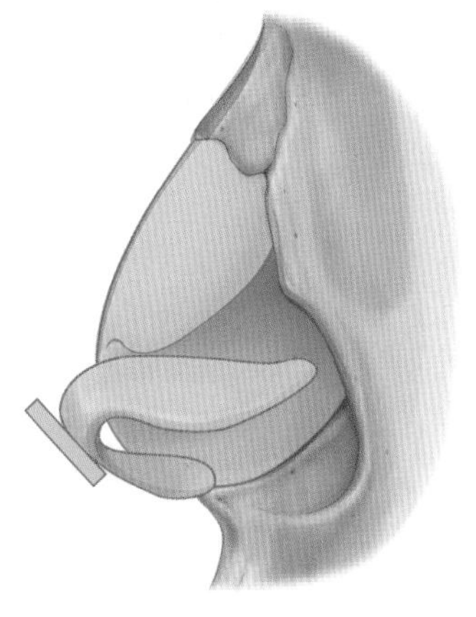

Figure 45 The leading edge of the shield graft must be slightly higher than the domal height.

However, it is not easy to obtain cartilage that is strong enough to push up thick skin when covered. Therefore, if the upper boundary is even slightly higher than the dome, the cartilage may be bent by the weight of the thick skin and result in cephalic bending, making the nose seem upturned. To prevent this, and to produce the desired effect, the following techniques can be used:

- ☑ Place a graft that supports the shield from the back of the shield graft *(Figure 46)* (cartilage backstop, backing graft, buttress graft).
- ☑ Support the shield graft on both sides with lateral crural onlay graft *(Figure 47)*.
- ☑ Make the columellar strut long and be exposed on the top of the dome to support the shield graft from behind *(Figure 48)*.
- ☑ Place the concave surface of conchal cartilage to be directed toward the caudal direction to exert a spring-like action *(Figure 49)*.

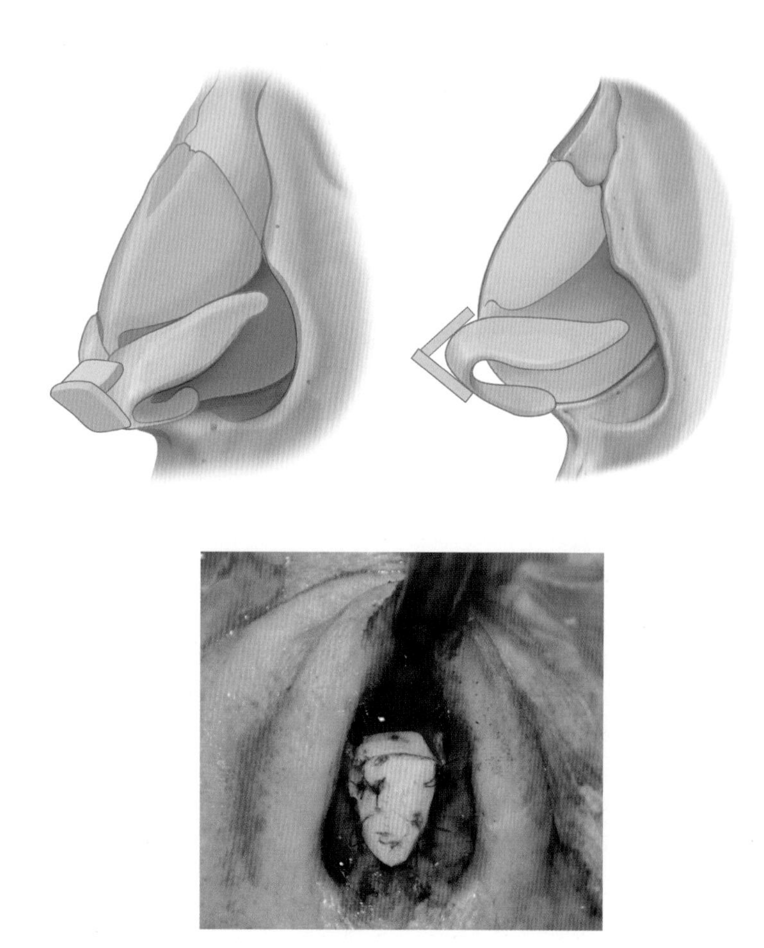

Figure 46 A buttress graft can be placed to prevent cephalic bending of the shield graft.

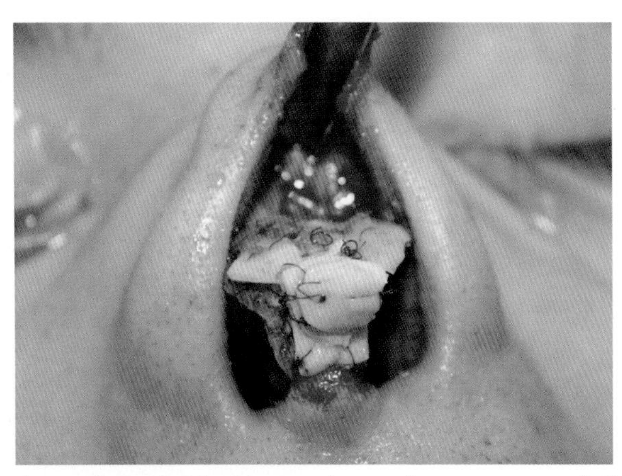

Figure 47 Lateral crural onlay grafts on both sides can be used to prevent cephalic bending of the shield graft.

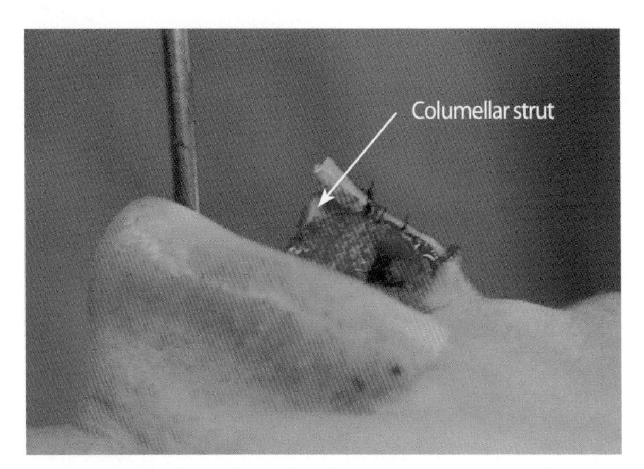

Figure 48 A columellar strut projected higher than the dome can be created to support the shield graft from behind, and prevent cephalic bending of the shield graft.

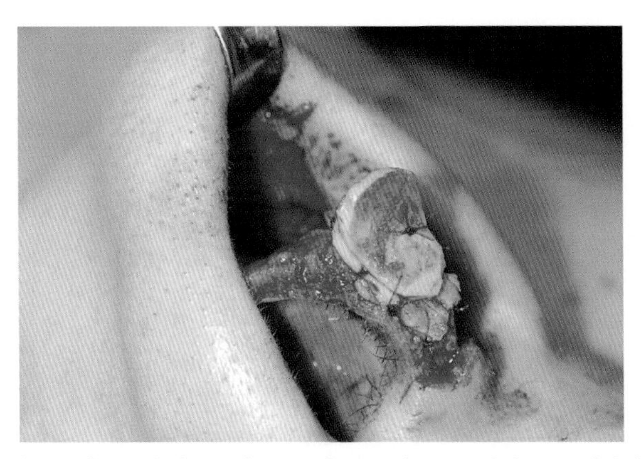

Figure 49 If the concave surface of conchal cartilage is directed toward the caudal direction when making the shield graft using conchal cartilage, it can produce the effect of a natural antero-caudal projection of the tip.

(3) Extended Columellar Strut-Tip Graft (Extended Shield Graft) *(Figure 50)*

Extended columellar strut-tip graft is a name for a very long shield graft that protrudes over the dome anteriorly, and extends close to the medial crural footplate posteriorly. Using this graft, one can expect to improve the tip support and tip definition. To perform this technique, the anterior end of the graft needs to be made round and thin so that the graft does not become overly visible through the skin. Using such a graft can lead to a loss of the infratip break, resulting in the columella taking on an unnaturally straight look.

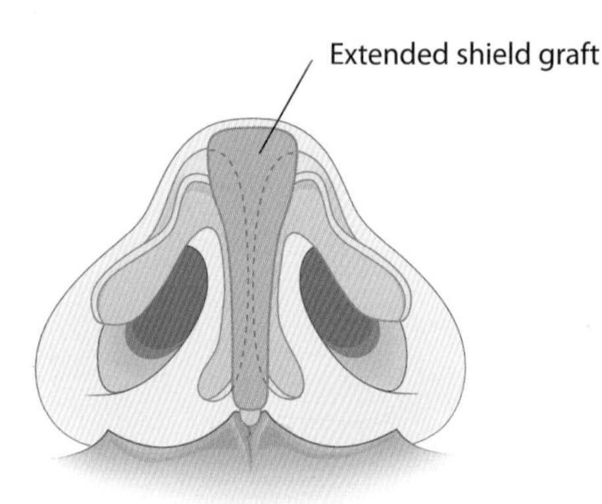

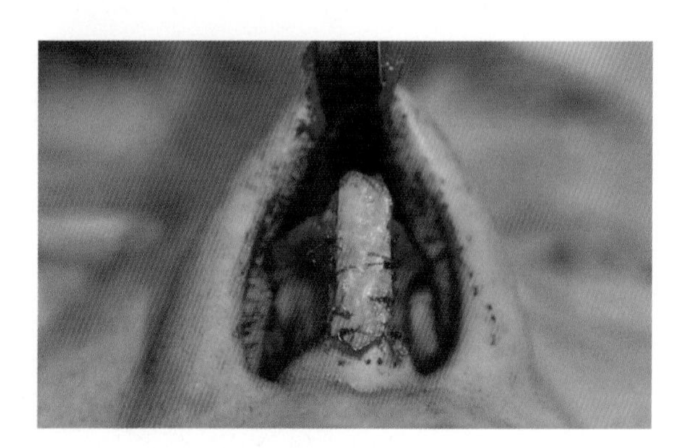

Figure 50 Extended columellar strut-tip graft (extended shield graft)

(4) Multilayer (Multi-Tier) Cartilaginous Tip Graft

As emphasized by the author many times, the antero-caudal projection of the tip cannot be obtained with only one shield graft. An underprojected tip often presents with a round tip contour, and a vertically oriented shield graft or onlay graft can actually worsen the nasal tip shape. Therefore, many shield grafts must be arranged in layers to create antero-caudal projection, and if a cartilage backstop graft is added, it is possible to create the "hill on the top of the mountain", or the "second tip" *(Figure 51)*. The multilayer cartilaginous tip-grafting technique maintains the

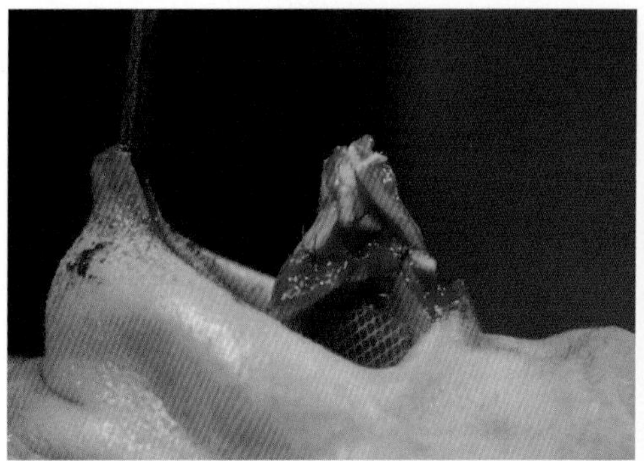

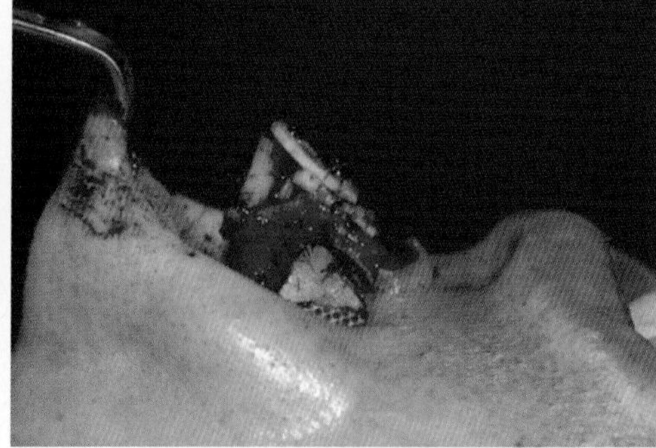

Figure 51 To overcome the round contour of the tip cartilage and to obtain a greater degree of tip projection, it is necessary to perform (creation of second tip or hill on the mountain) multilayer tip grafting with an intention to create another peak on a small mountain.

advantages of shield-shaped tip grafts, which help to improve nasal tip projection and definition, and overcomes issues relating to thick skin, soft tissue, and weak cartilaginous framework often encountered in Asian rhinoplasty patients.

This procedure has some distinct advantages.

- First, it is a very flexible approach in which the number of grafts required can be adjusted intraoperatively, thus allowing individual tailoring to different lower lateral cartilage shape and configurations, and it results in an aesthetically pleasing antero-caudal tip projection, without causing unwanted cephalic rotation.
- Second, good tip definition can be obtained even in patients with thick skin. It was found that this procedure can increase nasal tip projection and improve the nasolabial angle very effectively.

Multilayer cartilaginous tip-grafting technique has some potential drawbacks.

- A relatively large amount of cartilage is required for the tip framework. Hence, the procedure may be associated with donor site morbidity.
- There is a higher risk of tip graft visibility postoperatively.
- Use of multiple cartilage grafts may increase the risk of inflammation and secondary infection.

A. Surgical Technique

This procedure is conducted using an external approach. If required, septoplasty, hump resection, osteotomy, or inferior turbinectomy are performed before nasal tip refinement. Septal, conchal, tragal, and/or costal cartilage is harvested depending on the amount of cartilage required, and the quality and amount of nasal septal cartilage available in the patient. Where necessary, caudal extension of the septum, columellar strut placement, dome suturing, and/or trimming of skin–soft tissue envelope is performed prior to the multilayer tip grafting. Following these procedures, the first cartilaginous shield graft layer is placed on the dome and secured with 5-0 PDS suture. Additional shield graft layers are then placed on top of the first layer. The more caudal layer is placed so that its leading (superior) edge is always higher than the height of the existing dome and the layer(s) beneath it. The numbers of graft layers applied depends on how much projection is required, and is determined intraoperatively. The shield graft horizontal width is adjusted according to tip skin thickness. For thin skin, the horizontal width should be wider to provide better tip definition. For thick skin, a narrower width provided better results. Meticulous smoothing of graft margins with gentle carving is important to provide a smooth tip contour. For evaluation of the final tip shape, the tip skin is redraped with interim stitching of the columellar incision. When the tip skin is redraped, it would usually push the grafts backward and could distort the tip shape and orientation. In order to prevent cephalic bending of the grafts, one can use two techniques *(Figures 52, 53, 54)*:

- Grafting with conchal cartilage by facing the concave side caudally. This allows the natural antero-caudally directed spring-like effect to resist cephalic bending.
- For grafts that did not possess intrinsic curvature, such as septal cartilage, placement of a backing graft.

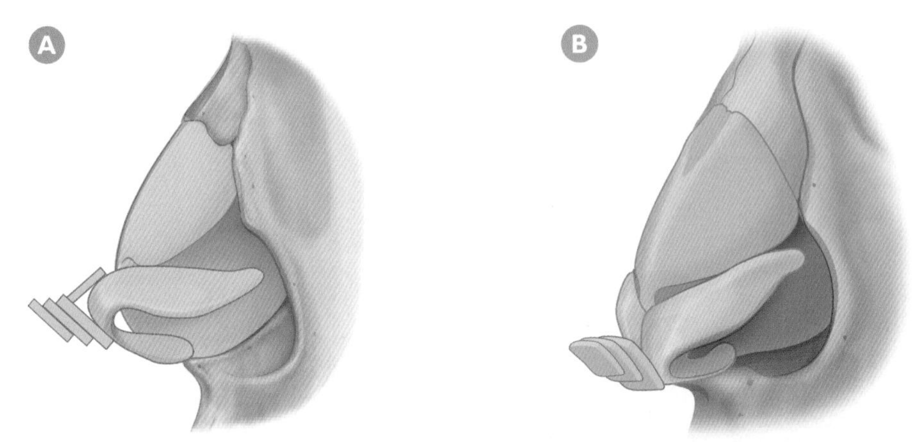

Figure 52 Multilayer tip graft with buttress grafting (A) and without buttress grafting (B).

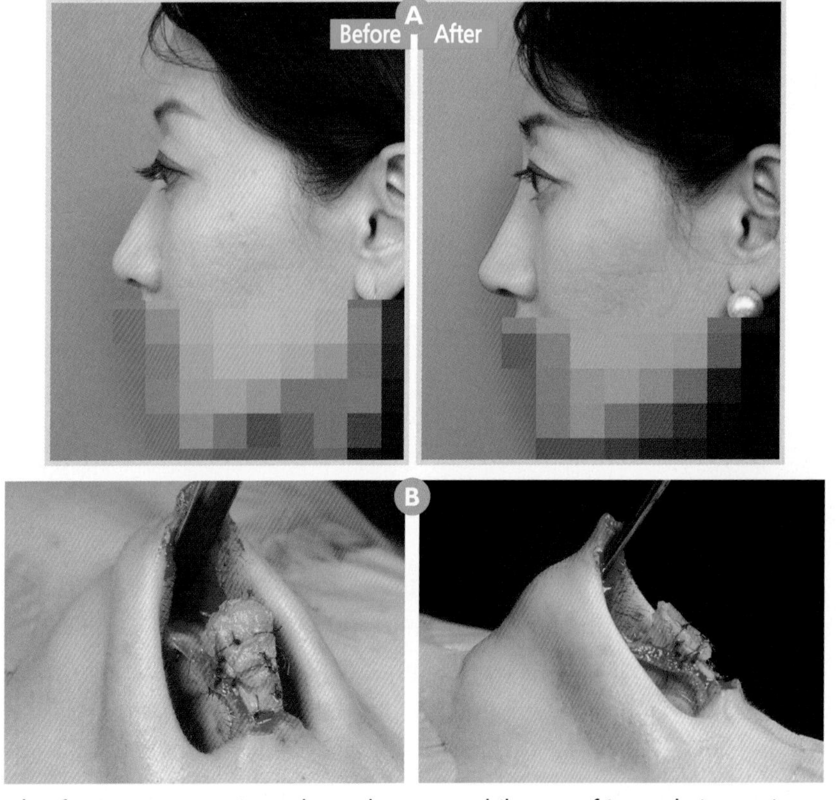

Figure 53 Example of a tip surgery patient who underwent multilayer grafting technique using septal cartilage (A) and intraoperative photos (B).

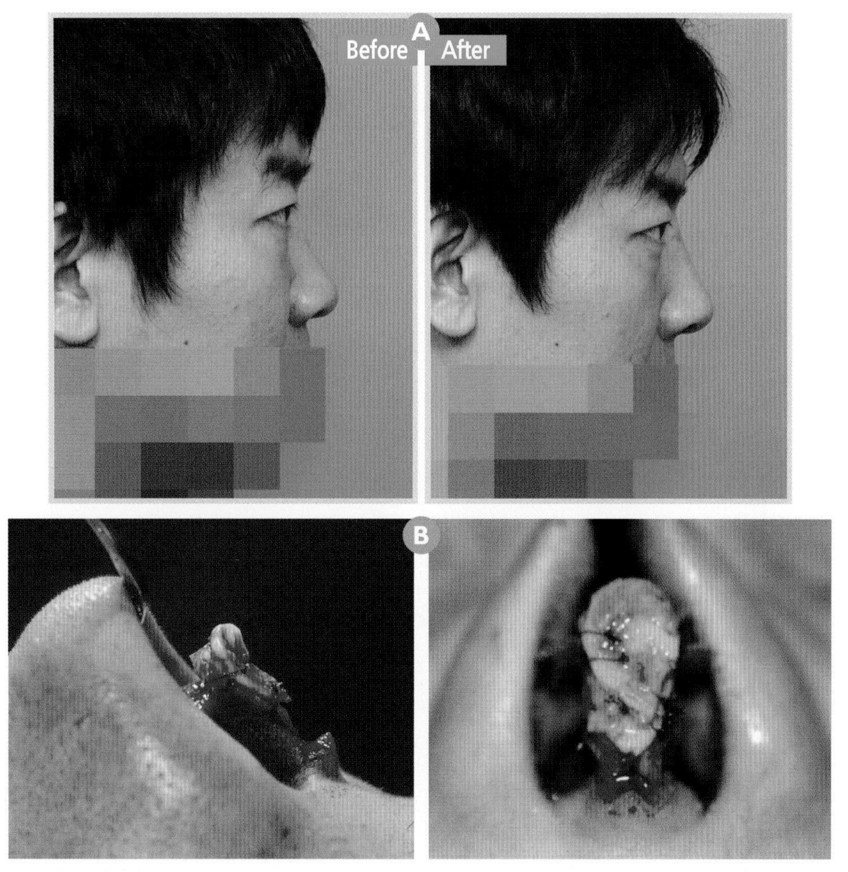

Figure 54 Photograph of the patient who received multilayer tip grafting technique using conchal cartilage (A) and the intraoperative photos (B).

If the tip grafts are too conspicuous (the phenomenon which is more likely to occur in patients with thin tip skin) perichondrium, fascia, or crushed cartilage is placed for smoothening of the graft edges *(Figure 55)*.

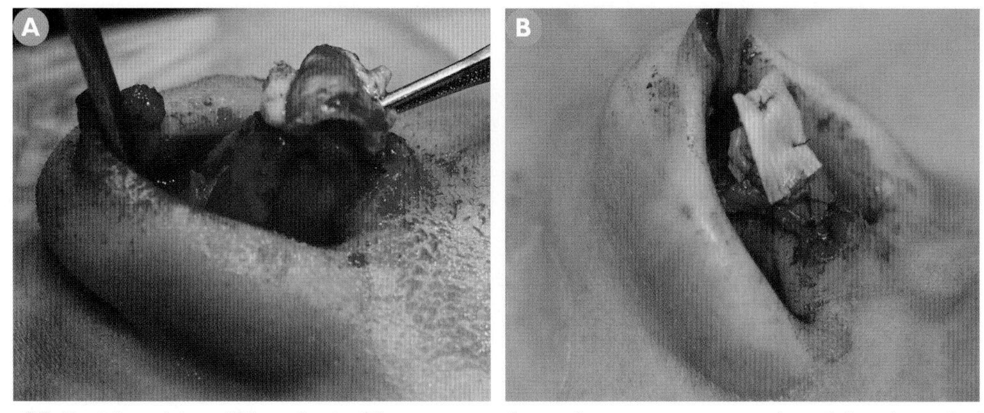

Figure 55 Perichondrium (A) or fascia (B) can cover the graft to prevent tip graft visibility through the skin.

(5) Tip Onlay Graft

Tip onlay grafting is a procedure that places one or several layers of graft horizontally on the dome of the tip *(Figure 56)*. While the shield graft is a vertically oriented cartilage graft, the onlay graft is a horizontal graft in which the width is greater than the height. This technique can be performed to increase the tip projection, or camouflage tip irregularities in patients with adequate tip support and a certain degree of projection. This graft must be fixed on the caudal margin of the dome. This graft softens the transition on the side from the dome to the alar lobule, increases tip projection, and improves definition *(Figures 57, 58)*. If the contour of the tip graft is too round and blunt, onlay grafting may not lead to an aesthetically pleasing result. Another type of tip onlay grafting is inserting cartilage pieces or crushed cartilage to obtain additional tip projection after suturing the transcolumellar incision in via an external rhinoplasty approach *(Figure 59)*. If several layers of onlay grafts are positioned on the tip, even though tip projection may be improved to some extent when viewed from the lateral side, the infratip lobule area can become excessively long when viewed from the basal side, and thus cause an unnatural appearance. Graft visibility is also a common complication.

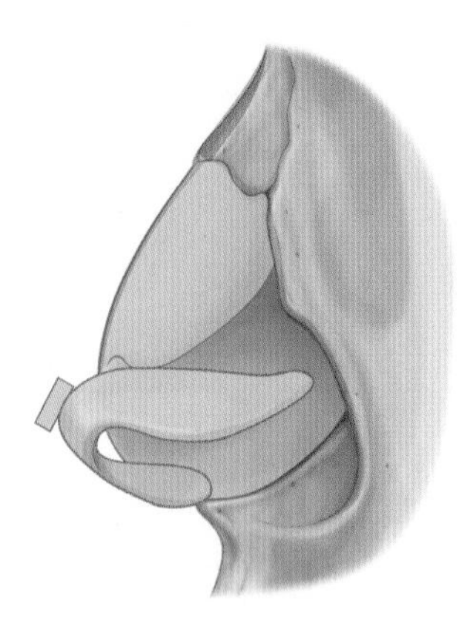

Figure 56 Tip onlay graft.

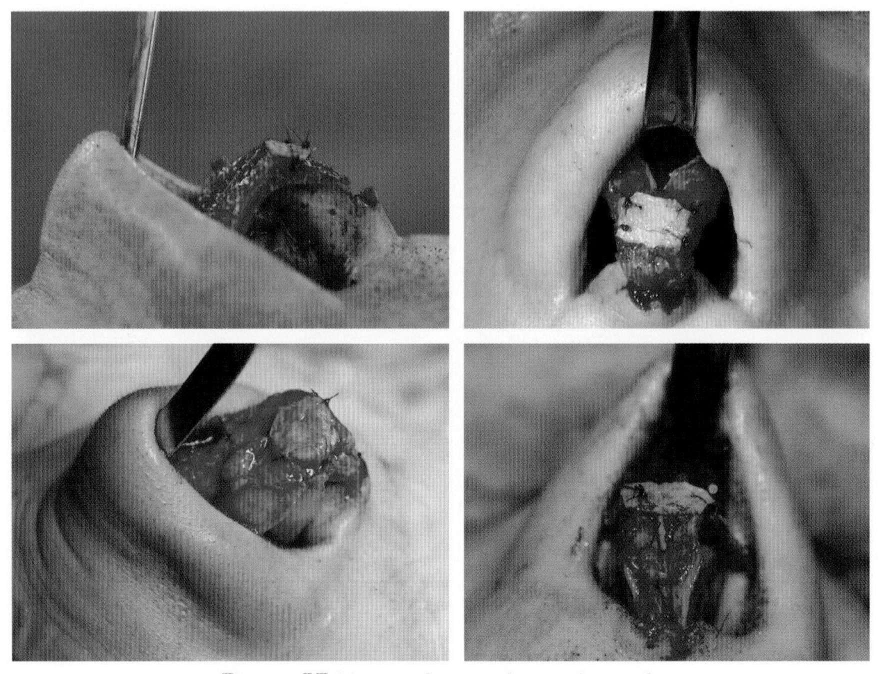

Figure 57 Various forms of tip onlay graft.

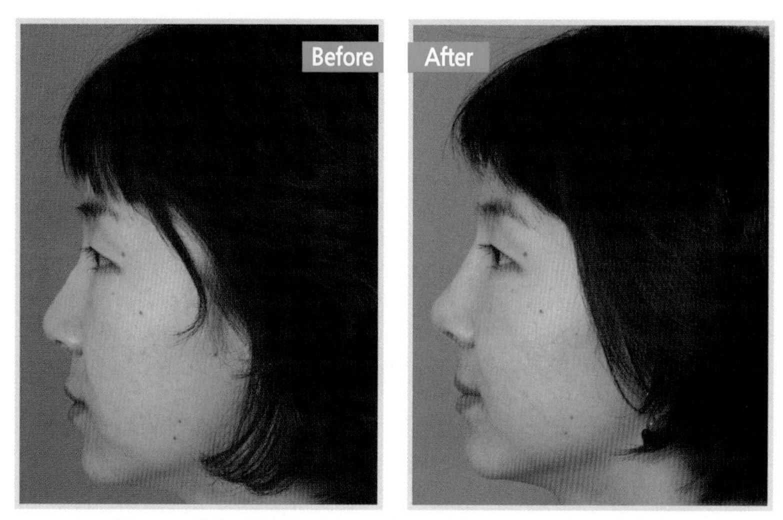

Figure 58 Change in tip shape after tip onlay grafting.

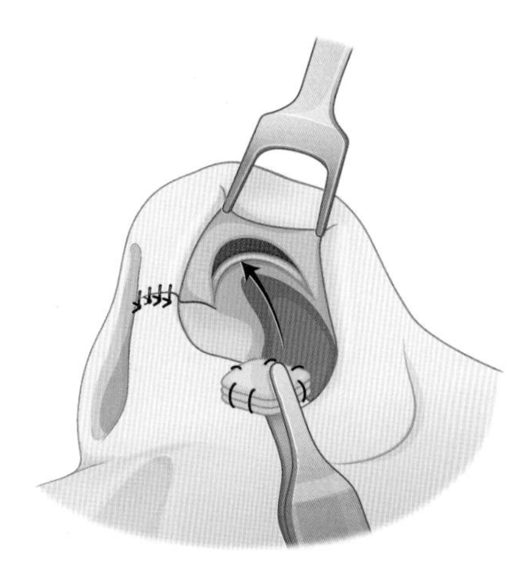

Figure 59 Performing tip onlay graft surgery to obtain additional tip projection after suturing the transcolumellar incision.

(6) Modified Vertical Dome Division Technique

Vertical dome division is one of the classical surgical techniques that have been used effectively to improve the nasal tip shape. Since Goldman described vertical dome division as a method of refining tip position without the use of columellar grafts, this technique has gained a degree of popularity and acceptance with various modifications. Vertical dome division can be used for various nasal deformities, including overprojection or underprojection, suboptimal rotation, disproportionate lobule ratios, and broad or asymmetric tips.

Although vertical dome division can dramatically change tip definition, concern exists about the risks of weakening the intrinsic tip support mechanism that can result in tip irregularities such as pinching, alar notching, and tent pole nasal tip. The classical vertical dome division is a technique in which the dome is excised including the skin, medialized, and sewn together at the midline *(Figure 60)*. This technique may damage a part of the lateral support in patients with thin skin and solid cartilage, resulting in lateral wall collapse, alar retraction, or unequal tip uplift. In many cases, it is difficult to obtain an ideal nasal tip with only the vertical dome division procedure. The author is using the modified vertical dome division technique, which is effective for patients with thick skin *(Figure 61)*.

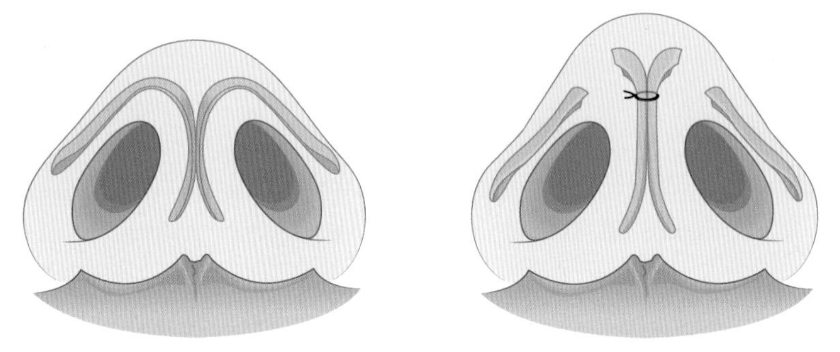

Figure 60 Typical vertical dome division technique. This procedure can produce tip projection by unifying the tip dome with the skin by incising it as shown in the figure.

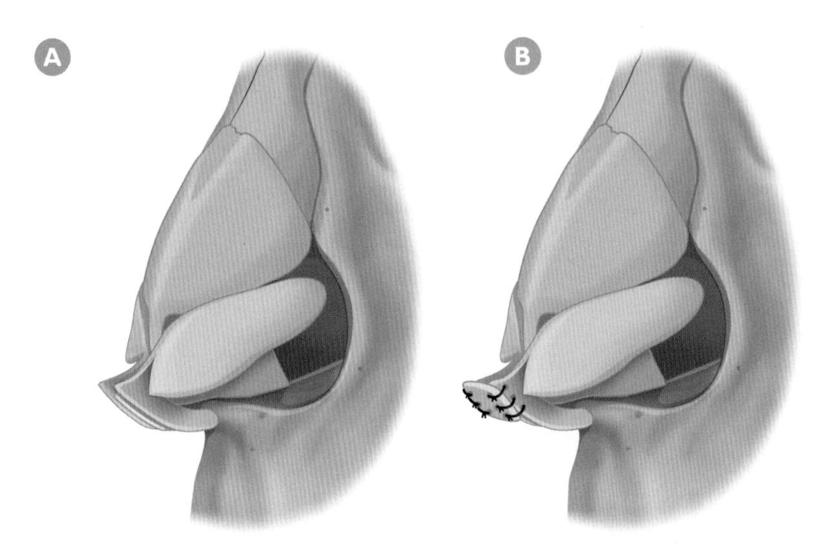

Figure 61 In the modified vertical dome division technique, cartilage graft mimicking, a columellar strut (A), is inserted after dome division, and additional shield shape graft is placed on the caudal location (B).

A. Surgical Technique

The incisions are performed on both domes, borrowing a large amount of cartilage from the caudal margin so that the lateral view of the medialized cartilage has a triangular projection shape towards the antero-caudal direction *(Figure 62)*. The vestibular skin is preserved by wide undermining along the medial and lateral crural surfaces. A cartilage strip, shaped like a columellar strut, is placed between both limbs of the divided dome, and is sewn together with the medialized domal portion of the lower lateral cartilages *(Figure 63)*.

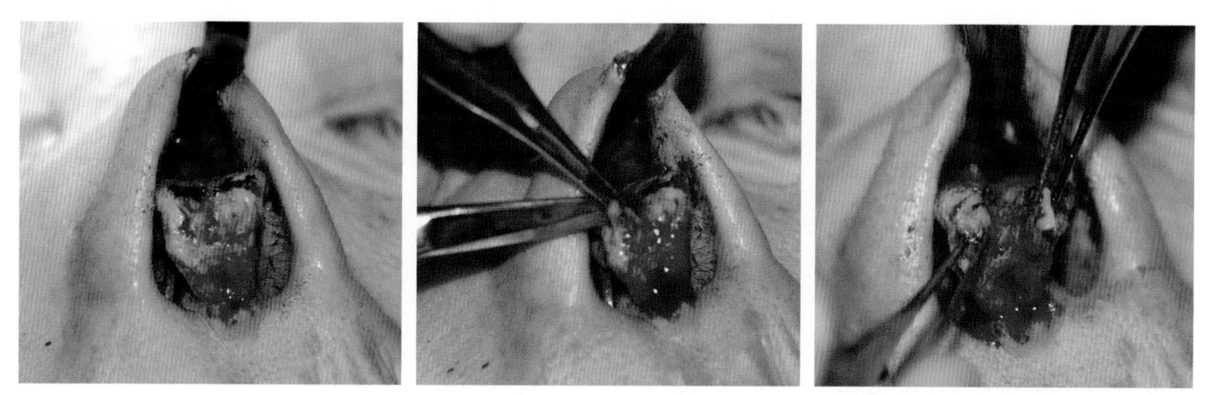

Figure 62 Modified vertical dome division. Both sides of the dome are incised while preserving vestibular skin, lifting up the cartilage.

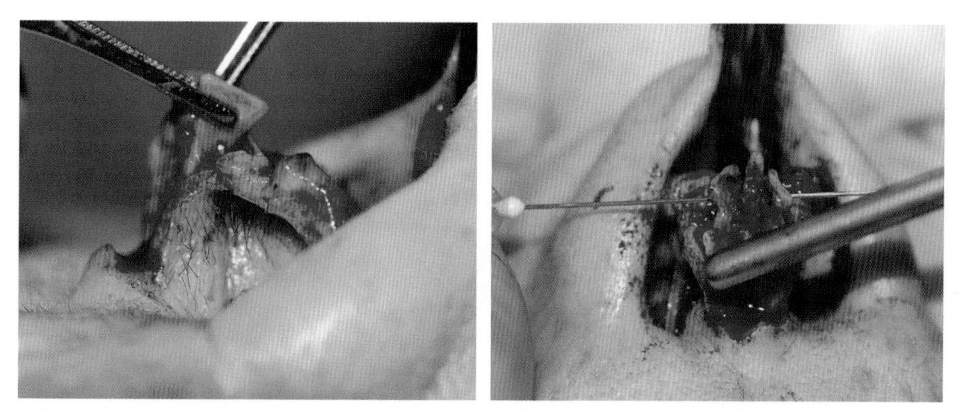

Figure 63 Modified vertical dome division. After placing the cartilage strip similar in shape with the columellar strut between both limbs of the incised dome, the surgeon sutures the medialized domal portion of the lower lateral cartilages.

A shield-shaped tip graft is placed just in front of the newly created cartilage-strut complex. The leading edge of the shield-shaped graft is adjusted according to the desired height of the new tip *(Figure 64)*.

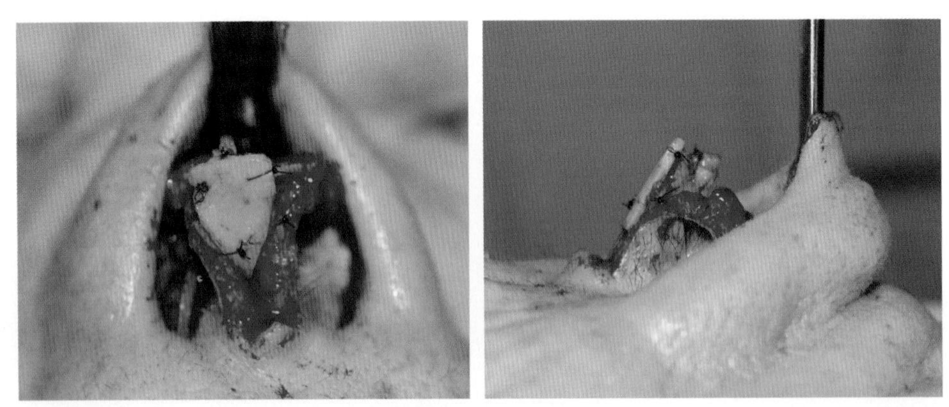

Figure 64 Modified vertical dome division. Shield-shaped tip graft is placed on the caudal aspect of cartilage-strut complex so that the leading edge of the shield-shaped tip graft forms a new tip with desired height.

B. Indications and Complications

Modified vertical dome division technique is aimed at patients with thick tip skin and relatively strong, well-developed lower lateral cartilages *(Figure 65)*. However, because it is difficult to accurately evaluate the degree of lower lateral cartilage development preoperatively, the author's patient selection for modified vertical dome division is determined intraoperatively in most cases. Excessive narrowing and asymmetry of the nasal tip may occur in some patients as a complication of the modified vertical dome division.

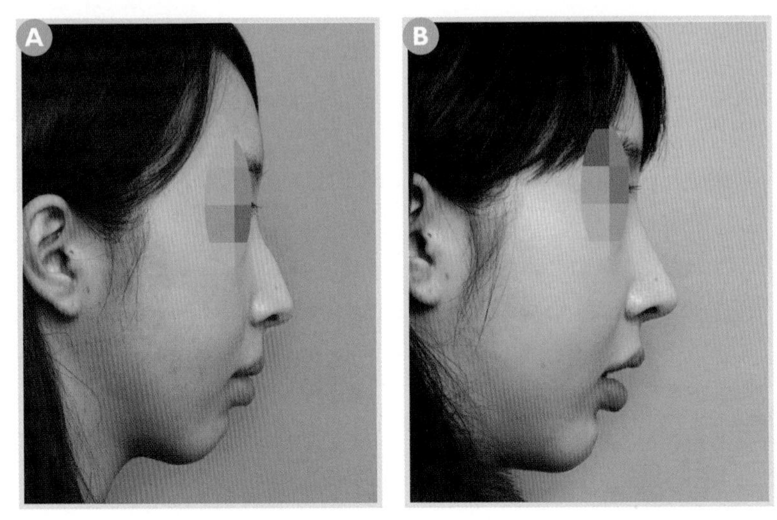

Figure 65 Photograph of the patient whose tip projection increased after applying modified vertical dome division technique. Before surgery (A) and after surgery (B).

(7) Lateral Crural Onlay Graft

This graft is placed on the lateral crus *(Figure 66)*. This technique can be applied in the following situations *(Figures 67, 68)*.

- ☑ To correct concavity of the lateral crus
- ☑ To correct irregularities of alar contour
- ☑ To reinforce the lateral crura with the effect of improving the collapsed external valve
- ☑ To prevent cephalic bending of a shield graft

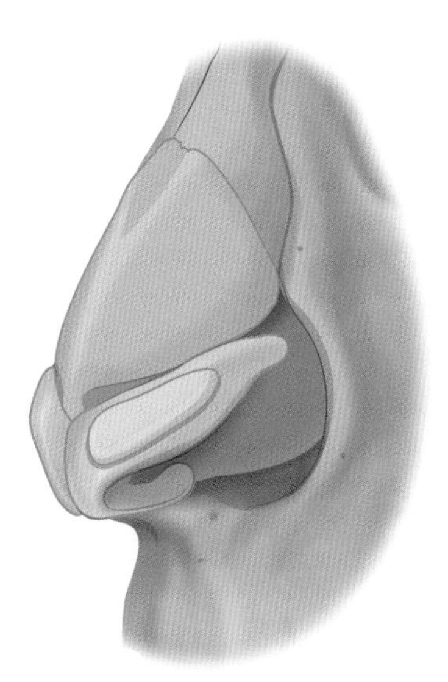

Figure 66 Lateral crural onlay graft.

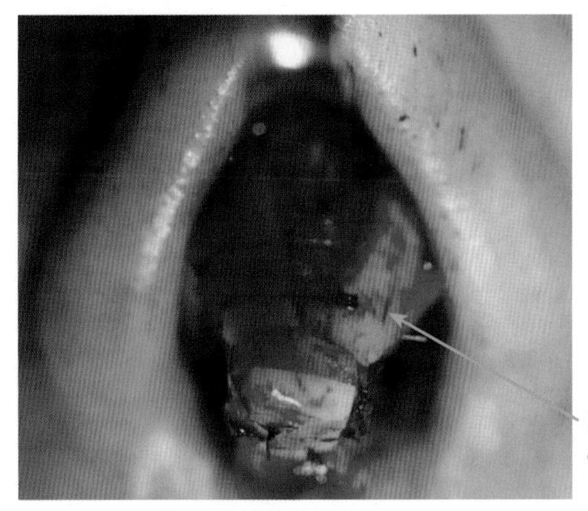

Figure 67 Lateral crural onlay graft.

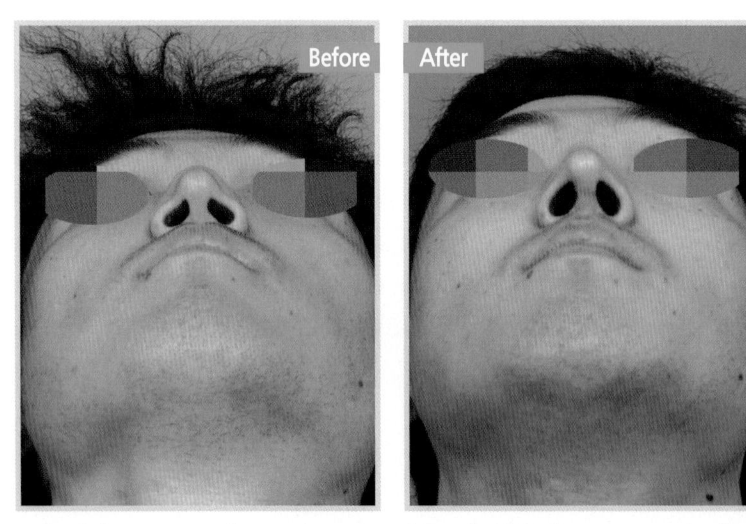

Figure 68 Photograph of the patient whose concavity of the alar lobule was improved by lateral crural onlay grafts.

(8) Lateral Crural Strut Graft

This is a surgical technique in which the surgeon creates a pocket between the vestibular skin and the lateral crus, and places the graft in this pocket. If needed, the lateral crus-strut graft complex can be caudally rotated, and fixed to the more caudally located soft tissue pocket at the inner side of the alar lobule *(Figure 69)*.

This technique can be applied to correct following situations:

- Alar retraction
- Alar rim collapse
- Concave lateral crura
- Boxy nasal tip
- Malpositioned lateral crura

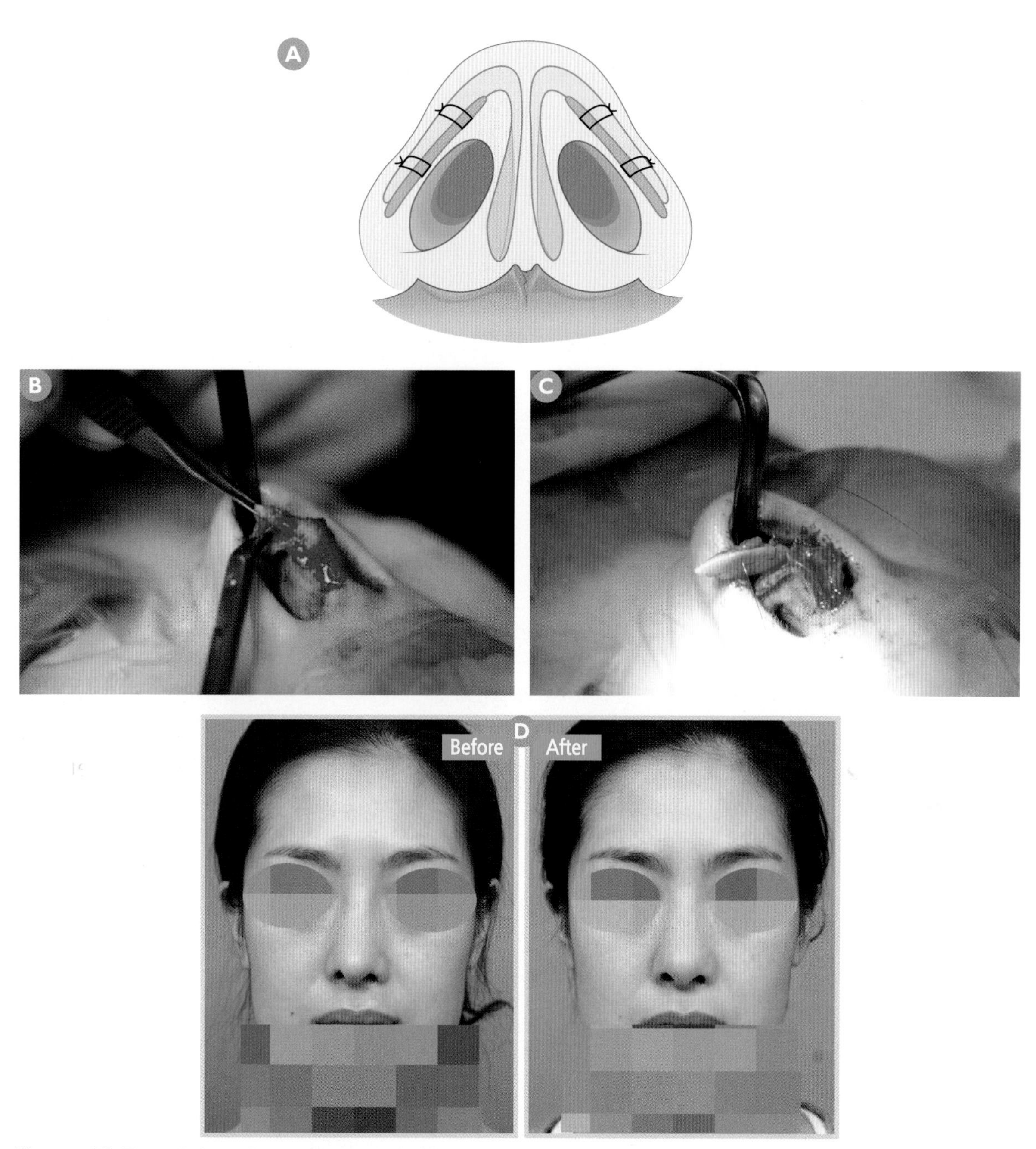

Figure 69 To apply lateral crural strut graft (A), the lateral crus in the photograph is dissected off from the vestibular skin (B), after which caudal rotation was performed by inserting septal cartilage (C), and fixed to a new pocket. As a result, nostril asymmetry by alar retraction was corrected (D).

(9) Columellar Plumping Graft

This graft is placed in front of the anterior nasal spine to correct the acute columellar-labial angle. To maximize the effect of this grafting, a big piece of costal cartilage can be carved and inserted. As it is not easy to fix the inserted cartilage, it is desirable to perform adequate dissection of a pocket suitable for the size of the graft. The surgery can also be performed using crushed cartilage *(Figure 70)*.

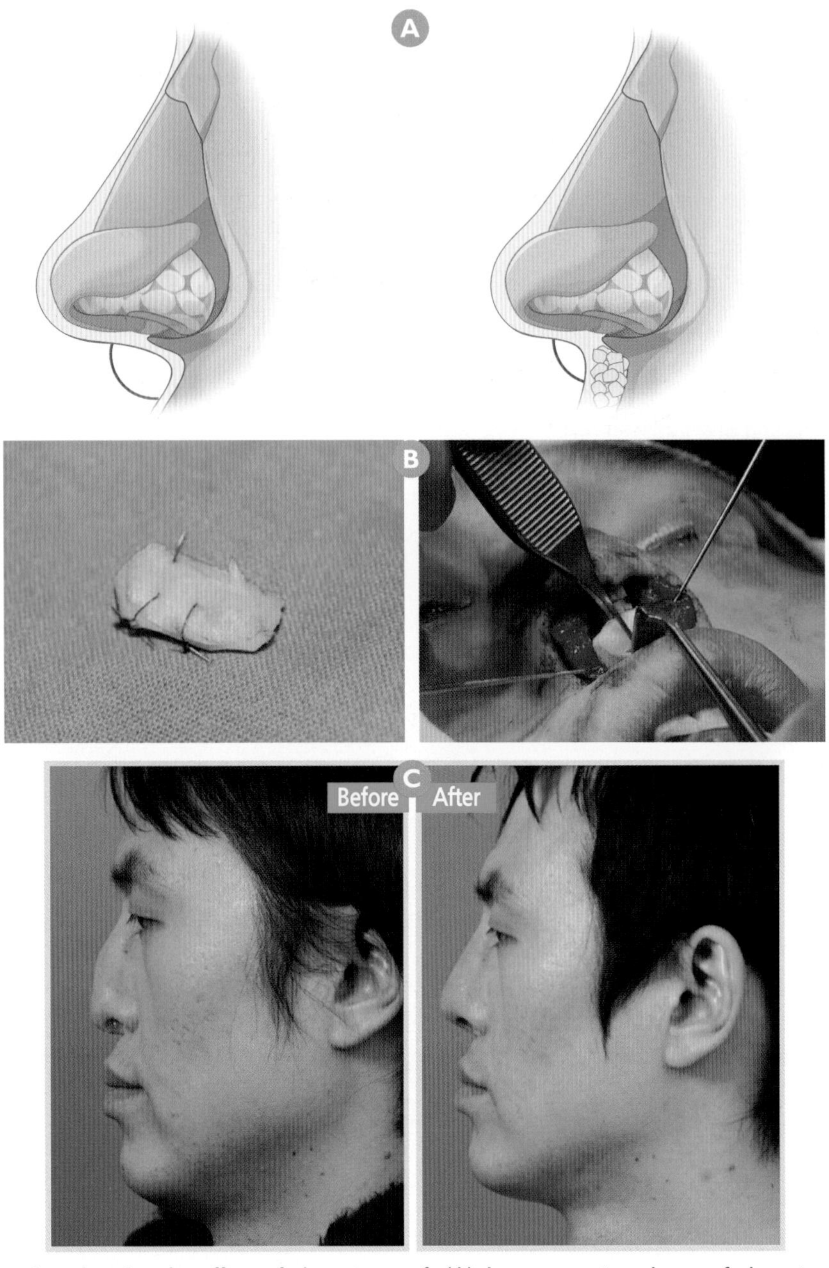

Figure 70 Illustration showing the effect of plumping graft (A). Intraoperative photo of plumping graft made of costal cartilage (B). The patient's columellar-labial angle improved after surgery (C).

V. Complications

1. Deprojection

This is a phenomenon in which projection obtained at an early stage of surgery declines over time owing to absorption of the tip graft or loosened sutures *(Figure 71)*.

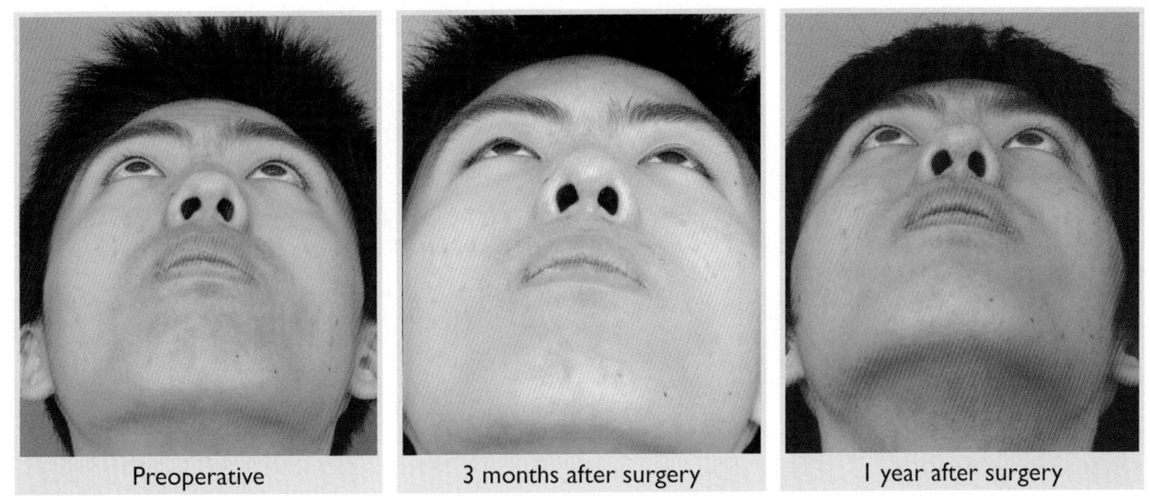

Figure 71 Example of a patient who experienced loss of the tip projection that was initially acquired by transdomal suture.

2. Infection

This complication occurs when too many cartilage pieces are used as tip grafts, or thick costal cartilage is used as a tip graft *(Figure 72)*. Another cause may be using a large quantity of suture material to fix the tip grafts.

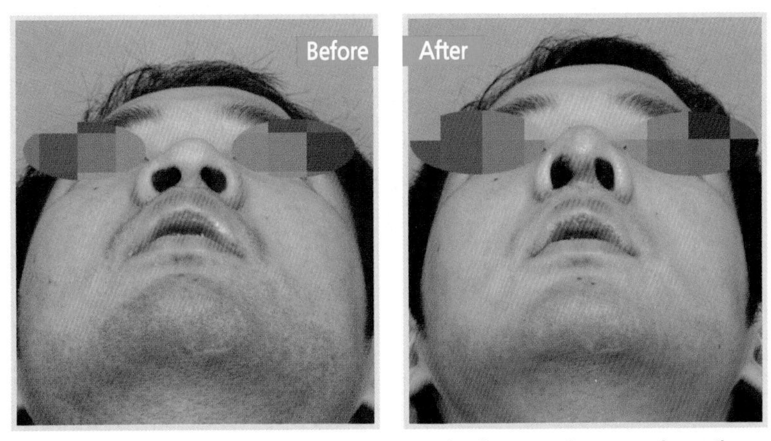

Figure 72 Photograph of a patient who experienced infection after costal cartilage tip grafting.

3. Graft Visibility, Migration, Deviation

This complication commonly occurs when tip grafting is performed on patients with relatively thin skin, or when the grafted cartilage margin is not trimmed smoothly *(Figure 73)*.

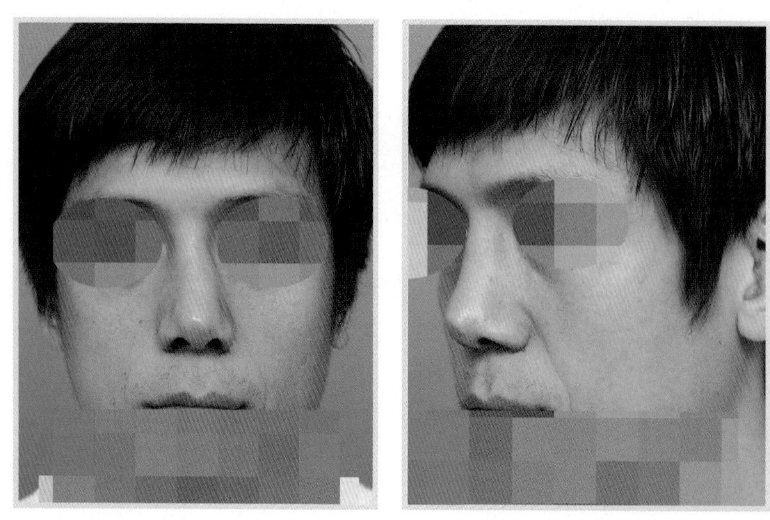

Figure 73 Example of a patient whose tip graft using conchal cartilage became visible through the skin a year after the surgery.

4. Overprojection

This complication is a problem of showing greater degree of tip projection more than desired by the patient. This complication occurs more frequently in patients with thin skin to which excessively aggressive tip grafting has been performed *(Figure 74)*.

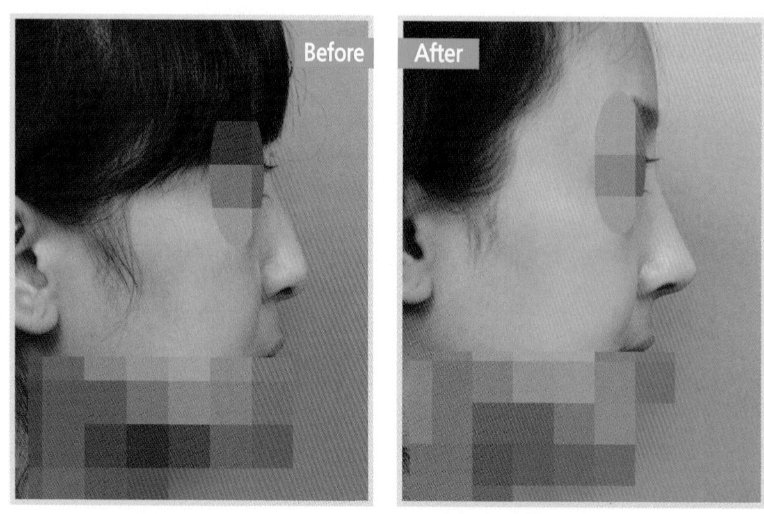

Figure 74 Example of a patient who expressed dissatisfaction due to the tip over projection after surgery.

References

1. Adamson PA. Open Rhinoplasty. Otolaryngol Clin North Am 1987; 20: 837-52.
2. Anderson JR. A Reasoned approach to the nasal base. Arch Otolaryngol 1984; 110: 349-58.
3. Behrbohm H, Tardy ME. Essentials of Septorhinoplasty. Thieme, 2004; 137-48.
4. Behmand RA, Ghavami A, Guyuron B. Nasal tip sutures, Part I: The evolution. Plast Reconstr Surg 2003; 112: 1125-9.
5. Cho GS, Kim JH, Yeo NK, Jang YJ. Nasal skin thickness measured using computed tomography and its effect on tip surgery outcomes. Otolaryngol Head Neck Surg 2011; 144: 522-7.
6. Daniel RK. Rhinoplasty. Little Brown Co, 1992; 677-704.
7. Gruber RP, Friedman GD. Suture algorithm for the broad or bulbous nasal tip. Plast Reconstr Surg 2002; 110: 1752-64.
8. Gunter JP, Landecker A, Cochran CS. Frequently used grafts in rhinoplasty: nomenclature and analysis. Plast Reconstr Surg 2006; 118: 14-29.
9. Hamra ST. Crushed cartilage grafts over alar dome reduction in open rhinoplasty. Plast Reconstr Surg 1993: 92: 352-6.
10. Hubbard TJ. Exploiting the septum for maximal tip control. Ann Plast Surg 2000; 44: 173-80.
11. Jang YJ, Min JY, Lau BC. A multilayer cartilaginous tip-grafting technique for improved nasal tip refinement in Asian rhinoplasty. Otolaryngol Head Neck Surg 2011; 145: 217-22.
12. Jang YJ, Yu MS. Rhinoplasty for the Asian nose. Facial Plast Surg 2010; 26: 93-101.
13. Min JY, Jang YJ. Use of 2-octylcyanoacrylate (Dermabond) tissue adhesive for tip graft fixation in open rhinoplasty. Otolaryngol Head Neck Surg 2011; 145: 737-41.
14. Pastorek NJ, Bustillo A, Murphy MR, Becker DG. The extended columellar strut-tip graft. Arch Facial Plast Surg 2005; 7: 176-84.
15. Rich JS. Friedman WH. Pearlman SJ. The effects of lower lateral cartilage excision on nasaltip projection. Arch Otolaryngol Head Neck Surg 1991; 117: 56-9.
16. Rohrich RJ, Adams WP. The boxy nasal tip: Classification and management based on lower lateral cartilage suturing techniques. Plast Reconstr Surg 2001; 107: 1849-63.
17. Yu MS, Jang YJ. Modified vertical dome division technique for rhinoplasty in Asian patients. Laryngoscope 2010; 120: 668-72.

Case 1

A 35-year-old male visited for a deformed nose with nasal obstruction. The patient underwent septoplasty 10 years ago.

Analysis

Frontal: Deviated nose, bulbous tip
Basal: Nostril asymmetry, poor tip projection
Lateral and Oblique: Acute nasolabial angle, ptotic tip
Endoscopy: Caudal septal deviation

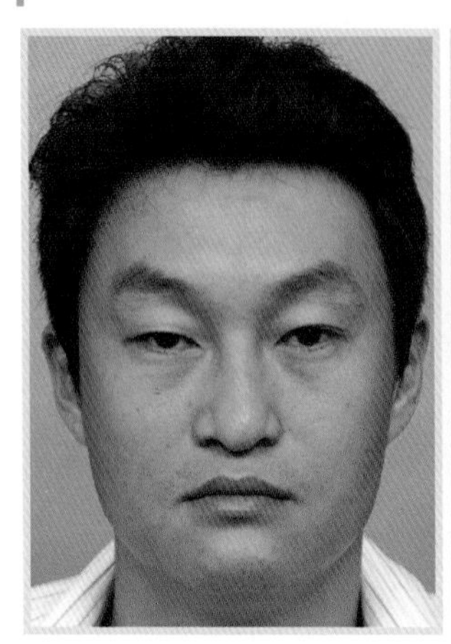
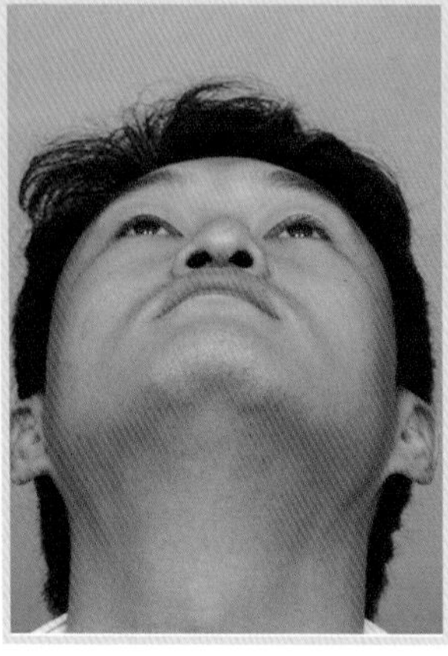
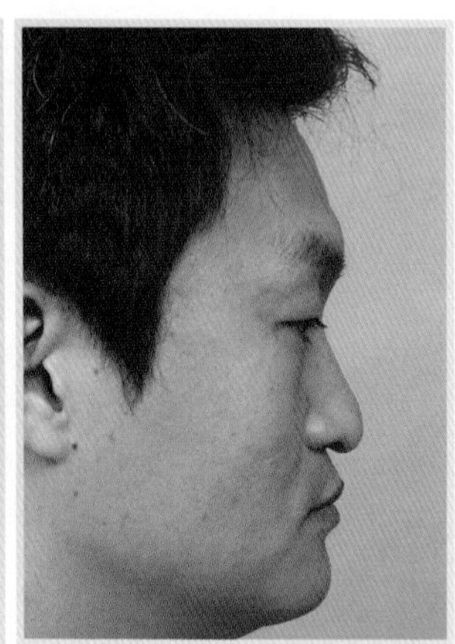

Operative Procedures

Open rhinoplasty approach
Septoplasty and harvesting of septal cartilage and bone
Costal cartilage harvest
Caudal septal cutting and suture
Caudal septal extension grafting using costal cartilage (bilateral)
Spreader grafting using costal cartilage (bilateral)
Multilayer tip grafting using costal cartilage
Tip graft covered with perichondrium
Dorsal augmentation using costal cartilage

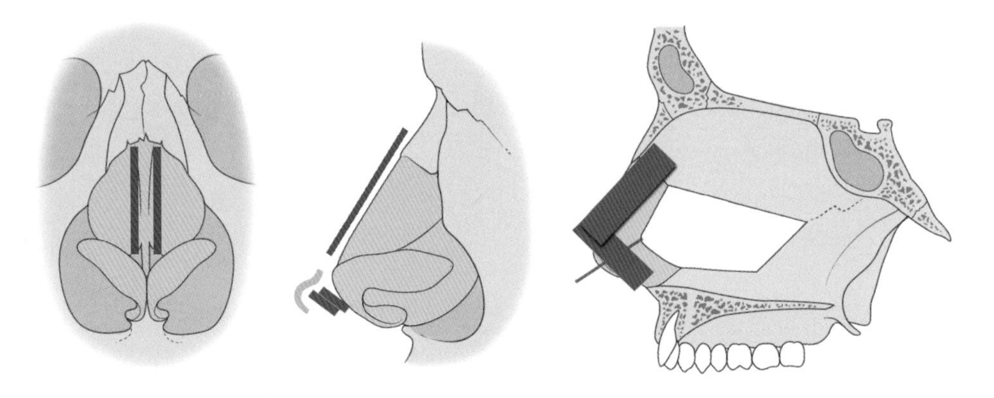

Postoperative Changes

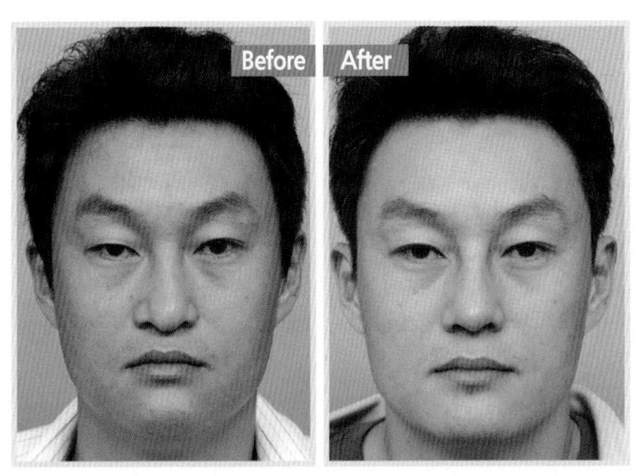

Frontal: Deviation was corrected. Blunt tip was defined. Columella and alar base levels were improved.

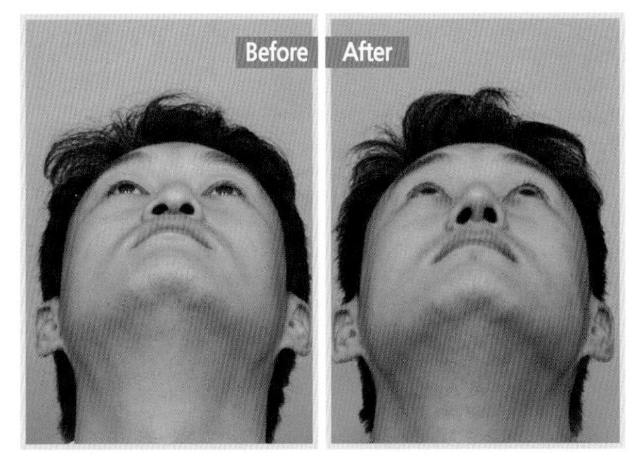

Basal: Tip projection was improved. Nostril asymmetry was corrected.

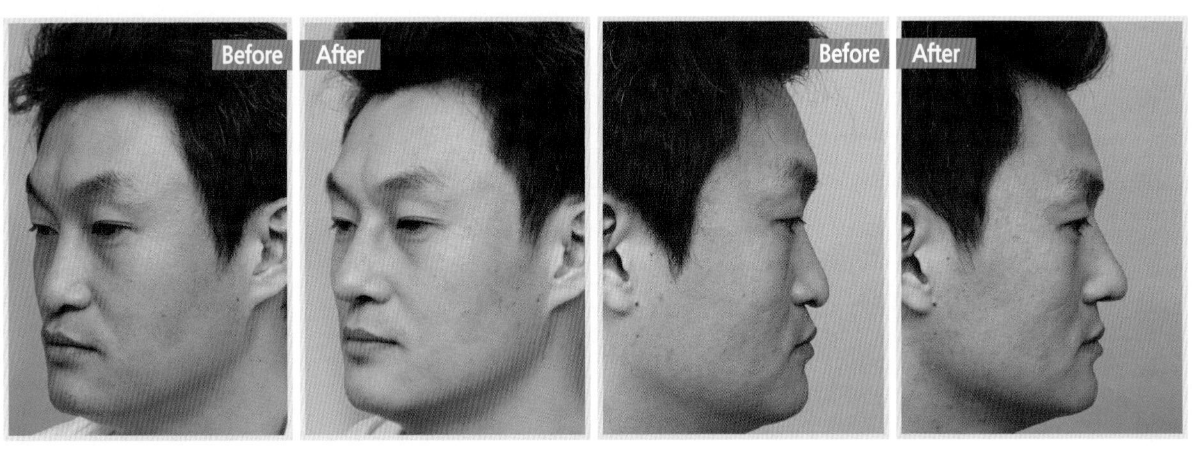

Lateral and Oblique: Nasolabial angle was widened after cephalic rotation of the ptotic tip. Tip projection was increased. Dorsal height was improved.

Case 2

A 21-year-old male visited for a flat nose deformity and wide dorsum.

Analysis

Frontal: Low dorsum, poor tip definition, thick skin
Basal: Poor tip projection, small nostril
Lateral and Oblique: Low dorsal height, low tip height

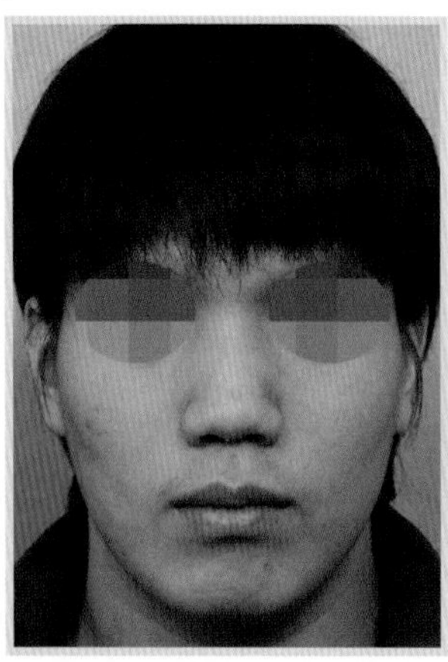
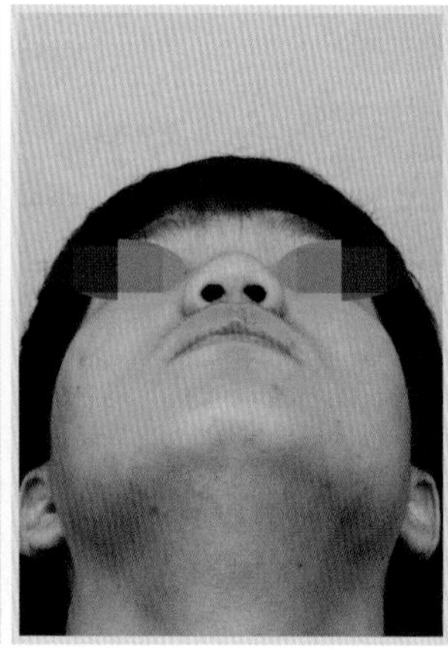
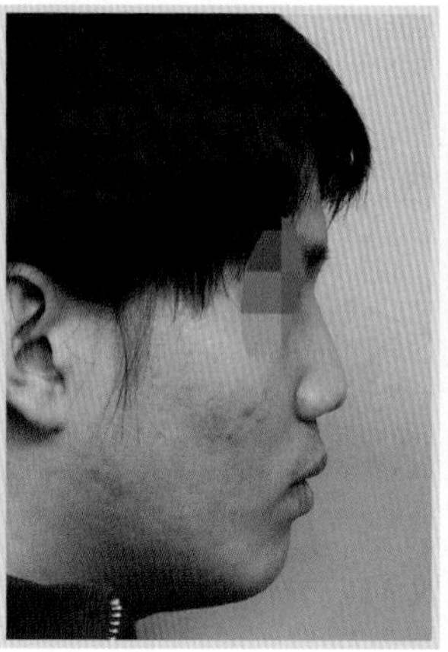
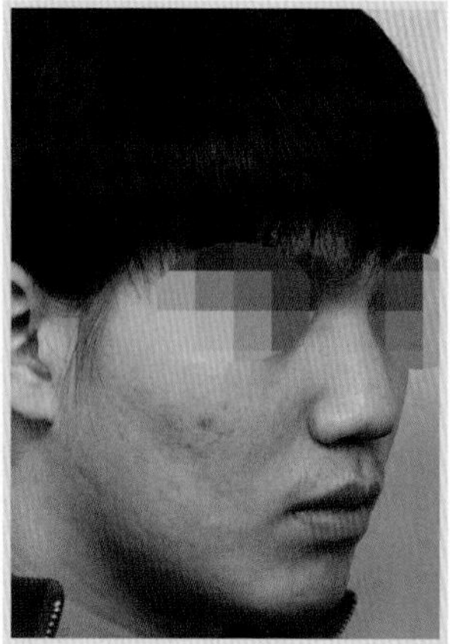

Operative Procedures

Open rhinoplasty approach
Septoplasty and harvesting of septal bone and cartilage
Costal cartilage harvest
Medial and lateral osteotomies
Caudal septal extension grafting using costal cartilage (left)
Backstop grafting using costal cartilage
Dorsal augmentation using crushed septal cartilage

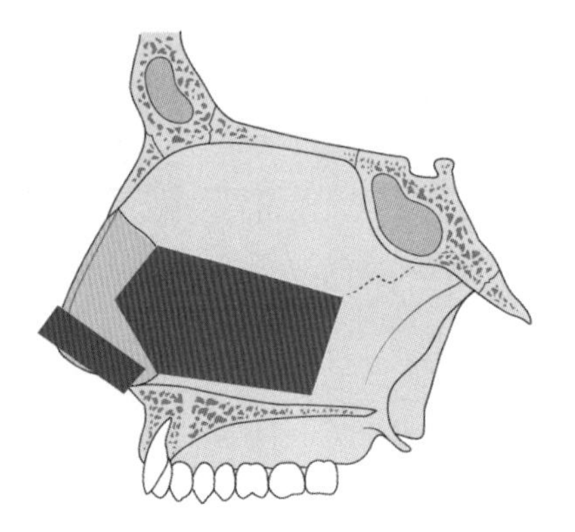
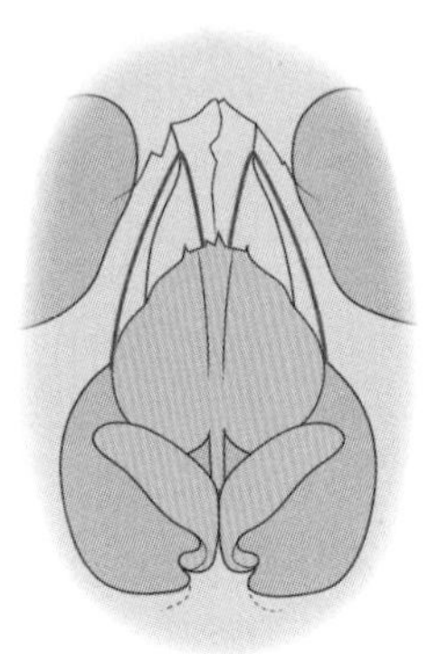
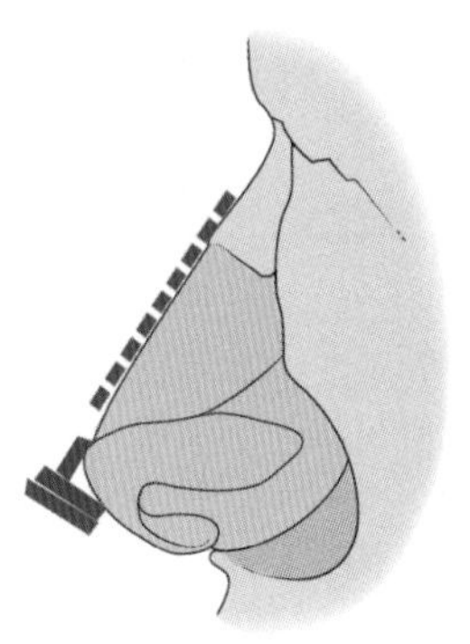

Postoperative Changes

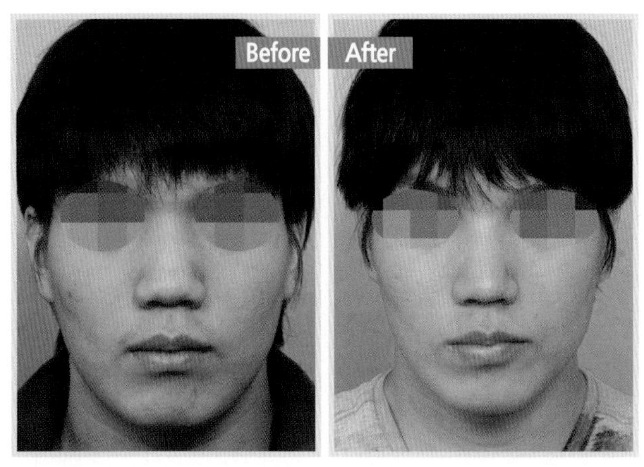

Frontal: Dorsal aesthetic lines were sharpened. Tip definition was improved.

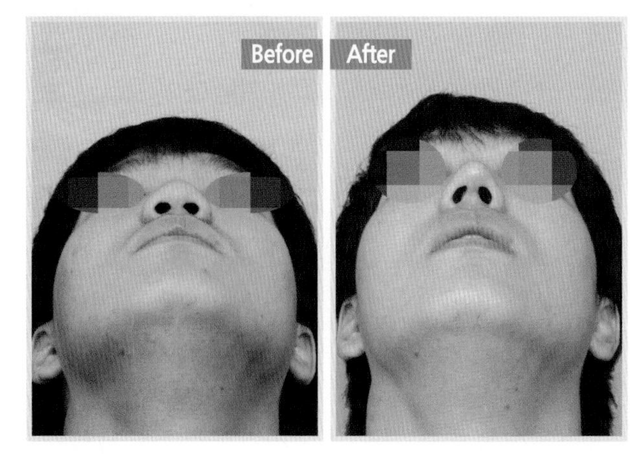

Basal: Tip projection and nostril shape were improved.

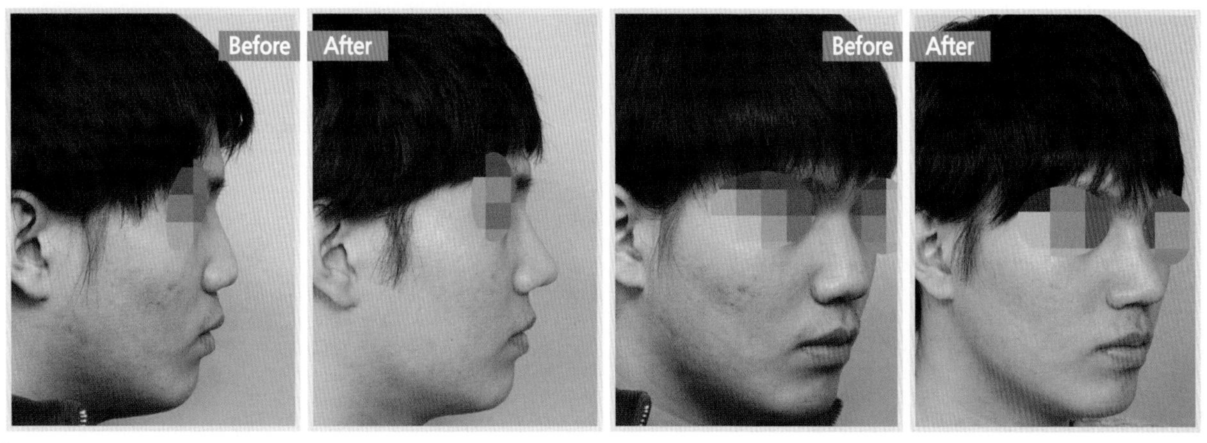

Lateral and Oblique: Dorsal convexity was improved by tip projection. Tip definition was improved.

Case 3

A 25-year-old female visited for a hump nose deformity.

Analysis

Frontal: Mild deviation
Basal: Poor tip projection, nostril asymmetry
Lateral and Oblique: Mild convexity of the nasal dorsum

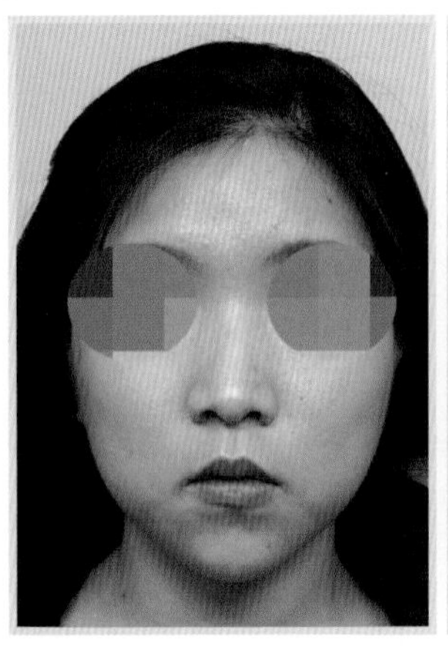

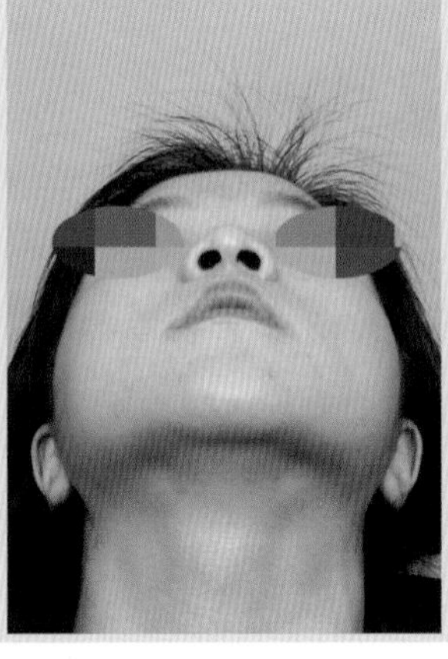

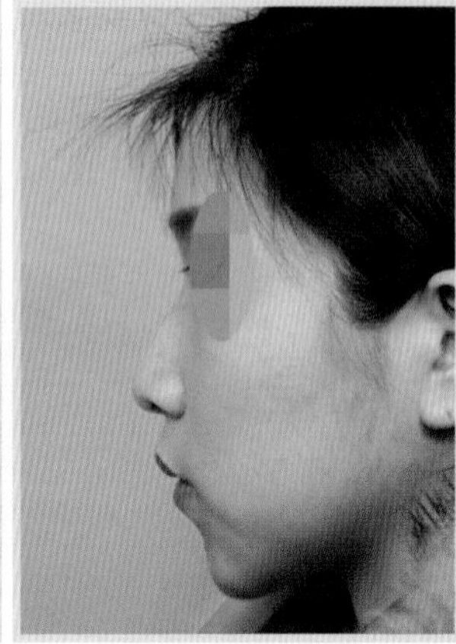

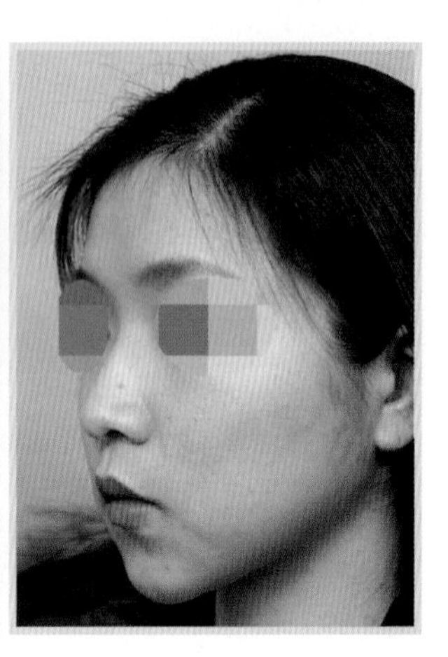

Operative Procedures

Open rhinoplasty approach
Septoplasty and harvesting of septal bone and cartilage
Hump rasping
Caudal septal extension grafting using septal cartilage
Spreader grafting using septal cartilage (bilateral)
Shield grafting using conchal cartilage
Backstop grafting using conchal cartilage
Dorsal augmentation using processed fascia lata and crushed cartilage

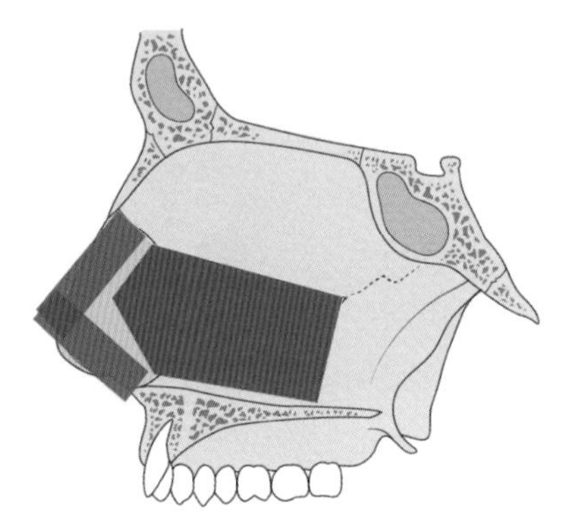

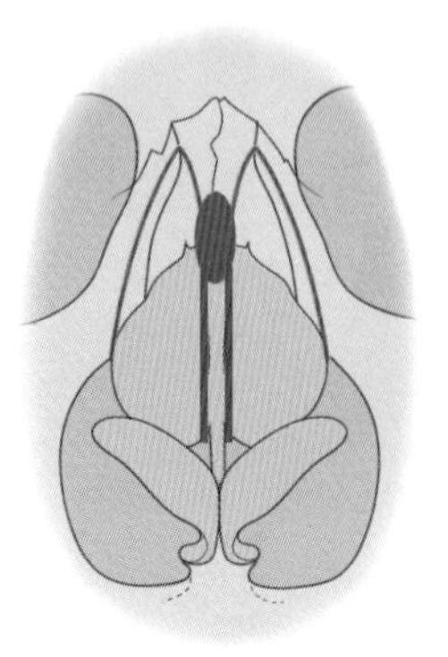

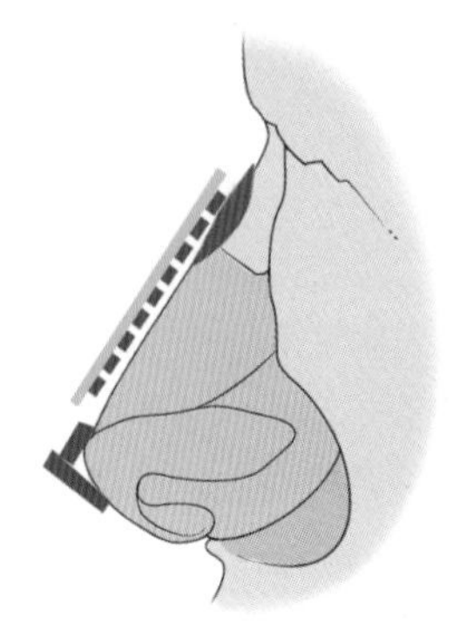

Postoperative Changes

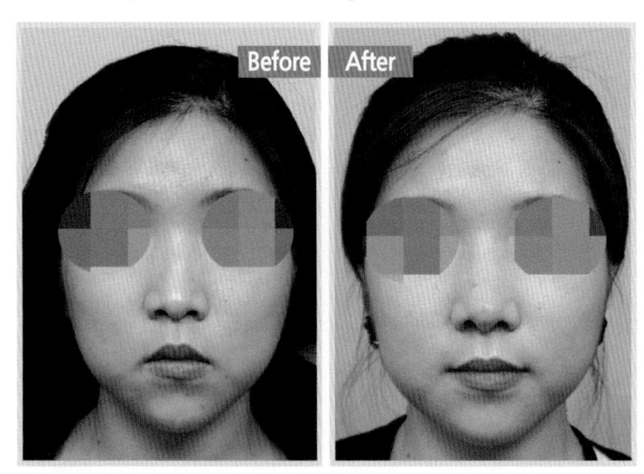

Frontal: Dorsal deviation was improved. Dorsal width was slightly increased.

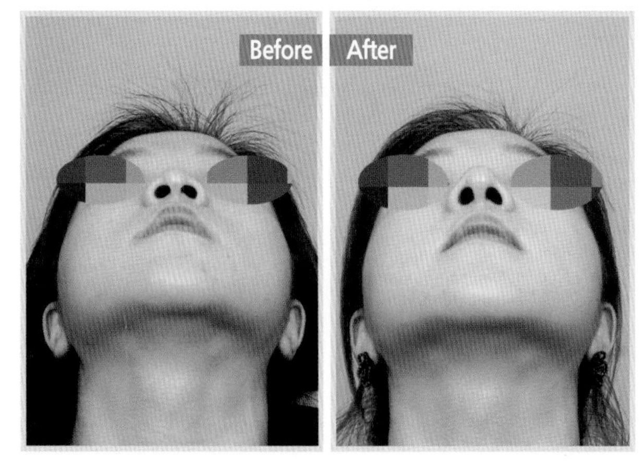

Basal: Tip projection was increased. Nostril shape was improved.

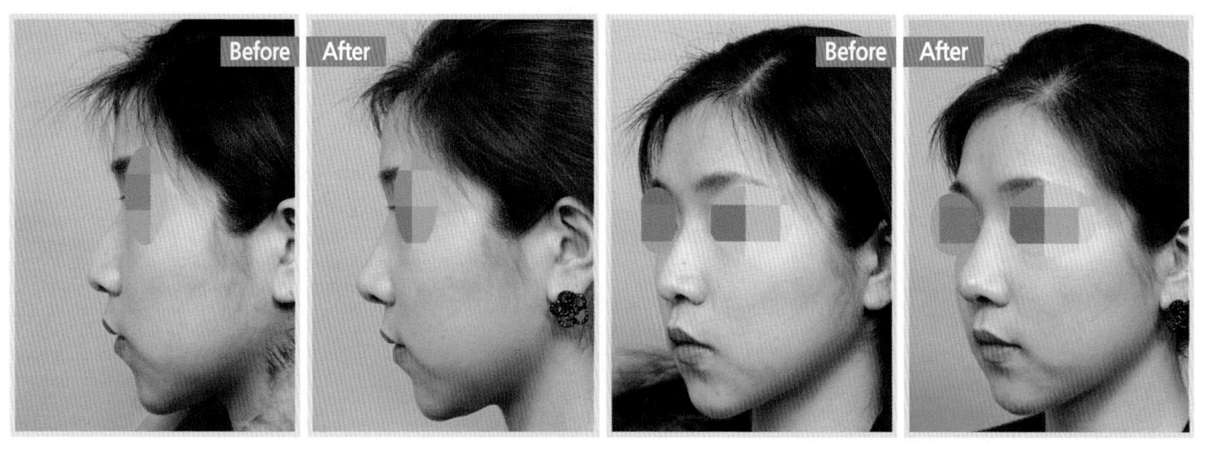

Lateral and Oblique: Hump was removed. Natural dorsal line achieved through tip augmentation.

Case 4

A patient visited for her dorsal irregularity and low tip projection. She had undergone injection rhinoplasty on her tip and radix.

Analysis

Small nostril

Dorsal irregularity, low radix

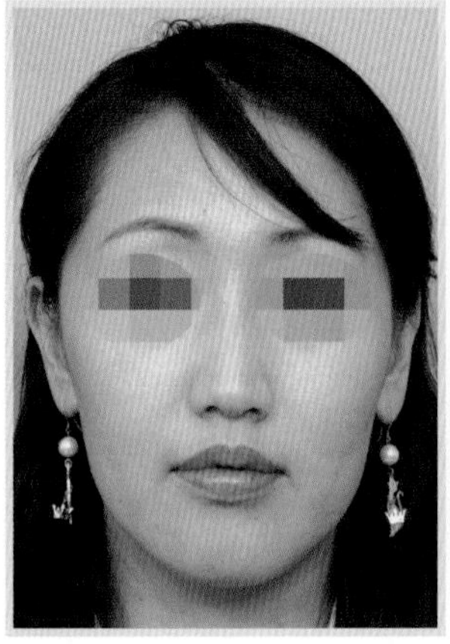
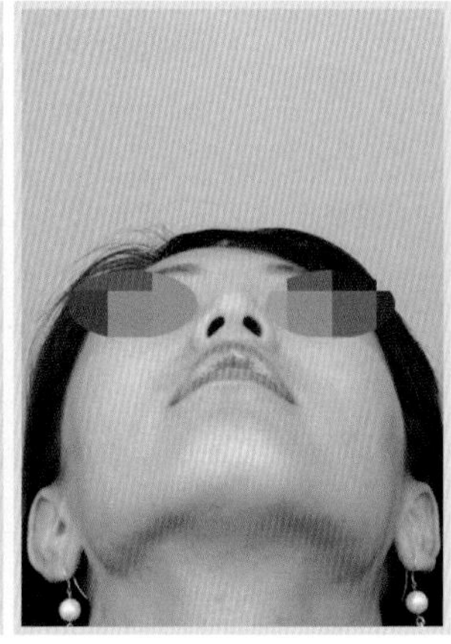
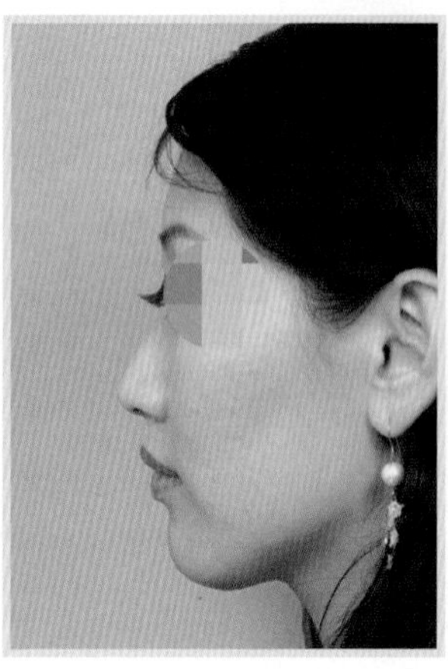
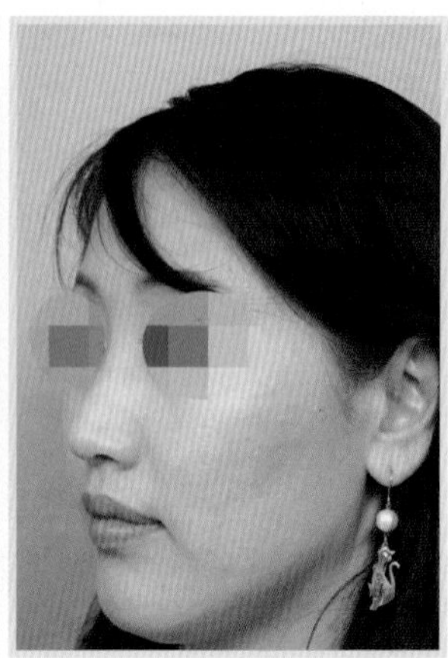

Operative Procedures

Open rhinoplasty approach

Hump rasping

Septoplasty and harvest of septal cartilage and bone

Multilayer tip grafting using septal cartilage

Backstop graft application

Supratip augmentation using crushed cartilage

Tip graft camouflaging using fascia lata

Dorsal augmentation using fascia lata

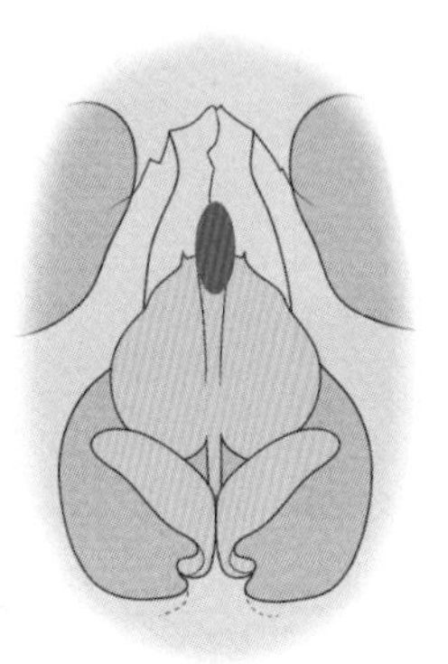
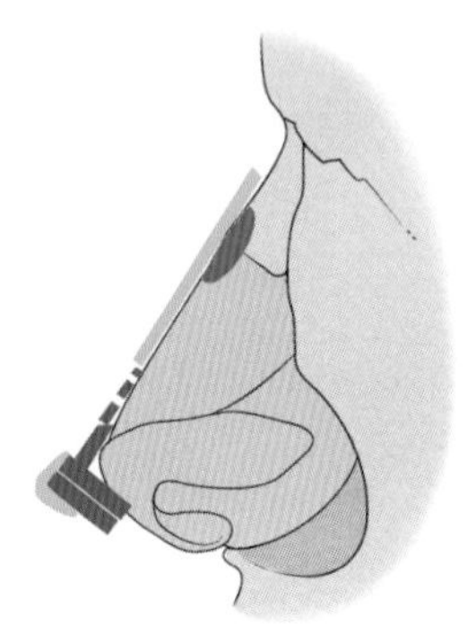

Postoperative Changes

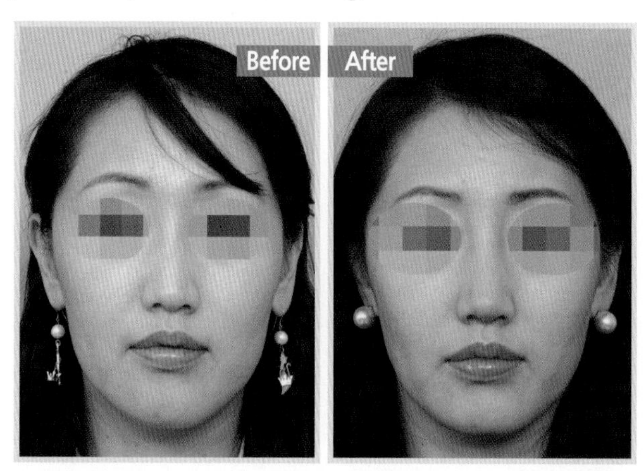

Frontal: Dorsal aesthetic lines were highlighted. Dorsal width was slightly widened.

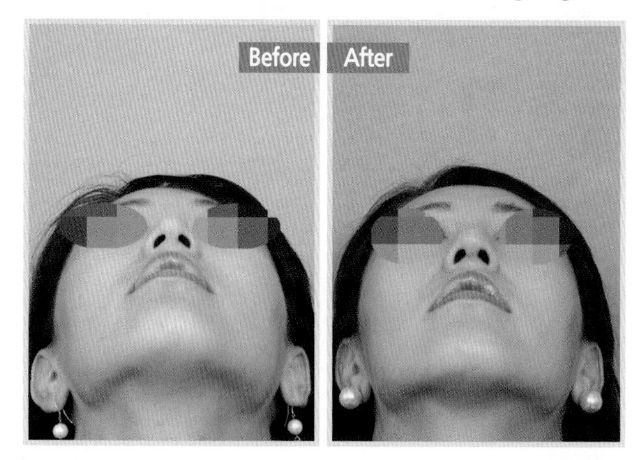

Basal: Nostrils were enlarged and the shapes were improved. Tip projection was improved.

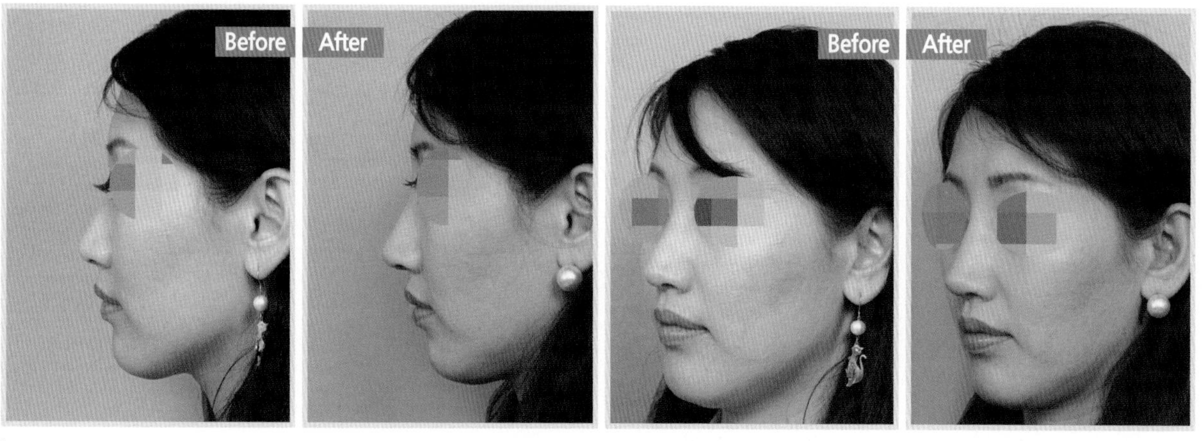

Lateral and Oblique: Dorsal irregularity was smoothened. Slightly concave dorsal line was formed by tip projection.

Case 5

A 31-year-old female visited for a deviated nose, bulbous tip, and convex dorsum.

Analysis

Frontal: Deviated nose, bulbous tip, thick skin
Basal: Poor tip projection and definition
Lateral and Oblique: Mild dorsal convexity

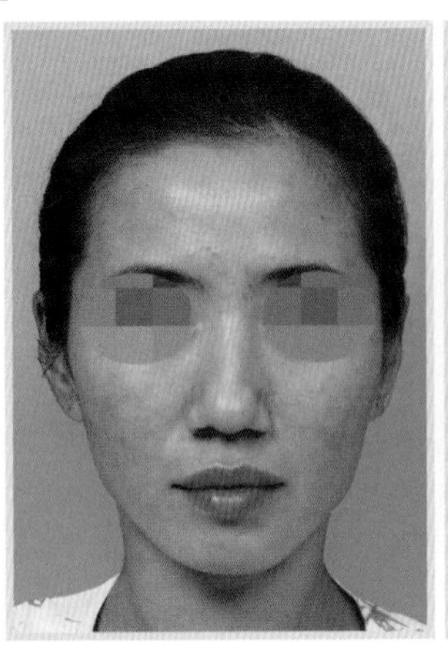
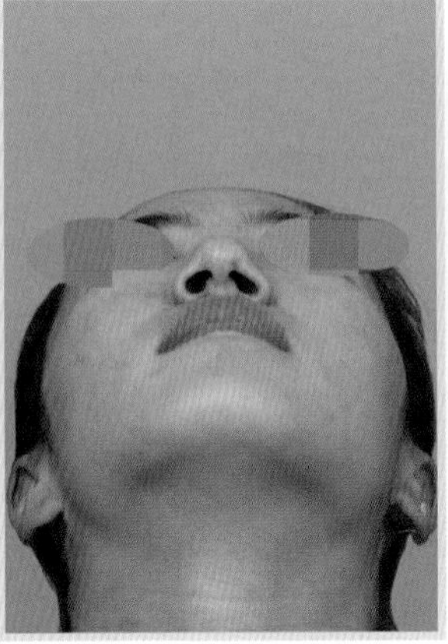
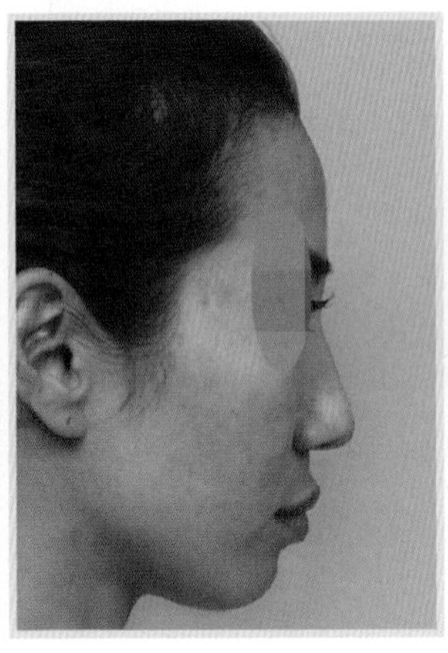
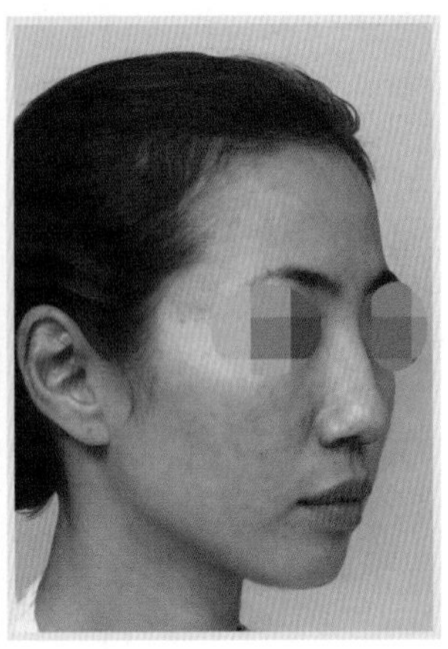

Operative Procedures

Open rhinoplasty approach
Septoplasty and harvesting of septal cartilage and bone
Medial, lateral, and percutaneous root osteotomies
Batten grafting using septal cartilage (left)
Modified vertical dome division
Columellar strut application
Double shield grafting using conchal cartilage
Backstop graft application
Tip graft camouflaging using processed fascia lata
Dorsal augmentation using Gore-Tex

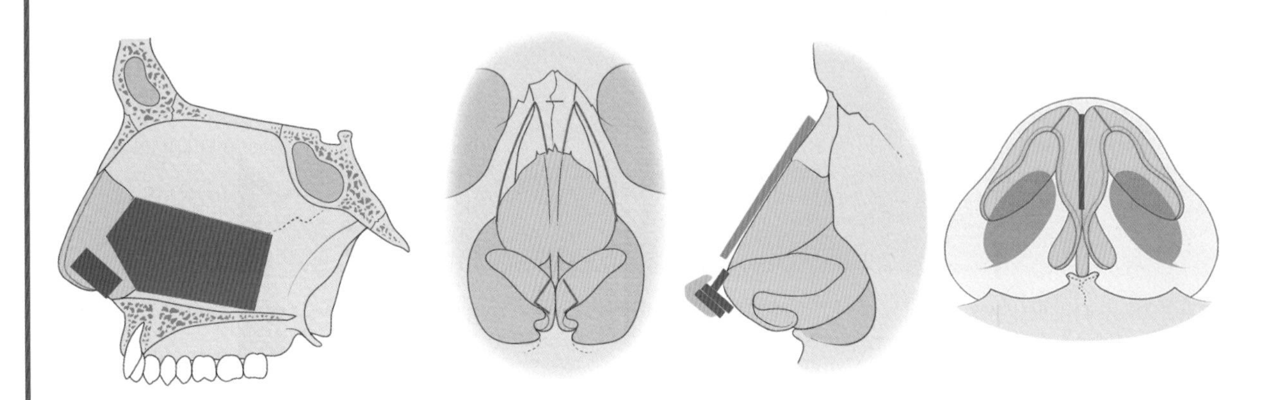

Postoperative Changes

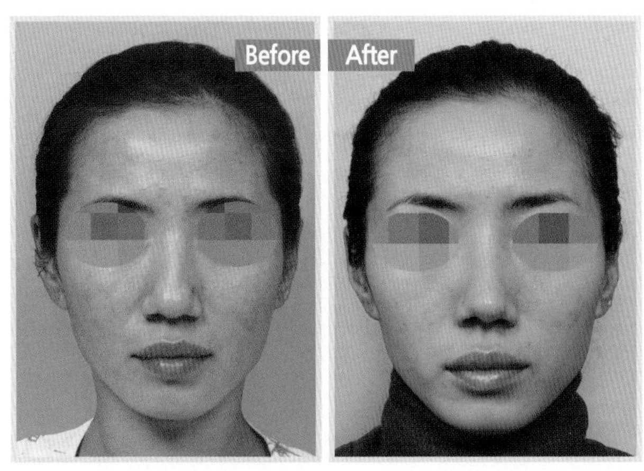

Frontal: Dorsal deviation was corrected. Tip definition was improved.

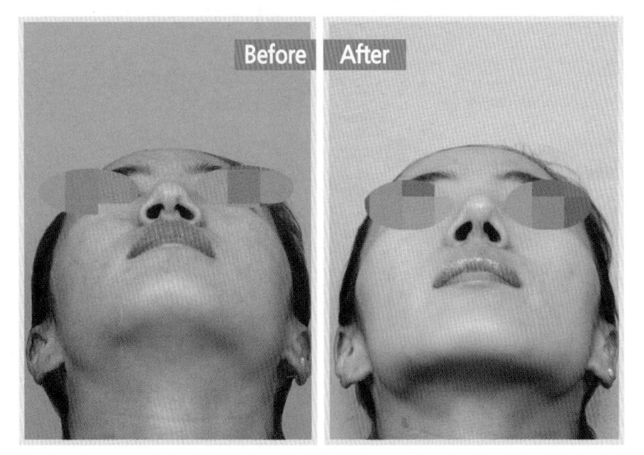

Basal: Tip projection was improved and nostril shapes became more natural looking.

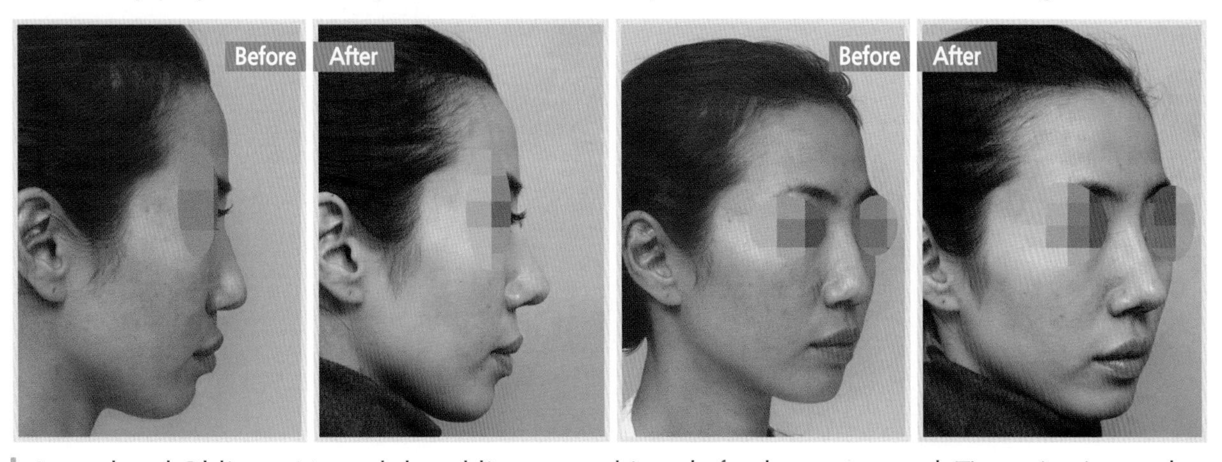

Lateral and Oblique: Natural dorsal line was achieved after hump removal. Tip projection and definition were improved.

Case 6

A 23-year-old male visited for a hump and a long nose deformity.

Analysis
Frontal: Ptotic tip
Basal: Poor tip projection, concave alar lobule
Lateral and Oblique: Low radix height, ptotic tip, acute nasolabial angle

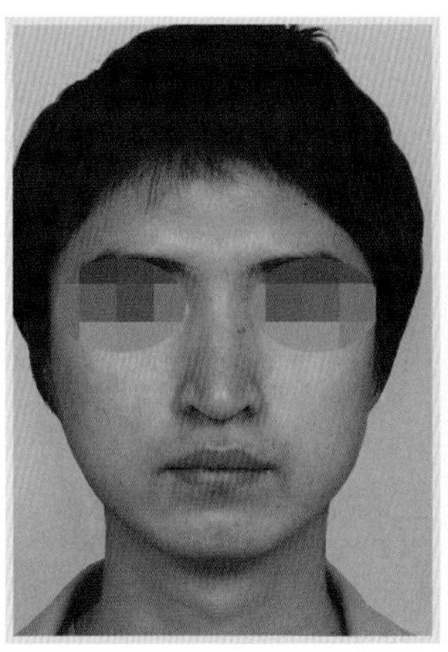 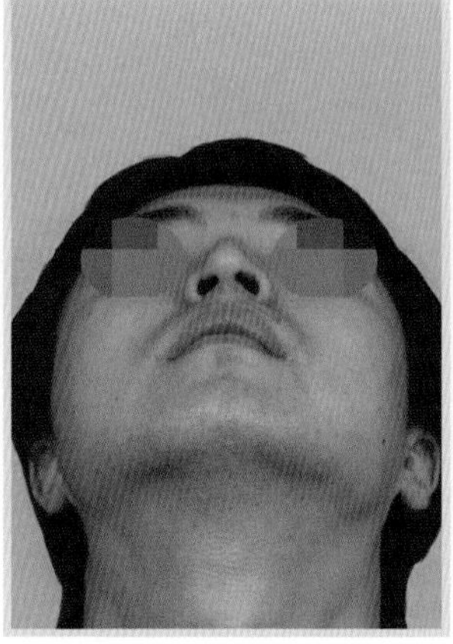 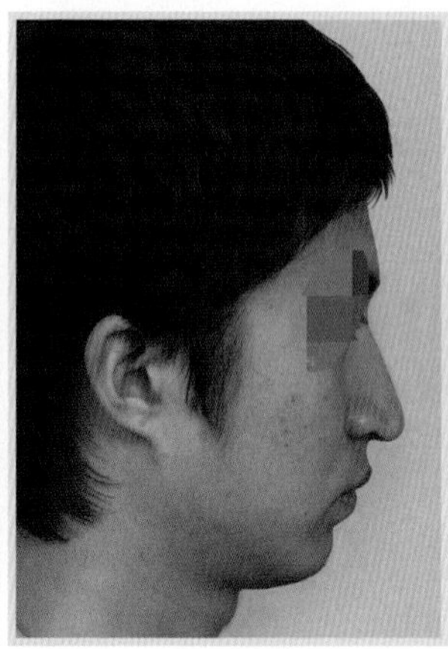 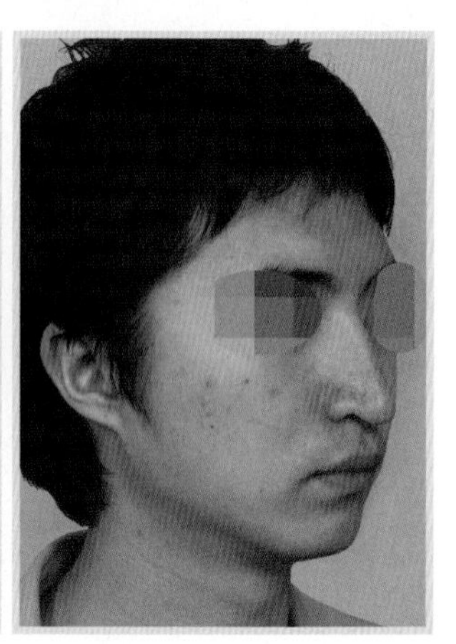

Operative Procedures

Open rhinoplasty approach
Septoplasty and harvesting of septal cartilage and bone
Hump rasping
Caudal septal extension grafting (bilateral)
Cephalic resection
Dome division
Shield grafting
Lateral crural overlay technique (bilateral)
Lateral crural onlay grafting (right)
Interdomal suturing
Dorsal augmentation using crushed cartilage and processed fascia lata

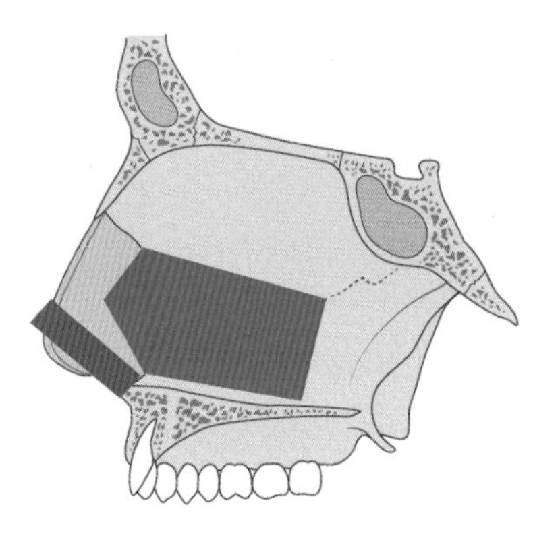 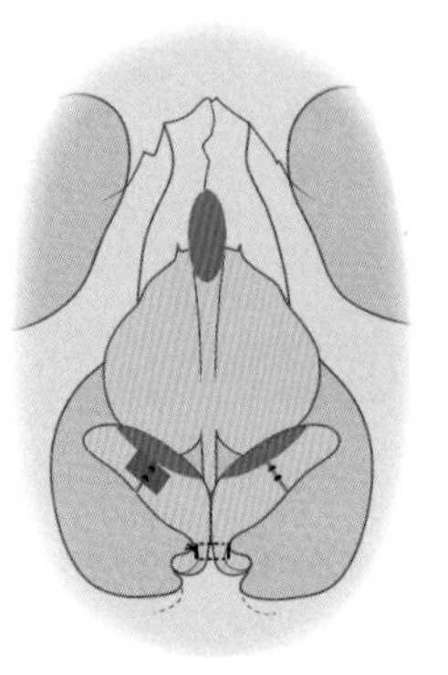 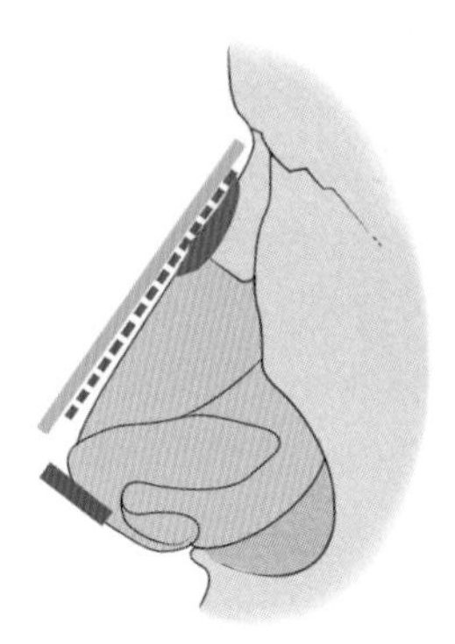

Postoperative Changes

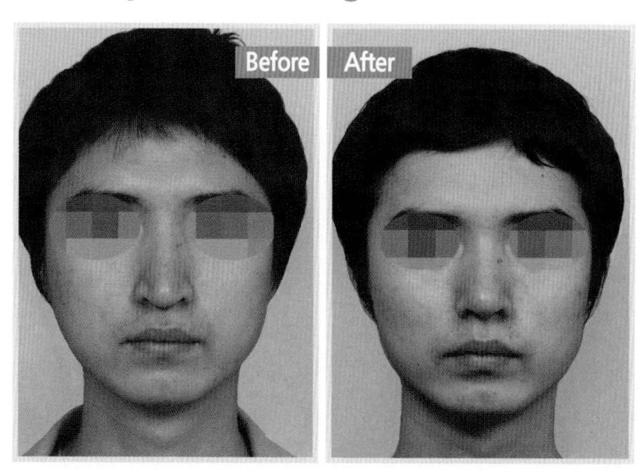

Frontal: Columellar show was improved after correction of the ptotic tip.

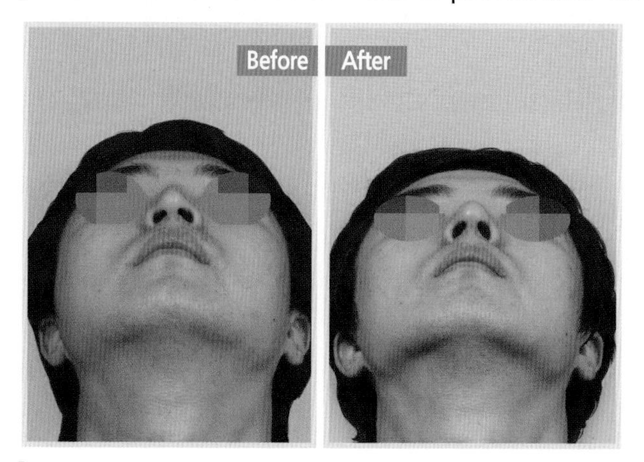

Basal: Nostril shapes were improved. Tip projection was increased. Alar lobule concavity was addressed, with a round contour achieved.

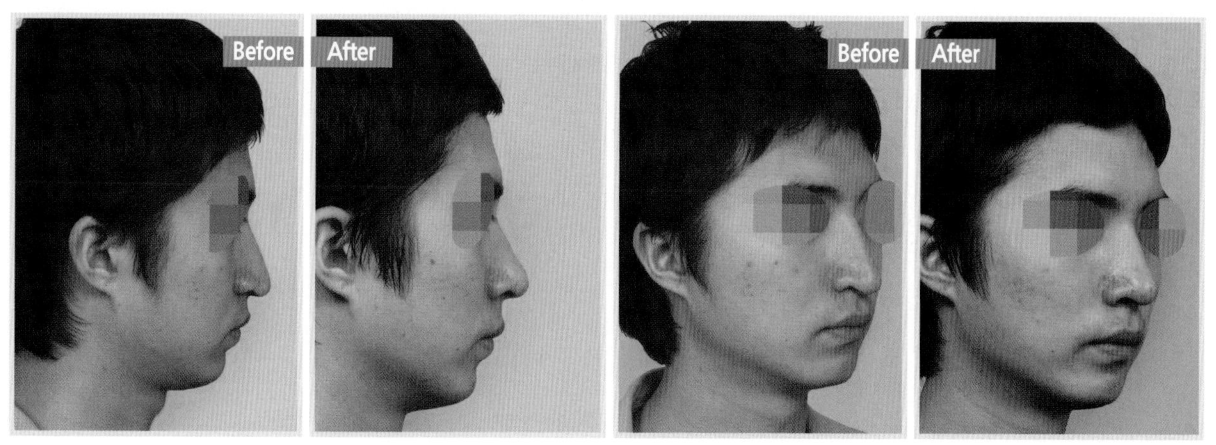

Lateral and Oblique: Increased nasal tip projection. Tip was cephalically rotated. Dorsal concavity was improved.

Case 7

A 24-year-old female visited for a hump nose and deviated nose deformity.

Analysis

Frontal: Mild deviation to right, bulbous nasal tip, wide alar base
Basal: Nostril asymmetry, poor tip projection
Lateral and Oblique: Convex nasal dorsum, ptotic tip, acute nasolabial angle

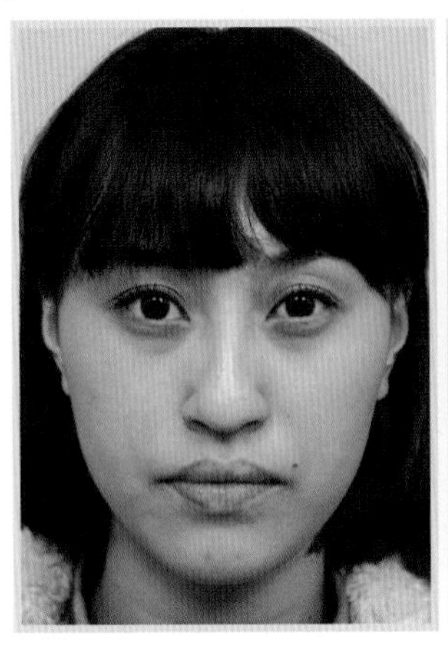

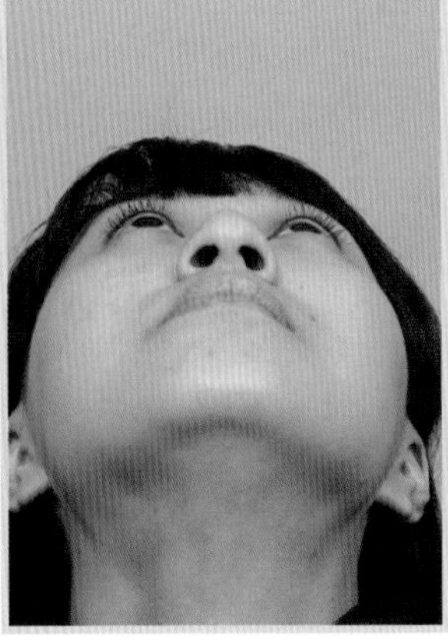

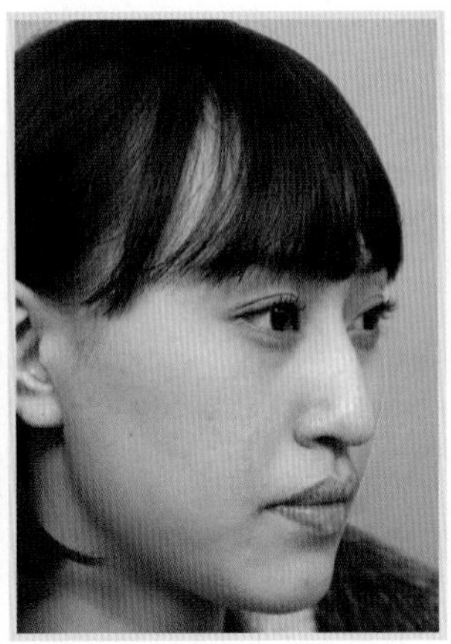

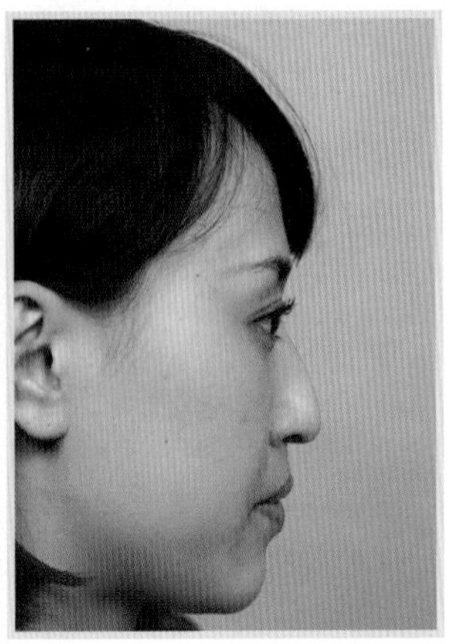

Operative Procedures

Open rhinoplasty approach
Septal cartilage harvest preserving an L-strut
Cartilaginous hump resection using #15 blade
Hump rasping
Medial, lateral, and percutaneous root osteotomies
Spreader grafting using septal cartilage (left)
Caudal batten grafting using septal cartilage (right)
Cephalic resection and transdomal suturing of the lower lateral cartilages
Multilayer tip grafting using septal cartilage
Dorsal augmentation using processed fascia lata
Alar base resection (bilateral)

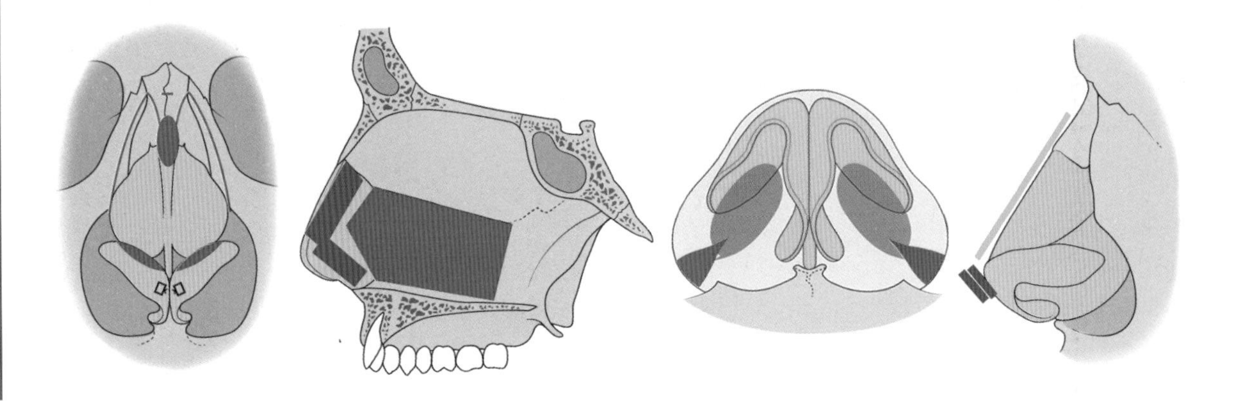

Postoperative Changes

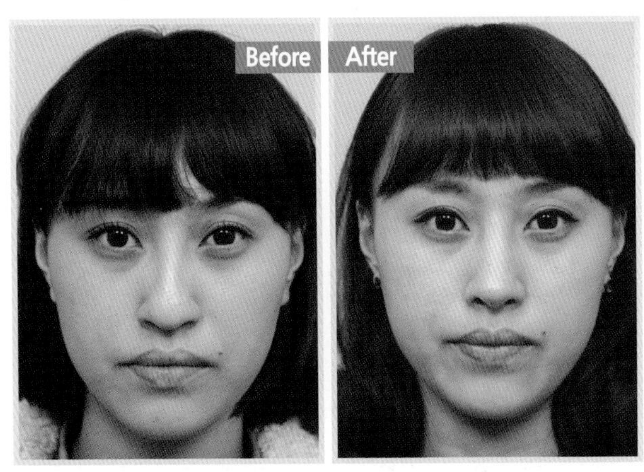

Frontal: Dorsal deviation was partially corrected. Tip definition was improved. Nostril show was increased as the tip rotated cephalically.

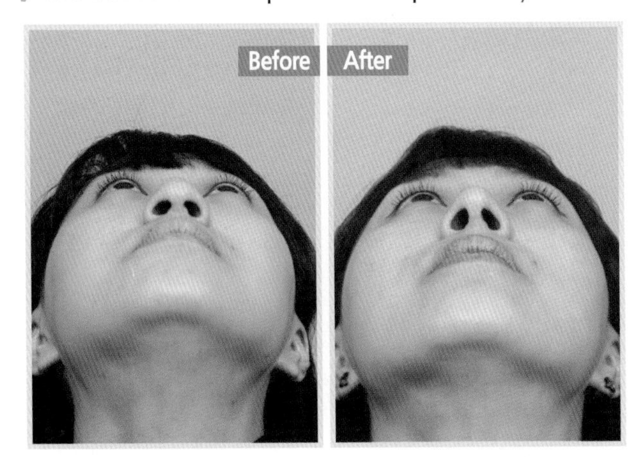

Basal: Ratio of columella and lobule changed to 2:1 after tip projection. The nostrils became larger. Asymmetry was not corrected completely.

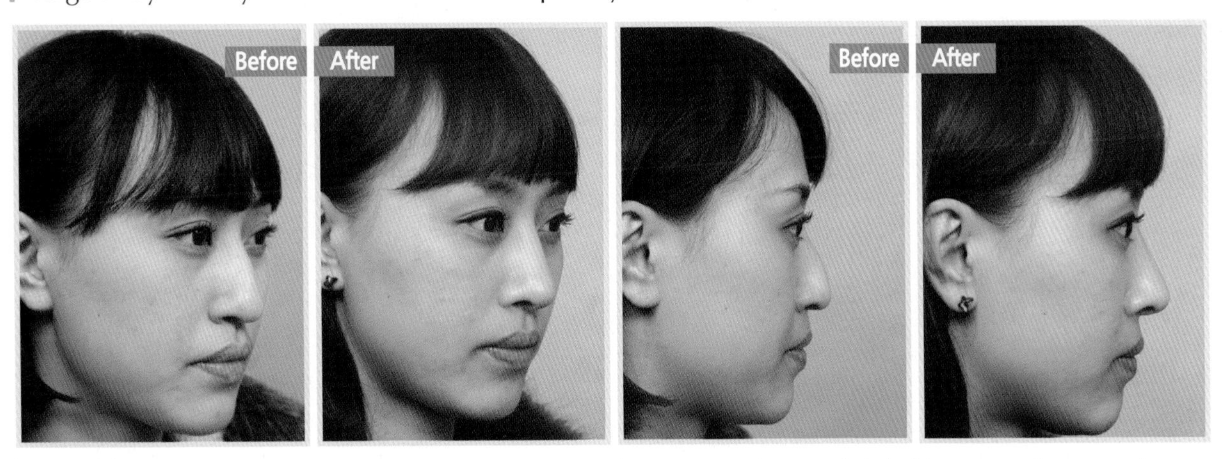

Lateral and Oblique: Radix height was augmented. Tip projection and definition were improved. Nasolabial angle was widened. An ideal dorsal line was achieved by correction of the dorsal convexity.

Septal Extension Graft

In Sang Kim · Yong Ju Jang

A septal extension graft is an additionally attached graft on the nasal septum, and is a surgical procedure designed to change the nasal shape by changing the size or shape of septal cartilage. This procedure can produce various effects such as reinforcement of tip support, adjustment of tip projection and rotation, extension of dorsal length, columellar advancement, and nasolabial angle improvement.

I. The Effects of a Septal Extension Graft

A septal extension graft can be used to create various effects. The shape, size, and direction of the graft can be adequately adjusted according to the intended effect *(Figure 1)*.

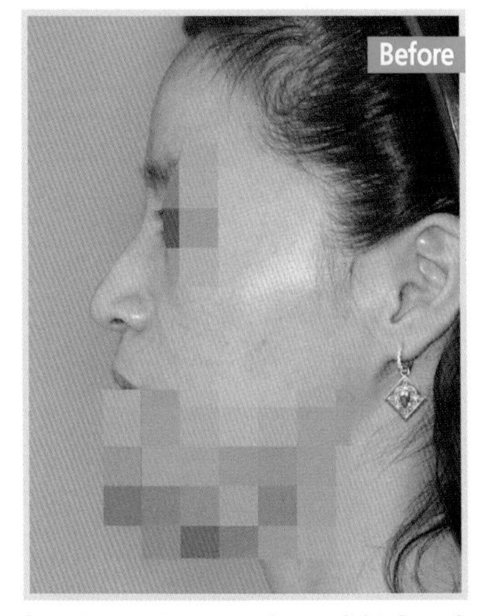

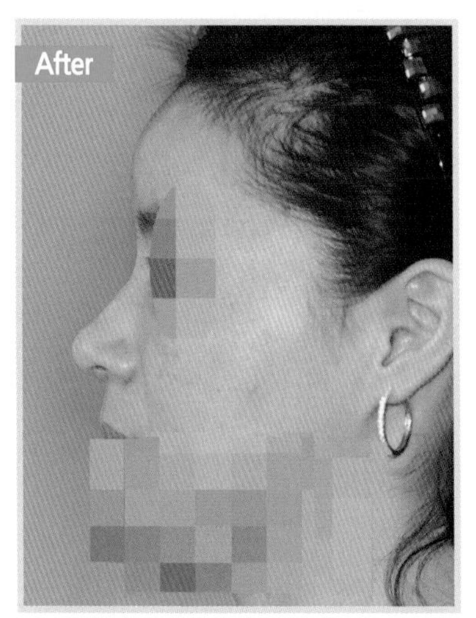

Figure 1 A case showing an improved nasolabial angle, tip projection, and rotation by septal extension grafting.

1. Reinforcement of Tip Support

A septal extension graft fixes the alar cartilages to the desired position and reinforces tip support by connecting the septal cartilage that has little flexibility and alar cartilages that has greater flexibility. Many Asians tend to have short and weak medial crura of the alar cartilages. This procedure is effective in reinforcing and extending the medial crus. However, in exchange for gaining a stronger tip support, the mobility of alar cartilage maybe reduced, making the nasal tip stiffer.

2. Adjustment of Tip Projection and Rotation

Using septal extension grafts, tip projection and rotation can be adjusted relatively easily and securely *(Figure 2)*. Septal extension grafts can easily adjust the direction and projection of the alar cartilages by adjusting the direction and length of the graft. It has the advantage of not creating an unnaturally long infratip lobule as seen in tip onlay grafting. Moreover, as it is hidden at the bottom of alar cartilages, it does not have the complications of graft visibility and skin thinning, complications commonly seen in tip grafting.

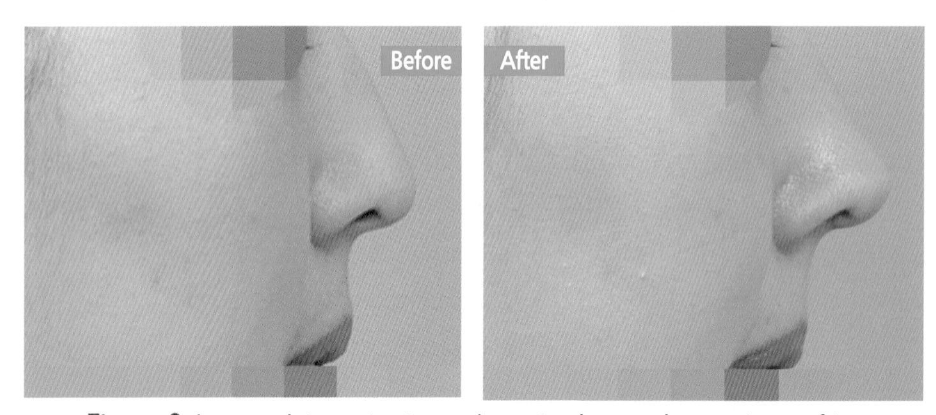

Figure 2 Improved tip projection and rotation by septal extension grafting.

3. Improvement of Nostril Shape

As a septal extension graft extends the nostril vertically, good aesthetic effects can be expected in the rhinoplasty of Asians who, in many cases, have a horizontal nostril axis *(Figure 3)*. Moreover, as a result of septal extension grafting, the vertical length of the columella also increases, improving the columellar-lobular ratio of Asians who have a relatively short columella and long infratip lobule.

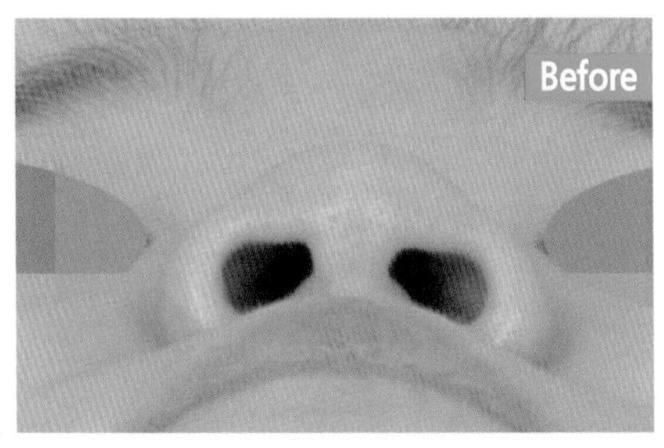

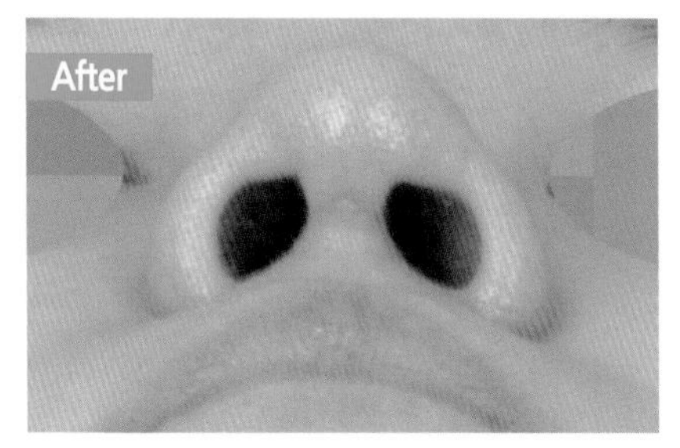

Figure 3 Improvement of nostril shape by septal extension grafting.

4. Columellar Advancement and Nasolabial Angle Improvement

If the septal extension graft is fixed at the caudal septum with the intention of pushing the base of the columella caudally, it has the effect of improving the acute nasolabial angle. If the shape of the graft is adjusted properly, it can also selectively advance the base or tip of the columella *(Figure 4)*.

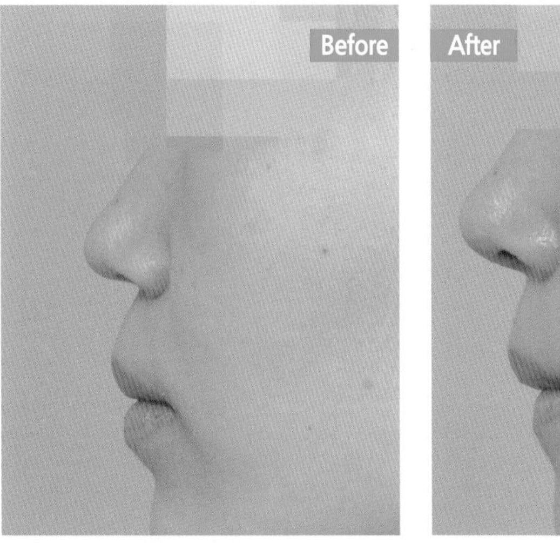

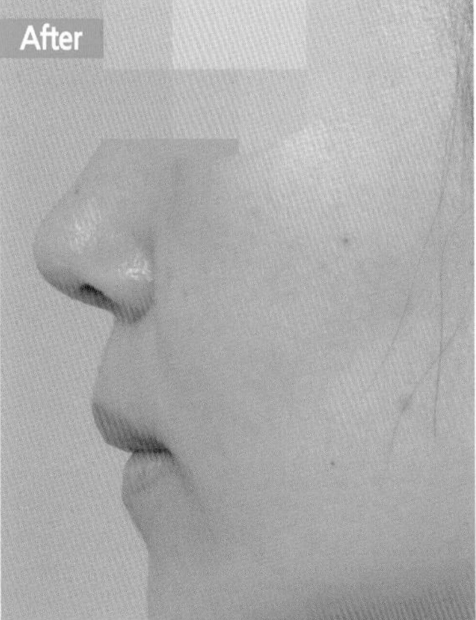

Figure 4 Nasolabial angle improvement and columellar advancement by septal extension grafting.

To improve the nasolabial angle, the graft must be located deeply and posteriorly near the premaxilla and the anterior nasal spine. If the main purpose of graft is columellar advancement, it is better to intend a lesser degree of reinforcement of tip projection or tip support. If maxilla is not fully developed and the columellar retraction is severe, the improvement of the nasolabial angle may not be achieved by septal extension graft alone. In such cases, additional premaxillary grafts or plumping grafts may be required.

5. Improvement of Symmetry between the Tip and Nostril

By pulling both alar cartilages together and fixing it on the septal extension graft, flaring of the middle crura and domal divergence of alar cartilages can be reduced, thus, the width of nasal tip can be narrowed, and the columellar shape can be improved. Nostril asymmetry can be improved in the process of fixing the asymmetrical alar cartilages on the septal extension graft, which consequently improves the symmetry between columella and the nostril. Deviation of the nasal tip can be improved to a certain degree by asymmetrically fixing the alar cartilages on the septal extension graft, and fixing the septal extension graft tilted slightly toward the direction to which the nasal tip is intended to move.

6. Extension of Nasal Length

A septal extension graft can extend the lower third of the nose, or tip-columella complex, in the caudal direction, which is effective in correcting a short nose or over-rotation of the nasal tip *(Figure 5)*. Septal extension grafts provide strong support for the extended tip. In order to reduce the excessive tension on the graft and surrounding tissues after placement of a septal extension graft for lengthening purposes, it is best to adequately dissect the areas around the alar cartilages such as the scroll area and pyriform ligament.

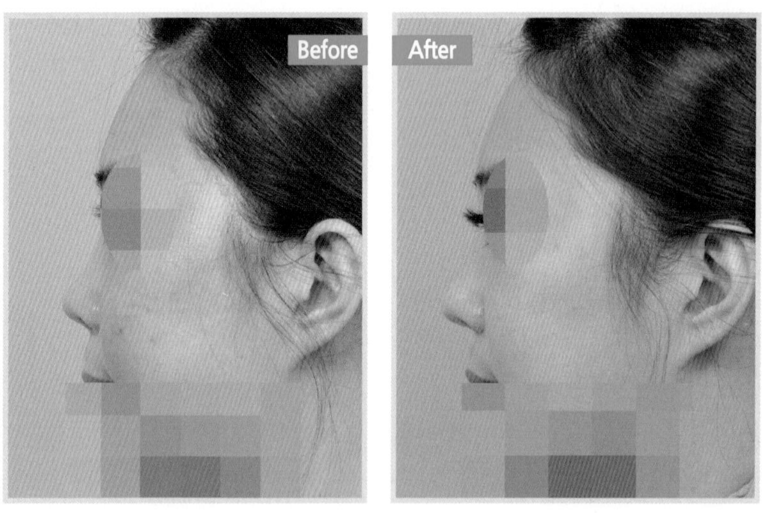

Figure 5 A case showing extension of nasal length by septal extension grafting.

II. Prerequisites for Successful Septal Extension Grafting

When performing septal extension grafting, the most important factor that makes a difference in the surgical effects is the condition of the septal cartilage, such as the size, strength, and shape of it. For successful septal extension grafting, the septal cartilage must be thick and strong. If the cartilage is weak, the cartilage harvested for grafting as well as the supporting L-strut is also weak, which gradually causes deformation of the grafted cartilage and the supporting L-strut, leading to deprojection and deformation of the tip. Moreover, the size of the harvested septal cartilage must be big enough and not distorted. It will not be effective enough if the harvested cartilage is small and abnormally shaped, which makes it difficult for it to be put in the right position and is likely to cause deviation of the nasal tip. There must be no deviation on the caudal septum that will recieve the extension graft. Better results can be expected using the septal extension graft if the degree of projection of the anterior septal angle and caudal extension of the septum are good.

III. Types of Septal Extension Grafts

Byrd, et al. categorized septal extension graft into three types: paired spreader, paired batten, and direct extension grafts. However, aside from these three types, grafts can be modified into various types according to surgical purpose, or according to the shape or size of the harvested graft.

1. Extended Spreader Graft Type

This is a type of spreader graft in which the graft is linearly extended towards the nasal tip along the dorsal septum, primarily used for extension of the nasal length and derotation of the nasal tip. Following a straight line extended along the dorsal septum, the middle crus or medial crus of the lower lateral cartilages can be found. If the surgical purpose is tip projection, it must be modified in such a way that the end of the graft is turned little bit upward and bends anteriorly above the extension line of dorsal septum. The location, length, and angle of the curve varies according to the desired shape of the nasal tip *(Figure 6)*.

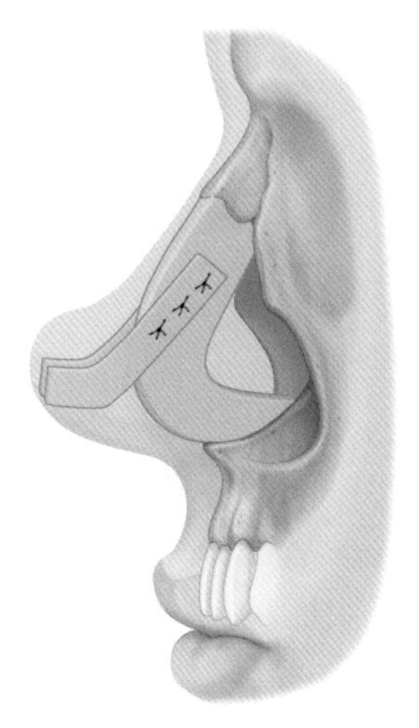

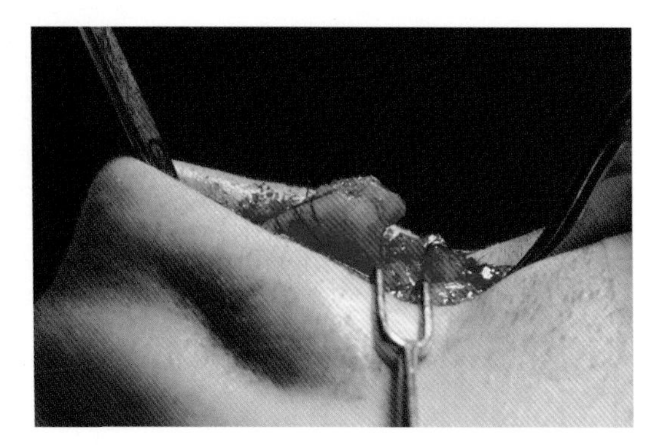

Figure 6 Septal extension graft of extended spreader graft type.

This extended spreader graft type has relatively little intranasal projection as the overlap with the nasal septum is located along the dorsal septum. However, using thick cartilage such as costal cartilage may cause nasal obstruction due to intranasal projection of the graft. This type of graft can provide strong support as the pressure on the graft is disturbed along the whole length on the dorsal septum with relatively lower possibility of bending and buckling, instead of exerting pressure on the caudal septum that is thin and weak.

2. Batten Type

A batten type septal extension graft is located diagonally across the remaining nasal septum towards the nasal tip, adjusting tip projection and rotation *(Figure 7)*. This type can obtain considerable tip projection when the extension graft is overlapped enough with the septal cartilage. If there is not enough overlap with the septal cartilage, the stability of the graft decreases. If it is fixed in a small overlapping area around the relatively thin anterior septal angle, there is an increased possibility of bending or buckling of the septal cartilage. Furthermore, less overlapping combined with longer extension increases the chance of distortion. Therefore, in order to gain enough stability, the batten type is best positioned and fixed to the posterior part of the relatively thick septal cartilage. This batten type septal extension graft is more likely to cause nasal obstruction due to the intranasal projection of the posterior part. Therefore, it is necessary to trim the graft meticulously around the overlapping area after it is fixed on the septum. The paired batten type septal extension grafts can be implanted so that they face each other on both sides of the septal cartilage.

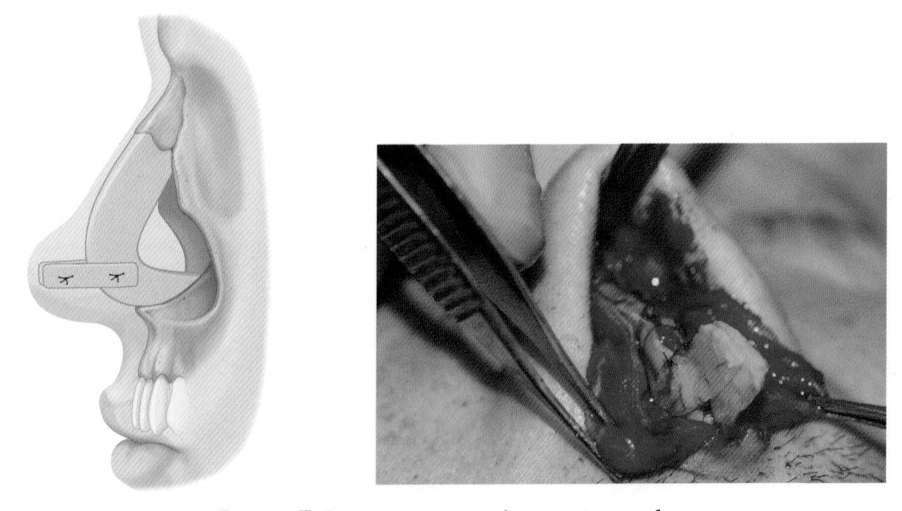

Figure 7 Batten type septal extension graft.

3. Spreader-Batten Type

This type of septal extension graft is a combination of an extended spreader graft on one side and a batten type septal extension graft on the other *(Figure 8)*. Here, the pressure placed on the graft can be distributed in two directions of the septal cartilage, resulting in stable fixation with the use of relatively smaller grafts. It is also advantageous in that it can adjust the degree of the nasal extension and tip projection by modifying the length and direction of the grafts on both sides.

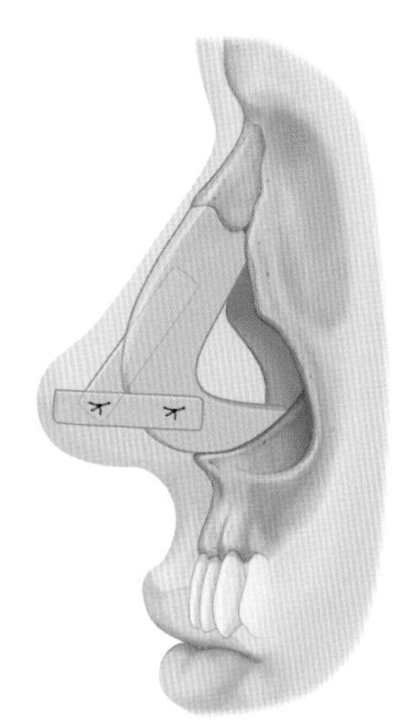

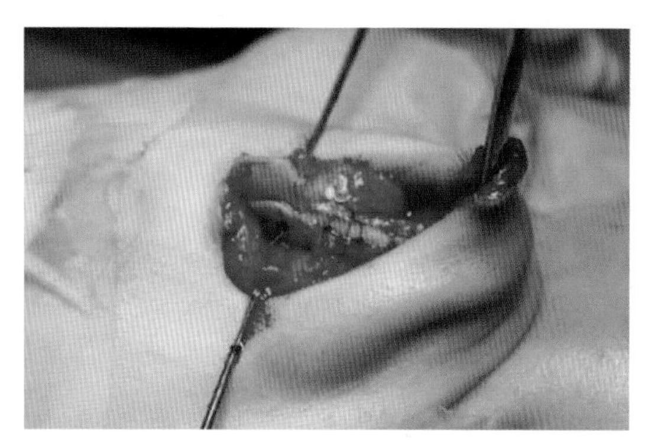

Figure 8 Spreader-batten combination.

4. Caudal Extension Type

In this type, the graft is overlapped and fixed over the entire caudal septum; thus, the caudal border of the septum is extended caudally *(Figure 9)*. This septal extension graft type is useful in correcting the retracted columella and acute nasolabial angle. Moreover, it is effective in increasing the nasal length and improving tip support. If the main purpose of this graft is to correct the nasolabial angle, the graft must be designed so that the basal part is more projected; if the main purpose is to extend the nasal length, it must be designed so that the anterior part is more projected. Large grafts are needed to simultaneously correct the retracted columella and underprojected tip. This grafting technique requires extreme care as the graft can be easily bent by skin tension, and may cause complications such as columellar deformation or intranasal projection, causing nasal obstruction.

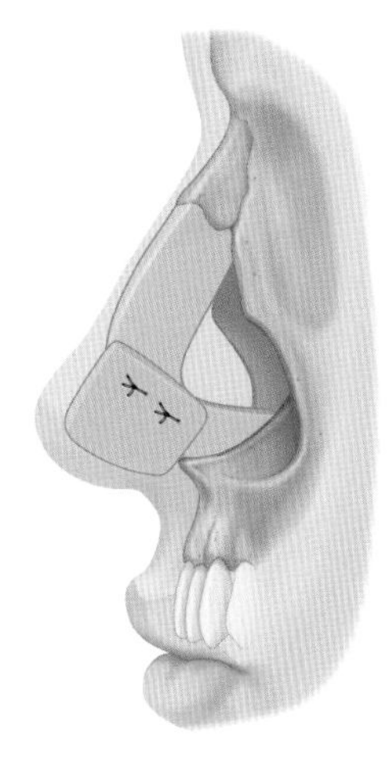

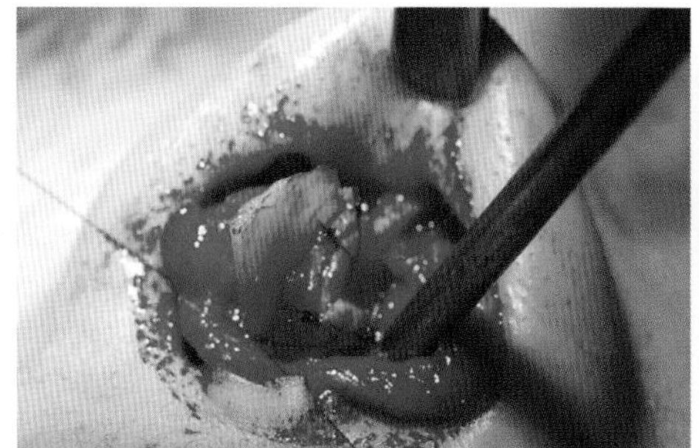

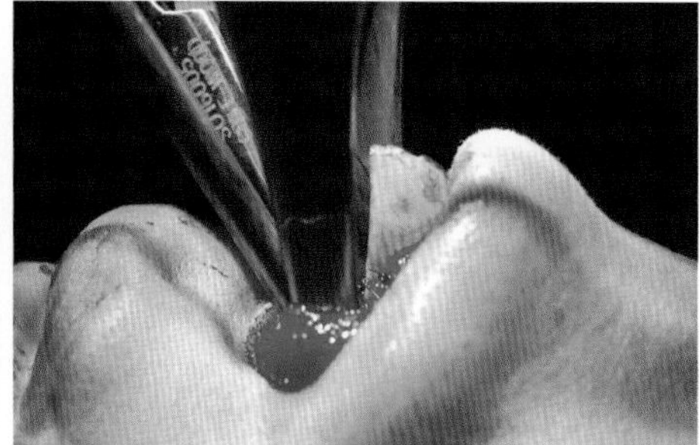

Figure 9 Septal extension graft of caudal extension type.

5. Anterior Extension Type

This type fixes the graft on the anterior part of the nasal septal L-strut closer to the nasal tip with the intention of greatly increasing tip projection *(Figure 10)*. This graft should be secured with a wide overlapping area with the remaining septal cartilage. The part that is projected higher than dorsal septum may cause supratip fullness; thus, it is better to be mindful to prevent this unwanted effect. Moreover, it is also necessary to closely examine the extended part towards the columella, and remove excess graft in that area to minimize asymmetry, distortion, and deformation of the columella.

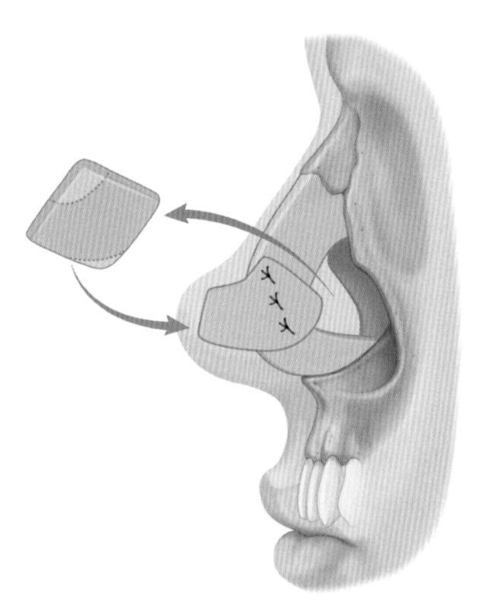

Figure 10 Septal extension graft of anterior extension type.

This grafting technique can result in considerable tip projection similar to the extended spreader type. This graft type requires extreme care in terms of stability as it exerts greater pressure on the caudal septum if greater tip projection effect is intended. It is better to have the graft overlapped on the posterior part of thicker nasal septum.

6. End-to-End Anastomosis Type

In this type, the septal extension graft is sutured to the caudal end of the L-strut in an end-to end fashion instead of overlapping *(Figure 11A)*. Using this technique, the direct tip projection effect is not that good, but this technique reinforces tip support by stabilizing the medial crura of alar cartilages and the membranous septum. If properly placed at the midline, this technique does not cause columellar asymmetry, and also does not exert undue tension to the overlying tip skin, or pressure on the remaining septal cartilage. Therefore, it is less likely to cause weakening and distortion of the septal cartilage in the long run. The main purpose of this type is to provide a stable foundation for additional control of tip projection using tip grafts such as onlay grafting. It is also effective in columellar advancement and nasolabial angle correction. To fix the graft to the caudal septum, "figure of 8" sutures using non-absorbable suture material is used. This graft can further be reinforced with transmucosal sutures using absorbable suture material. For stronger fixation, it can also be occasionally used together with an extended spreader graft or batten graft *(Figure 11B)*.

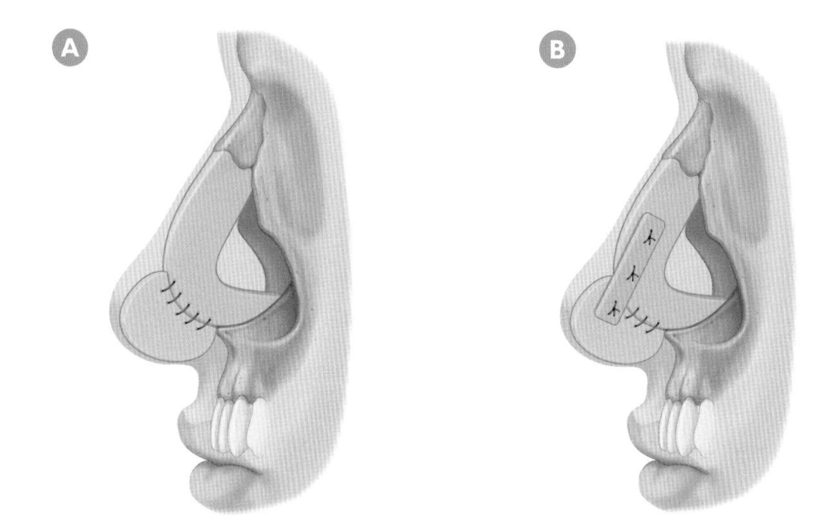

Figure 11 End-to-End anastomosis type (A) and end-to-end anastomosis type combined with extended spreader graft (B).

IV. Surgical Procedures of Septal Extension Grafting

1. Septal Cartilage Harvesting

In general, septal cartilage is harvested preserving at least 1 cm of dorsal strut and 1 cm caudal strut. Some argue that the width of the remaining L-strut must be over 1.5 cm, but others argue that 7-8 mm is enough. Therefore, 1 cm is not the absolute standard, and requires adjustment as the thickness and size of the septal cartilage varies among patients. Asians, especially women, tend to have extremely thin septal cartilage; in this case it is safer to leave as much width as possible, and it is best not to perform septal extension grafting if the septal cartilage will not permit it. If septal extension grafting is planned, the load exerted on the remaining septal cartilage must be considered. It is advisable to harvest the graft with bigger remaining cartilage at the areas that greatly affect the structural stability of the nose, such as the bone-cartilage junction near the keystone area, corner of the L-strut, and the region in which the caudal strut meets the maxillary crest *(Figure 12)*.

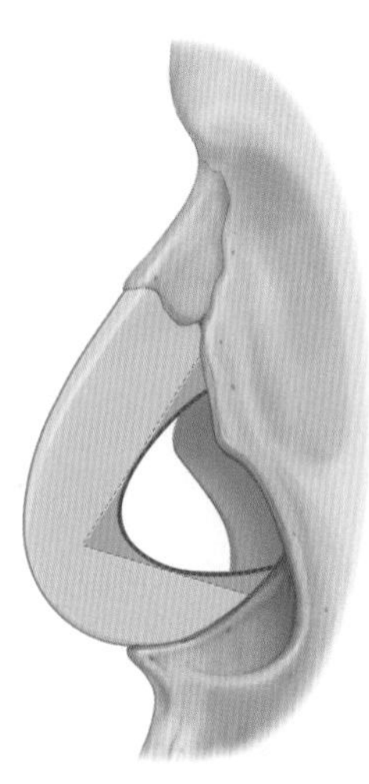

Figure 12 It helps to harvest the cartilage by leaving a little more cartilage in the areas that greatly affect structural stability.

Another thing to consider in harvesting septal cartilage is that patients with weak tip support, thick soft tissue at the nasal tip, and columellar retraction generally require bigger grafts to gain a greater degree of tip projection. However, these patients tend to have smaller and weaker septal cartilage. Therefore, it is better to harvest the septal cartilage as conservatively and safely as possible rather than weaken the nasal septum that is already small and weak. Furthermore, it is more effective and safer to consider additional surgical procedures such as tip grafting using conchal cartilage, rather than relying only on the septal extension graft. When harvesting the septal cartilage, the bony septum can be taken together with the cartilage. This bone graft can be used to reinforce the remaining L-strut.

2. Alignment of Grafts

Verifying precise alignment is important before fixing the septal extension graft to the septal cartilage. It is important to locate the septal extension graft at the midline, while adequately aligning it with the nasal dorsum and nasal tip along the ideal line. To fix the septal extension graft in the ideal position, the thickness of each part of the graft, location of the caudal septum, curvatu re of the septal cartilage and graft, and degree of overlap in the anterior-posterior and cephalo-caudal directions must be considered. It is necessary to attempt combinations of various directions, depths, and overlap configurations of sides before selecting the most appropriate combination.

If the septal extension graft is not located at the proper position, tip deviation is likely to occur *(Figure 13)*. Moreover, it increases the possibility of nasal obstruction owing to the intranasal projection of the graft. The size of overlap between the septal extension graft and septal cartilage is also an important matter to consider. If the area overlapped is small and is relatively slender, the stability of the septal extension graft decreases, and it is more likely to be distorted. On the other hand, if the area overlapped is wide, the stability increases but it is more likely to cause nasal obstruction, making it difficult to obtain intended degree of septal extension. Moreover, if the graft is implanted on the posterior part too close to the anterior nasal spine or maxillary crest, the anterior-posterior movement of the graft is extremely limited. If the extension graft is too small, it may be difficult to get the intended effect; on the contrary, if it is too big relative to the bearing capacity of caudal septum, the strength and bearing capacity of caudal septum is overwhelmed by the increased tension of the nasal tip, deviating and distorting the entire septum-graft complex *(Figure 14)*.

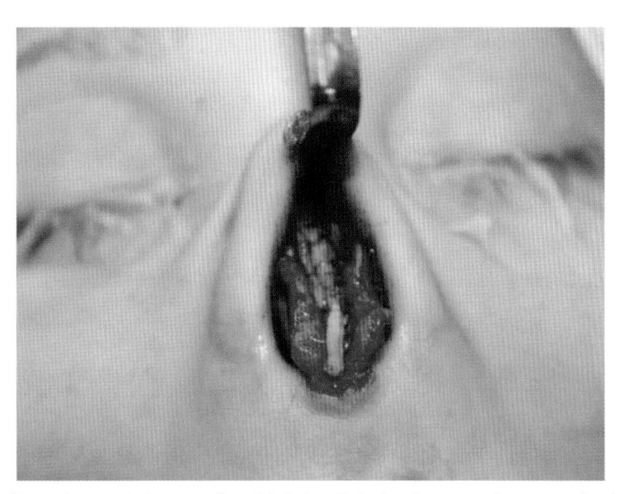

Figure 13 Septal extension graft which is slightly distorted towards the right side.

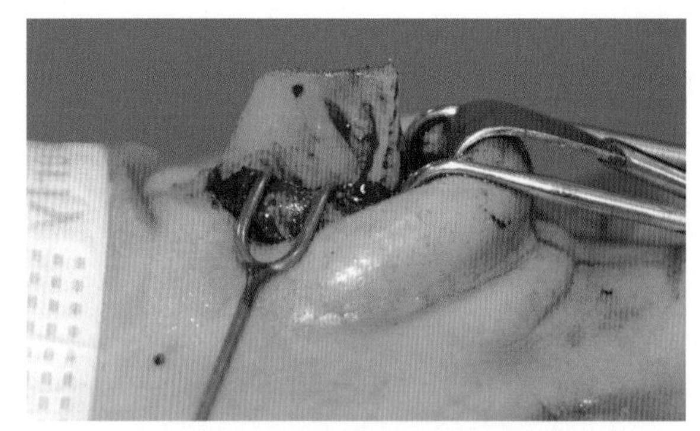

Figure 14 Overly large septal extension graft.

Toriumi, et al. stated that, in order to build the ideal supratip shape, patients with thick skin require the gap of 8-10 mm while those with thin skin require 6-8 mm between the domes of alar cartilages and the anterior septal angle. Asians have relatively low projection of the anterior septal angle and mostly require sufficient projection of at least 8 mm to get an ideal profile. If too much tip projection is achieved by the septal extension graft, a supratip depression may occur. This problem can be solved by implanting a supratip onlay graft or performing dorsal augmentation simultaneously.

3. Fixation between the Septal Cartilage and Extension Graft

5-0 Nylon or 5-0 PDS are used to fix the septal extension graft to the septal cartilage. 3-4 stitches are usually enough, but a locking suture is occasionally required at the transitional area of dorsal septum and caudal septum in order to prevent rotation of the graft in an antero-caudal direction. After suturing, the surgeon must gently press the graft with a finger to test the strength of the fixation. It is better to trim or remove parts of the graft that are not useful for fixation and may cause nasal obstruction.

4. Fixation between the Septal Extension Graft and the Alar Cartilages

When fixing the septal extension graft to the alar cartilages, the graft is generally fixed to the domal segments of both sides of the middle crura. If this fixation suture goes down to the level of the medial crura, the width of columella becomes narrower, and the possibility of columellar deformation increases. Thus, it is desirable to fix the graft on the middle crura or above the middle crura. The caudal end of the septal extension graft is usually connected to the caudal border on both sides of the alar cartilages, but it can also be connected to the cephalic border or the middle part of the alar cartilages if needed. 1 or 2 buried sutures using non-absorbable suture, material such as 5-0 Nylon are usually enough for proper fixation. Using absorbable suture such as 4-0 Vicryl at the membranous septum to further fix the graft will result in stronger fixation and can remove dead space. However, transmembranous sutures can cause inflammation, and thus must be observed with great care in the postoperative follow up. After fixing the alar cartilages, the excess cartilage projecting towards the supratip or columella must be trimmed *(Figure 15).*

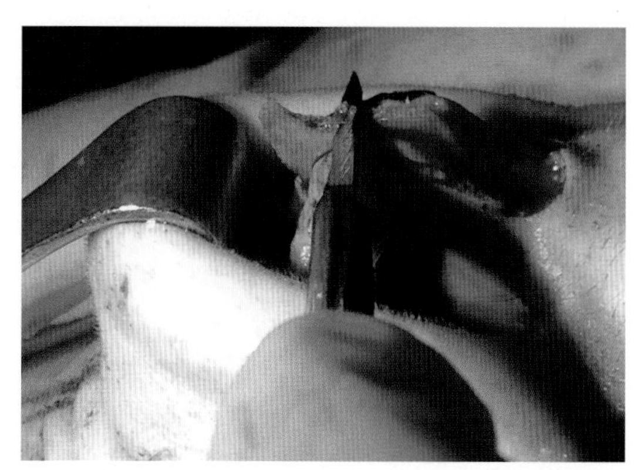

Figure 15 The process of trimming excess cartilage after fixing septal extension graft.

V. Limitations and Complications of Septal Extension Grafting

While the septal extension graft has many advantages, it also has numerous limitations. This graft frequently creates supratip projection, which may be due to excess projection of the graft's anterior part towards the supratip. It is necessary to remove the extra part if seen. On the other hand, a relative supratip depression may occur as a result of improved tip projection. The most critical disadvantage of the septal extension graft is that this does not change the fundamental form of the alar cartilages while changing the dimension of the alar cartilages. Therefore, fine adjustments on the definition of the nasal tip or tip-lobule relationship must be achieved by additional tip grafting procedures. Other than the limitations mentioned, septal extension grafting may be associated with the following complications.

1. Stiffness of the Nasal Tip

Some forms of septal extension grafts can replace the membranous septum with rigid cartilage, thus abolishing the membranous septum. If membranous septum is lost, the patients will lose mobility of the nasal tip, and thus may feel uncomfortable.

2. Nasal Obstruction

Another common problem in septal extension grafting is that the graft can be projected towards one side of the nasal cavity, causing nasal obstruction or asymmetry of the nostrils. These problems may occur if the overlapping parts of the graft are not trimmed adequately. Furthermore, the graft can also be projected toward one side of the nasal cavity if the graft is too thick, there is preexisting caudal septal deviation, the fixation is loosened, or if there is septal buckling.

3. Septal Buckling

Buckling is one of the most common complications of septal extension grafting. This occurs when a heavy load exceeding the capacity that the caudal septum can support is exerted on the caudal septum, causing the cartilage to bend or be distorted *(Figure 16)*. Septal buckling presents with several aesthetic and functional issues including deviation of the columella and nasal tip, nostril asymmetry, short nose deformity, and nasal obstruction *(Figure 17)*. This complication is likely to occur if excessive tip projection was intended using a septal extension graft. It is especially more likely to occur if the caudal septum is thin and weak, or if there is caudal septal deviation. If there is a preexisting caudal septal deviation, the surgeon must fix the graft on the most stable location on which the end of the graft will not easily bend towards one side maintaining a midline location. However, if a procedure to weaken caudal septal cartilage is necessary to correct a caudal septal deviation, it is better not to use the septal extension graft for tip projection purposes. If septal buckling occurs, the graft must be removed, and the alar cartilages should be realigned to the proper position by revision surgery.

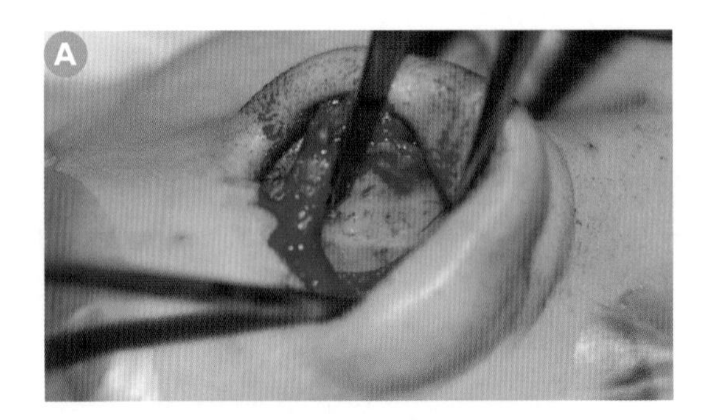

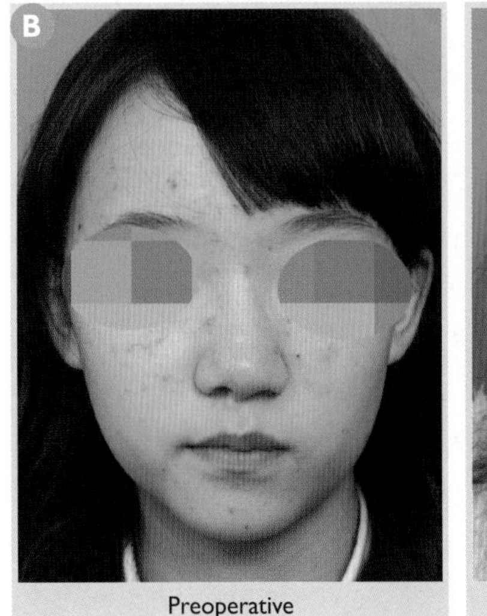

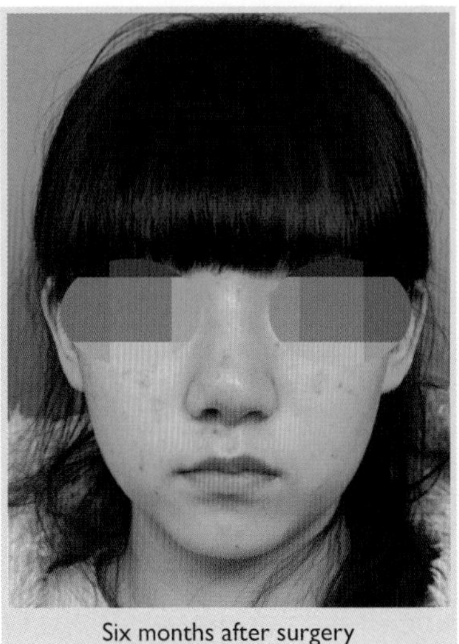

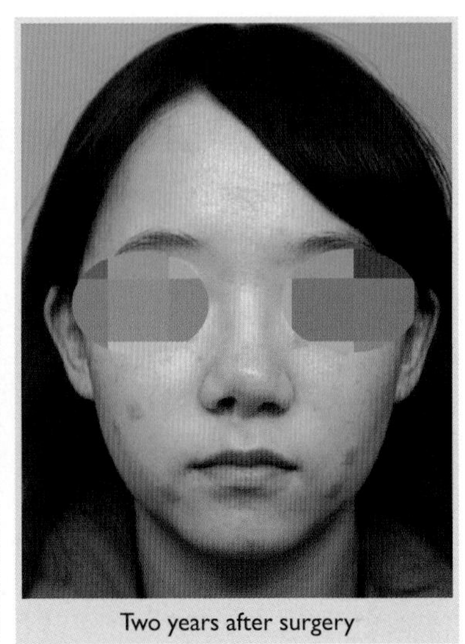

Figure 16 Septal buckling (A). This patient underwent septal extension grafting and showed no problems until 6 months after surgery. Two years later, the patient developed nostril deformity (B).

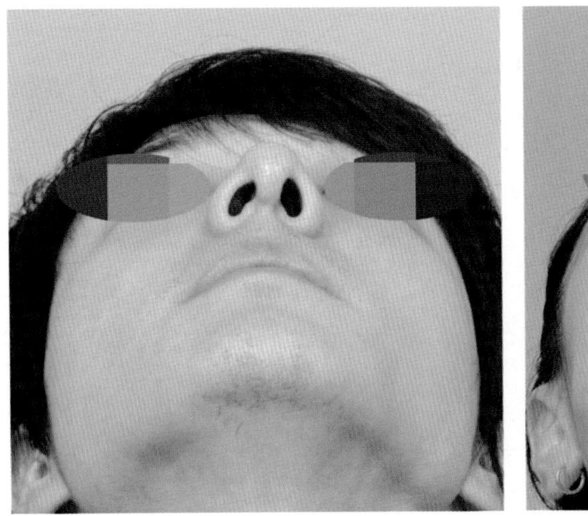
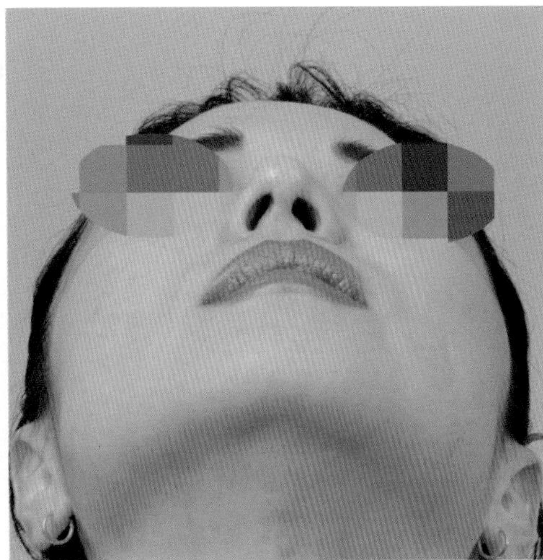

Figure 17 Septal buckling as a complication of septal extension grafting.

4. Deprojection and Rotation of the Nasal Tip

Several months or years after septal extension grafting, the tip projection that was initially achieved by septal extension grafting may be lost, or the tip may show cephalic rotation. This is mostly due to the deformation, weakening or atrophy of the septal cartilage or the septal extension graft itself. Another cause may be the loosening of the sutures, and pressure or ischemic necrosis of the cartilage *(Figures 18, 19).*

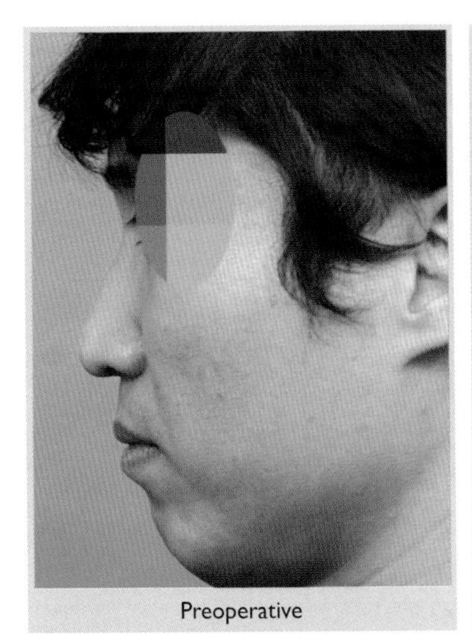

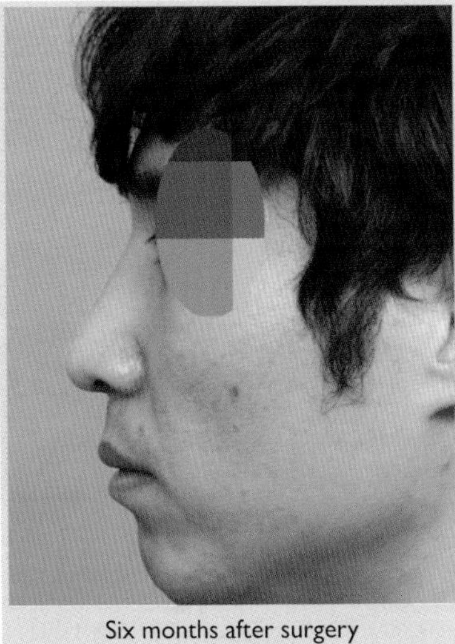

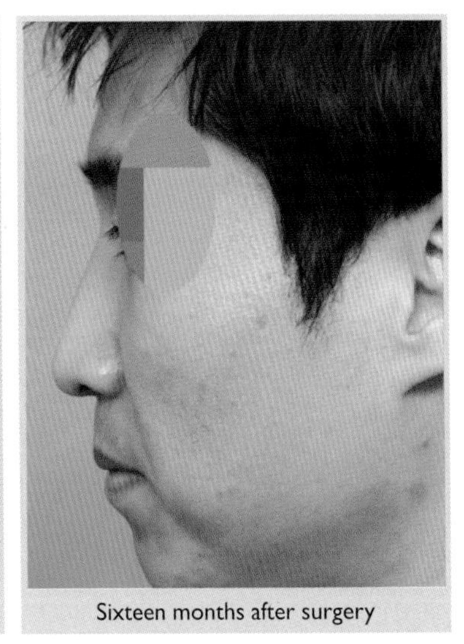

Figure 18 This patient showed good tip projection until 6 months after septal extension grafting. The patient showed signs of reduced tip projection 16 months after surgery.

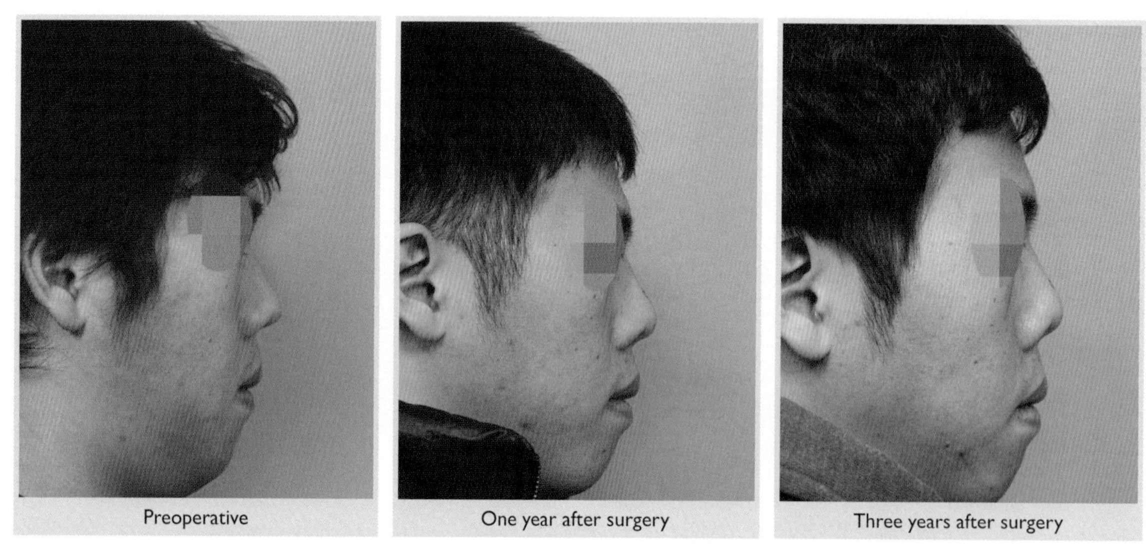

Figure 19 This patient underwent septal extension grafting and showed no problems until 6 months after surgery. Three years later, the patient showed a short nose deformity.

VI. Other Precautions for Septal Extension Grafting

If there is a need for a substantial degree of nasal tip projection or nasal length extension which can exert excessive tension on the tip skin, it may be necessary to perform wide dissection of the area surrounding the alar cartilages to reduce tension on the nasal skin. This can be done by adequately extending the marginal incision laterally and dissecting the fibrous connections between the pyriform aperture and the alar cartilages. Moreover, it may be necessary to dissect the scroll area between upper lateral and alar cartilages. Occasionally, dissection of the middle crus and medial crus from the vestibular skin may be helpful. In many cases, the septal extension graft is fixed on one side of septal cartilage, but it needs to be fixed on both sides to increase the stability of the graft. In conclusion, septal extension grafting is one of the most important surgical techniques to be mastered in rhinoplasty for Asians. However, as much as it is effective, the complications and risks are also not uncommon.

References

1. Byrd HS, Andochick S, Copit S, Walton KG. Septal extension grafts: a method of controlling tip projection shape. Plast Reconstr Surg 1997; 100: 999-1010.
2. Huang J, Liu Y. A modified technique of septal extension using a septal cartilage graft for short-nose rhinoplasty in Asians. Aesthet Plast Surg 2012; 36: 1028-38.
3. Hwang SH, Hwang K. Supporting strength of septal extension grafts. J Craniofac Surg 2011; 22: 2323-6.
4. Han K, Jeong JW, Kim JH, Son D, Kim S, Park SW, Choi J, Choi TH. Complete septal extension grafts using porous high-density polyethylene sheets for the westernization of the Asian nose. Plast Reconstr Surg 2012; 130: 106e-15e.
5. Koch CA, Friedman O. Modified back-to-back autogenous conchal cartilage graft for caudal septal reconstruction: the medial crural extension graft. Arch Facial Plast Surg 2011; 13: 20-5.
6. Kang JG, Ryu J. Nasal tip surgery using a modified septal extension graft by means of extended marginal incision. Plast Reconstr Surg 2009; 123: 343-52.
7. Seyhan A, Ozden S, Ozaslan U, Sir E. A simplified use of septal extension graft to control nasal tip location. Aesthet Plast Surg 2007; 31: 506-11.
8. Jung DH, Chang GU, Shan L, Liu DL, Wang ZJ, Tian HJ, Chen C, Han WW. Pressure necrosis of septal cartilage associated with bilateral extended spreader grafts in rhinoplasty. Arch Facial Plast Surg 2010; 12: 257-62.
9. Toriumi DM. New concepts in nasal tip contouring. Arch Facial Plast Surg 2006; 8: 156-85.

Case 1

A 23-year-old female visited for a flat nose deformity with nasal deviation.

Analysis
Deviated nose
Low radix
Low dorsum
Poor tip projection
Endoscopy: Septal deviation

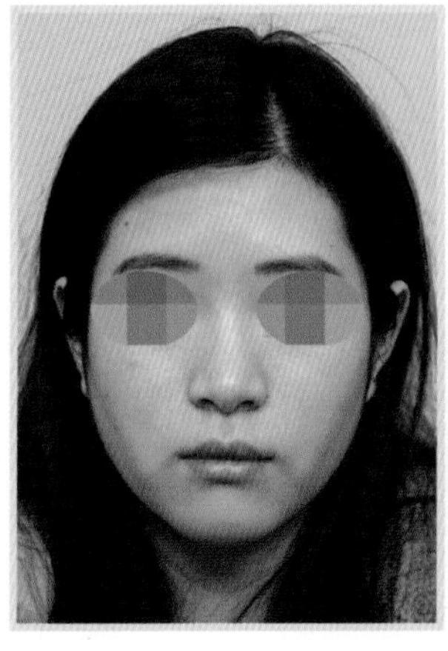
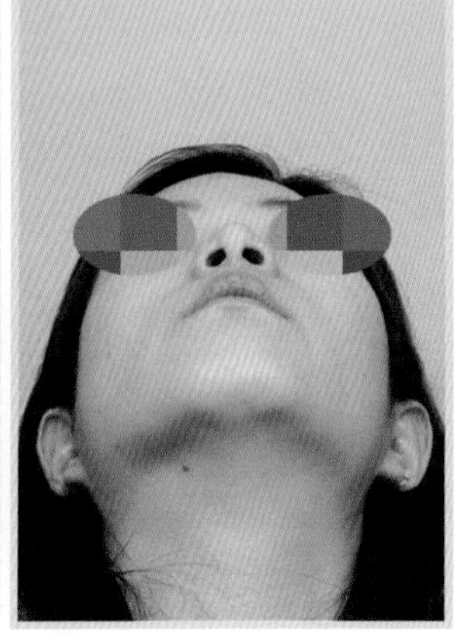
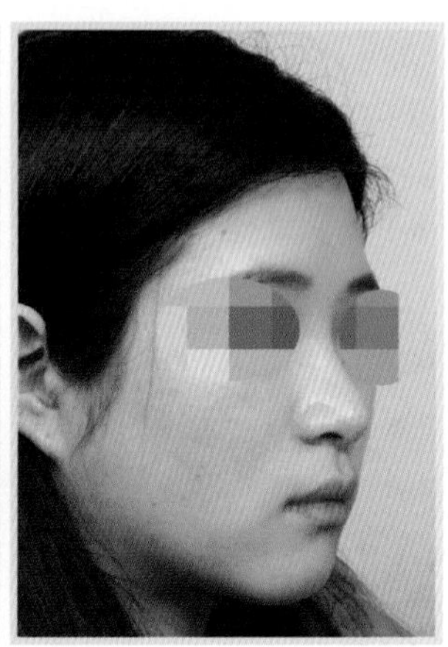

Operative Procedures

Open rhinoplasty approach
Septoplasty and harvest of septal cartilage and bone
Cutting and suture technique for caudal septal correction
Medial and lateral osteotomies
Caudal septal extension grafting using septal cartilage (right)
Spreader grafting (right)
Dorsal augmentation using Gore-Tex

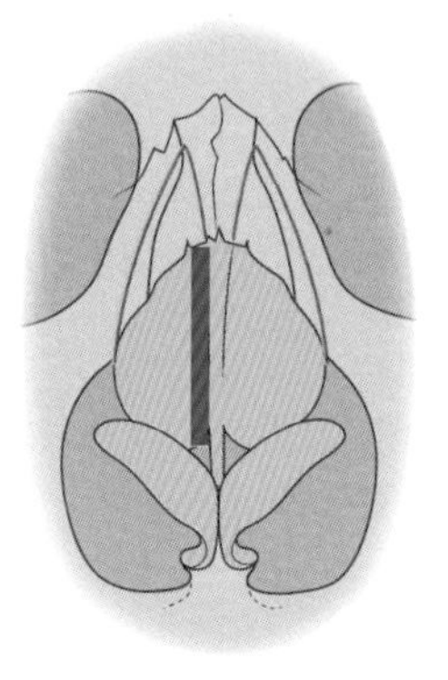
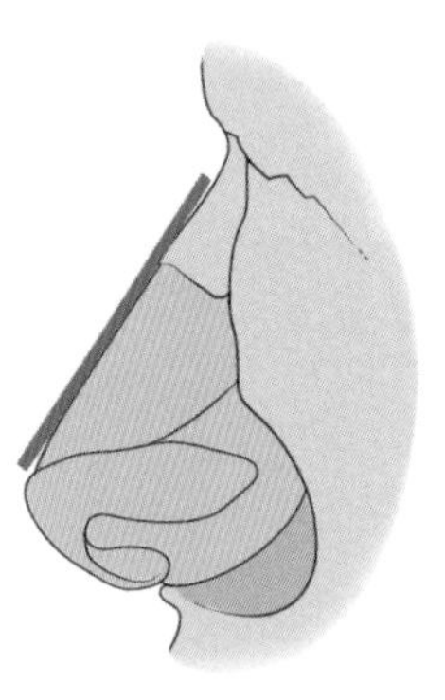
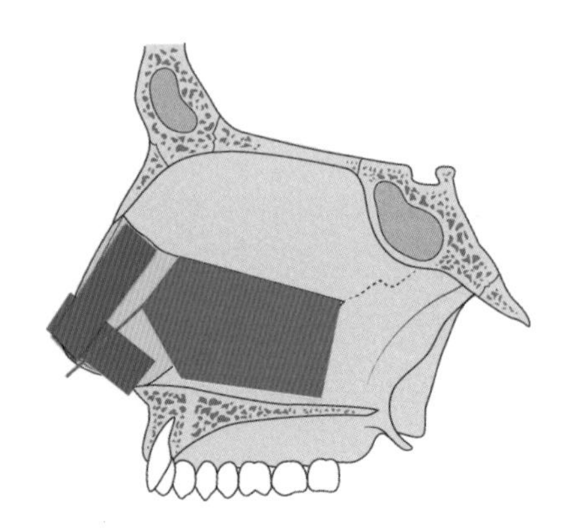

Postoperative Changes

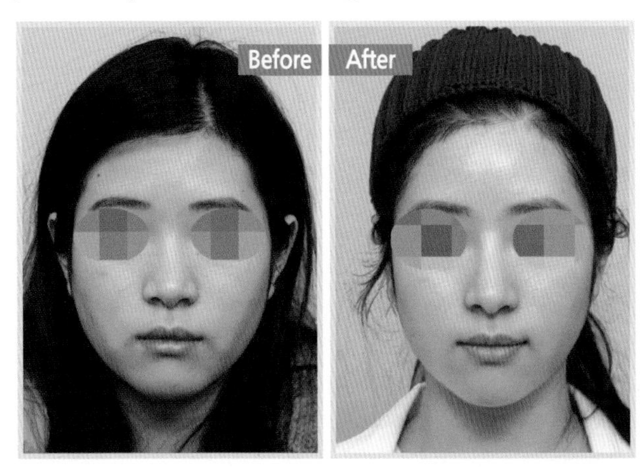

Frontal: Dorsal deviation was corrected. Heights of the dorsum and tip were increased.

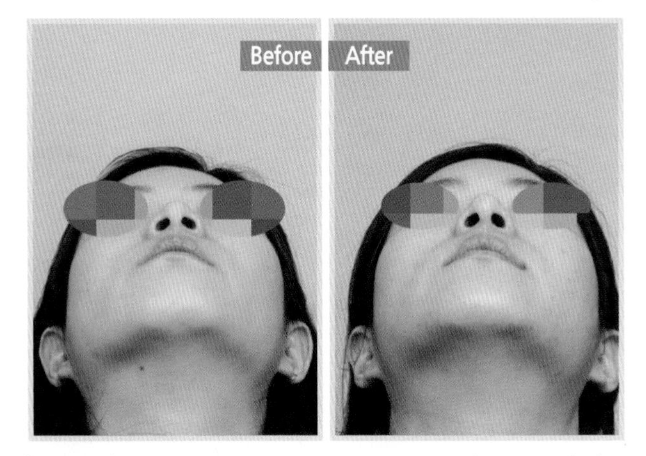

Basal: Tip projection was improved. Nostril shape became more natural.

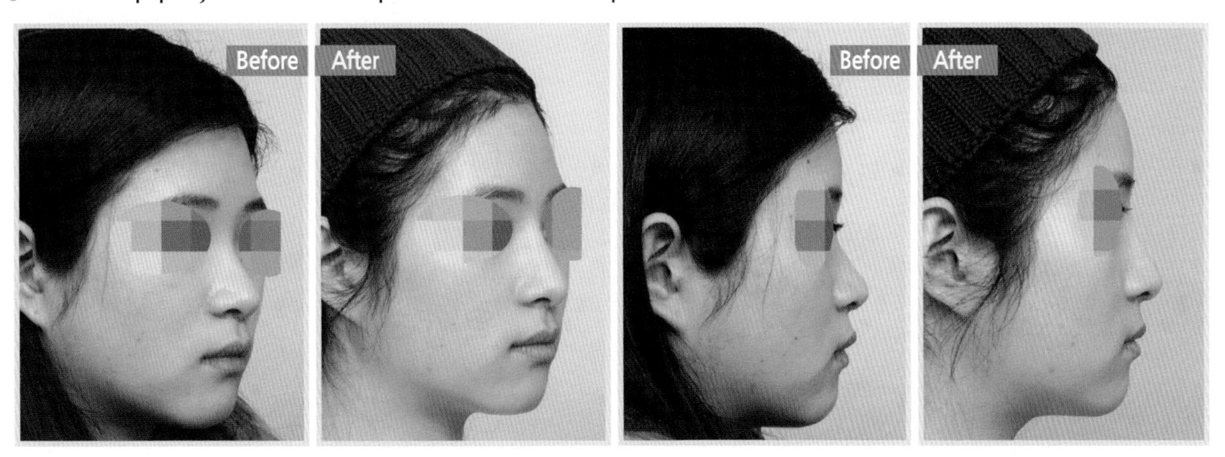

Lateral and Oblique: Radix height was augmented. Tip projection was improved.

Case 2

A 20-year-old female visited for a deviated nose with associated nasal obstruction.

Analysis

Deviated nose
Convex dorsum
Wide columellar-lobular angle
Poor tip projection
Endoscopy: Caudal septal deviation

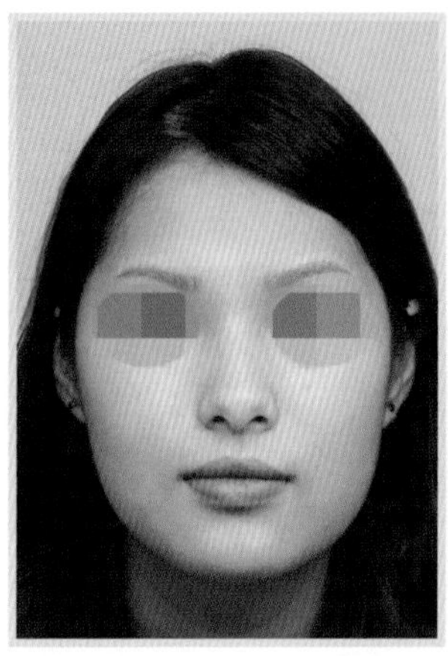 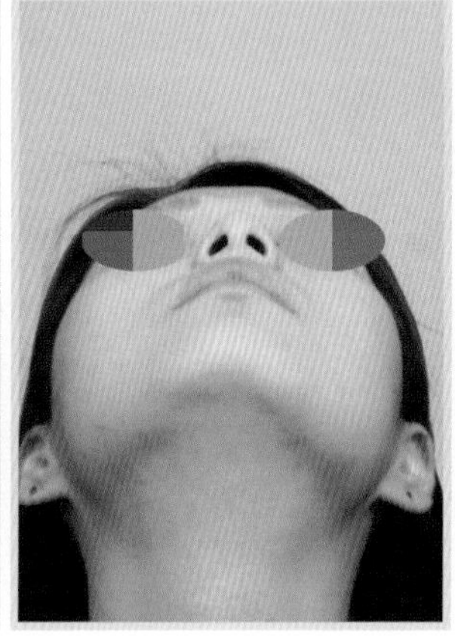 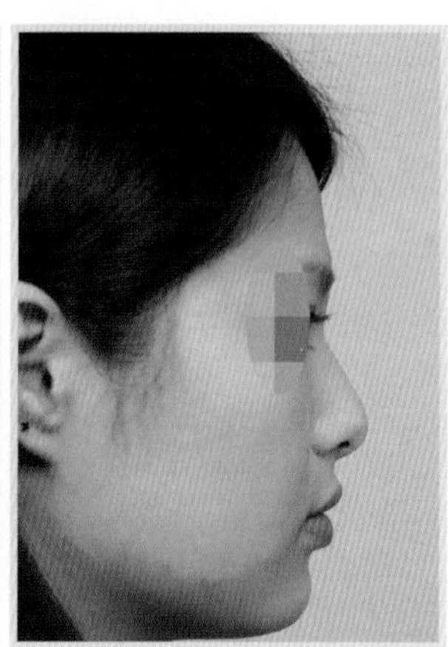

Operative Procedures

Open rhinoplasty approach
Septal and conchal cartilage harvest
Caudal septum repositioning (left to right)
Spreader grafting using septal cartilage (bilateral)
Caudal septal extension grafting using septal cartilage (right)
Medial and lateral osteotomies
Interdomal and transdomal suturing of the alar cartilages
Dorsal augmentation using Gore-Tex
Multilayer tip grafting with backstop using conchal cartilage
Camouflaging of supratip graft using crushed cartilage

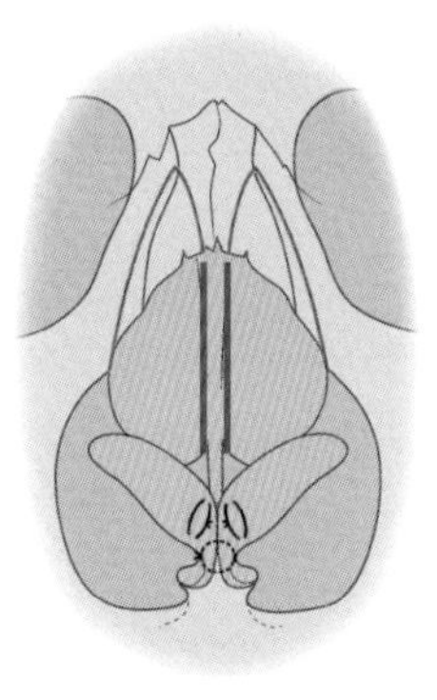 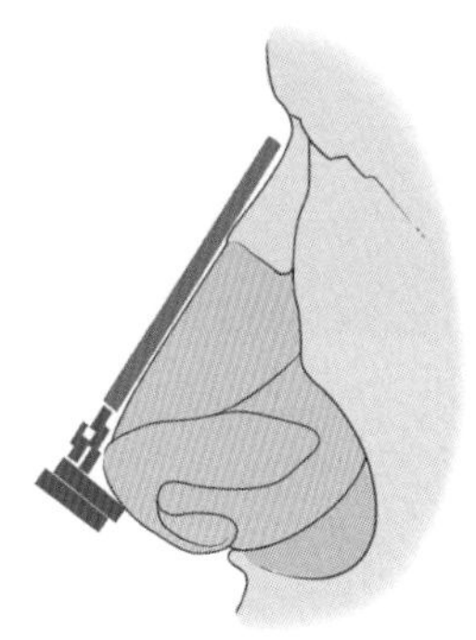 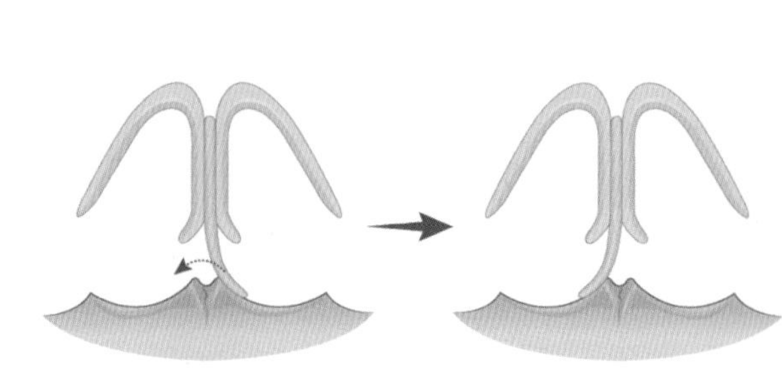

Postoperative Changes

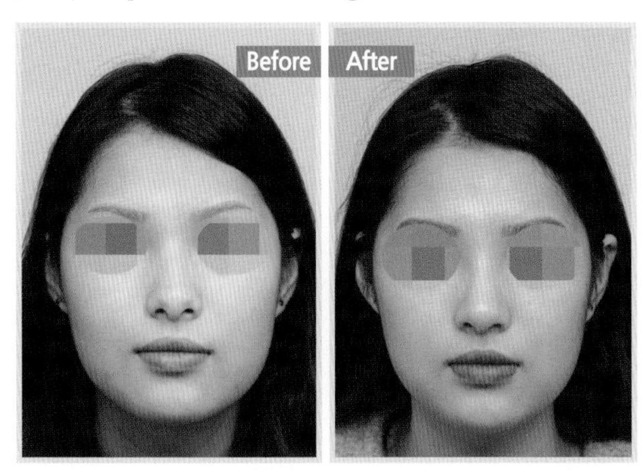

Frontal: Dorsal deviation was corrected. Nostril show was decreased.

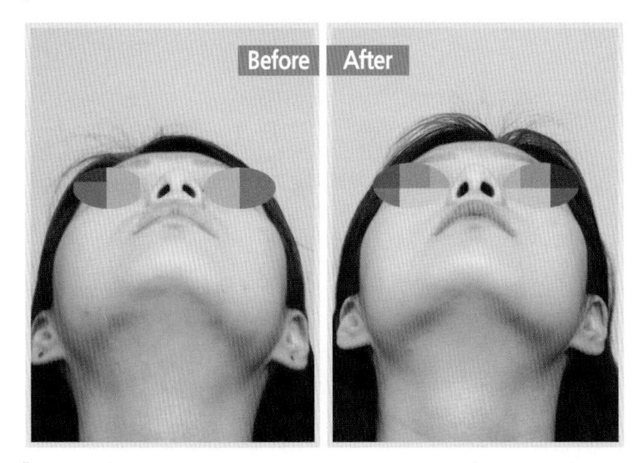

Basal: Tip projection was improved. Nostrils were widened.

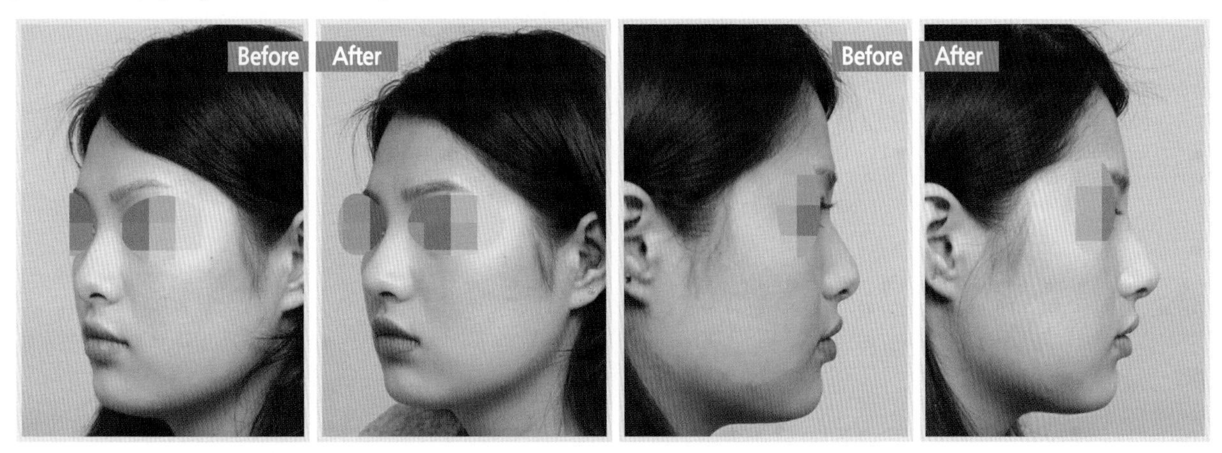

Lateral and Oblique: Dorsal convexity was corrected. Radix height was augmented. Tip projection was improved.

Chapter 24 Alar Base Surgery

Yong Ju Jang

Alar base surgery is a very important supplementary surgical technique, the purpose of which is the construction of a cosmetically balanced nasal base. Most alar base surgeries are performed to reduce the width of the nose, and are known by various terms such as alar base reduction, alar base resection, and alar wedge resection. Whether the alar base surgery is a done on the alar lobule or the nostril sill, it can be classified as either alar wedge excision or a nostril sill excision. Alar base surgery can be classified according to the surgical technique. It can be divided between alar base resection, which resects soft-tissue, and alar cinching suture technique, which utilizes a suture.

I. Anatomy

The nasal base is composed of the alar lobule, alar lobule and cheek junction, alar lobule and upper lip junction, nostril, nostril sill and upper lip junction, and columellar-labial junction *(Figure 1)*. The alar lobule is made up of fibro-areolar tissue of varying density; the skin covering this area is thicker compared to other parts of the nose and has much more sebaceous glands. Furthermore, this area receives abundant blood flow compared to other regions.

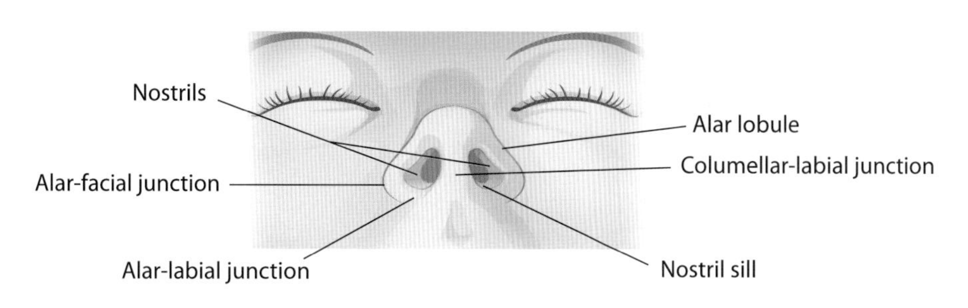

Figure 1 Topographic anatomy of the nasal base.

II. Aesthetic Considerations

Observed from the front, the ideal width of the broadest area of the ala should be equal to that of the width of the eyes or the space between the eyebrows. Also, it is ideal for the width to be about 70% of the distance between the nasion to the tip-defining points. Seen from the basal view, it is recommended that the tip lobule, alar lobule, nostril sill, and the columellar base form an equilateral triangle. It is also desirable that the nostrils maintain an oval shape. In addition, it is better that the width of the tip lobule does not exceed 75% of that of the alar base *(Figure 2)*. However, as the shape of the alar base among Asians varies greatly, it is inappropriate to apply this cosmetic ratio on all patients and establish it as surgical objectives.

When the distance between the ala is excessively wide giving a funnel-like appearance, it is termed as alar flare. The contributing factors of alar flare include excessive subcutaneous fat, thick skin, wide and flat crura, and poor tip support *(Figure 3)*.

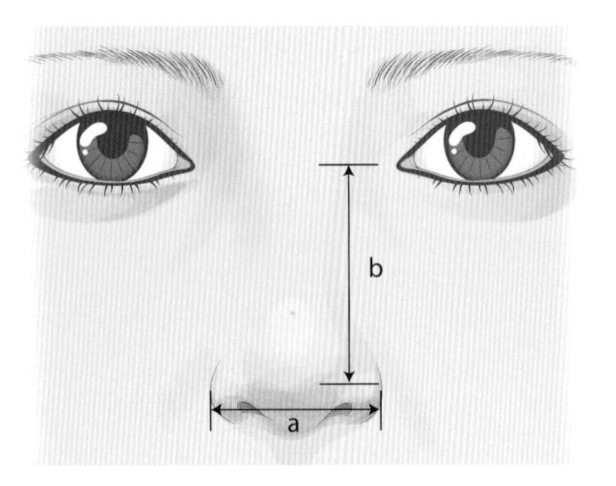

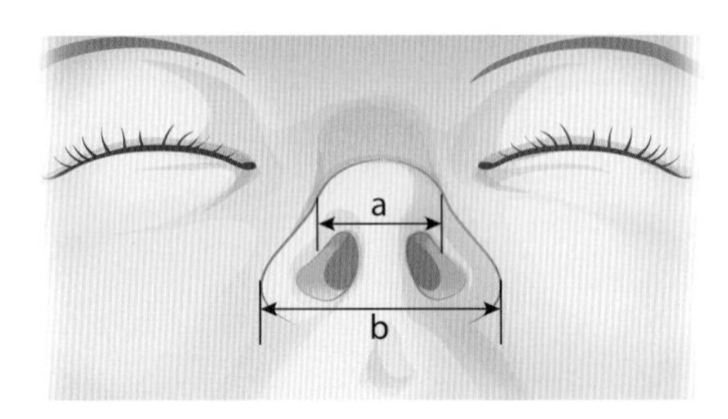

Figure 2 Ideal shape of alar base. Relative to the length of the nose, the ideal width of the alar base is about 70% that of the former (a/b). In the basal view, it is recommended that the width of the tip lobule does not exceed 75% of the alar base.

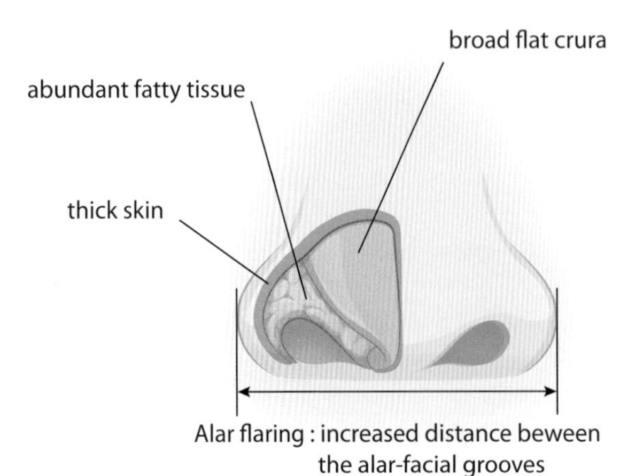

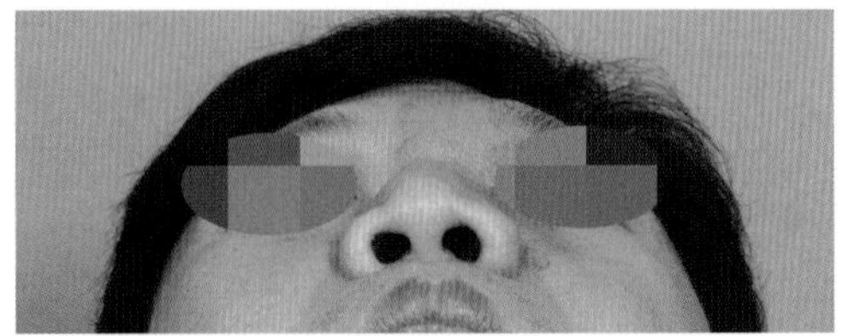

Figure 3 Alar flaring: an increased distance between the alar-facial grooves. The determining factors of alar flare include excessive subcutaneous fat, thick skin, wide and flat crura, and poor tip support.

III. Alar Base Resection

1. The Dynamics of Alar Base Resection

Alar base resection involves three variables: location, shape, and amount. The interaction of these factors is responsible for a variety of changes. Changes following alar base surgery can be expected from the perspective of the horizontal axis and vertical axis. The horizontal axis can be thought of as a line that passes across the nostril sill, and the vertical axis can be presumed to be a line that runs parallel to the columella from the base to the tip. While the horizontal tissue resection of the nostril sill can narrow the nasal base, it can slightly increase the alar flare thereby making the nostrils look more open (because the procedure alters the horizontal axis without changing the vertical axis, it can cause the alar rim to bend further outward). However, if the vertical axis is resected, the alar flare can be reduced but the height of the tip can be slightly lowered *(Figure 4)*. Once the location and shape of the resection is decided upon, another decision must be made on the size of resection to be performed. This matter needs to be approached in a very careful manner. If the surgical result is unsatisfactory due to inadequate resection, it is possible to perform revision surgery. However, in cases of excessive resection, it is extremely difficult to undo. It is therefore recommended that, the extent of resection not exceed 5 mm.

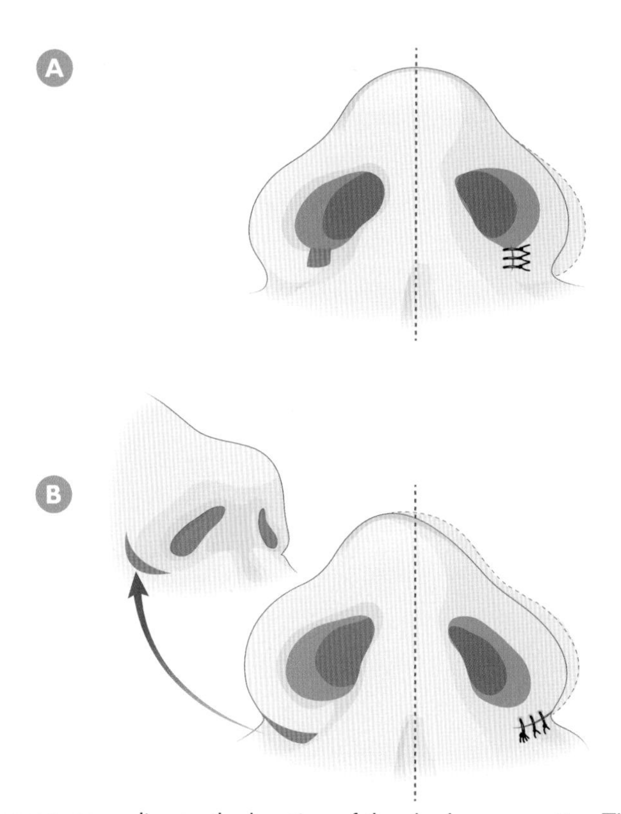

Figure 4 The effect of surgery according to the location of the alar base resection. The resection of the nostril sill can change the shape of the nostril and increase the alar flare (A). If only the lower part of the alar lobule is resected, the alar flare can be reduced but the height of the tip can be lowered slightly (B).

2. Selection and Application of Surgical Technique

On the basis of understanding the above listed dynamics of surgery, we can examine the specific patterns of surgical application. The alteration sought by the surgeon through alar base surgery can vary according to the intrinsic shape of the patient's alar base. Various possible objectives are as follows:

- ☑ Reducing the alar flare
- ☑ Narrowing of the nostril sill
- ☑ Reducing the size of the alar lobule
- ☑ Changing the attachment of the alar lobule
- ☑ Enhancing the harmony between the alar rim and the tip-columella complex

We can simplify the above objectives into three:

- ☑ Alar flare reduction
- ☑ Nostril size reduction
- ☑ Combination of alar flare reduction and nostril size reduction

1) Alar Flare Reduction (Alar Wedge Excision)

When the size of the nostril is close to normal but there is an alar flare, an elliptical wedge resection is recommended. During the resection, a wedge can be removed 2-5 mm in thickness 1 mm above the alar crease. This technique is also termed as alar wedge excision *(Figure 5).*

2) Nostril Size Reduction (Nostril Sill Excision)

In cases where the nostril is wide and the alar flare isn't severe, a sill excision is performed. In this procedure, the resection must be carried out in such a manner that both the ala and vestibular skin are included in the resection. In this case, the wedge is located in a perpendicular direction to the nostril floor in 2-4 mm thickness and must not bent sideways. Moreover, the resected skin must be located at the lateral aspect of the nostril sill *(Figure 6).* In real surgical practice, however, it's not common to perform a nostril sill excision alone. In most cases, a combined sill/alar excision is performed.

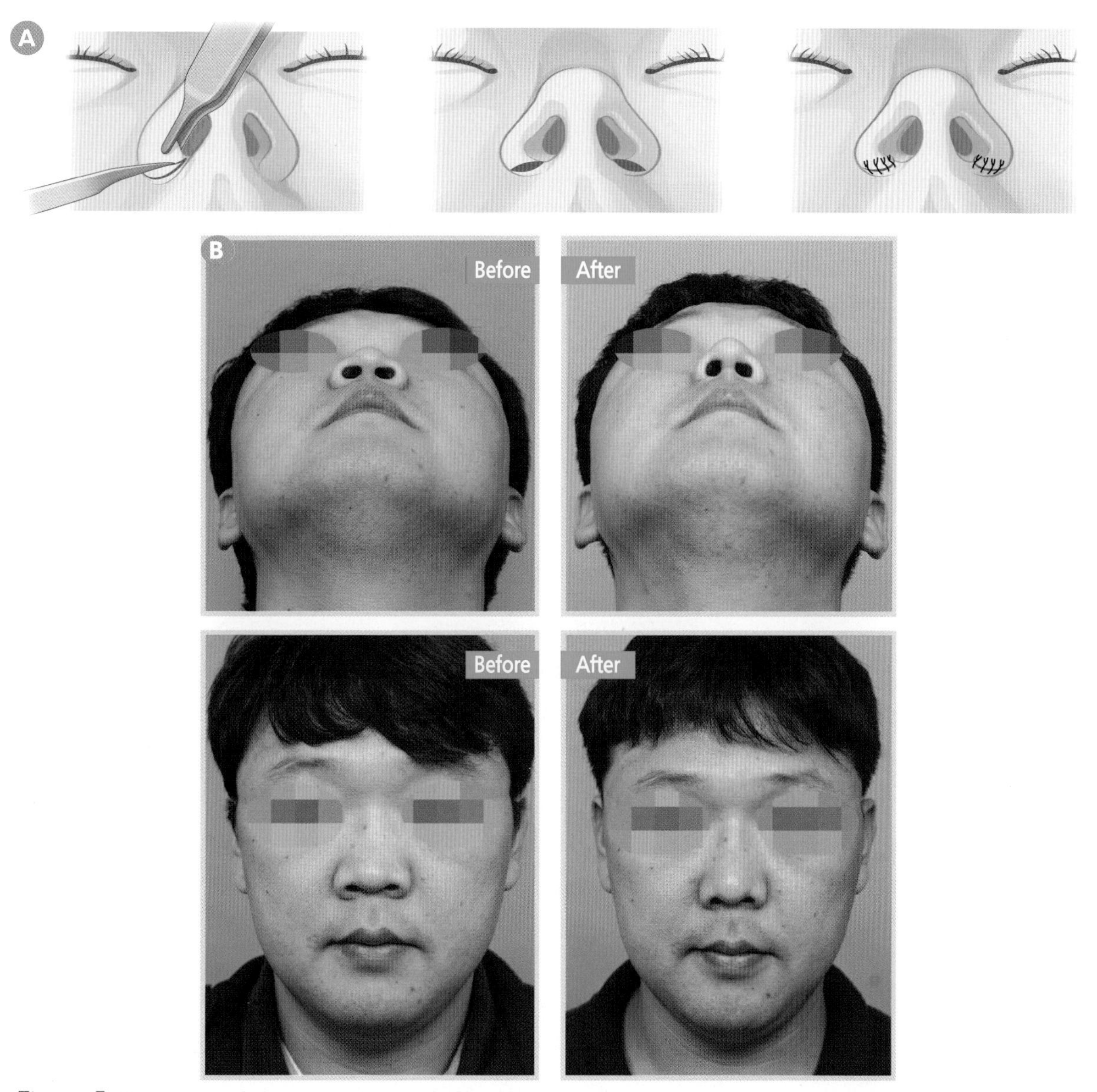

Figure 5 Illustration of alar wedge excision (A) and photographs of a patient who underwent this technique (B).

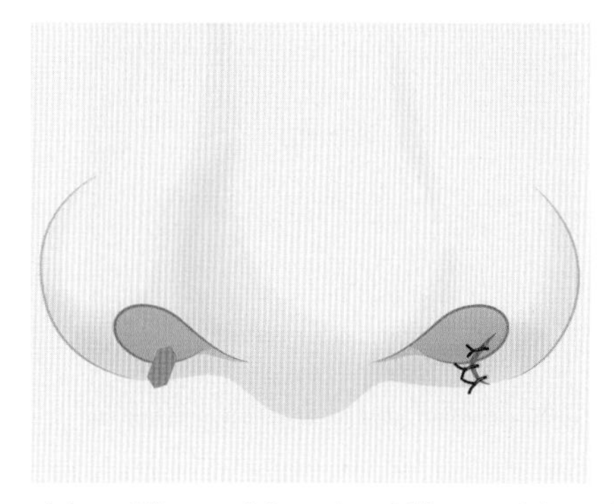

Figure 6 Nostril sill excision. The excision should be positioned as laterally as possible.

3) Combination of Alar Flare Reduction and Nostril Size Reduction (Combined Sill/ Ala Excision)

When the nostril is wide and there is an alar flare, sill excision and alar wedge resection is performed simultaneously. Such a method is also called the combined sill/ala excision *(Figure 7)*. In addition to the methods described above, the shape of the wedge resection can be altered in various different shapes. This technique can also be used to correct asymmetric nostil *(Figure 8)*.

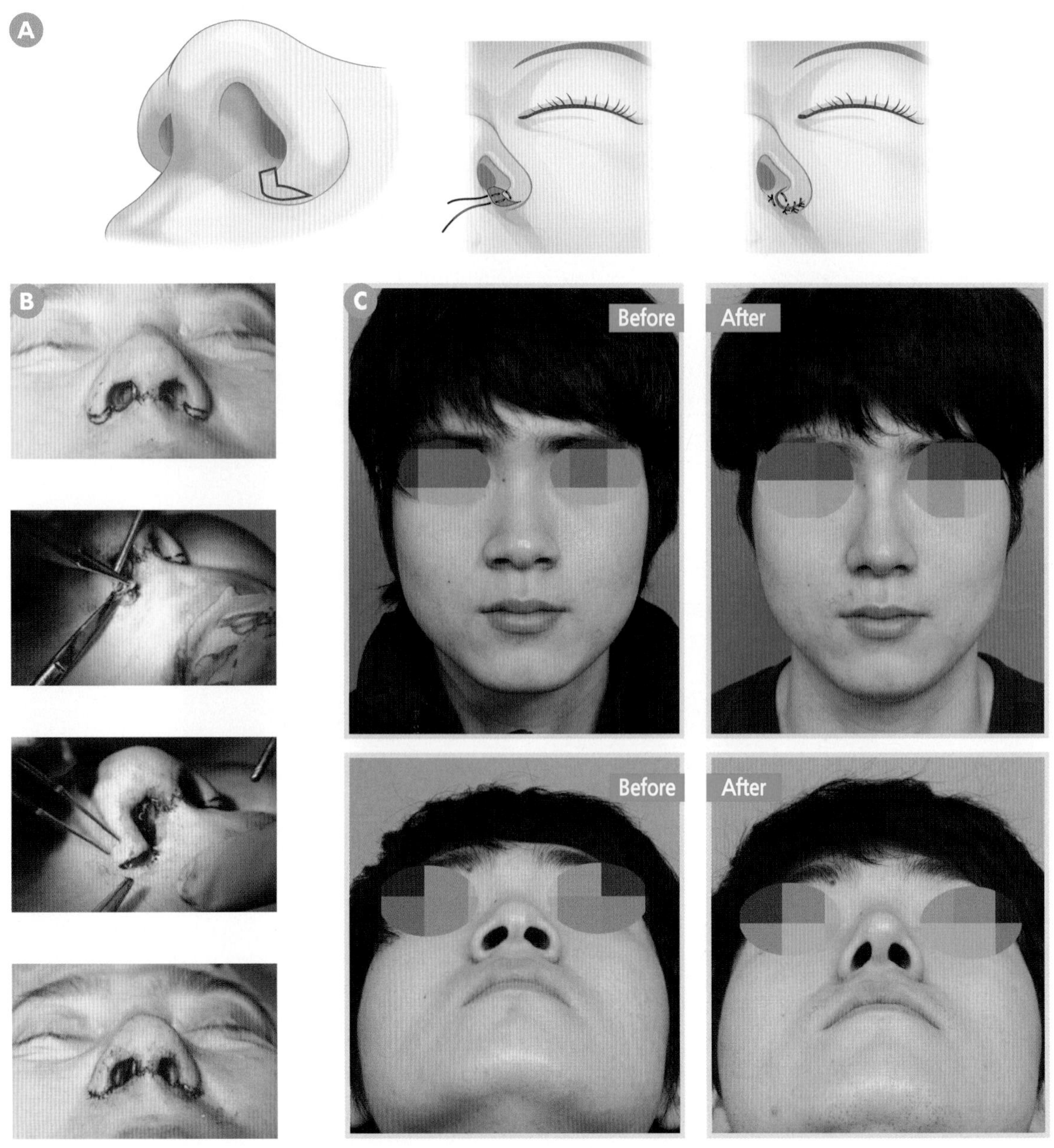

Figure 7 Combined sill/ala excision. Illustration (A), intraoperative photographs (B), and patient who underwent combined sill/ala excision using this technique (C).

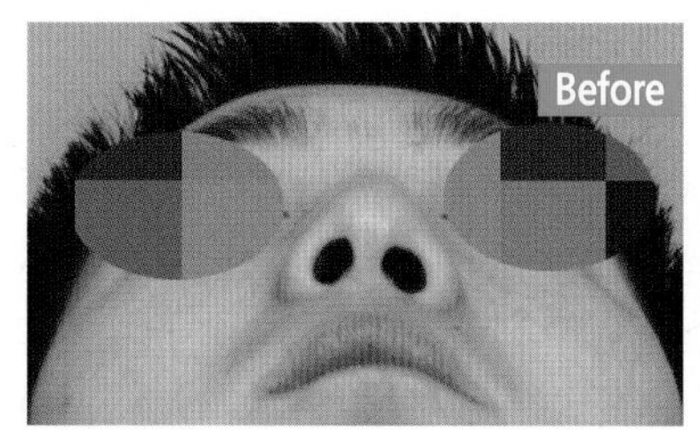

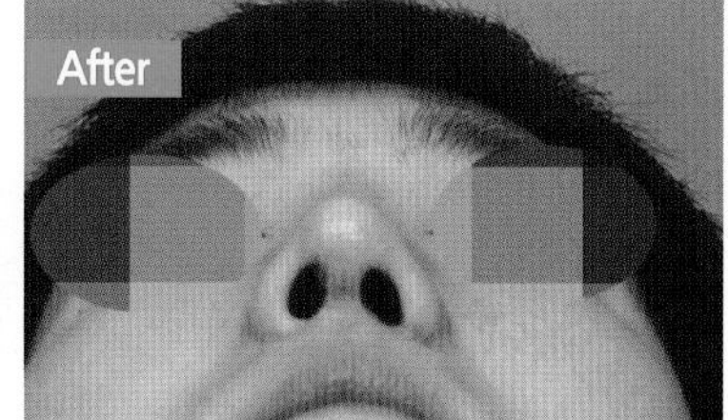

Figure 8 Surgical example of a combined sill/ala excision at left side for correction of nostril asymmetry.

3. The Order of Surgery and Detailed Surgical Techniques

1) Order of Surgery

In most cases, alar base resection is carried out as the final step of rhinoplasty after the tip surgery has been concluded. The reason for this is, if the alar base surgery is performed first and then surgery on the tip or dorsum next, there is a risk of loosening the alar base sutures or unnecessary tension exerted on the alar skin closure wound. More importantly, it is much more ideal to determine the extent of the alar base modification in accordance to the altered tip shape following tip surgery. In rhinoplasty, tip surgery can improve the projection of the tip, and its relation to the nasal base can be transformed into an equilateral triangle. In such cases, even though alar base reduction was included in the initial plan for surgery, the need for such a procedure may disappear as a result of the altered shape of the nasal tip.

2) Surgical Techniques

First, mark the targeted area for resection on the skin, then inject a local vasoconstrictor solution. Because the skin of the ala can be easily bruised or scarred if it is picked up with forceps, the surgeon should hold the alar lobule securely with the fingers and perform resection using a sharp blade. When excising the skin inside the vestibule, giving a slight inclination on the margin of the nostril helps to facilitate tight approximation of the skin while suturing. If the resection of the lower part of the ala is located at the groove of the alar-facial junction, closure of the resected margins can become a little more complicated. Therefore, locate the incision line slightly above it at the lobule area. For closure, use 5-0 Catgut or 6-0 Vicryl® at the vestibular side and a 6-0 Nylon on the skin of the ala. Suturing must be performed very carefully, and even after removal of the stitches, it is a good idea to apply Steri-Strips. The vestibular skin need not be over-meticulously sutured; this has the effect of draining residual blood.

IV. Suture Technique (Alar Cinching Suture)

Alar base resection by itself cannot provide adequate correction for patients with a wide alar base along with a broad columellar base. Such a problem needs to be solved by using a semi-permanent suture (alar cinching suture). The basic concept of this maneuver is the narrowing the nasal base without resection of alar base tissue. It is performed after making an incision at the junction of the nostril sill and ala, or nostril sill excision has been carried out. To detach the alar base away from the maxilla below, as well as to maintain the narrowed alar base in the long run, extensive undermining of the soft-tissue of the alar base must be done prior to performing the suture. This involves creating a soft-tissue tunnel along the nasal floor from one side of the alar wound to the other side using tenotomy scissors. Along this tunnel, particularly in a vertical direction, separating an adequate amount of soft tissue attachment is required. When this has been completed, and the alar base can move easily, the ala can be brought together without tension using the suture technique.

With the completion of the tunnel, the two alar incisions are approximated with 2-0 Nylon which is then passed through the tunnel. This first suture is pulled and tied until the desired width of the nostril floor is achieved. The same procedure is done on the opposite side with another 2-0 Nylon suture. This suture is also passed through the tunnel. The second suture acts to narrow the gap created while binding the first suture as well as to provide additional supports *(Figure 9)*. These two sutures not only keep hold of the ala, but acts to narrow the nasal base as well. When both alae are pulled in this fashion, a slight tip projection can be achieved.

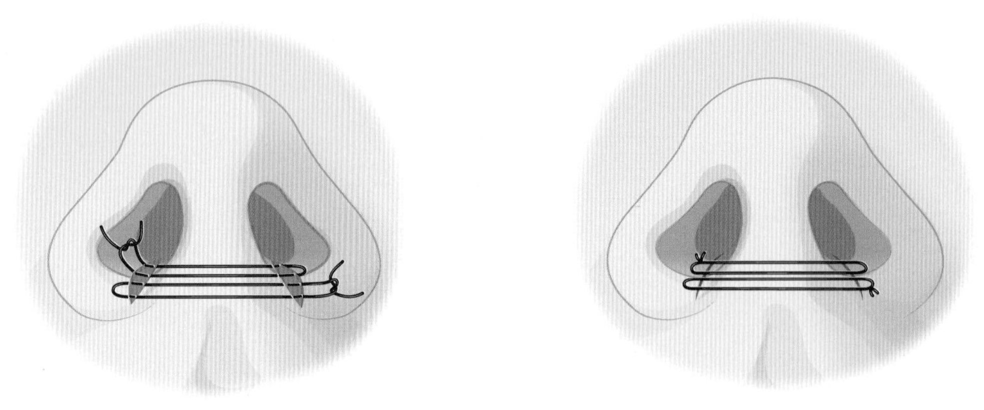

Figure 9 Alar cinching suture.

V. Complications

The following complications can occur while performing alar base surgery.

- Asymmetry of nostril size and alar lobules
- Imbalance between the two sides of the ala
- Obvious scarring
- Notching of the nostril sill
- Nostril deformity

Patients who have thick skin with abundant sebaceous glands are in particular risk of developing scarring. There is a high probability of nostril asymmetry when alar cinching is performed, and there is a risk of unsightly scarring when alar base resection is carried out *(Figure 10)*. Notching of the nostril sill (tear drop like shape) can occur, and this arises when lateral extension is performed insufficiently during alar soft tissue excision.

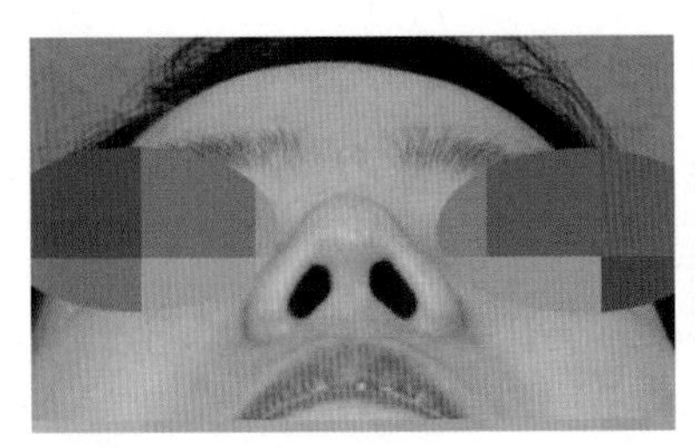
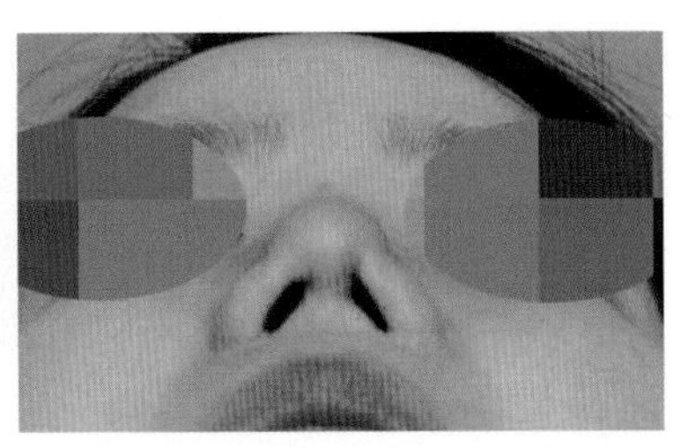

Figure 10 A patient showing nostril stenosis and asymmetry after alar base surgery.

References

1. Adamson PA. Alar base reduction. Arch Facial Plast Surg 2005; 7: 98-101.
2. Becker DG, Weinberger MS, Greene BA, Tardy ME. Clinical study of alar anatomy and surgery of the alar base. Arch Otolaryngol Head Neck Surg 1997; 123: 789-95.
3. Bennett GH, Lessow A, Song P, Constantinides M. The long-term effects of alar base reduction. Arch Facial Plast Surg 2005; 7: 94-7.
4. Bohluli B, Moharamnejad N, Yamani A. Nasal base surgery. Oral Maxillofac Surg Clin North Am 2012; 24: 87-94.
5. Foda HM. Alar base reduction: the boomerang-shaped excision. Facial Plast Surg 2011; 27: 225-33.
6. Gilbert SE. Alar reductions in rhinoplasty. Arch Otolaryngol Head Neck Surg 1996; 122: 781-4.
7. Guyuron B, Behmand RA. Alar base abnormalities. Classification and correction. Clin Plast Surg 1996; 23: 263-70.
8. Guyuron M, Crosby DR, Wolford LM. The alar base cinch suture to control nasal width in maxillary osteotomies. Int J Adult Orthodon Orthognath Surg 1988; 3: 89-95.
9. Kriedel RW, Catellano RD. A simplified approach to alar base reduction: a review of 124 patients over 20 years. Arch Facial Plast Surg 2005; 7: 81-93.
10. Kim EK, Daniel RK. Operative techniques in Asian rhinoplasty. Aesthet Surg J 2012; 32: 1018-30.

Case 1

A 20-year-old male visited for a wide nasal dorsum with nasal obstruction. He had undergone septoplasty 5 years ago.

Analysis

Frontal: Wide dorsum, deviated nose
Basal: Wide alar base, poor tip projection
Lateral and Oblique: Hanging columella, low dorsal height

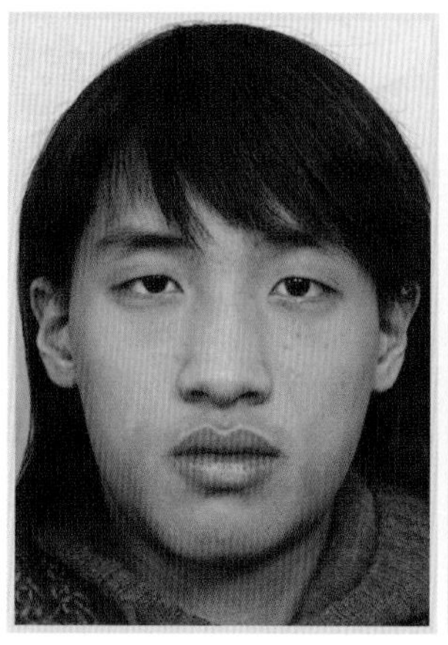
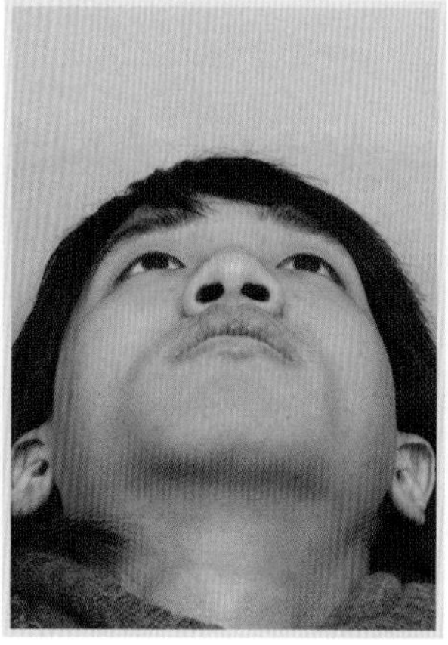
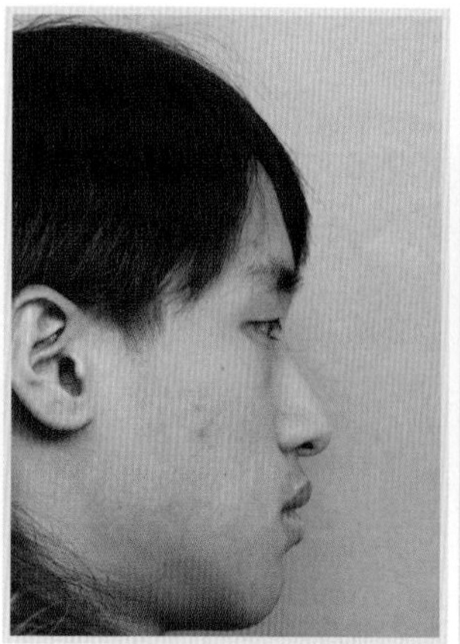
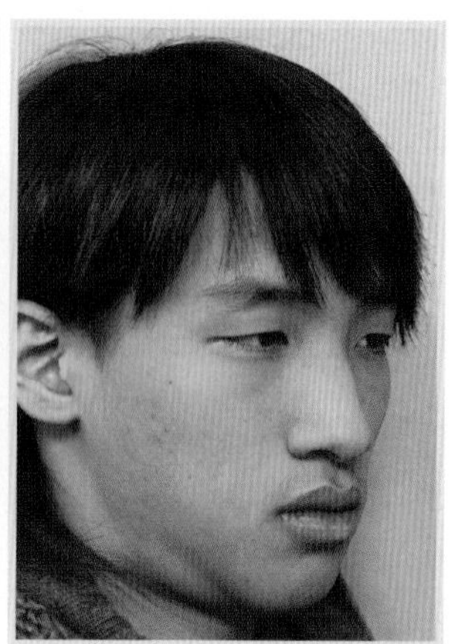

Operative Procedures

Open rhinoplasty approach
Remaining septal cartilage harvest
Conchal cartilage harvest
Medial, lateral, and percutaneous root osteotomies
Cutting and suture technique of the caudal septum
Caudal septal extension grafting (right)
Spreader grafting (right)
Multilayer tip grafting using conchal cartilage
Interdomal suturing
Dorsal augmentation using processed fascia lata and crushed cartilage
Camouflaging of tip graft using processed fascia lata
Alar base resection (bilateral)

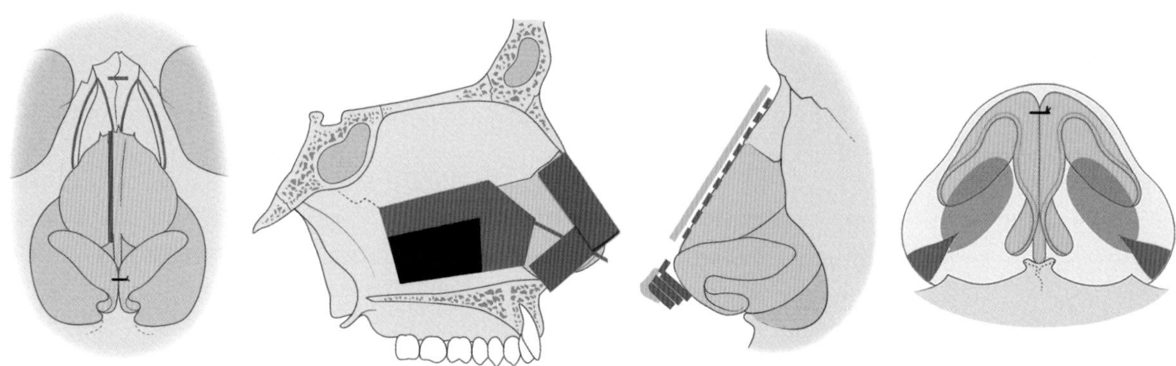

Postoperative Changes

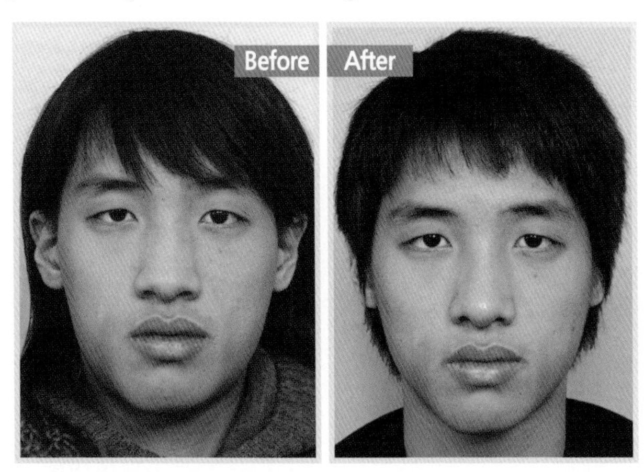

Frontal: The dorsal aesthetic lines were highlighted. Wide dorsum was narrowed.

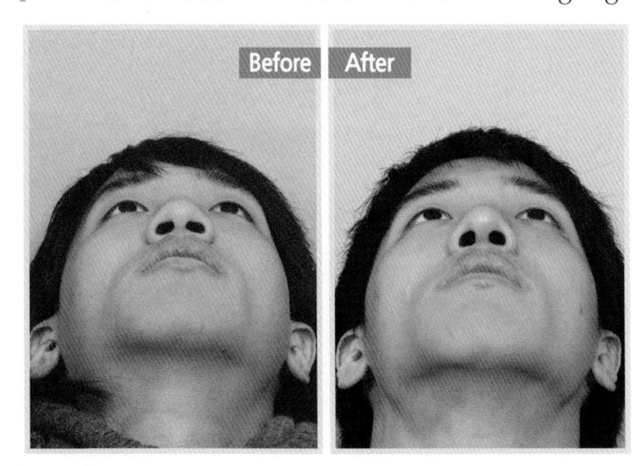

Basal: Tip projection was improved. Alar base width was reduced.

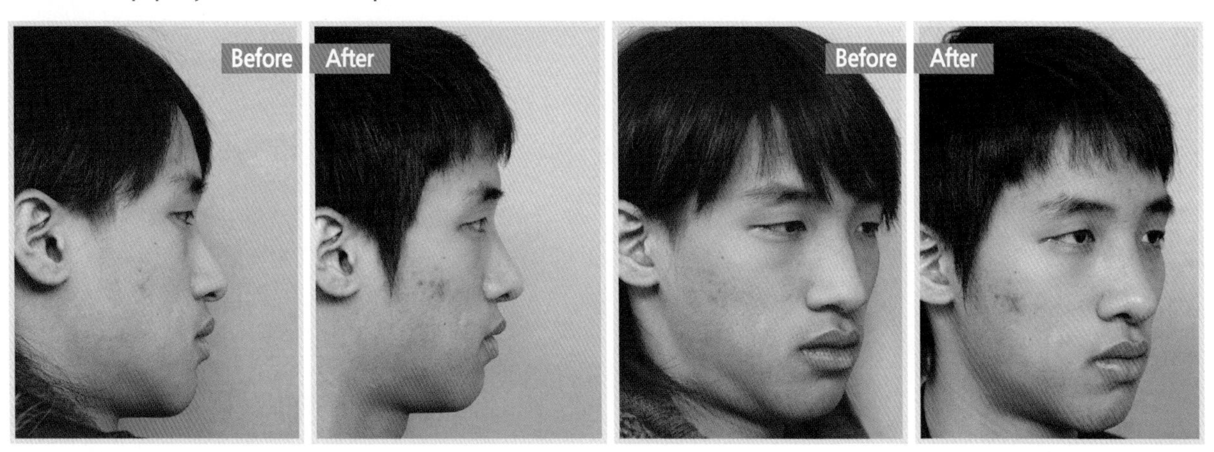

Lateral and Oblique: Dorsal height was increased. Tip projection was improved. Nasolabial angle was widened.

Alar-Columellar Relationship

Yong Ju Jang

The height and shape of the dorsum or tip are major factors for a balanced and attractive nose. However, equally important is the shape of the nasal base with a particular emphasis on the nostril, columella, and ala as it appears in lateral and frontal views. The shape of the nasal base created by the relationship between the columella and the ala is known as the alar-columellar relationship.

I. Aesthetic Considerations

As observed from a frontal photograph, the cosmetically desirable alar-columellar relationship is one that takes on the shape of a gull wing. It is desirable that the vertical distance between the columellar-lobular angle and the tip defining point be bisected by a horizontal line that connects the apices of the alar rims *(Figure 1)*. From a lateral view, a cosmetically desirable nostril takes on an oval outline. The alar rim constitutes the upper half of this egg-like shape and the lower half is made up of skin, connecting tissue of the vestibular skin, and columellar rim. The line that connects the foremost and the rearmost parts of this oval shape is the long axis of the nostril and this line divides the oval shaped lateral nostril into the upper and lower parts as previously mentioned. Aesthetic analysis of the alar-columellar relationship is determined by the distance between nostril long axis to the alar rim, or columellar rim.

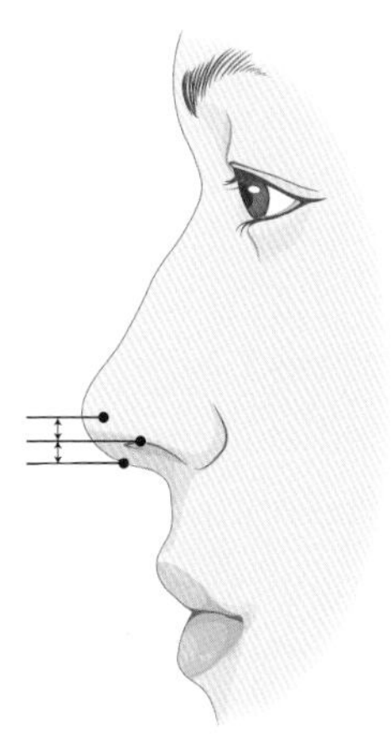

Figure 1 It is desirable that the vertical distance between the columellar-lobular angle and the tip defining point be bisected by a horizontal line that connects the apices of the alar rims.

II. Classification of Alar-Columellar Relationship and Treatment

1.Classification

If the alar-columellar relationship is classified using the long axis of the nostril as a reference line, and applying its distance to the alar rim of the upper part and the columellar rim of the lower part, it is possible to classify the alar-columellar relationship into roughly six different types *(Figure 2)*. Types I-III are characterized by an increased columellar show with a greater display of columellar skin and mucosa while types IV-VI are related to a reduced columellar show.

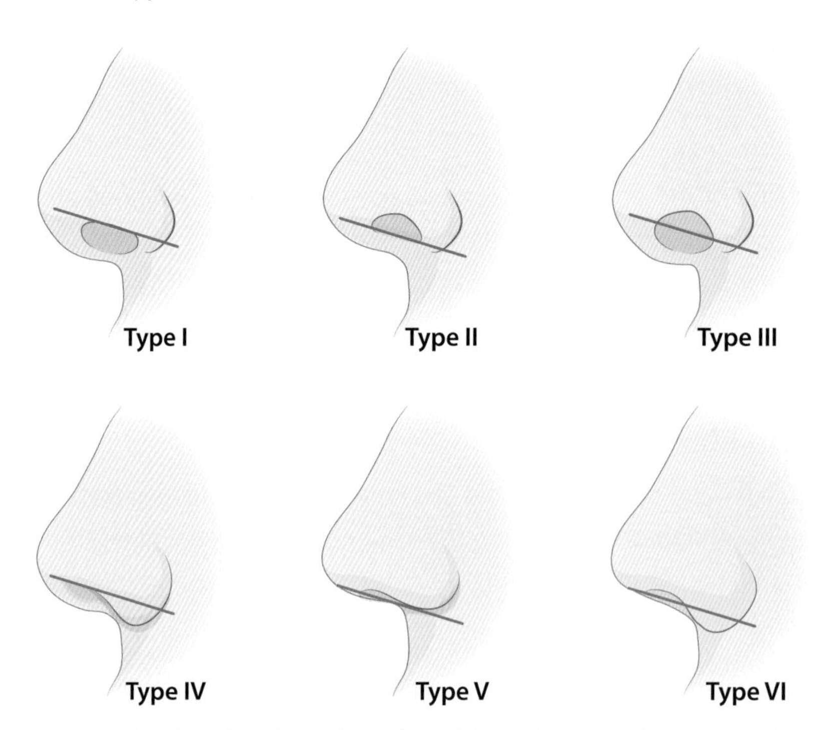

Figure 2 Classification of the alar-columellar relationships. Type I, hanging columella; Type II, retracted ala; Type III, combination of; Types I and II, Type IV, hanging ala; Type V, retracted columella, and Type VI, combination of Types IV and V.

2.Treatment

1) Type I (Hanging Columella)

This type is called as hanging columella wherein the distance between the long axis and the columellar rim of the nostril is more than 2 mm and the distance to the alar rim is 1-2 mm. To solve this problem, resection of the membranous septum, both inclusive and exclusive of the caudal septum can be performed. If the columella is severely exposed due to the expanded width of the medial crura, resection of the vestibular skin covering it can be carried out, and the columellar border relocated cephalically. In addition, medial crural overlay or lateral crural overlay techniques can be performed to change the shape of lower lateral cartilage. The tongue-in-groove technique by which the surgeon can pull the medial crura cephalically and connect them with the caudal septum is another good technique to correct a hanging columella *(Figure 3)*.

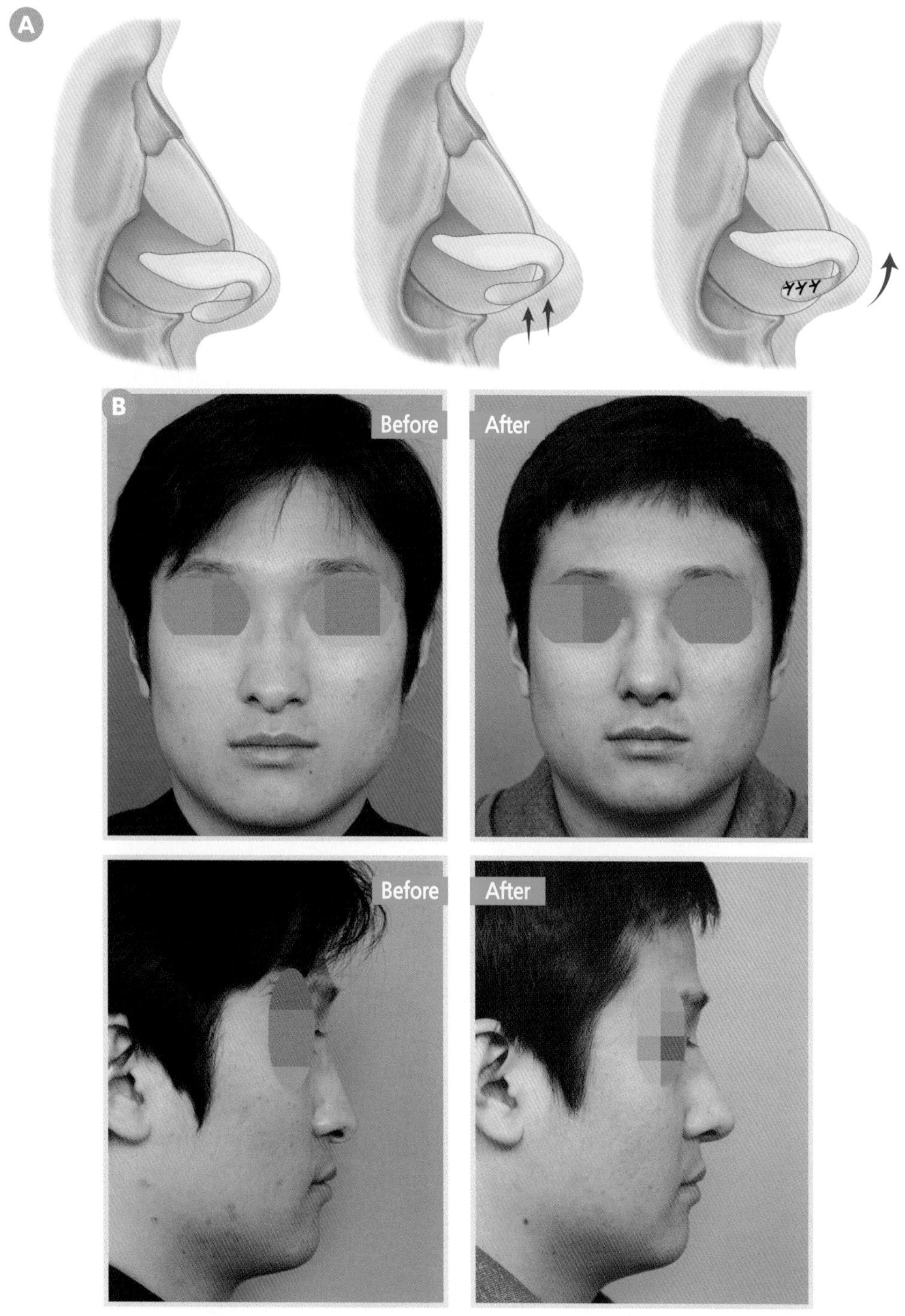

Figure 3 Tongue-in-grove technique (A). A patient showing improved hanging columella by the use of tongue-in-groove technique (B).

2) Type II (Retracted Ala)

This deformity is also known as a retracted ala. In this type, increased columellar show is mainly due to alar retraction. The retracted ala can be managed with following techniques:

(1) Composite Conchal Cartilage Graft

This method is applicable for lowering the alar rim, correcting vestibular stenosis, and reconstructing the internal valve. The graft is usually obtained from the ipsilateral cymba concha. An area of 10 mm in width is dissected from the skin of this area. Excising out the skin too broadly will cause difficult primary skin closure in some cases. In that case, a skin graft using the postauricular skin is required. A piece of cartilage larger than the covering skin needs to be resected followed by primary skin closure. In lowering the height of the alar rim, an incision of the area 2-3 mm interior to the area with the most severe notching needs to be performed and then the skin spread open vertically. This procedure should be carried out not with the aim of creating a pocket but with an intention to push the skin downward from the caudal edge of the lateral crura. Suturing is then performed first on the skin of the composite graft to the alar rim followed by the lower part. The size of the composite graft should be slightly bigger than needed to overcome the secondary contracture of the wound *(Figures 4, 5)*. Occasionally, the graft contour can be seen as a bulge inside of the nostril. The possibility of this complication should be informed to the patient.

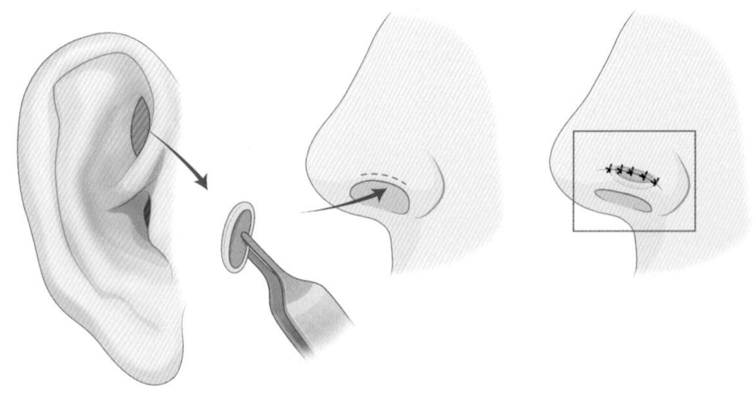

Figure 4 Method of correcting a retracted ala using a composite conchal cartilage graft.

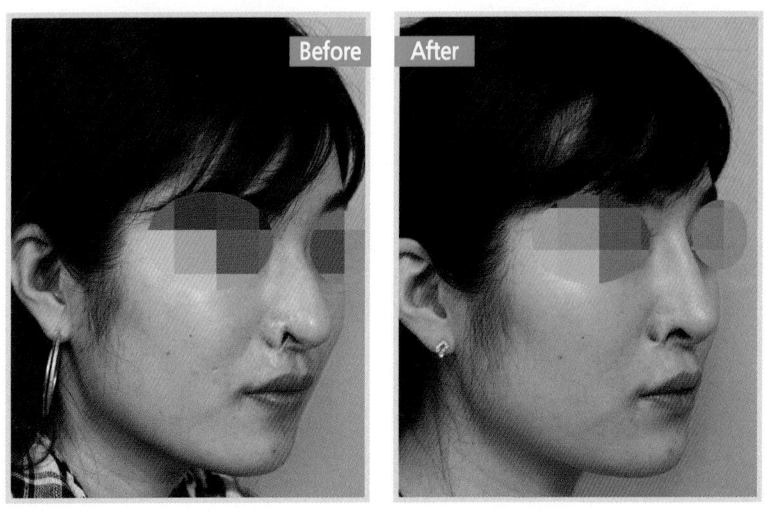

Figure 5 A patient showing improved alar retraction after placement of a composite conchal cartilage graft.

(2) Alar Rim Graft (Alar Strut Graft)

An alar rim graft procedure using septal or conchal cartilage is one of the useful techniques for treating patients with a retracted ala or when alar retraction is expected after surgery. This method is useful in patients requiring revision surgery, in particular for those with notching of the alar rim due to excessive resection of the lateral crura. As a composite graft of conchal cartilage is overly thick and easily visible from the outside, this graft is problematic for use on minor alar retraction. For patients showing only a minor degree of alar retraction, the use of an alar rim graft is recommended. Various types of suture techniques used in tip surgery have a tendency to induce postoperative notching of the alar rim. Performing alar rim grafts during tip work on such patients can prevent notching of the alar rim. This method involves first carving a septal cartilage piece, 10-14 mm long and 2-4 mm wide. Then a horizontal skin incision of about 4 mm in size is made at the inner lower part of the alar rim. If a marginal incision is already made for the external approach, dissection needs to be carried out on the alar rim soft tissue remaining around the caudal area of the marginal incision. Next, using small scissors, a pocket parallel to the alar rim is created and the graft inserted in this pocket, and then the incision closed *(Figure 6)*. If a greater extent of correction is called for, it is better to use a composite graft or lateral crural strut graft.

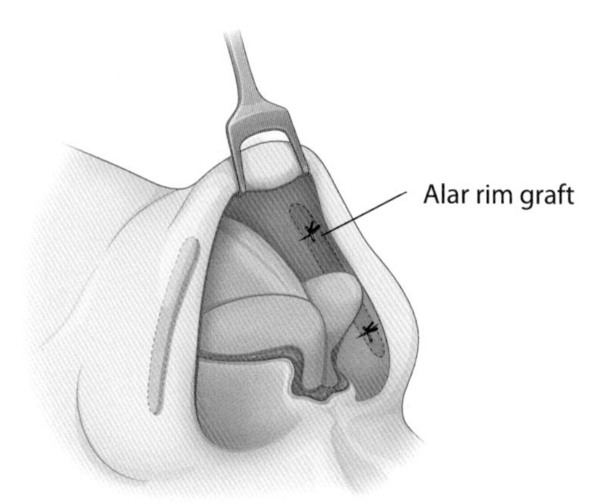

Figure 6 Surgical technique of alar rim grafting.

(3) Lateral Crural Strut Graft

In correcting a retracted ala, a lateral crural strut graft is even more effective than a composite graft. To perform this, the lateral crus should be freed from the underlying vestibular skin. Septal cartilage or other forms cartilage graft is sewn under the lateral crus, and the lateral crus-graft complex is rotated caudally. The lateral end of the graft is inserted into a more caudally located soft tissue pocket *(Figure 7)*.

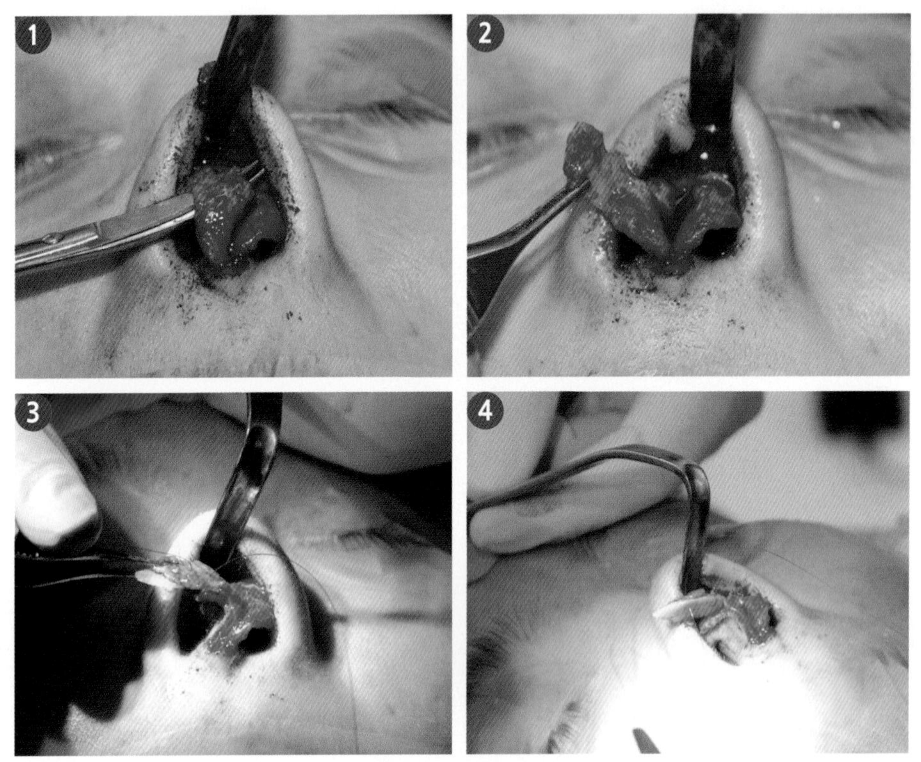

Figure 7 Serial intraopertive photos of lateral crural strut grafting.

3) Type III (Combination of Hanging Columella and Retracted Ala)

A Type III deformity combines Type I and Type II deformities. Such a compound deformity is characterized by a hanging columella and retracted ala, and the proper treatment must be selected from among the above mentioned treatments to correct the two deformities.

4) Type IV (Hanging Ala)

The Type IV alar-columellar relationship, one of the most common alar-columellar discrepancies found in Asians, is also called a hanging ala, in which the distance between the long axis of the nostril and the alar rim above becomes so shortened that the columella becomes almost invisible laterally.

Prior to treating a hanging ala, the columella needs to be examined to verify if it is properly located in the caudal area. The reason for this is because the maximum the alar rim that can be surgically lifted up is 2-3 mm. The most common surgical procedure used is performing an excision of about 3 mm of the vestibular skin in an oval shape at the inner part of the alar lobule; then suturing the excision margin *(Figure 8)*. The shape of the excised skin can be modified according to the desired shape of the alar lobule. For example, if the lower part of the alar lobule needs to be raised more, one can excise the skin in the shape of a wide-based triangle *(Figures 9, 10)*.

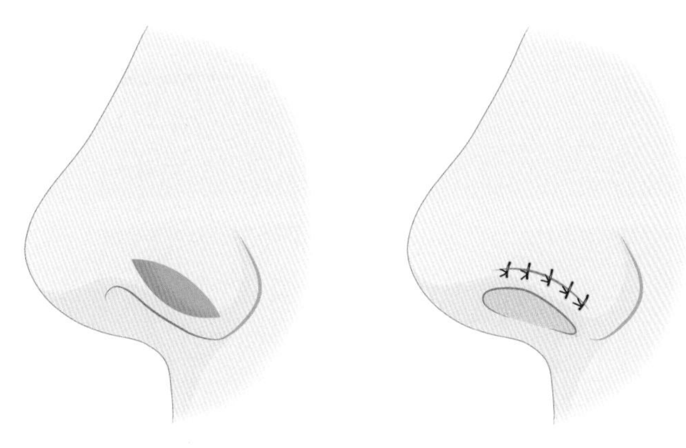

Figure 8 Excision of vestibular skin, which is performed to correct a hanging ala.

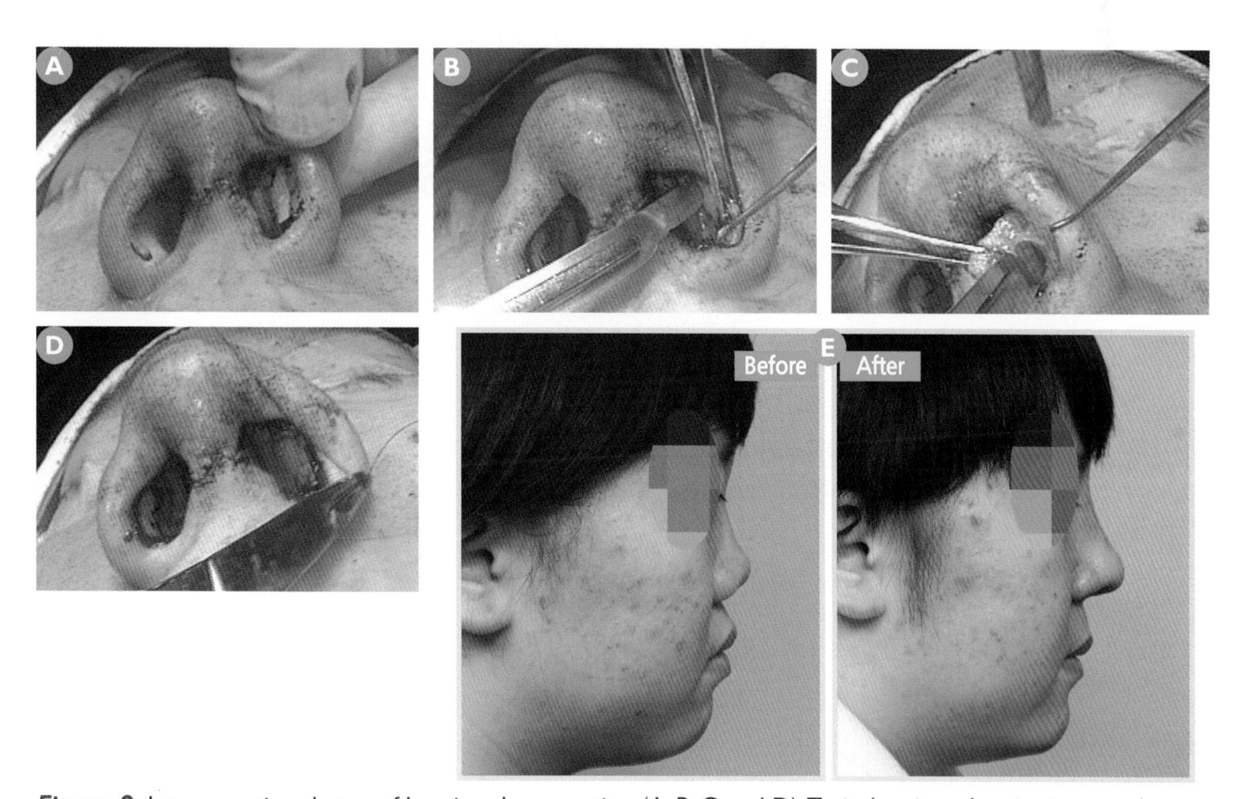

Figure 9 Intraoperative photos of hanging ala correction (A, B, C, and D). Typical patient showing improved hanging ala after excision of vestibular skin (E).

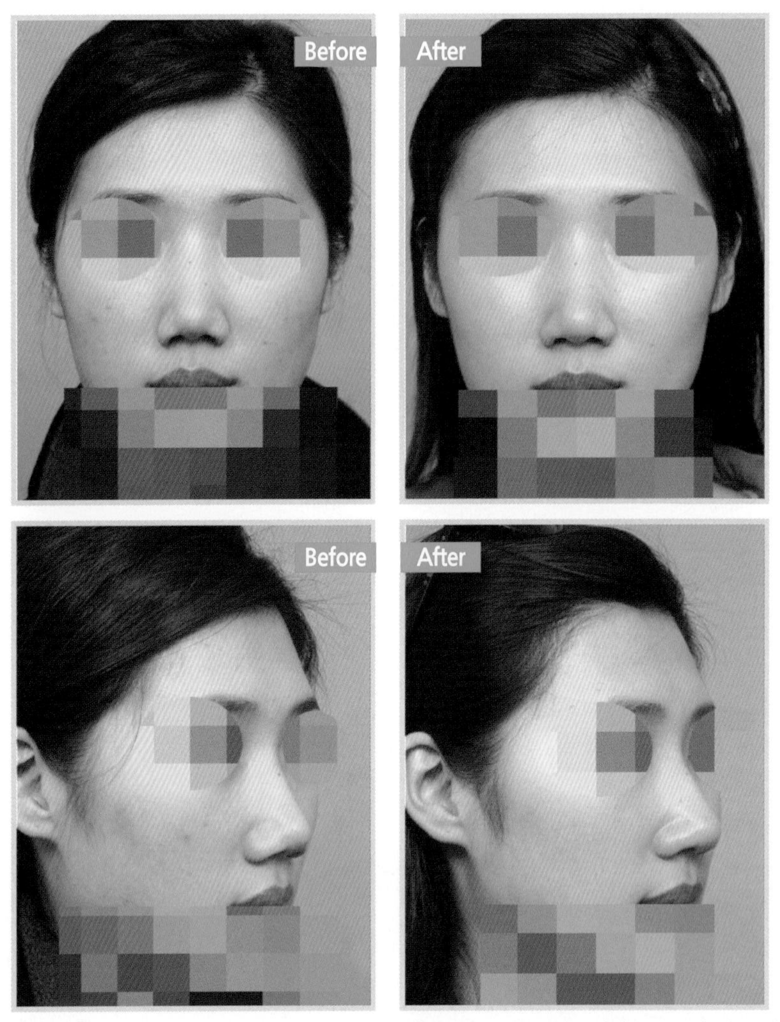

Figure 10 Improved hanging ala after performing excision of the vestibular skin.

If the excision of the skin is excessive, the alar rim can take on an unnaturally curled shape, or lose its naturally round contour. In severe hanging ala cases, the excision can include the skin of the alar rim and alar lobule. This technique results is dramatic change, however carries the risk of visible scar formation and nostril deformity *(Figures 11, 12, 13)*.

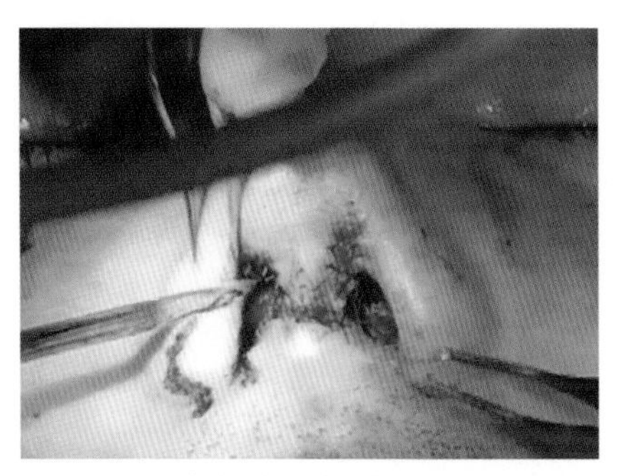

Figure 11 Direct excision of alar lobule skin to correct a severe hanging ala.

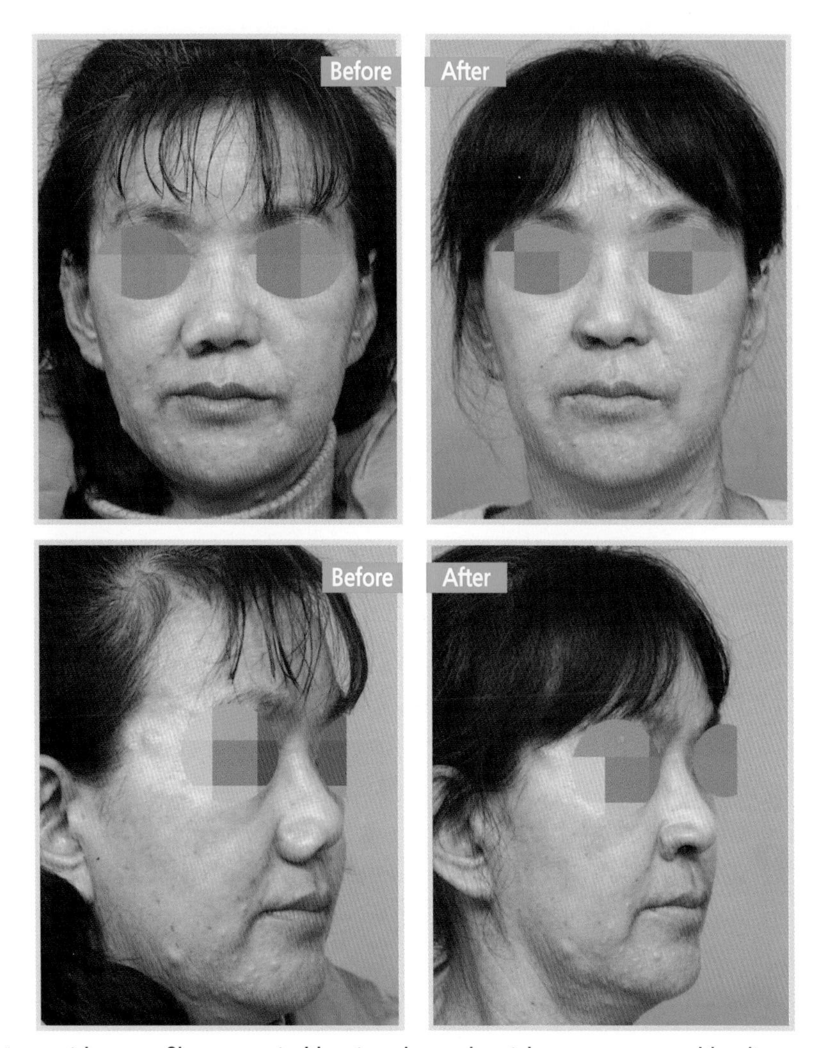

Figure 12 A patient with neurofibromatosis. Hanging ala on the right was corrected by direct excision of skin on the alar lobule.

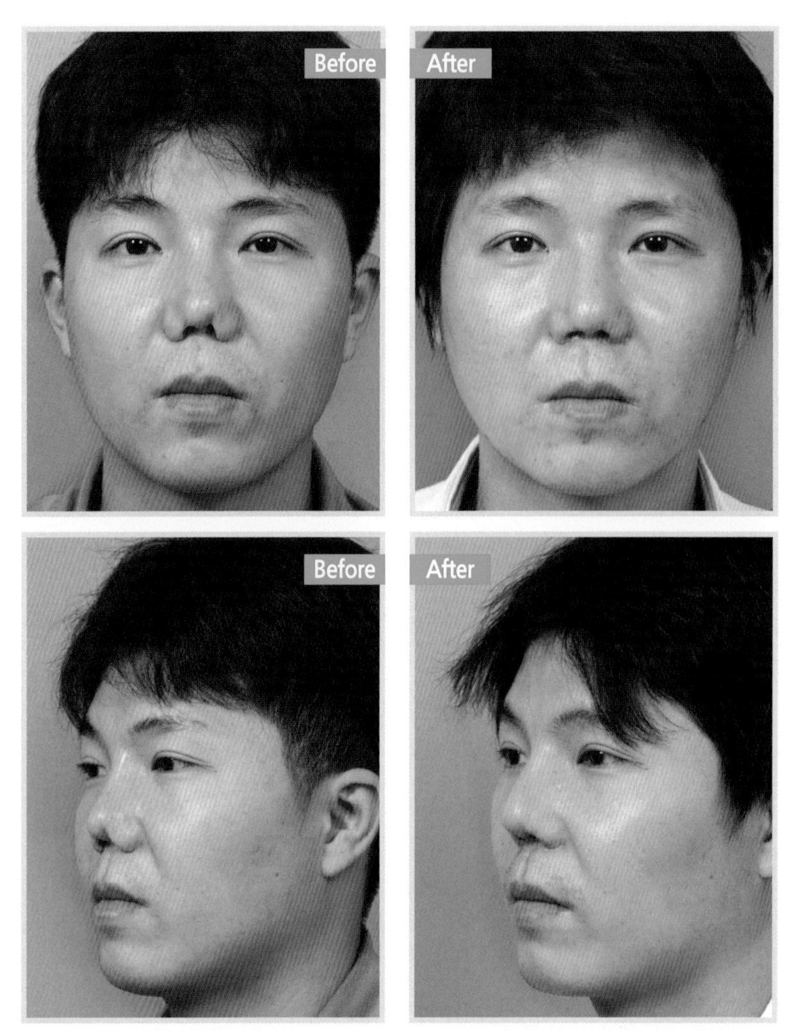

Figure 13 A patient showing dramatic improvement of hanging ala after direct excision of alar lobule skin.

5) Type V (Retracted Columella)

Type V deformity or retracted columella is a condition wherein the distance between the long axis of the nostril and the columella has become shortened. Correction of such a deformity can be attempted by placement of a caudal septal extension graft. If necessary, the extension graft can be designed to modify the columellar-labial angle. A retracted columella is frequently associated with an acute nasolabial angle. It is therefore necessary to place plumping grafts or premaxillary grafts on these patients. Placement of one or two layers of shield grafts at the space between the columellar skin and the medial crura can be another option to treat a retracted columella *(Figure 14)*. However, caution must be exercised when inserting multiple layers of grafts because they increase the risk of graft-related infection and may prohibit easier closure of the transcolumellar incision, especially in revision cases.

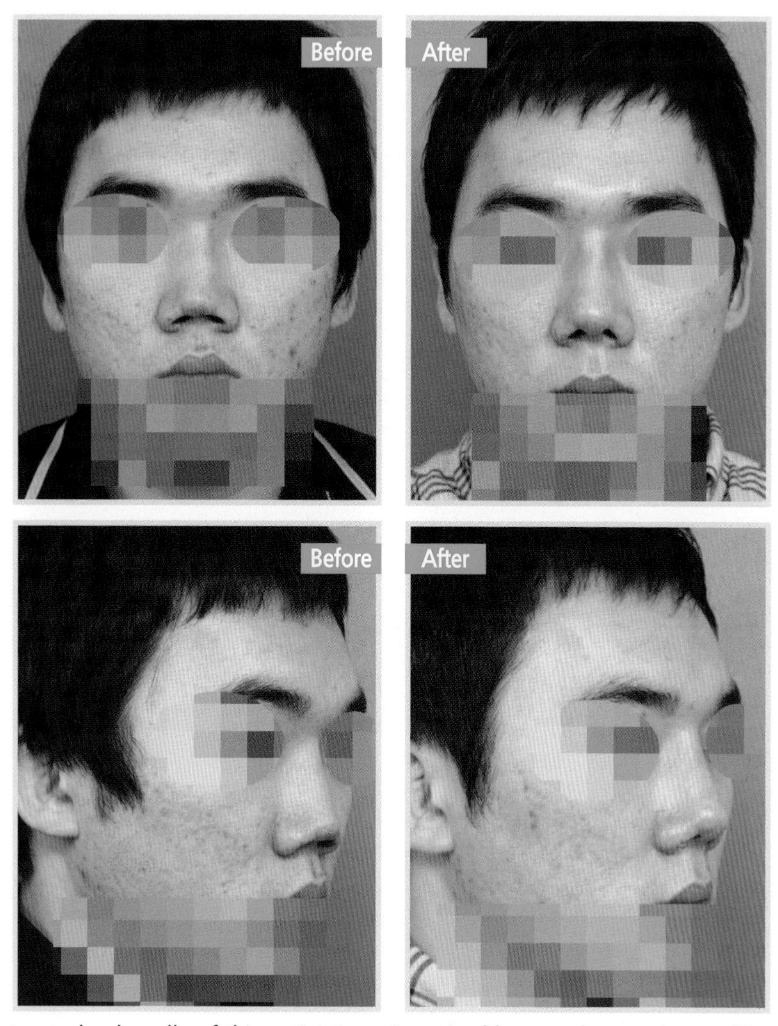

Figure 14 The retracted columella of this patient was improved by septal extension grafting and shied grafting.

3. Complications

During a composite conchal cartilage-skin graft procedure to correct a retracted columella, there may be cases where the dissection of the recipient area for the graft may not be carried out sufficiently. In such a situation, the transplanted composite graft can protrude toward the nasal vestibule during recovery. Such a result can lead to nasal blockage due to narrowing of the external valve. In addition, the graft can become visible through the nostril. Excision of vestibular skin for hanging ala correction may result in unnatural sloping of the alar lobule and nostril asymmetry *(Figure 15)*.

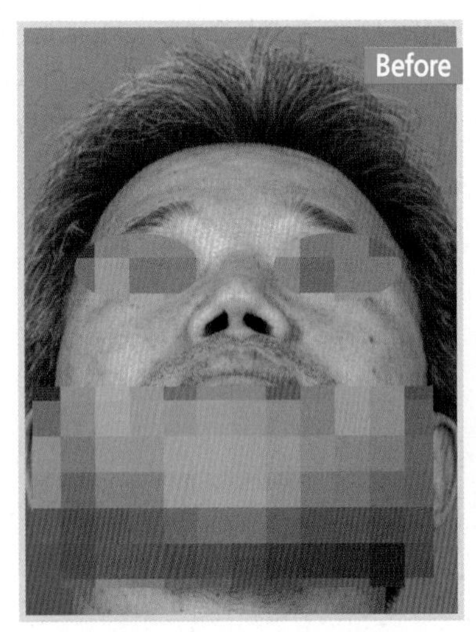

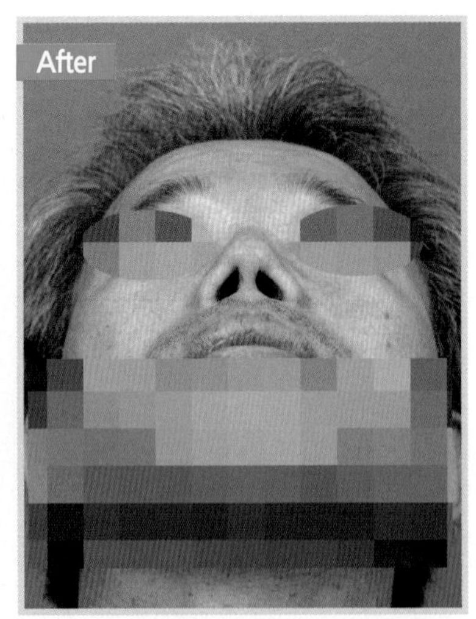

Figure 15 A patient showing unnatural sloping of the alar lobule as a result of vestibular skin excision.

References

1. Adamson PA. Anatomic considerations in the management of the hanging columella. Arch Facial Plast Surg 2000; 2: 178-9.
2. Bilen BT, Aytekin AH, Erbatur S, Geyik Y. Correction of true hanging columella using medial crural tuck-up technique. Aesthet Plast Surg 2013; 37: 210-5.
3. Guyuron B. Alar rim deformities. Plast Reconstr Surg 2001; 107: 856-63.
4. Hafezi F, Naghibzadeh B. Prevention of hanging columella in open rhinoplasty. Ann Otol Rhinol Laryngol 2004; 113: 839-42.
5. Matarasso A, Greer SE, Longaker MT. The true hanging columella: simplified diagnosis and treatment using a modified direct approach. Plast Reconstr Surg 2000; 106: 469-74.
6. McKinney P, Stalnecker ML. The hanging ala. Plast Reconstr Surg 1984; 73: 427-30.
7. Silver WE, Sajjadian A. Nasal base surgery. Otolaryngol Clin North Am 1999; 32: 653-68.
8. Williams EF. Alar-columellar disharmony using the tongue-in-groove maneuver in primary endonasal rhinoplasty. Arch Facial Plast Surg 2012; 14: 283-8.
9. Yap E. Improving the hanging ala. Facial Plast Surg 2012; 28: 213-7.

Chapter 26 Nostril Deformity

Yong Ju Jang · Sung Bu Lee

The shape of the nostril seen from the basal view has less aesthetic importance than the shape of the dorsum and nasal tip as seen from the profile view. However, a severe nostril deformity identifiable even from the frontal view can be catchy to one's attention; thus the symmetry and shape of the nostrils can be an important aesthetic consideration in patients. The shape of the nostril is determined by the original shape of the lower lateral cartilages and the surrounding skin-soft tissue envelope. An ideal interplay between the lower lateral cartilages and skin-soft tissue envelope of appropriate thickness can bring about a beautiful nostril of kidney bean shape *(Figure 1)*. Conversely, abnormally shaped lower lateral cartilages will result in an abnormally shaped nostril *(Figure 2)*. This Chapter will deal mostly with the surgical correction of asymmetric nostrils and small nostrils.

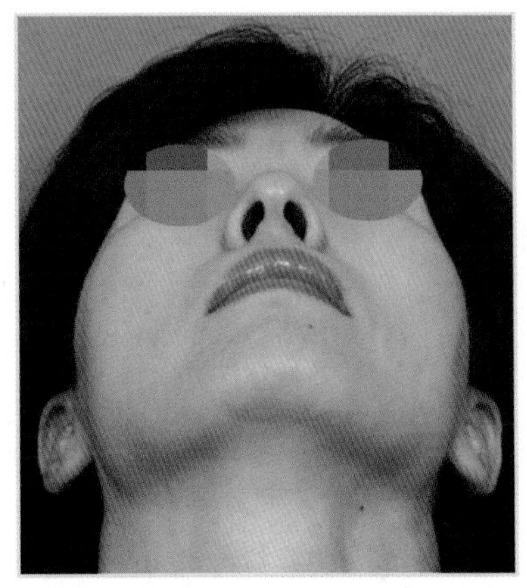

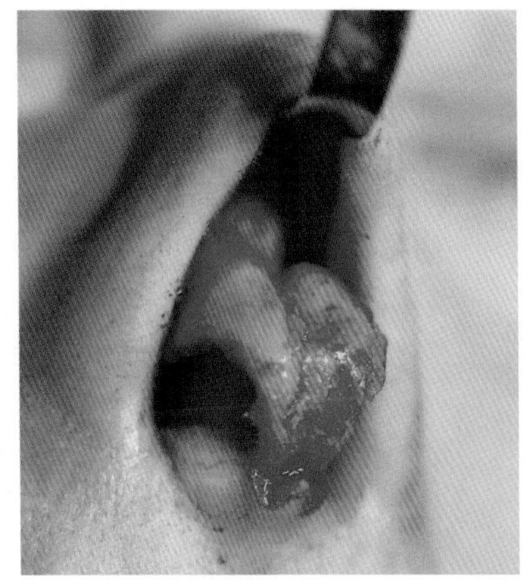

Figure 1 The ideal shape of the nostril as determined by the lower lateral cartilages.

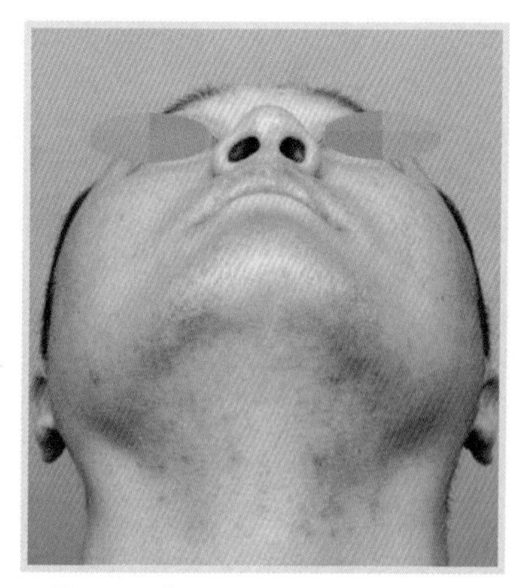
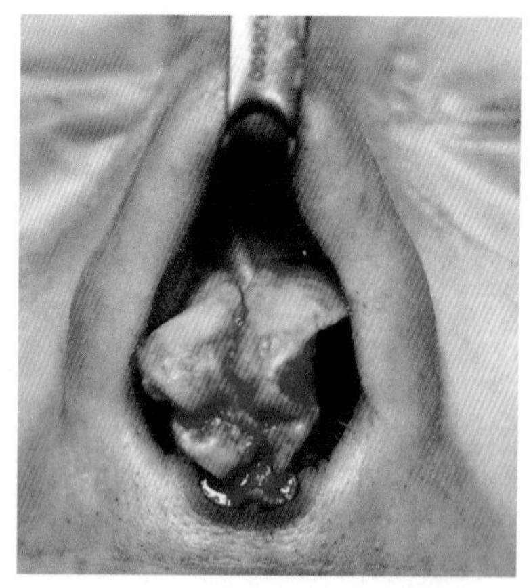

Figure 2 Nostril deformity due to deformed lower lateral cartilages.

I . Classification and Treatment Strategy

The authors classify the nostril deformities into primary deformities and secondary deformities.

Primary nostril deformities include:

- ☑ Primary asymmetric nostril without sill deformity: asymmetric nostril due to intrinsic deformity of lower lateral cartilages, not associated with deformed septum and upper lateral cartilages
- ☑ Cleft lip nose-like deformity
- ☑ Small nostril

Secondary nostril deformities include:

- ☑ Nostril deformity due to caudal septal deviation
- ☑ Nostril deformity in patients with a deviated nose
- ☑ Cleft lip nose deformity
- ☑ Nostril deformity due to scar contracture
- ☑ Nostril stenoisis

There are other forms of nostril deformities that do not exactly fit in above-mentioned classification, but they can be corrected by applying the following treatment techniques.

1. Primary Nostril Deformities

1) Primary Asymmetric Nostril without Sill Deformity

This type of deformity is relatively common, and is characterized by mildly asymmetric nostrils without a difference on the level of both nostril sills. In order to correct this deformity, one can apply a medial crural overlay or lateral crural overlay technique that can bring about symmetry of the alar cartilages. Further adjustment can also be achieved by the use of a columellar strut. Persisting asymmetry after implementation of the above can be corrected by execution of additional techniques such as lateral crural onlay, lateral crural strut grafting, lateral crural flip-flop, and shield grafting *(Figure 3)*.

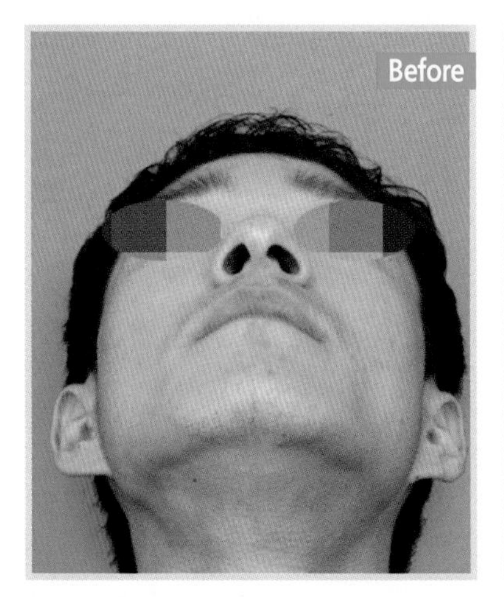

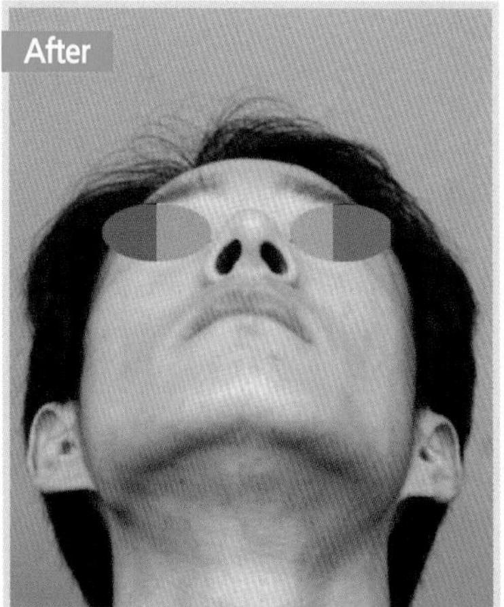

Figure 3 A patient with primary asymmetric nostril. Asymmetric nostrils were improved by applying a lateral crural overlay technique, columellar strut, and footplate modification.

2) Cleft Lip Nose-Like Deformity

In clinical practice, we can find a subset of patients who demonstrate nostril deformity mimicking those of cleft lip nose patients, but not having a definite cleft lip *(Figure 4)*. These patients typically show a unilaterally under-developed nostril sill, decreased convexity of the alar lobule on the same side, and an increased width of the nostril base. This deformity is quite similar to the nostril deformity seen in cleft lip nose patients. One of the most difficult tasks in correcting this type of deformity is to equalize the different vertical levels of the nostril sills. This can be corrected by augmentation of the deficient nostril sill through a sublabial approach or a subcutaneous tunnel created at the lateral aspect of columellar base. However, the aesthetic outcome of any kind of surgical maneuver is usually disappointing. The big discrepancy between the horizontal width of nostril base can

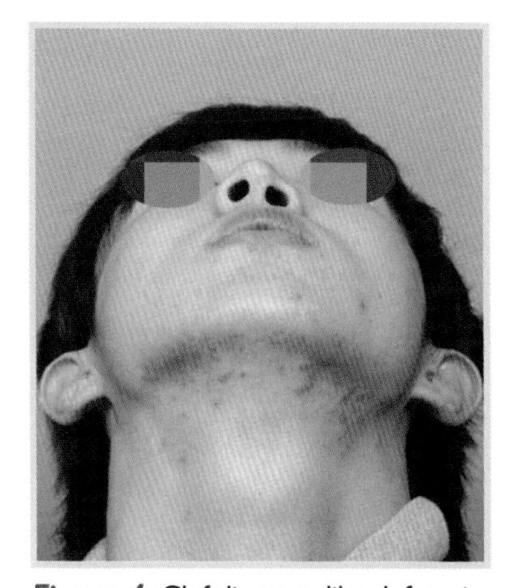

Figure 4 Cleft lip nose-like deformity.

be corrected by unilateral alar base narrowing *(Figure 5)*. The abnormal contour of the alar lobule, characterized by a linear sloping or abnormal concavity, can be corrected by using columellar strut, alar rim graft, lateral crural onlay graft, and lateral crural strut graft *(Figure 6)*. This type of the

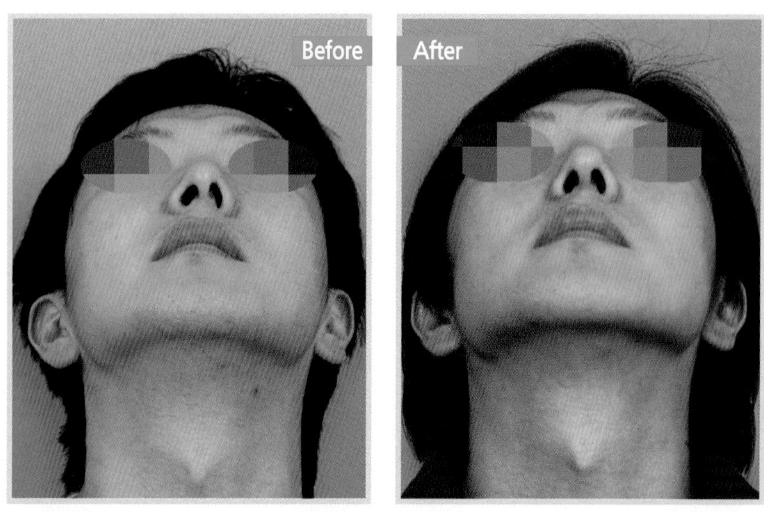

Figure 5 If there is much difference in horizontal width of the nostril base, unilateral alar base narrowing will be helpful. In this patient, a right alar base resection was performed.

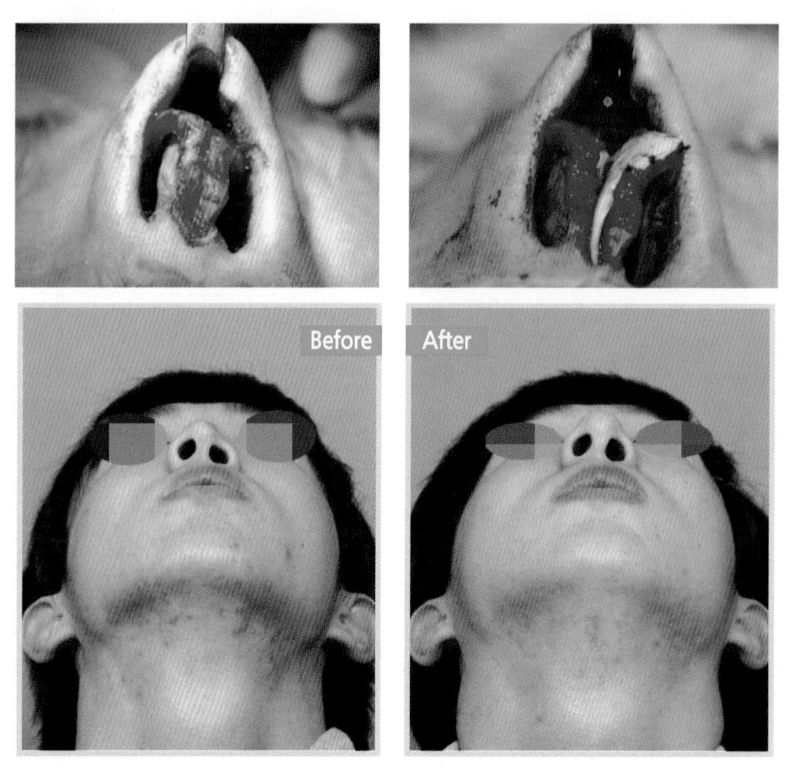

Figure 6 The left lower lateral cartilage dimension is different from the right in this cleft lip nose-like deformity patient. Grafting with lateral crural onlay and columellar strut graft at the same time was made using costal cartilage to improve these dysmorphic features.

nostril deformity usually presents with different heights of the nostril apex, which can be perceived as alar notching observable from the frontal view.

3) Small Nostril

There are no absolute aesthetic standards that define the ideal size of the nostril. However, too small a nostril can cause impaired nasal breathing; furthermore it gives an infantile nose-like appearance, thus mandating adequate correction when indicated. In patients with small nostrils, if the patient experiences easier nasal breathing after pinching the columellar base using forceps to widen the nostril, the surgeon can predict a favorable outcome in nostriloplasty in improving nasal breathing.

The underlying anatomic abnormalities of small nostrils are:

- ☑ Hypoplastic lower lateral cartilages
- ☑ Laterally bulged, hyperplasic footplate of the alar cartilages
- ☑ Excessive alar soft tissue

To adequately correct the small nostril, the authors usually expose the entire alar cartilages through an external rhinoplasty approach, followed by diagnosis of the underlying anatomical issues. Laterally bulged hyperplastic footplates should be partially resected and sewn together medially to widen the nostril *(Figure 7)*.

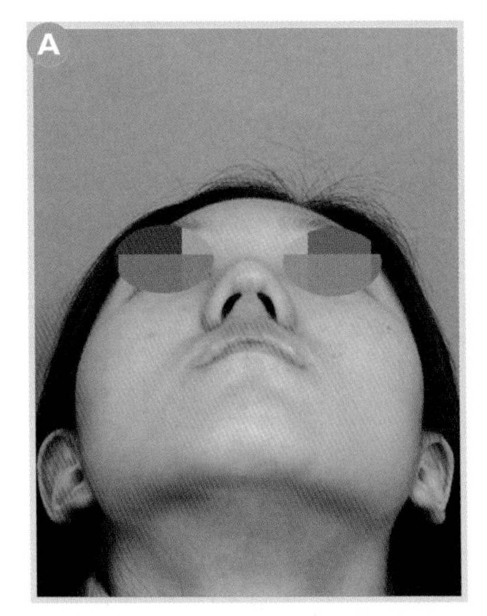

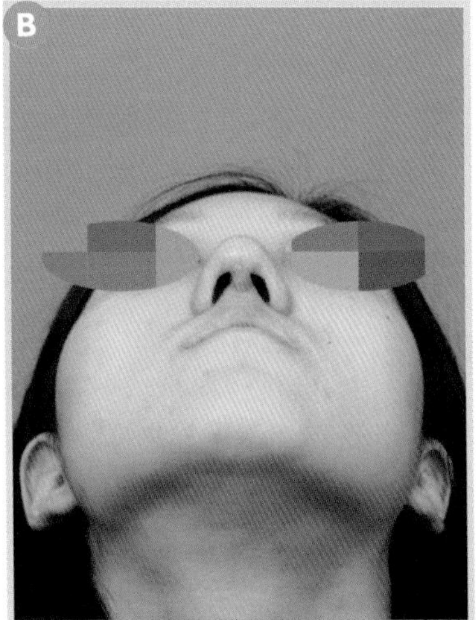

Figure 7 Small nostril operation. Preoperative (A) and postoperative photo (B). Nostrils were enlarged partially by removing the lateral projection of the footplates, and medializing both medial crura by suturing.

In some patients, severely underdeveloped and hypoplastic lower lateral cartilages are the underlying anatomical cause of the small nostrils. In this scenario, after dissection of the lower lateral cartilages from the underlying vestibular skin, the columellar height and lateral crural dimension is expanded using a big columellar strut or lateral crural onlay graft aiming to create a bigger skeleton for the nostril. For that purpose, one can use costal cartilage if the septal cartilage is not strong and thick enough to serve as a sound framework to withstand the skin-soft tissue envelope *(Figure 8)*.

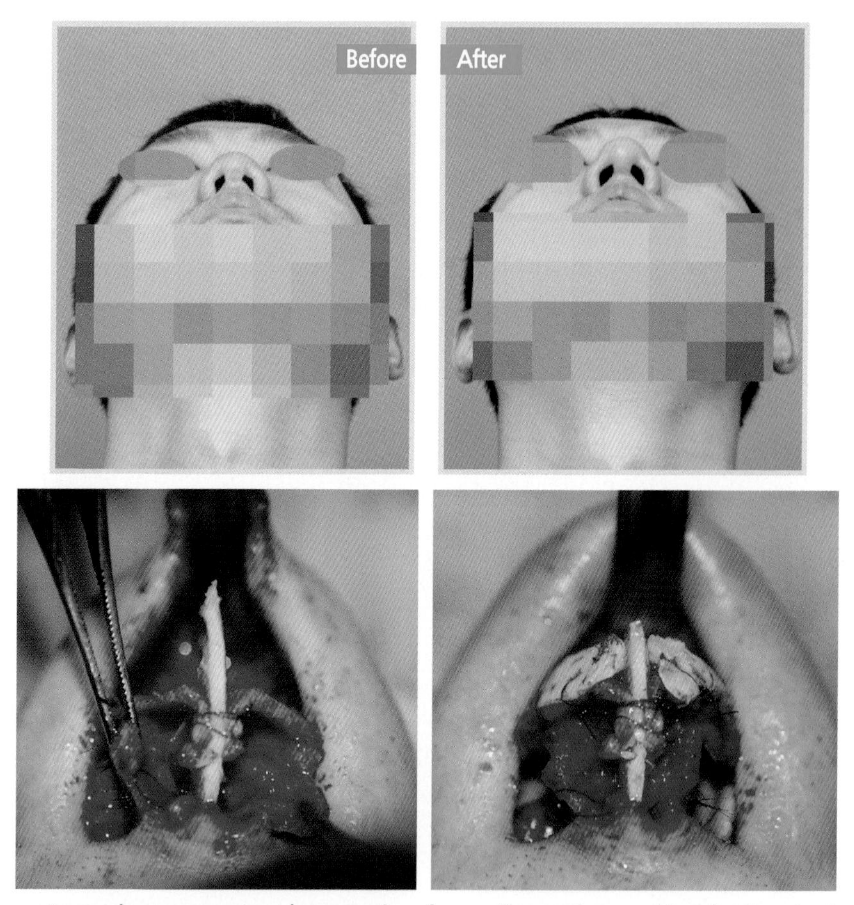

Figure 8 Preoperative and postoperative photographs of a small nostril case. After freeing the lower lateral cartilages from the underlying vestibular skin, a strong and long columellar strut and lateral crural onlay graft using costal cartilage was inserted, making a new framework for the nostril.

2. Secondary Nostril Deformities

1) Nostril Deformity Secondary to Caudal Septal Deviation.

A severely deflected caudal septum toward one direction can narrow the horizontal width of the nostril, which can result in a nostril deformity. This can be corrected by straightening the caudal septum. In most cases, there is excess cartilage in the caudal septum. The excess cartilage should be resected; and the displaced caudal septum repositioned at the midline. A deviated anterior nasal spine should also be corrected by reshaping and fracturing *(Figure 9)*.

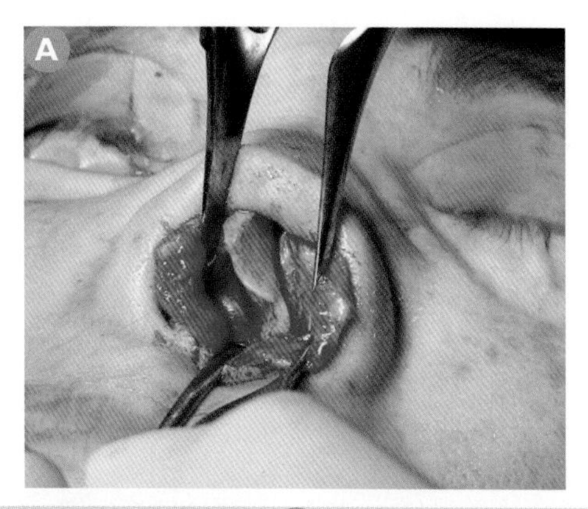

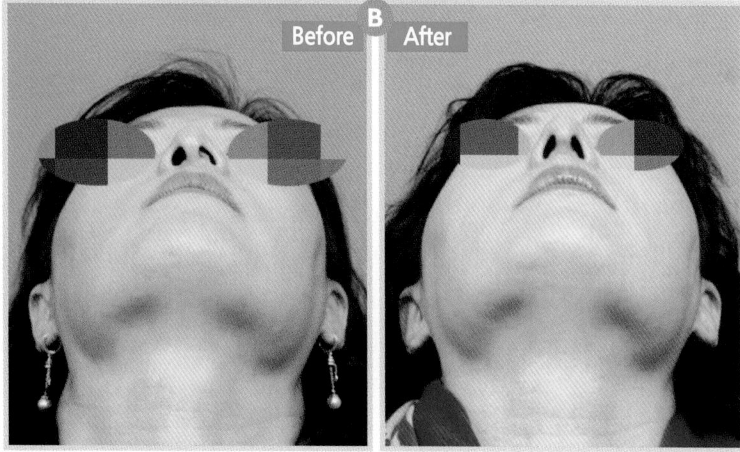

Figure 9 Nostril deformity secondary to caudal septum deformity (A). Improved deformity after surgery (B).

2) Nostril Deformity Secondary to a Deviated Nose

Patients with deviated nose frequently demonstrate a unilateral concave upper lateral cartilage and a concave contour of the alar lobule on the ipsilateral side. This type of nostril deformity can easily be corrected if the deviated cartilaginous dorsum is adequately corrected by septoplasty, spreader graft, or other techniques designed to correct cartilaginous deviation *(Figure 10)*. Persisting deviation after proper correction of the deviated cartilaginous dorsum can be further managed using techniques applicable to the correction of primary nostril deformity.

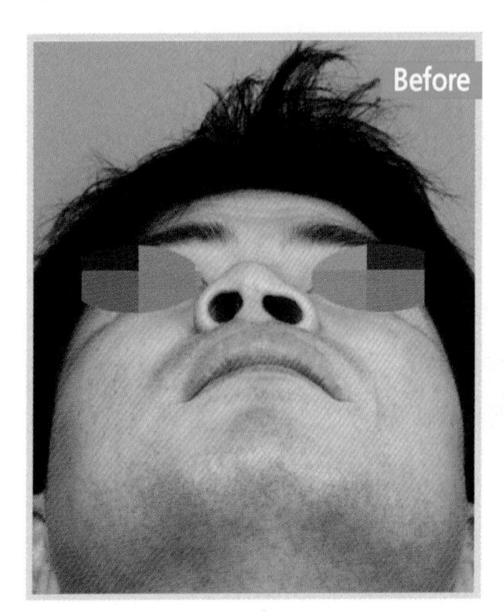

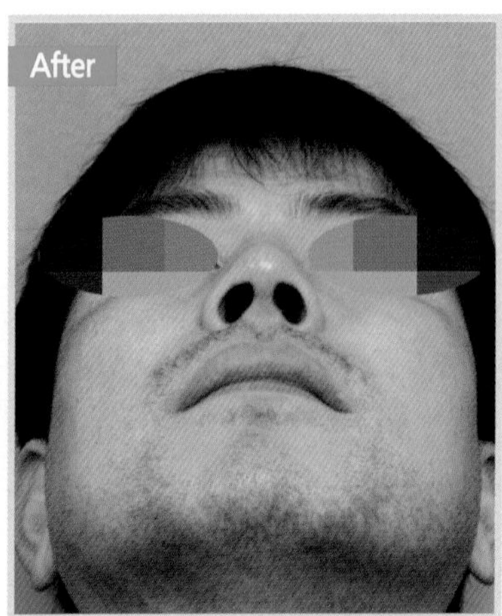

Figure 10 Nostril asymmetry secondary to a deviated nose was corrected after treatment of the deviated nose.

3) Cleft Lip Nose Deformity

Cleft lip, especially unilateral cleft lip, is accompanied by a nostril deformity in most cases. The typical characteristic of a unilateral cleft lip nose deformiy is a three-dimensional asymmetry of the nasal tip and alar base. The columella and the caudal septum of these patients are always deviated to the contralateral side of the cleft. Asymmetric development of the orbicularis oris muscle often underlies the formation of the nostril deformity. The cleft alar base is asymmetric and ala is directed laterally and inferiorly. The nasal tip is also asymmetric, because the medial crus of the cleft side is shorter and lateral crus of the cleft side is longer compared to the non-cleft side *(Figure 11)*.

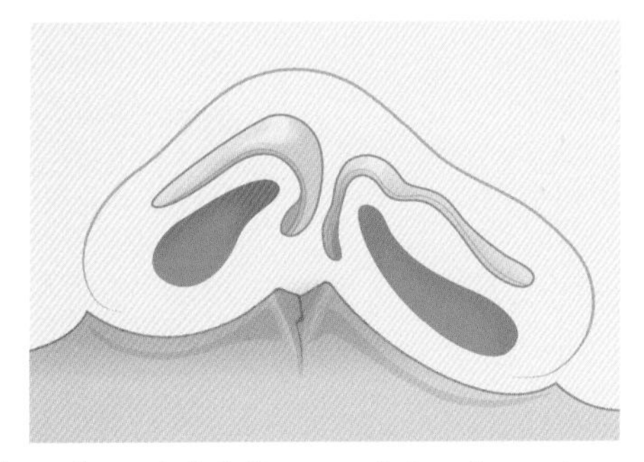

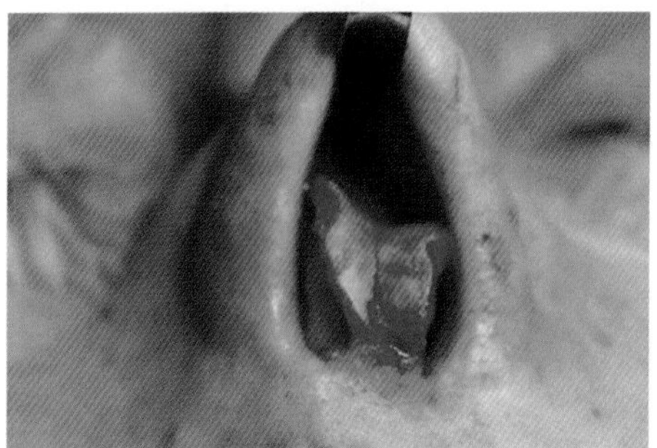

Figure 11 In unilateral cleft lip nose deformity patients, the cleft side alar cartilage has shorter medial crus and longer lateral crus compared to the non-cleft side.

Since the lower lateral cartilage of the cleft side is weak and abnormally shaped, the nostril is usually wide and horizontally oriented. The main reason for the asymmetric alar base in the cleft lip nose is deficient skeletal supporting structure of the alar base in the cleft side. The deformed skeletal structure around the pyriform aperture of the cleft side provides insufficient support on the medial and lateral aspect of the alar base *(Figure 12).*

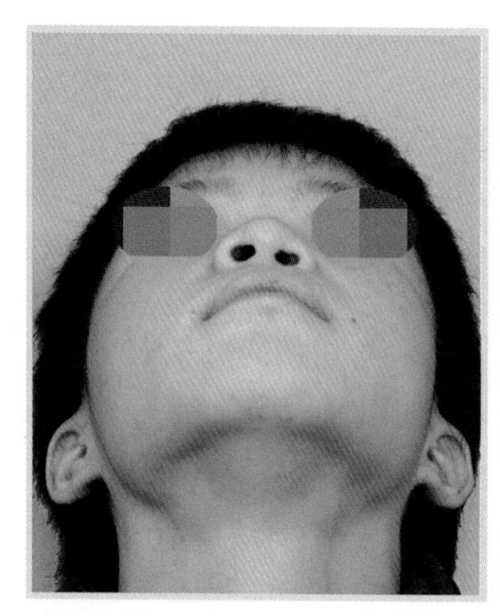

Figure 12 The cause of the alar base asymmetry in the unilateral cleft lip nose deformity is lack of skeletal supporting structures in the cleft side alar base.

The successful correction of a nostril deformity in a cleft lip nose deformity depends on proper execution all the rhinoplasty maneuvers required for cleft lip nose correction. The first objective is stabilization of the caudal septum and securing three dimensional symmetry of the alar base. Placement of a columellar strut is useful in improving symmetry and providing further support for the nasal tip *(Figure 13)*. In order to gain symmetry, the medial crus of cleft side should be mobilized in an anterior-posterior or cephalo-caudal direction. To correct alar hooding, the alar cartilage of the cleft side has to be mobilized more anteriorly compared to that of non cleft side. For a stable long-term correction, the use of thick and strong cartilage as graft material is advisable. For the equalization of the domal height of the lateral crura, a lateral crural steal technique can be used effectively. The dome division technique is also helpful in creating a new dome with equal height on both sides *(Figure 14).*

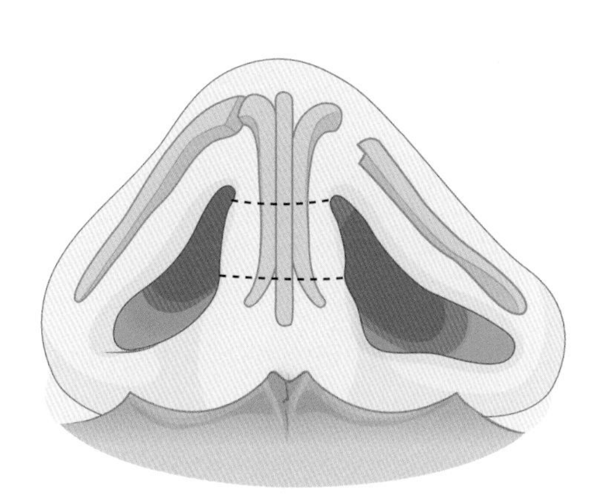

Figure 13 The columellar strut can be effectively used for nostril deformity correction in cleft lip nose deformity patients.

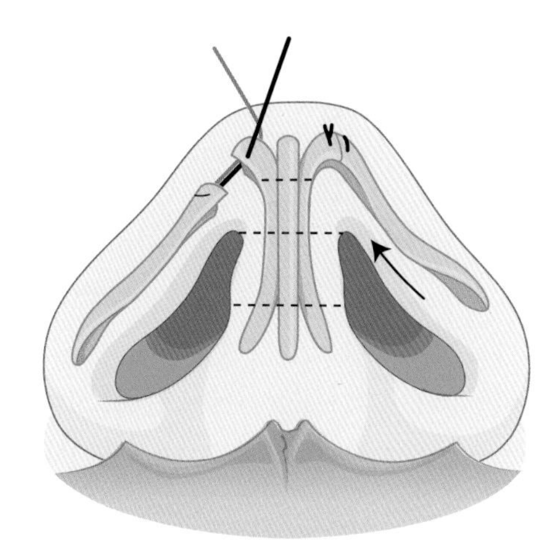

Figure 14 Discrepant level of the domes can be equalized by the use of the dome division technique.

It is advisable to place a lateral crural onlay graft at the cartilage-void area remaining after the dome division technique. Correction of alar hooding persisting after dome division can be achieved by suture fixation of the the lateral crus to the caudal end of upper lateral cartilage *(Figure 15)*. After correction and stabilization of the lower lateral cartilages, one can apply tip grafting, through a shield graft or only graft, which can improve tip support and provide better tip definition. This can further correct irregular surfaces and the remaining asymmetry *(Figure 16)*. A number of options are available to correct the concave lateral crus. One useful technique is upside down placement of the lateral crus after dissection from the vestibular skin (flip-flop of the lateral crus) *(Figure 17)*. Placement of a lateral crural strut graft is one other technique that can effectively correct a concave lateral crus.

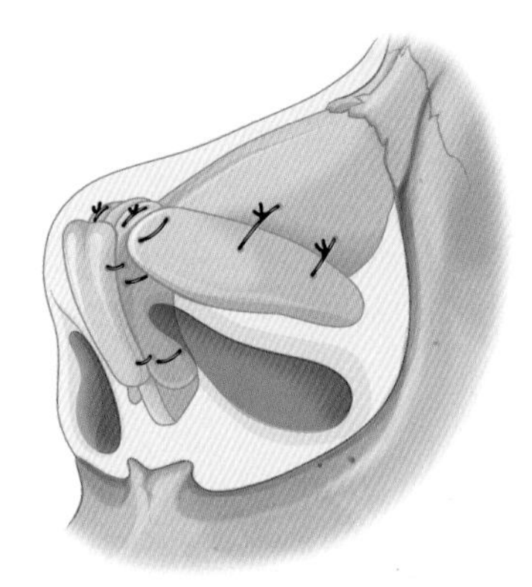

Figure 15 Cephalic margin of the lateral crus on the cleft side can be sutured to the upper lateral cartilage in order to correct drooping of the alar lobule (alar hooding).

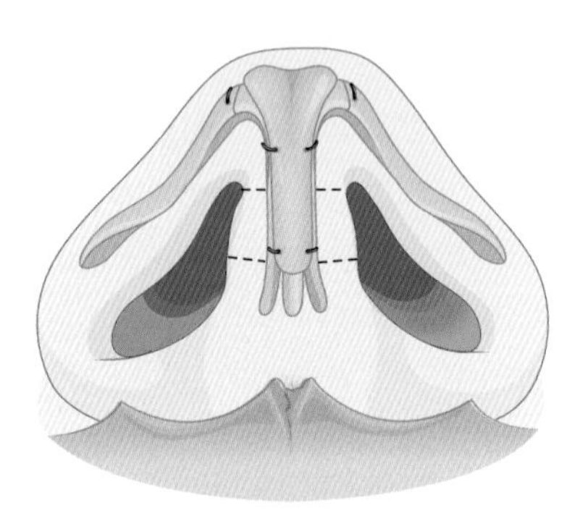

Figure 16 Tip graft applied in order to further stabilize the alar cartilages.

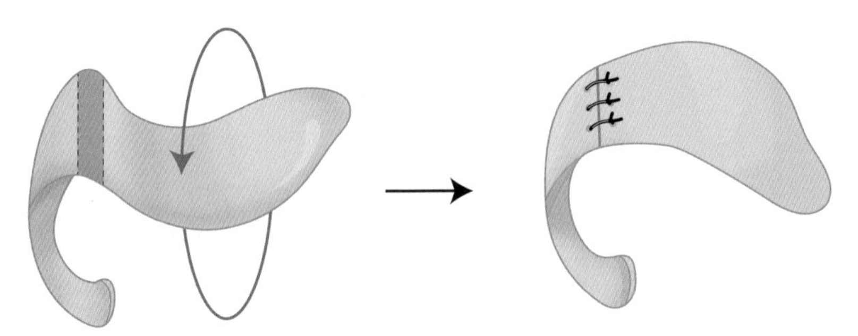

Figure 17 Flip-flop of the lateral crus.

Correction of the alar base deformity is the most challenging aspect in cleft lip nose rhinoplasty *(Figures 18, 19)*. The alar base of the cleft side is deficient towards the posterior, lateral, and inferior directions. The shape of the nostril thus looks abnormal. This deformity can be partially corrected by placement of multiple cartilage grafts on the base of the nostril sill or by doing a layered repair of the nostril sill. Cartilage grafts can be inserted through subcutaneous tunneling via an incision adjacent to the transcolumellar incision on the ipsilateral side.

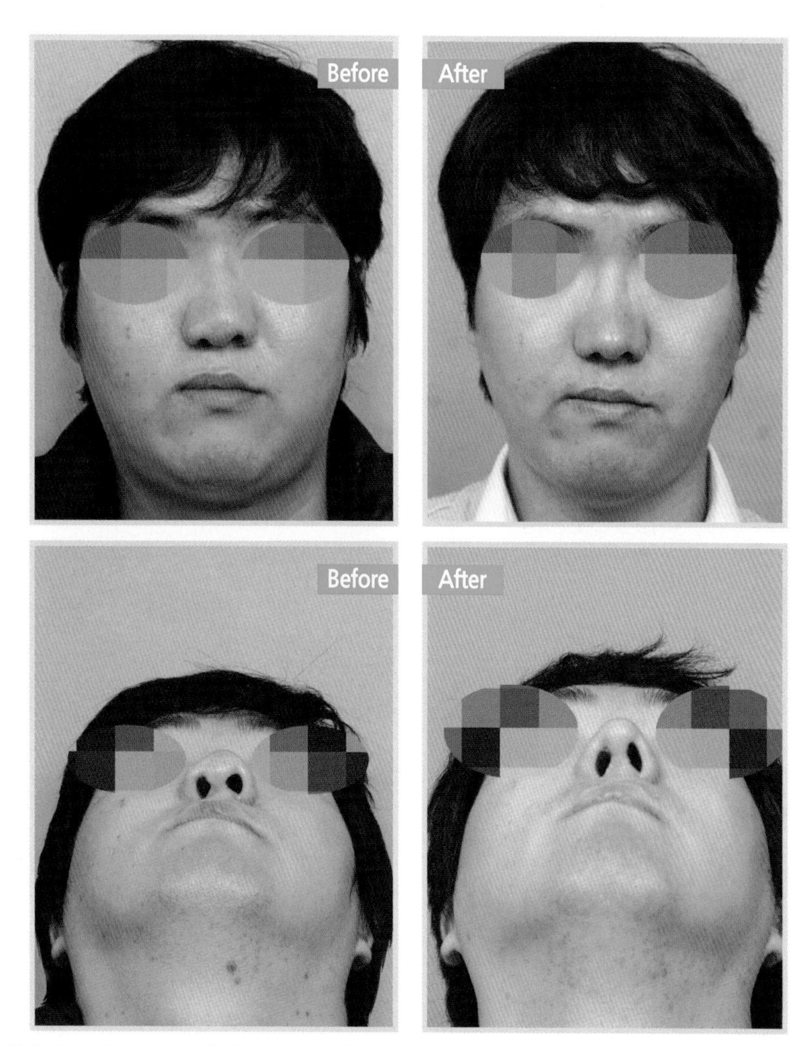

Figure 18 Nostril deformity in a cleft lip nose deformity patients. After surgery, the right alar concavity was improved, but differences in the height of nostril sill and nostril size were not greatly improved.

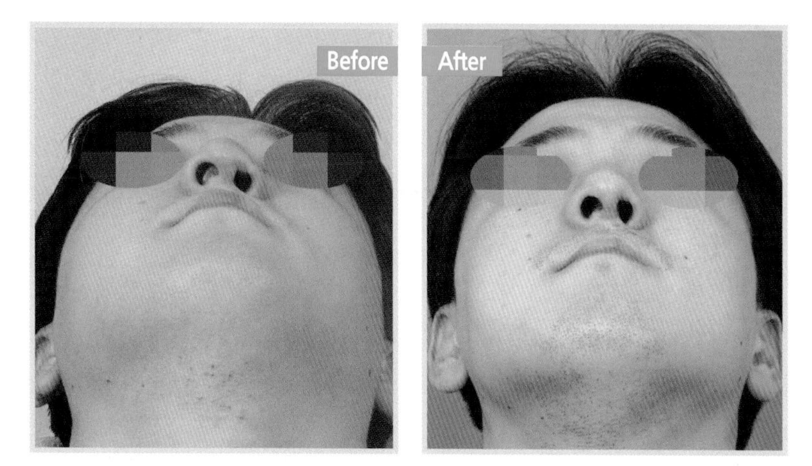

Figure 19 Nostril deformity in a cleft lip nose deformity patient. The nostril shape, height of both nostril apices, and the alar base symmetry have been improved.

4) Nostril Deformity due to Scar Contracture

A variety of nostril deformities can be formed depending on the different types of trauma and injuries to the nose. Minor scars and related nostril contour irregularities can be corrected by combining Z-plasty with an alar rim graft. For correction of a moderate alar contour deformity with notching, the use of a composite conchal cartilage graft may be useful *(Figure 20)*. The ultimate solution of a rather severe scar deformity of the nostril is reconstruction of the alar soft tissue using a forehead flap.

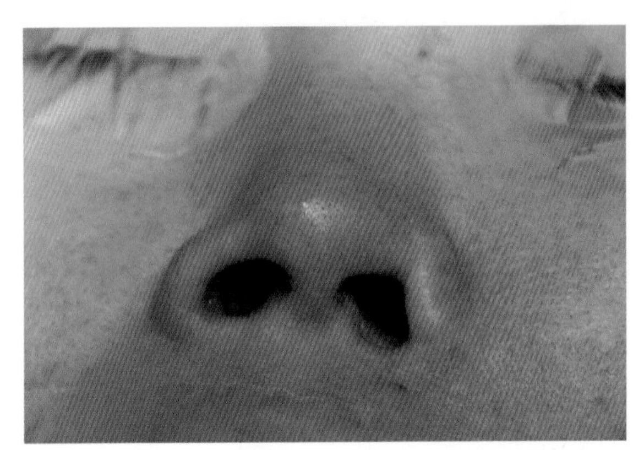
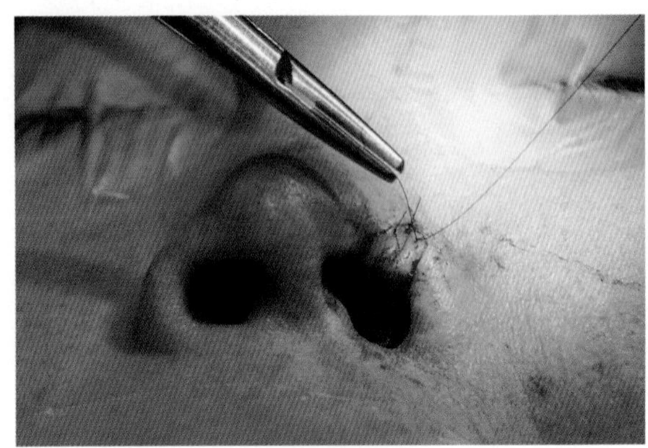

Figure 20 Intraoperative view of a composite cartilage graft designed to correct on alar contour deformity

5) Nostril Stenosis

A stenotic nostril is caused by scarring after smallpox infection, burns, laceration of the alar soft tissue deep in the nasal cavity, and nostril skin injury secondary to excessive nasal packing. Nostril stenosis usually involves circular scar contracture encompassing alar lobule, columella, and nostril sill. Numerous surgical techniques using W-plasty, Z-plasty, V-Y plasty, full thickness skin grafts, composite chondrocutaneous grafts, nasolabial flaps, and mucous membrane grafts have been introduced to correct stenotic nostrils *(Figure 21)*. The basic principle of the surgery is using the stenotic skin as the inner lining after designing it into various types of flaps, or using a conchal

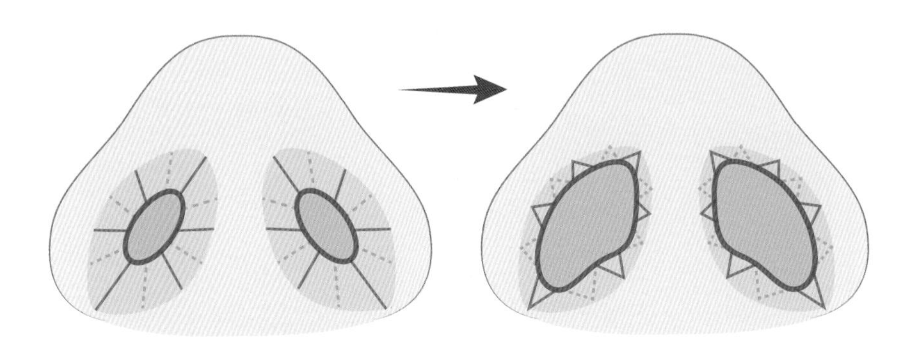

Figure 21 Running V-Y plasty for the treatment of nostril stenosis. Stenosis is corrected by running Y closure of 12 trianglular Y-flap after 6 inner incisions (dotted lines) and 6 outer incisions (solid lines).

cartilage composite graft to serve as framework for the nostril, or to supplement deficient skin areas to widen the nostril *(Figure 22)*. Despite the use of several techniques, the treatment outcome is generally not so satisfactory. Nostril retainers may be helpful to improve the surgical outcome of this perplexing problem.

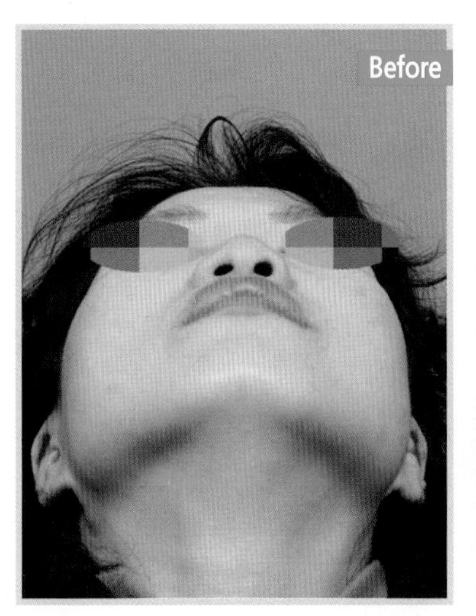

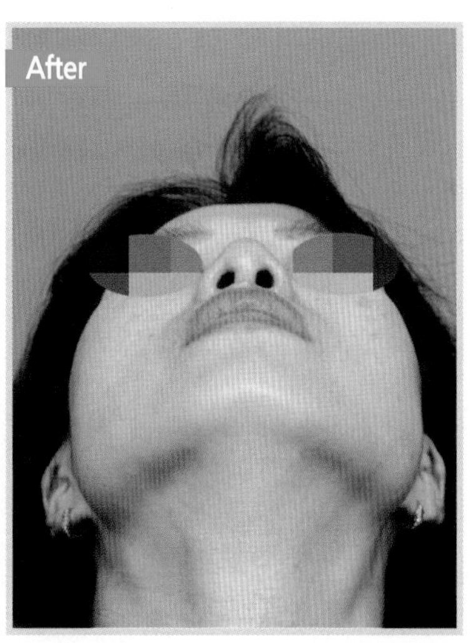

Figure 22 Right nostril stenosis due to scar contracture was improved by using a composite conchal cartilage graft. The narrowed nostril was somewhat expanded after surgery, but not to the size of the contralateral side.

References

1. Adamson PA. Anatomic considerations in the management of the hanging columella. Arch Facial Plast Burrm JS, Yang WY. Modification of running Y-V plasty to correct bilateral nostril stenosis with a circular, linear contracture. J Plast Reconstr Aesthet Surg 2011; 64: 1665-8.
2. Dines SM, Hamilton GS, Mobley SR. A graduated approach to repairing the stenotic nasal vestibule. Arch Facial Plast Surg 2010; 125: 332-8.
3. Gosla Reddy S, Devarakonda V, Reddy RR. Assessment of nostril symmetry after primary cleft rhinoplasty in patients with complete unilateral cleft lip and palate. J Craniomaxillofac Surg 2013; 41: 147-52.
4. Lu TC, Lam WL, Chang CS, Kuo-Ting Chen P. Primary correction of nasal deformity in unilateral incomplete cleft lip: a comparative study between three techniques. J Plast Reconstr Aesthet Surg 2012; 65: 456-63.
5. Sykes JM, Jang YJ. Cleft lip rhinoplasty. Facial Plast Surg Clin North Am 2009; 17: 133-44.

Case 1

A 20-year-old male visited for an aesthetic deformity. He had undergone surgery for the correction of a cleft lip.

Analysis

Frontal: Cartilaginous dorsum deviation, left alar retraction, alar asymmetry, bulbous tip, wide dorsum

Basal: Tilted columella and tip, nostril asymmetry, bulbous tip, wide alar base, nostril sill level difference

Lateral and Oblique: Supratip blunting, poor tip projection and definition

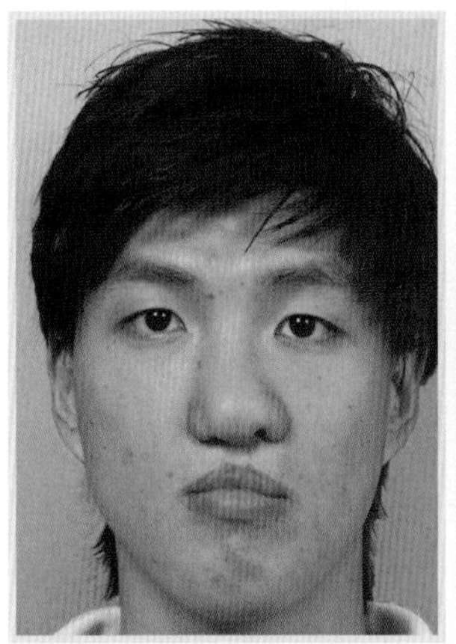
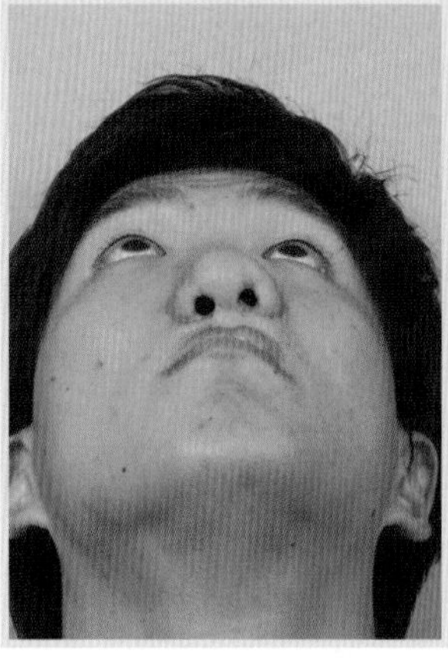
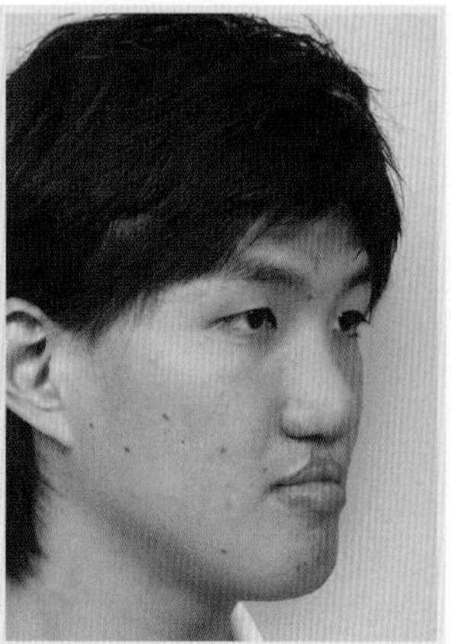
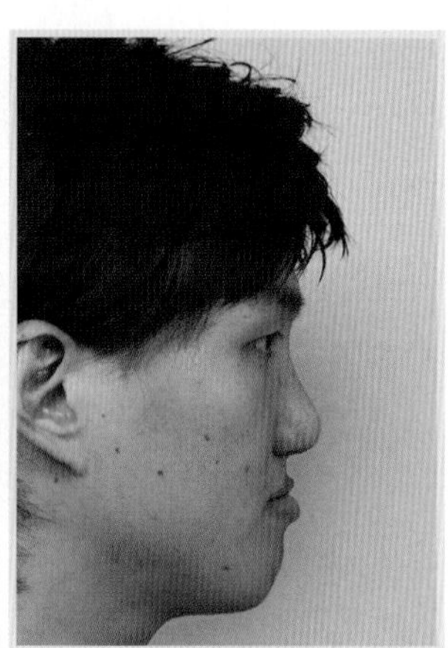

Operative Procedures

Open rhinoplasty approach
Medial and lateral osteotomies
Harvest of septal and conchal cartilage
Cephalic resection
Modified vertical dome division
Columellar strut application
Multilayer tip grafting
Alar base resection (left)
Nostril apex soft tissue excision (bilateral)

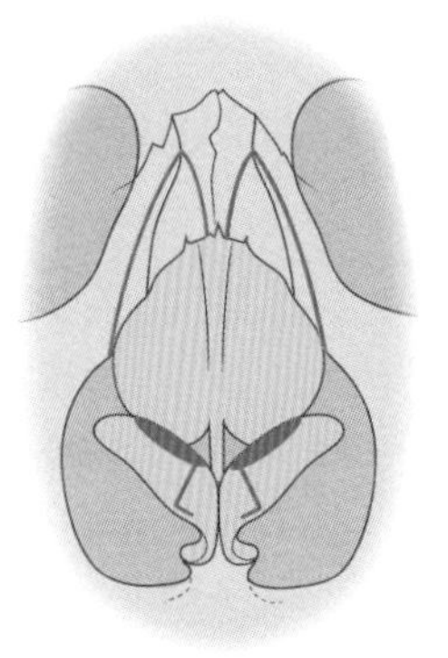
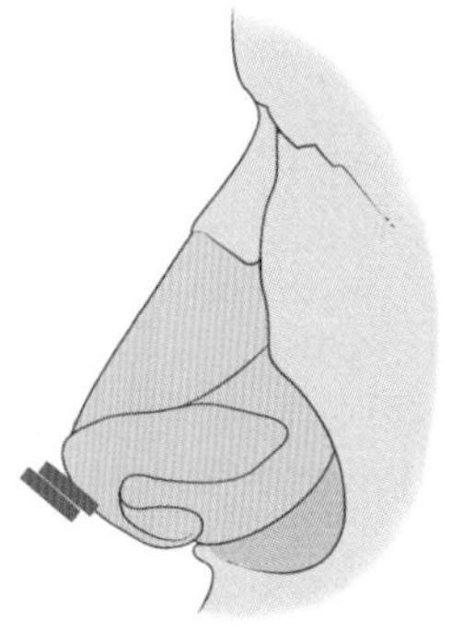
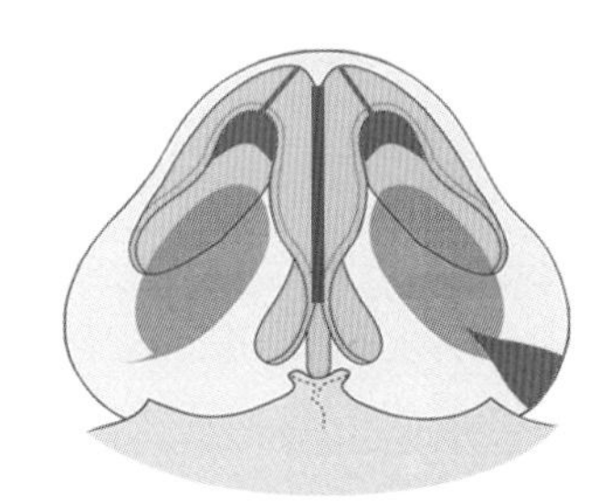

Postoperative Changes

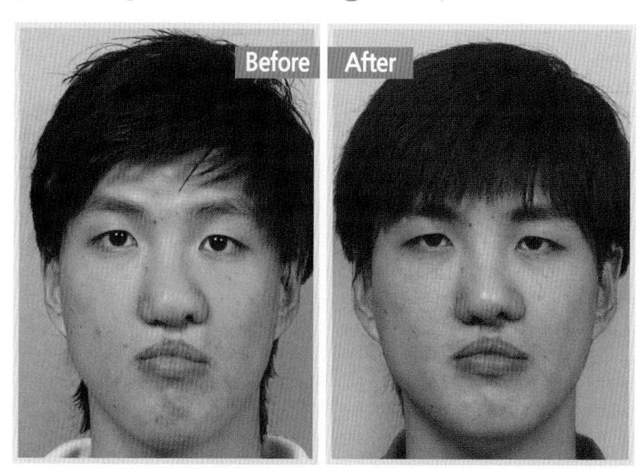

Frontal: Dorsal deviation was corrected. Although the dorsal width was not changed much, the aesthetic lines were improved. Tip definition was improved.

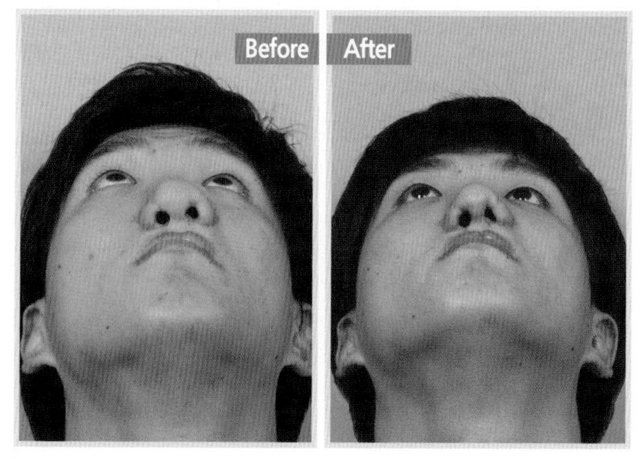

Basal: Tip projection was improved. Nevertheless the nostril sill level difference was not improved. Tilted tip was corrected.

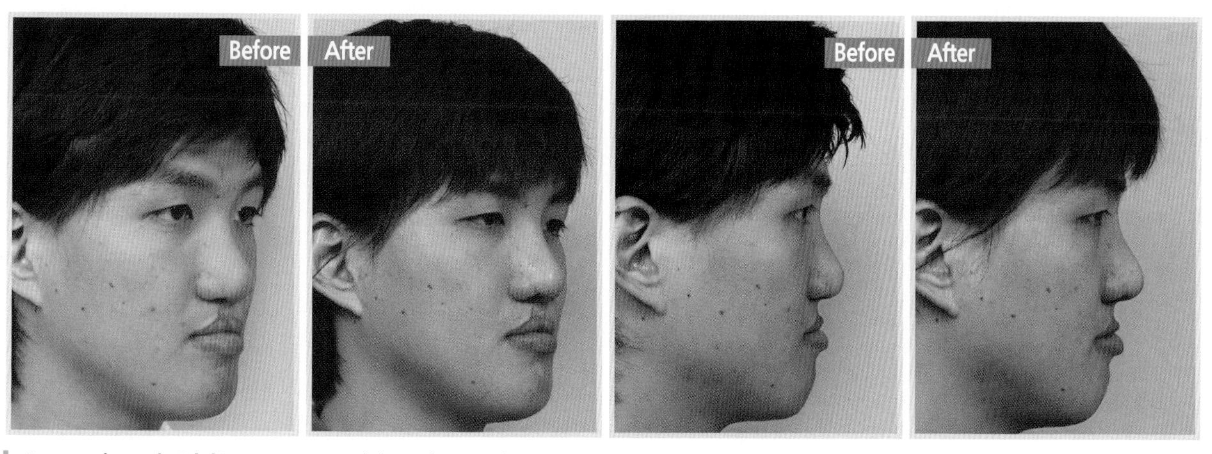

Lateral and Oblique: Dorsal height and tip projection were improved.

Case 2

A 29-year-old male visited for a deviated nose. He had undergone surgery for a cleft lip.

Analysis

Cleft nose deformity
Nostril asymmetry
Alar lobule asymmetry
Deviated nose
Narrow nasolabial angle

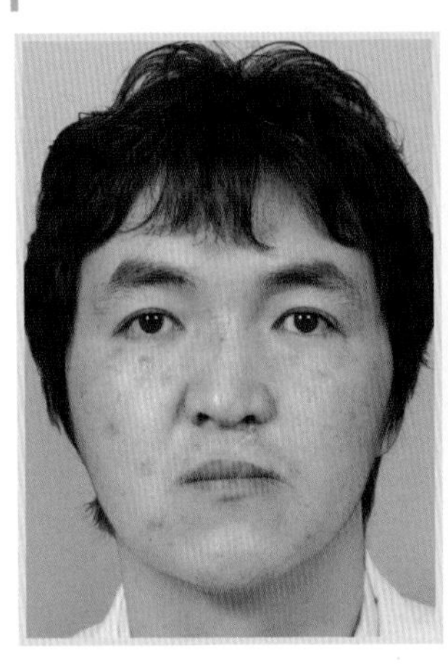
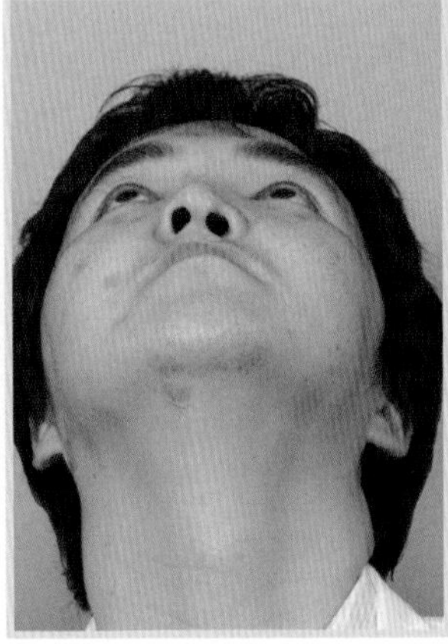
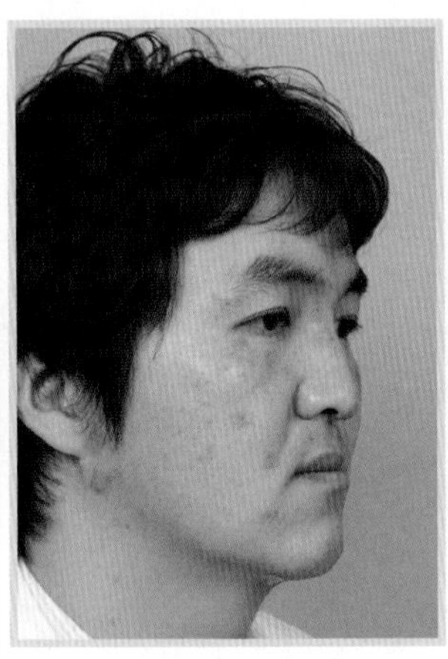
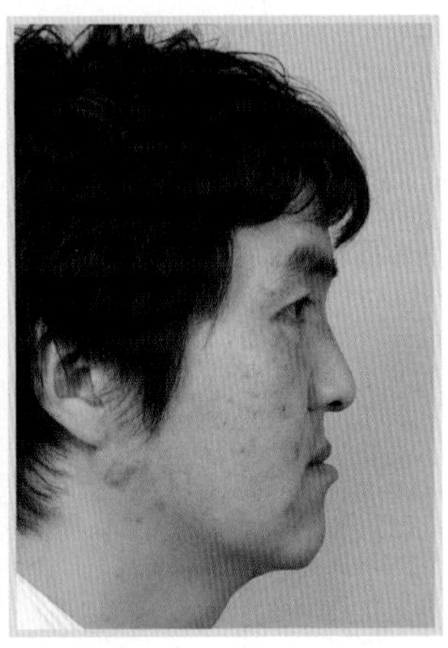

Operative Procedures

Open rhinoplasty approach
Septoplasty and harvest of septal cartilage and bone
Medial and lateral osteotomies
Spreader grafting (right)
Septal extension grafting (bilateral)
Lateral crural overlay (right)
Lateral crural onlay grafting (left)
Tip onlay grafting
Dorsal augmentation using crushed cartilage and processed fascia lata

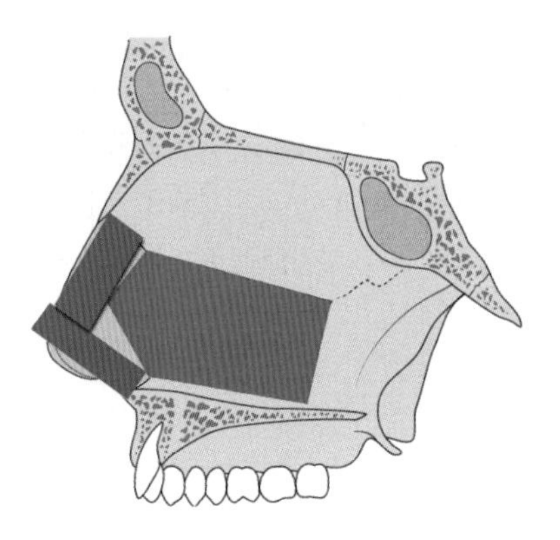
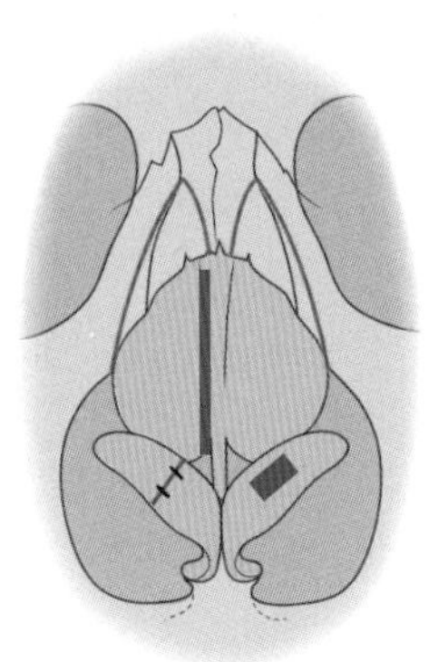
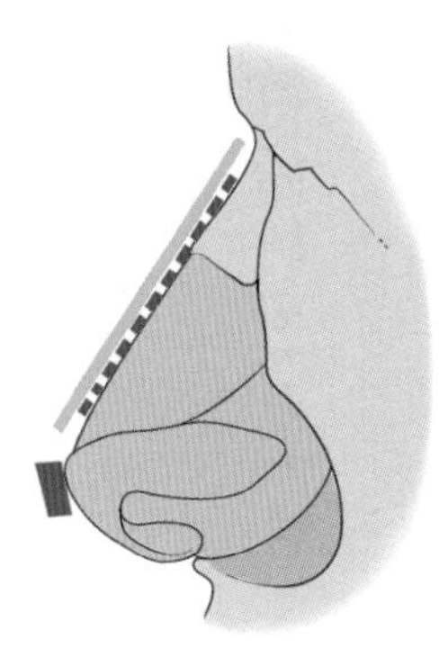

Postoperative Changes

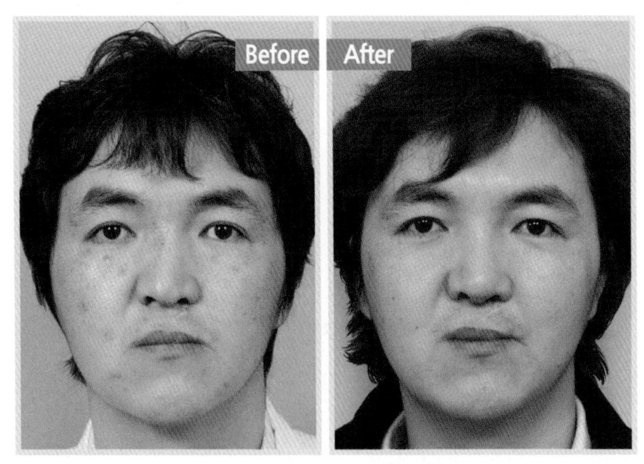

Frontal: Deviation was corrected. Tip definition was improved.

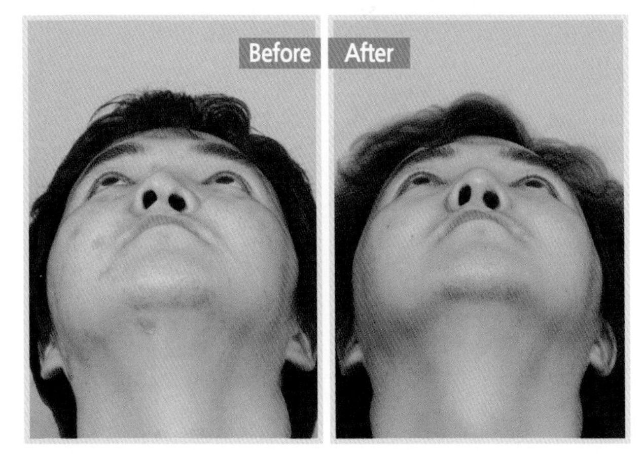

Basal: Left alar concavity was improved. Nostril asymmetry was corrected. Nasal sill level difference remained.

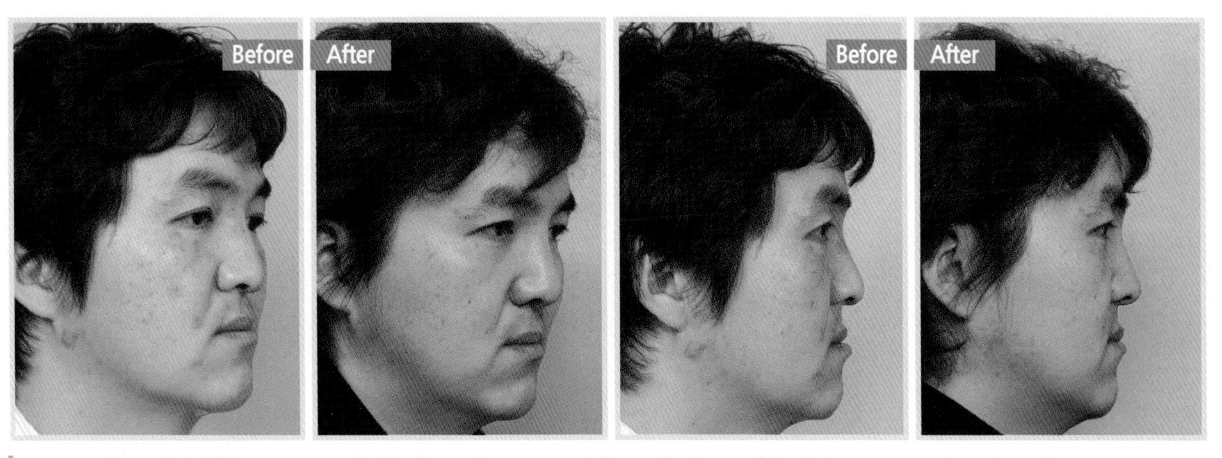

Lateral and Oblique: Nasolabial angle was widened. Dorsal height was maintained.

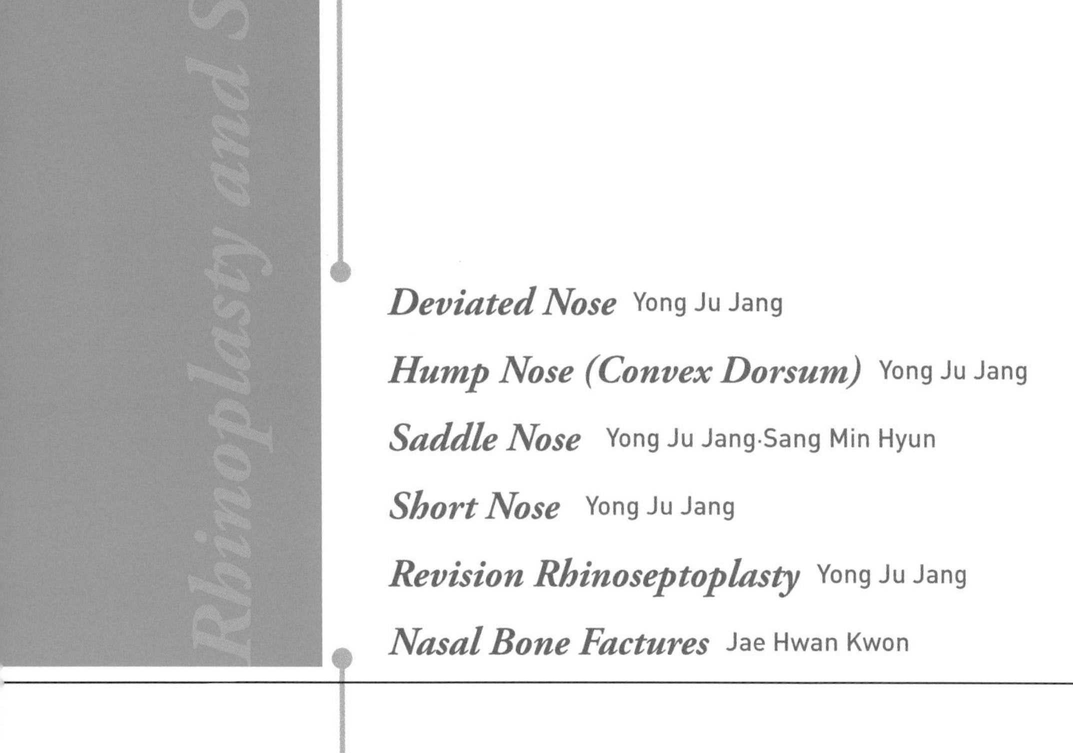

Section 06 *Problem-oriented Rhinoseptoplasty*

Deviated Nose

Yong Ju Jang

A deviated nose is a condition signified by the axis of a nose not being located at the very center of the face; terms such as twisted nose, crooked nose, hooked nose, asymmetric nose, scoliotic nose, and deflected nose are used to describe the condition. Some refer to noses that are twisted from the start to the tip linearly as deviated noses, while S and C shaped deformities are referred to as scoliotic noses, and crooked noses, respectively. At present, there is no established consensus in regard to the definition of these terms.

I. Causes

Causes for deviated noses include congenital deformities *(Figure 1)*, injury during childbirth, indistinct repetitive trauma, obvious external nasal trauma, complication of surgery, infection, etc. However, generally, the most important cause of deviated noses is external nasal trauma. Patients

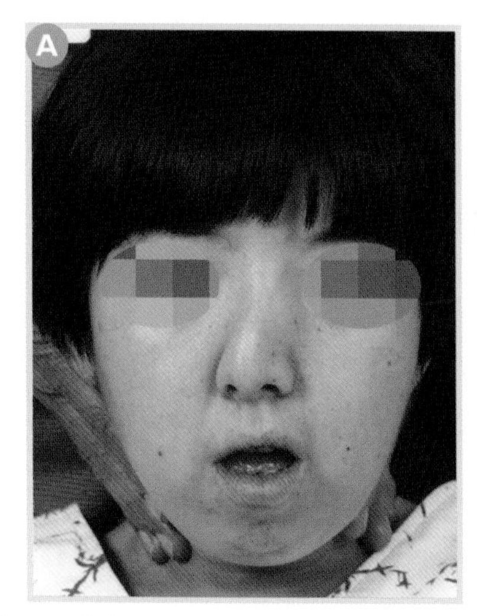

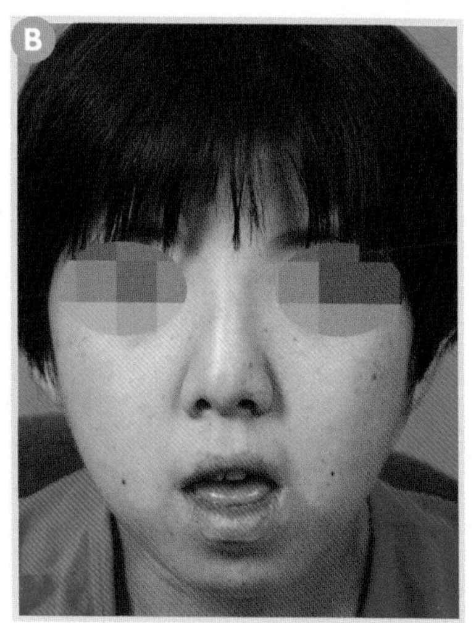

Figure 1 Patient having Rubinstein-Taybi syndrome, characterized by mental retardation and deviated nose. Before operation (A) and after operation (B).

who received closed reduction procedure for nasal bone fracture show a high occurrence of a deviated nose. The reason being is that closed reduction in itself is inadequate for treating damage to the cartilaginous area, thereby completing structural restoration of the bone. Also, traumatized bone is bound to show secondary deformity during its healing. For these reasons, nasal trauma suffered during infancy to early childhood may stay hidden, only to manifest itself as an obvious nasal deformity with the rapid facial growth during adolescence. Furthermore, minute facial trauma in early childhood could result in a severe deformity later on with the continual growth of the chondrocyte.

II. Classification

The author categorizes deviated noses into five different types *(Figure 2)*. The following classification system, based on the author's personal experience, divides the nasal dorsum into the bony and cartilaginous parts, and makes the distinctions according to the directions of each part in relation to the facial midline.

Type I: A straight tilted bony pyramid with a straight tilted cartilaginous vault in the opposite direction *(Figure 2-A)*.

Type II: A straight tilted bony pyramid with a concavely or convexly bent cartilaginous vault *(Figure 2-B)*.

Type III: A straight bony pyramid parallel to the facial midline and a tilted cartilaginous vault *(Figure 2-C)*.

Type IV: A straight bony pyramid parallel to the facial midline and a bent cartilaginous vault *(Figure 2-D)*.

Type V: A straight tilted bony pyramid and a tilted cartilaginous dorsum in the same direction *(Figure 2-E)*.

The above classification is useful in establishing the treatment plan prior to surgery. In the case of Type I deviations, a successful surgical outcome can be obtained simply through osteotomy. In Types III and IV deviations, osteotomy may not be required due to the axis of the nasal bone having no deviation. Types II and IV deviations show severe deformation of the cartilaginous dorsum, which means that the proper treatment of it is quintessential in a successful surgery. Type V deviations are difficult to treat, and the appropriate correction of the caudal septum is the decisive factor for successful correction. These classifications can be applied by analyzing the frontal photograph of the patient prior to surgery. However, more complex deviations may be observed during the actual surgery, and the appropriate application of surgical techniques based on intraoperative diagnosis is very important.

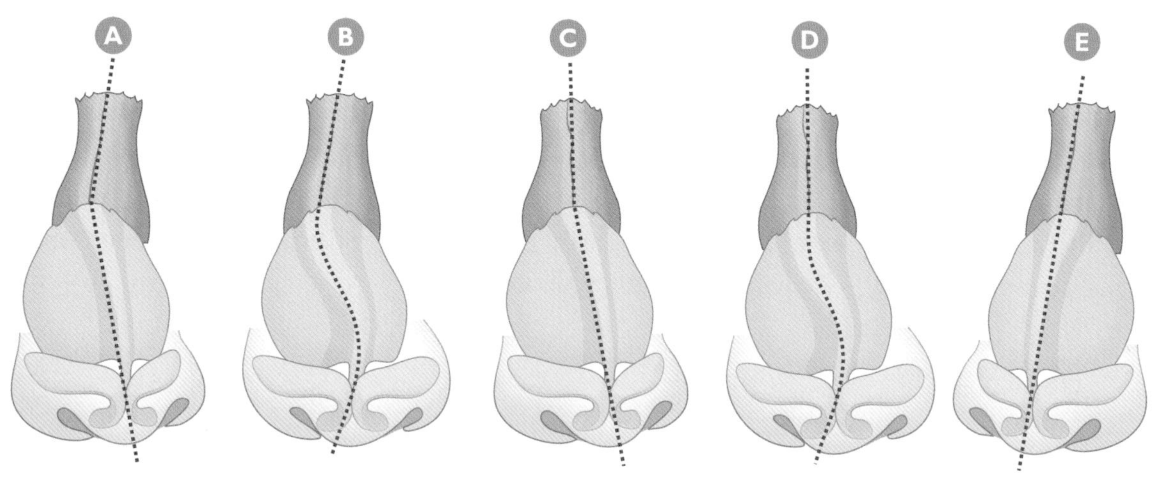

Figure 2 Classification of deviated nose. Type I (A), Type II (B), Type III (C), Type IV (D), and Type V (E).

III. Pathophysiology

1. Deviated Nose Inducing Forces

Deviated noses can be induced by external forces in the form of an asymmetrical attachment of the bone or cartilaginous parts; specifically the bony pyramids, upper lateral cartilages, lower lateral cartilages, or septum. Then there are internal nasal factors responsible for the deviation through the congenital or acquired deformity of the quadrangular cartilage. The first step of correcting the deviation is to remove the external force by separating the junction between septal cartilage and upper lateral cartilages, and the junction between both lower lateral cartilages. The nasal bone needs to be separated through osteotomies. Then the connections between these external factors should be restored through suture techniques or grafting, and the intrinsic deviation of the septal cartilage corrected using the various methods that will be described later in this Chapter.

2. Nasal Obstruction in Deviated Nose Patients

Almost all patients with a deviated nose have an accompanying septal deviation of different degrees. However, not all these patients suffer from nasal obstruction. According to a study conducted by the author, nearly 80% of patients with a deviated nose complained of nasal obstruction. Thus, prior to surgery, surgeons need to keep in mind that there are patients with no symptoms of nasal obstruction; to these patients, surgeons need to explain thoroughly that nasal obstruction can occur as a result of surgery. The most common cause of nasal obstruction among deviated nose patients is the deviation of the nasal septum. There are different forms of nasal septal deviation, including caudal deviation, dorsal deviation, mid-segment deviation, and bony deviation. These forms of deviation require different forms of treatment according to their characteristics. In addition, turbinate hypertrophy, disorder of the internal nasal valve caused by the collapse and deviation of the upper lateral cartilage, deviation of the nostril due to caudal septal deformity, and dynamic collapse during inspiration arising from a weakened lower lateral cartilage also cause nasal obstruction *(Figure 3)*. For precise surgical planning, surgeons need to make the correct diagnosis regarding the actual cause of the nasal obstruction prior to surgery. They also need to keep in mind that in some cases, the correction of structural deformities might not suffice for solving the underlying causes of nasal obstruction.

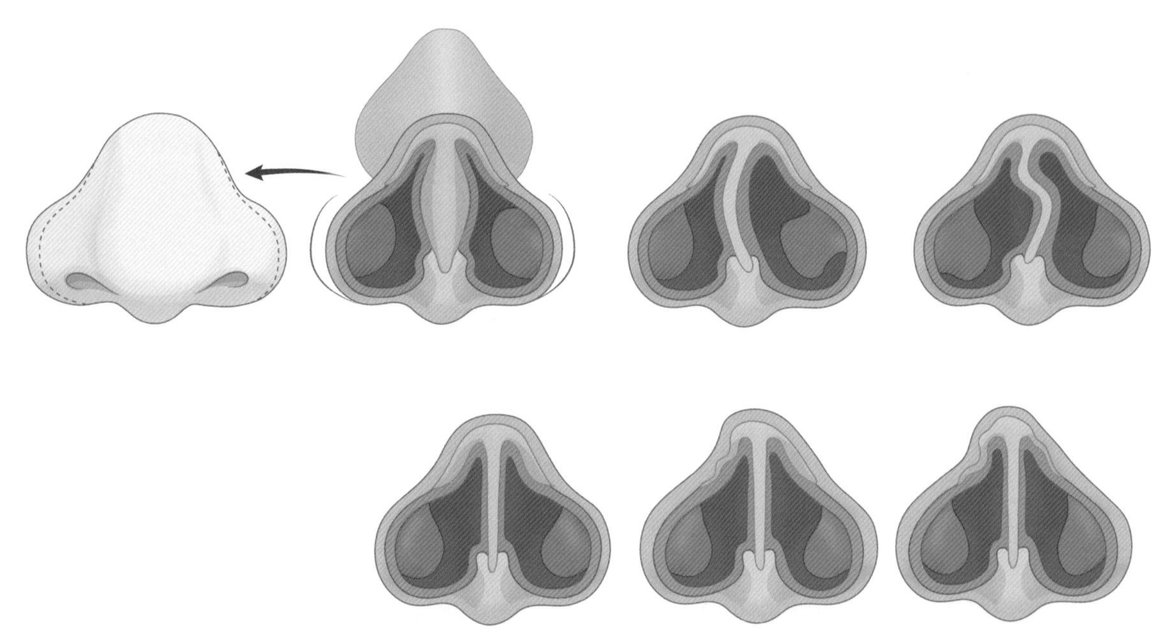

Figure 3 In deviated nose patients, several anatomical factors such as septal deviation, turbinate hypertrophy, and abnormally shaped upper lateral cartilages can be the causes for the subjective sensation of nasal obstruction.

IV. Preoperative Diagnosis and Examination

1. Physical Examination

In conducting a physical examination of deviated nose patients, the surgeon must first listen carefully to the patient's medical history and then perform inspection and palpation from the glabella to the central incisors. Then, an endoscopic photograph of the nasal cavity should be taken, followed by acoustic rhinometry and olfactory function testing in order to evaluate the function of the nose.

2. Photography

Prior to surgery, medical photos of the patient must be taken. These photos must include the frontal, oblique, lateral, and basal views *(Figure 4)*.

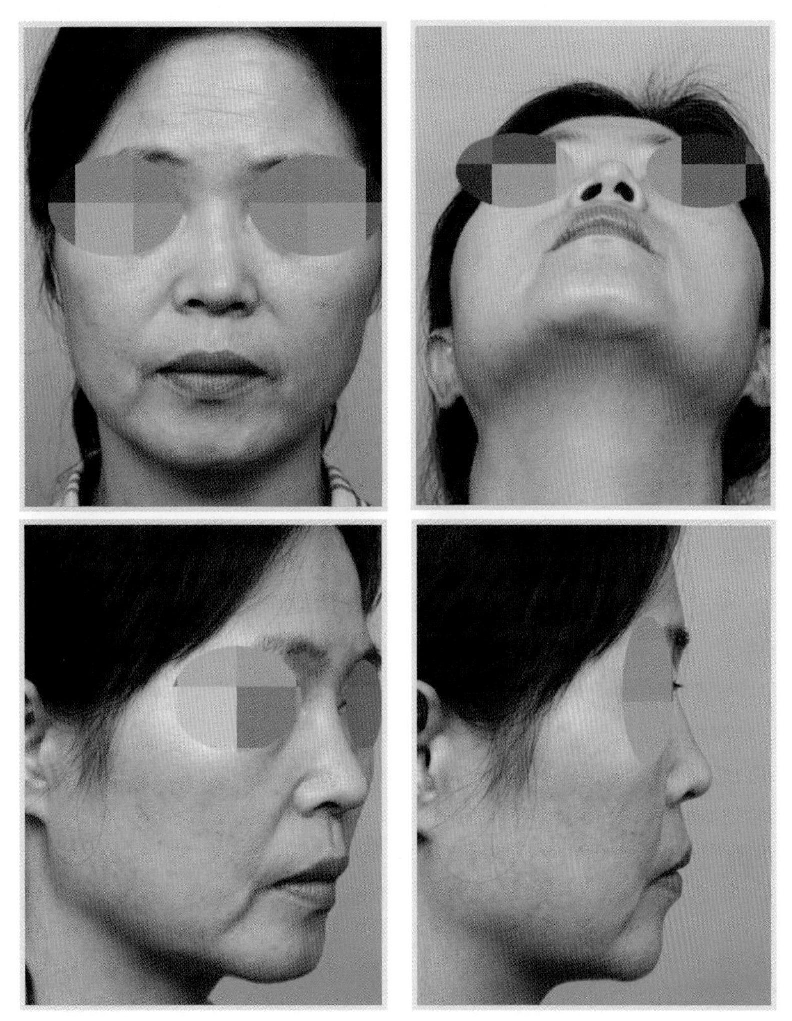

Figure 4 For proper evaluation of the deviated nose patient, facial photographs from frontal, basal, oblique, and lateral views should be obtained.

3. Aesthetic Analysis

To analyze the deviation and the asymmetry of the patient, the patient's nose can be divided into three, consisting of the upper, middle, and lower thirds, to be evaluated with regard to the central facial axis. The upper third consists of the bony pyramid; the middle third of the dorsal septum and the upper lateral cartilages; and the lower third of the alar cartilage, the caudal septum, and alar base. Many patients seeking correction of their deviated noses have unnoticed facial asymmetry of different degrees. With these patients, correcting the deviation will not guarantee harmony between the nose and the overall face, and their nose still can appear deviated even after a well-conducted rhinoplasty *(Figure 5)*. Also, these patients with facial asymmetry often show disharmony in the level of their alar base. This means that these patients' overall satisfaction will most likely be lesser than those without facial asymmetry. Thus, it is important to have a thorough consultation regarding the possible outcome of surgery in patients that have facial asymmetry, and inform the limitation of the surgery in achieving a straight-looking nose. In patients with severely asymmetric faces, it is better to suggest the patient undergo orthognathic surgery first to correct facial asymmetry. Rhinoplasty can be perfomed as a second operation for them. Technically, it is very difficult to make the nose look perfectly straight in these facial asymmetry patients; on the other hand, improved deviation of the nose after rhinoplasty can improve the asymmetric look of the overall face to some degree *(Figure 6)*.

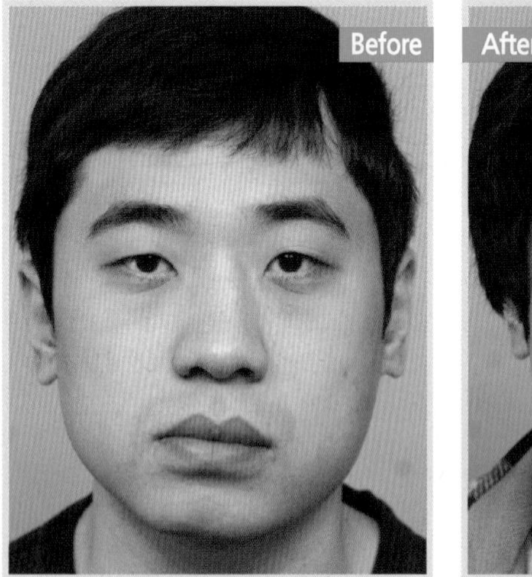

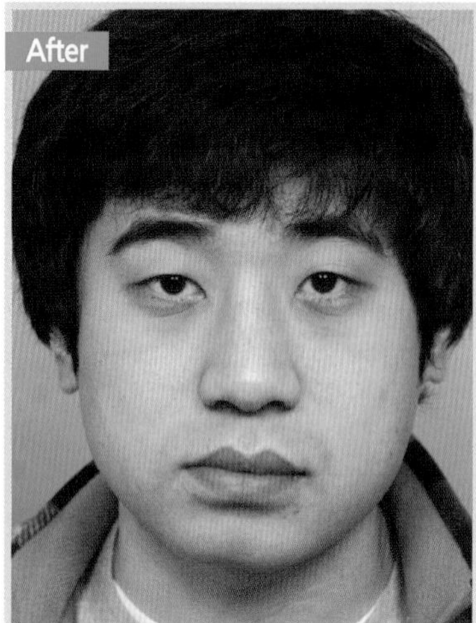

Figure 5 Before and after photographs of a patient who has lower face asymmetry and deviated nose. Despite successful correction of deviated nose, his nose does not look that straight because of underlying facial asymmetry.

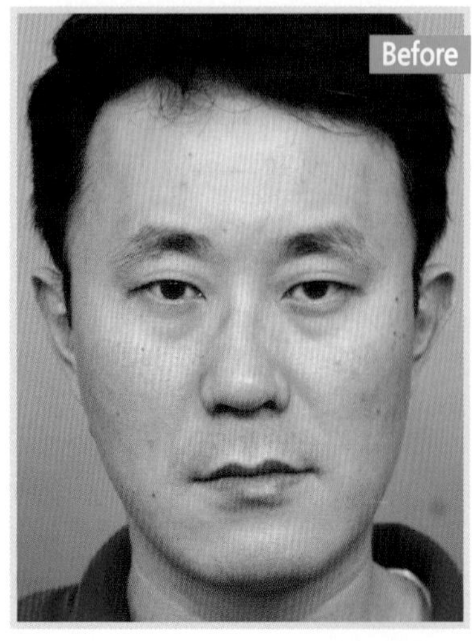

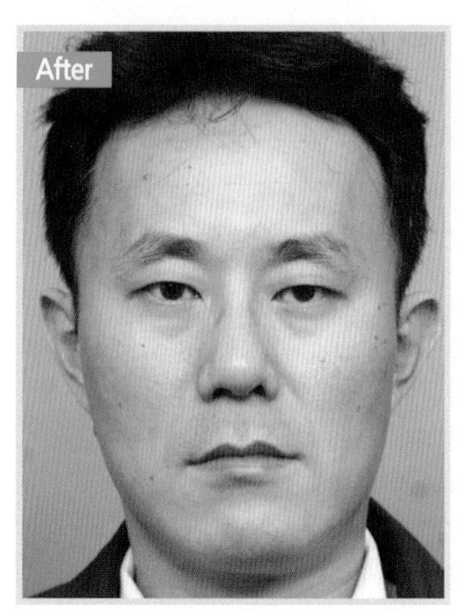

Figure 6 In this patient with deviated nose and facial asymmetry, improved deviation of the nose after rhinoplasty could improve the asymmetric look of the overall face to some degree.

4. Essential Elements in Preoperative Planning and Consultation

During a preoperative consultation, the patient must be informed of the surgical technique, possible complications, and the cost of the operation. Also, it is important to check whether the patient has nasal obstruction or not. The most important factor during consultation with patients is to have them fully understand the fact that perfect correction of the deviated nose is technically difficult; therefore there is a theoretically high risk of imperfection and recurrence. Excessive optimism will likely cause troubles for both the patient and the surgeon after the operation. The consultation should help the patient set a realistic goal. The surgeon should also advise the patient against having unreasonable expectations that their nasal obstruction can be 100% corrected.

V. Surgical Treatment

1. Principles and Objectives

Essentially, the objective of surgery is to achieve symmetry of the nasal airway and the external appearance. However, obtaining symmetry does not necessarily guarantee a successful surgery. For the surgery to be a success, the different parts of the nose such as the nasal dorsum and nasal tip must be in good aesthetic harmony based on the secured symmetry. In correcting deviated noses, the first fundamental rule to follow is to obtain maximum surgical exposure. The second rule is to eliminate the external forces that cause deviation of the septum. The third rule is to make sure that the nasal supporting structures are not damaged by the surgery.

2. Surgical Approach

1) Closed Approach

A closed approach in correcting a deviated nose can be performed using an intercartilaginous incision to access the nasal dorsum, a hemitransfixion incision to access the septum, and a marginal incision to manipulate the tip. When performing a medial osteotomy for correcting bony deviation, the first step is to elevate both sides of the septal mucosa. Then the upper lateral cartilage and the septal cartilage needs to be separated from each other, and through that gap an osteotme is inserted *(Figure 7)*.

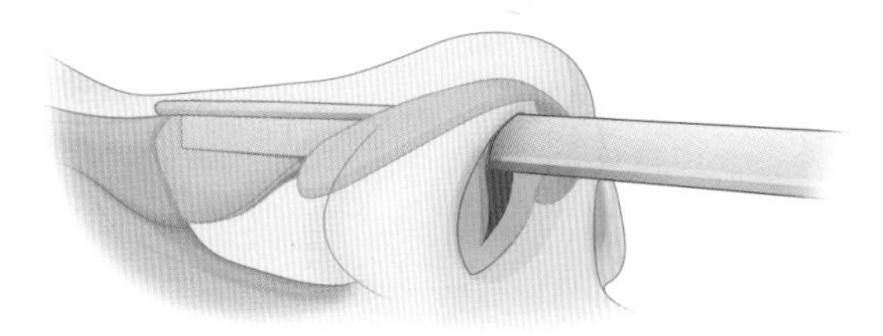

Figure 7 Medial osteotomy via closed approach for rhinoplasty

A lateral osteotomy is performed using the conventional method described in the Chapter "Osteotomy". Correction of the caudal septum can be performed by using relocation sutures of the caudal septum, cutting and suture techniques of the caudal septum, and septal batten grafts. In a closed approach, it is difficult to place a spreader graft, but not impossible. This is done by dissecting a mucosal pocket at the top of the septum, big enough for the graft to be inserted, and inserting the graft into the gap between the upper lateral cartilage and septal cartilage created by an incision in the endonasal route. While it is possible to separate the upper lateral cartilages from the septal cartilage using a closed approach, restoring the connection of both cartilages using sutures is not an easy task. For easier suture reconstruction of the nasal dorsum, wide undermining of nasal dorsal soft tissue using an extended marginal incision maybe useful. Because of this technical difficulty, trimming the convex area of the nasal dorsum and creating a pocket at a concave area of the dorsum to insert a camouflage graft made of cartilage or Gore-Tex are the more commonly performed surgical procedures in the closed approach. Using a closed approach for correcting deviated noses has its limits, in that it is difficult to fully execute the various surgical procedures required for correcting the deviation, in particular (in cases of severely deviated dorsal septum), the various structural reconstruction and suture techniques required.

2) External Approach (Open Approach)

Applying the external approach has the advantage in that it is easier to diagnose the anatomical problems causing the deviation, and that the cartilage can be exposed more extensively – making the surgery much easier *(Figure 8)*. The author highly recommends using the external approach in correcting deviated noses. The various surgical techniques to be described are usually performed under the external approach.

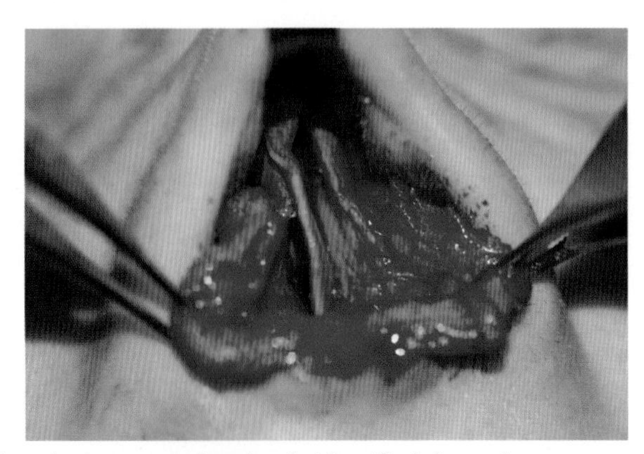

Figure 8 Deviated dorsal septum can be clearly identified through an external rhinoplasty approach.

3. Correction According to Anatomical Location

1) Correction of the Bony Pyramid

Among the surgical procedures used for correcting the upper third of the bony dorsum are osteotomy, rasping, and onlay grafting.

(1) Osteotomy

To correct the deviated bony pyramid, it is important to properly execute osteotomies to mobilize the nasal bone. The objective of the osteotomy in the correction of deviated nose is fracturing the deviated bony vault in order to reconstruct and reshape it into the desired form *(Figure 9)*.

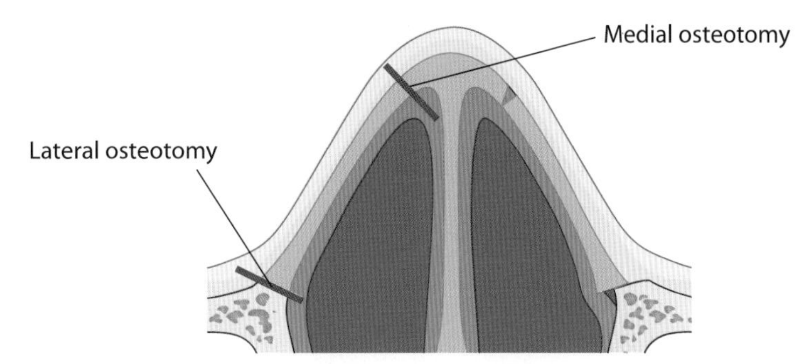

Figure 9 The nasal bony dorsum can be mobilized by performing medial and lateral osteotomies.

A) Medial Osteotomy

Medial osteotomies are used for correcting a broad bony dorsum or severely asymmetric bony pyramid. The bony dorsum must be incised to enable the nasal bone to be separated and mobilized, while maintaining the height.

B) Lateral Osteotomy

Lateral osteotomies ares used to make the lateral outline of the bony pyramid symmetrical. If a greenstick fracture occurs during the correction in question, there is high risk of the recurrence of the original deviation after surgery. Thus, an execution of complete osteotomy ensures a predictable postoperative result.

C) Root Osteotomy

A root osteotomy is used for mobilizing the central bony area into the midline, executed by horizontally incising the space between both sides of the medial osteotomy right under the nasion. In correcting deviated noses, a medial osteotomy is executed and then connected with a lateral osteotomy. The middle part of the nasal bone manifests as a triangular shaped bony septum. If the bony septum's direction is deviated and not corrected, the axis of the nose cannot be placed at the center. If the surgeon uses fingers to fracture the middle part to correct it, the fracture might not occur in the right place, and tend to occur in an area close to the keystone area *(Figure 10)*. Therefore, percutaneous root osteotomy can be executed to mobilize the middle part to the desired location *(Figure 11)*. This is executed by using a 2 mm osteotome at the intercanthal level. This should be done after the dorsal part of the cartilaginous septum is separated from the upper lateral cartilages. There is a chance of saddle nose deformity after the procedure, but can be prevented if the relationship between the caudal septum and the anterior nasal spine is well maintained.

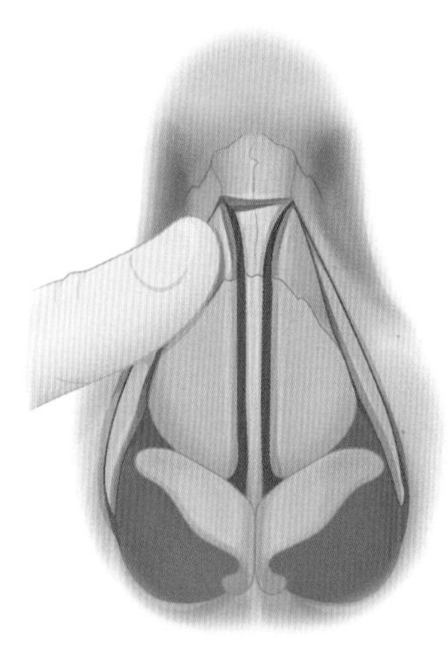

Figure 10 The deviated cental bony part remaining after medial and lateral osteotomies should be fractured to be mobilized at the midline position.

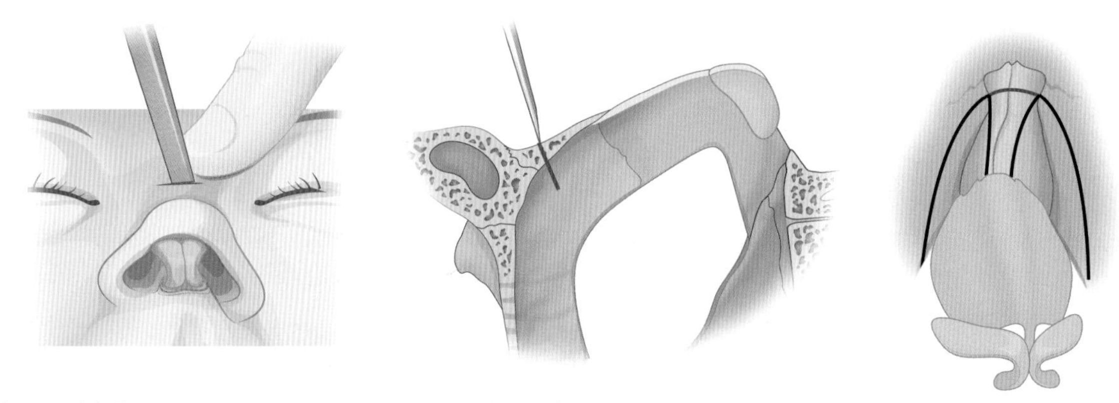

Figure 11 Percutaneous root osteotomy is performed to make a controlled fracture at the midline bony segment remaining after medial and lateral osteotomies.

(2) Rasping

Rasping can be performed on any partially protruding bone or asymmetry following an osteotomy. If rasping is performed after undergoing osteotomy, the bone fragments might fall out. Therefore, whenever possible, it is highly recommended to perform rasping before carrying out the osteotomy

(3) Onlay Grafting

Even after the axis of the nasal bone has been straightened after an osteotomy, irregularity from an uneven skeletal surface can still take place. In such a situation, an onlay graft can be positioned at the partially concave area. Materials for onlay grafts include the ethmoid bone harvested during septoplasty, septal cartilage, fascia, or Gore-Tex *(Figure12)*. If the cartilage is too thick, it needs to be slightly crushed before use. When there are only localized concavities of the nasal bone, onlay grafting will suffice, obviating the need for osteotomy.

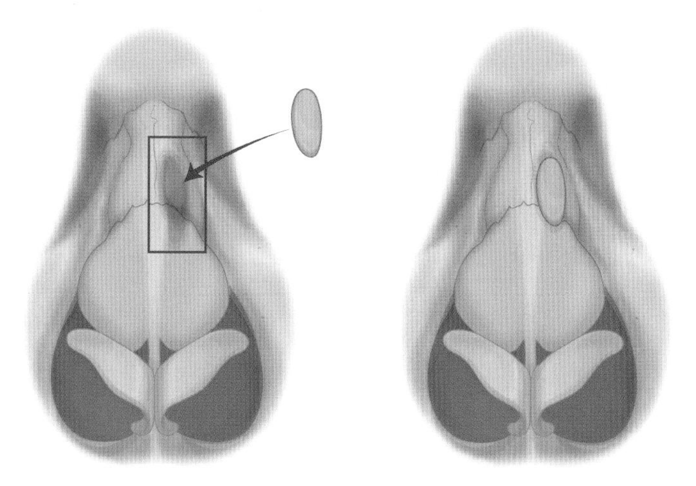

Figure 12 Partial concavity of the bony dorsum can be corrected with onlay grafting

2) Correction of the Septal Cartilage, Upper Lateral Cartilages, and Lower Lateral Cartilages

Correction of the nasal septum is the most important, yet difficult procedure in deviated nose surgery. The nasal septum is located at the center of the nose and plays a decisive role in maintaining structural integrity. Including the septal cartilage, all cartilages have a tendency of maintaining their preexisting shape, thus it is very difficult to correct cartilaginous deviations. The correction of the deviated nasal septum primarily can be achieved by means of a traditional septoplasty using the unilateral transfixion incision. However, it is more reasonable to correct the septum of a deviated nose patient using the open approach because this approach will allow the surgeon a very good surgical exposure through which multitude of different surgical techniques designed to straighten the septum can be applied.

(1) Correction of Septal Cartilage

The author divides the corrective techniques of septal cartilage into two categories *(Table 1)*. In situ correction is a method that involves degloving the septal cartilage, and then making an L-strut, utilizing various techniques in straightening the L-strut of the septal cartilage which is left unresected. Extracorporeal septoplasty involves a near total removal of the severely deviated septal cartilage from its original position for correction, and putting it back where it was after correcting it extracorporeally.

Table 1 Techniques for Septal Straightening

In Situ Technique	Spreader graft Dorsal L-strut cutting and suture Caudal batten graft Caudal L-strut cutting and suture Paired batten graft Resection of the posterior angle and reconnection to the anterior nasal spine Caudal L-strut relocation suture
Extracorporeal Septoplasty	Extracorporeal septoplasty

A) In Situ Septal Correction

(a) Spreader Grafts

A spreader graft is a linear cartilaginous graft inserted between the separated upper lateral cartilages and the dorsal septal cartilage. It is useful when the patient's nasal valve is narrow, as it widens the middle third of the nose – keeping the dorsal line natural. It can also be used to straighten and maintain the supporting structure of the nasal septum over an extended period of time. More than anything else, a spreader graft is most useful in correcting the deviated dorsal septum. It is probably the most commonly used technique in correcting deviated noses *(Figure 13)*. A spreader graft is made from the central part of the septal cartilage that was harvested leaving an L-strut. However, it is often difficult to fashion a cartilage long enough to be used as a spreader graft from patients with small septal cartilages. Even if the cartilage is long enough, there are cases where the cartilage is too crooked for making a suitable spreader graft. When the cartilage is not sufficient in its quantity, the graft is placed only on one of either the concave side or the convex side. However, to widen the nasal valve angle and to keep the dorsal septum straight, it is highly recommended to place grafts on both the concave and convex sides. The graft to be placed on the concave side should be thicker than the one placed on the convex side. If the spreader graft is long enough, it is best to place it through the gap created by the incision of the bone via medial osteotomy, to the anterior septal angle. If the graft is short, it needs to be placed on the left and right sides of the deviated cartilaginous area, to enable optimal correction of the deviation. If a cartilage bent in the opposite direction of the bend of the dorsal strut is used as a unilateral spreader graft, the two cartilages will straighten out after suturing – which means that a bent cartilage is sometimes more suitable to straighten curved dorsal L-strut. The fixation between the spreader graft and the dorsal strut of the septum is done using 5-0 or 4-0 PDS, and the fixation between the upper lateral cartilage and the spreader graft septal cartilage complex is done using 4-0 PDS *(Figure 14)*.

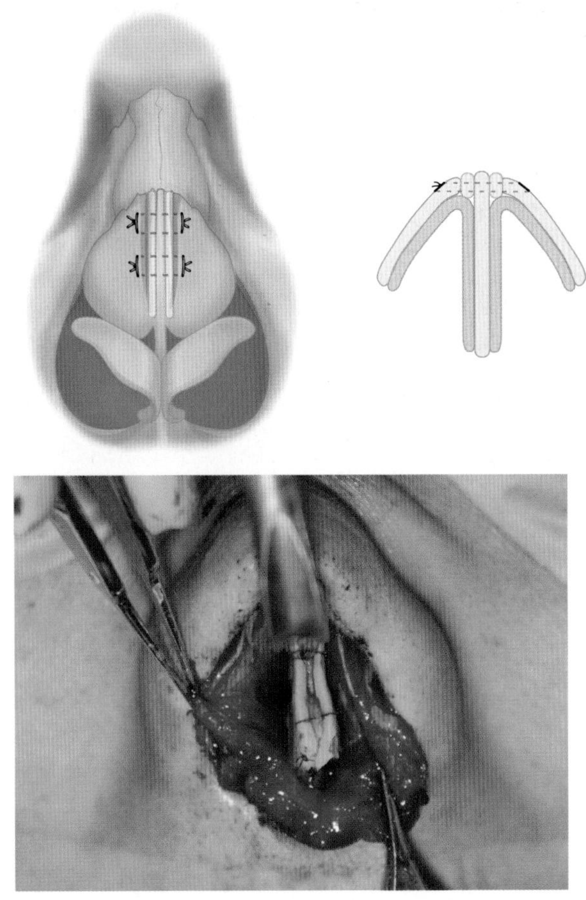

Figure 13 Spreader grafts placed on the both sides of the dorsal septum can straighten and stabilize the dorsal septal cartilage.

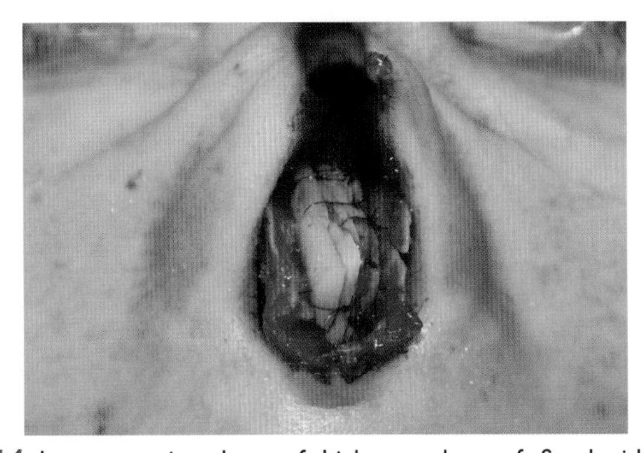

Figure 14 Intraoperative photo of thick spreader graft fixed with 5-0 PDS.

It is also possible to do scoring on the concave side of the L-strut before inserting the spreader graft, or to insert the spreader graft without scoring incision. Sometimes, scoring can weaken the cartilage and cause secondary deformities. If the spreader graft is too thick, it will cause mid vault widening, making the nose not aesthetically pleasing *(Figure 15)*.

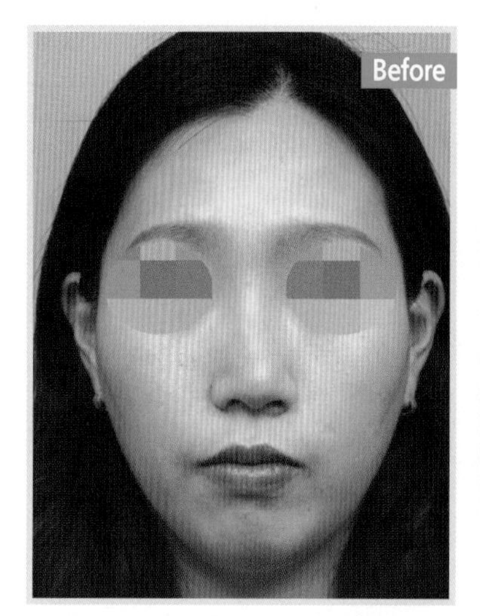

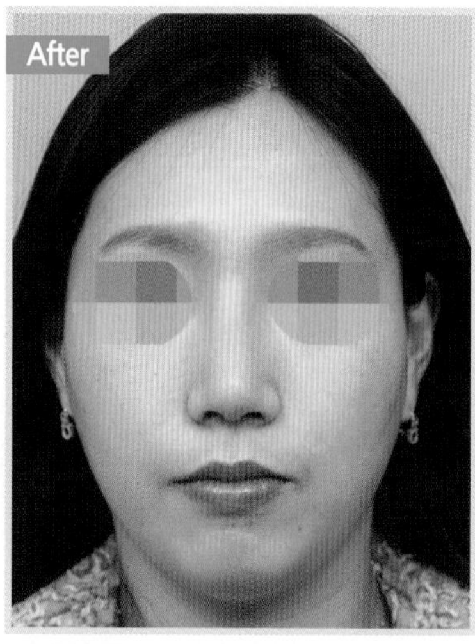

Figure 15 Placement of the spreader grafts may result in a wide nasal dorsum as demonstrated in this case.

(b) Dorsal L-strut Cutting and Suture Technique

When the dorsal L-strut is severely bent, spreader grafts alone will not overcome the intrinsic elasticity of the cartilage, which results in incomplete correction. In these situations, a dorsal L-strut cutting and suture technique can be applied to correct the severe cephalocaudal convexity of the dorsal L-strut *(Figure 16)*. This surgical technique preserves the keystone area and involves cutting the mid-section of the dorsal septum and reconnecting it using overlapping sutures. Theoretically, this technique can shorten the length of the dorsal septum, thereby increasing the cephalic rotation of the tip. However, this adverse effect can be prevented by inserting an extended spreader graft on one side or both sides of the L-strut *(Figure 17)*.

(c) Septal Batten Graft

The author believes that the strength of the caudal septum is the most important factor in the support of the nose. Furthermore, deformities in the caudal septum is most responsible in the formation of nasal obstruction. This means that straightening and strengthening the caudal septum is the most important step in a functionally and aesthetically successful surgery for deviated noses. Placement of a septal batten graft made from the cartilage of the mid-part of the septum at the caudal L-strut with or without scoring on the concave side of the caudal septum is a very effective technique in correcting caudal septal deviation. When placing a batten graft without scoring, suturing cartilage bent in the opposite direction of the caudal septal deviation can help straighten the cartilaginous deviation *(Figure 18)*. The batten graft should be placed on the concave side,

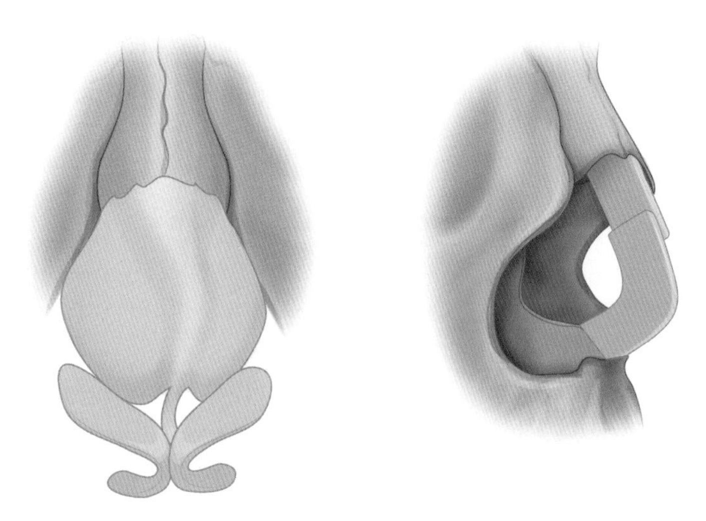

Figure 16 Cutting and suture technique to correct severely bent dorsal L-strut

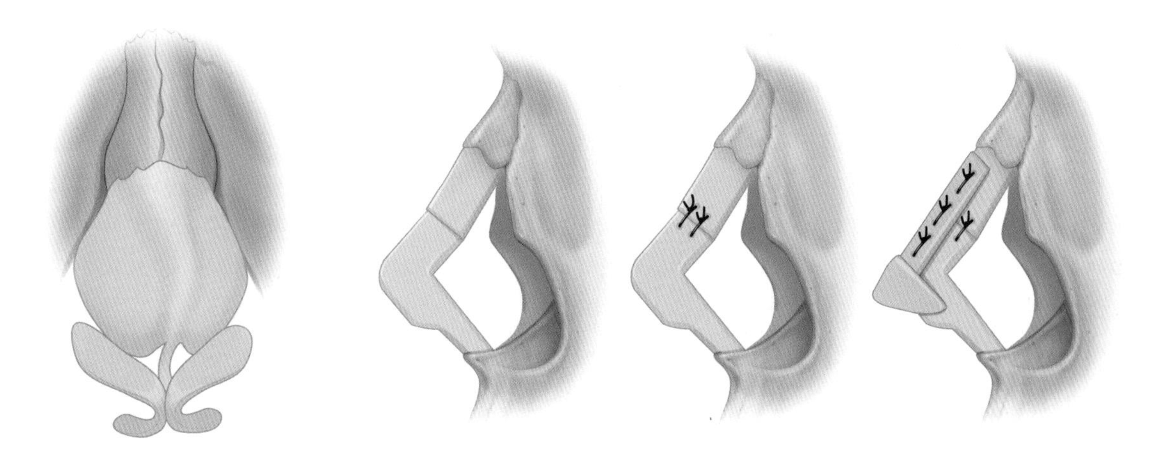

Figure 17 Shortening of the dorsal L-strut after cutting and suture technique can be prevented by the placement of an extended spreader graft.

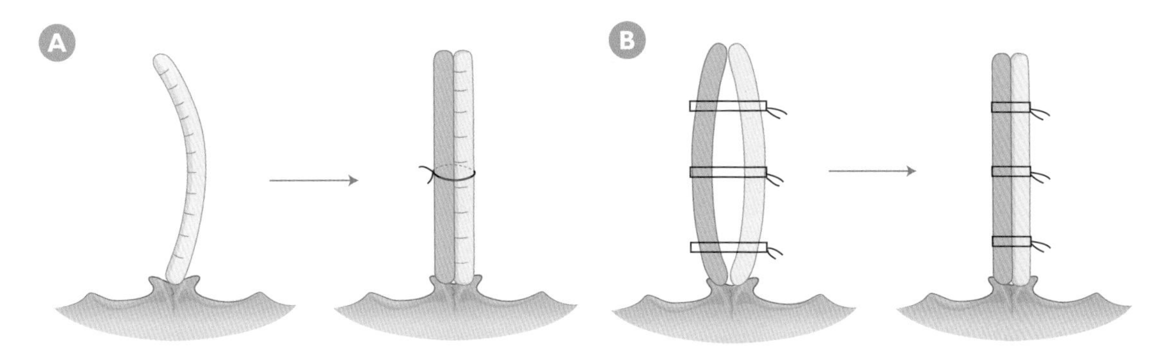

Figure 18 Septal batten graft placed at the concave side of the caudal septum after scoring (A). Placement of a septal batten graft bent in the opposite direction of the caudal septal deviation (B).

otherwise a batten placed on the convex side can further narrow the nasal airway. The length of the septal batten graft will differ according to the size of the cartilage available. If the batten graft is extended to the caudal or the anterior direction to induce change in shape of the tip, this can be called a caudal septal extension graft.

(d) Use of Septal Bone for Correction of the Caudal Septum

To apply a septal batten graft or a spreader graft, septal cartilage wide and long enough is required. In some cases, the quantity of the septal cartilage will not be sufficient for septal batten grafting or spreader grafting. Furthermore, the harvested septal cartilage is very useful in tip surgery, which means that the surgeon needs to secure enough cartilage for both septal straightening and tip work. The insufficiency of septal cartilage can be solved through harvesting the costal cartilage, but this will lengthen the time required for surgery and can induce an increase in morbidity. Performing septoplasy for deviated noses involves removing the central part of the quadrangular cartilage, and the perpendicular plate, and parts of the vomer of the ethmoid bone. The removed bones are usually disposed. However, if the surgeon uses the removed bones for grafting purposes, enough cartilage for tip work can be saved. This will ensure that the surgeon has decreased need for harvesting additional cartilage like conchal or the costal cartilages.

In order to get a nice bony piece suitable for use, the surgeon needs to remove the perpendicular plate from both the vomer and the ethmoid bone in one piece, using septal scissors. To prevent damage to the cribriform plate, the surgeon must be careful not to rock the bone when cutting. Using scissors and a drill, the harvested bone graft is designed to the appropriate size and shape. Then a number of holes need to be drilled, which will ensure easier suturing *(Figure 19)*. The author performs quilting mattress sutures or through and through sutures with a 5-0 PDS to fix the bone graft to the L-strut. These methods will ensure sturdy fixation of the graft to either one or both sides of the caudal or dorsal part of the L-strut *(Figures 20, 21)*.

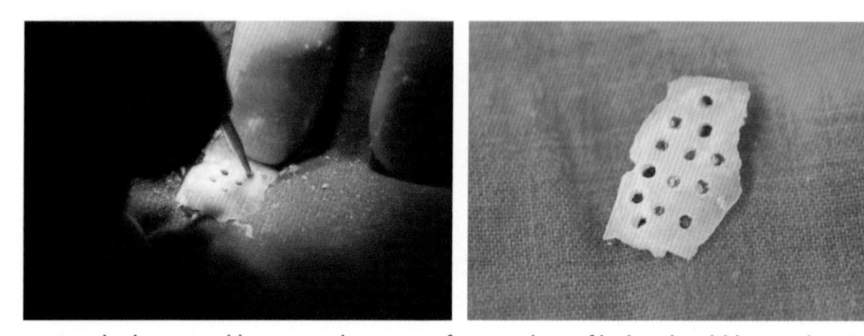

Figure 19 Before using the harvested bone as a batten graft, a number of holes should be made using an ear surgery drill.

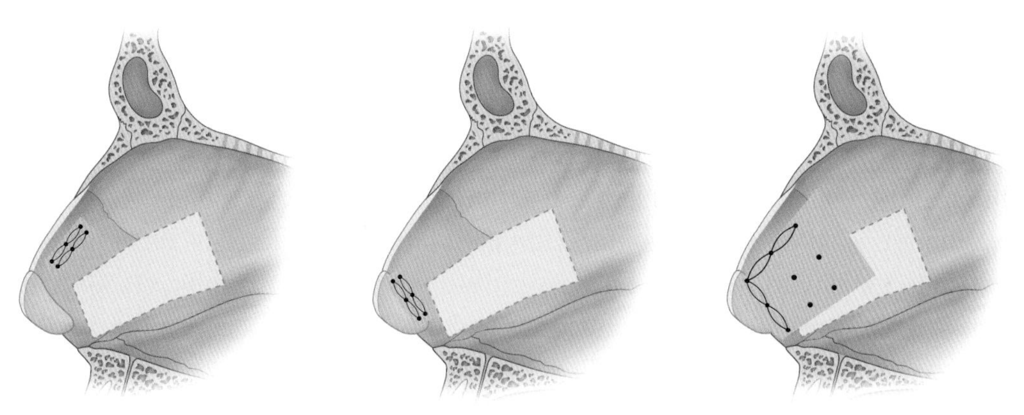

Figure 20 Bone grafts can be applied at various locations in various shapes.

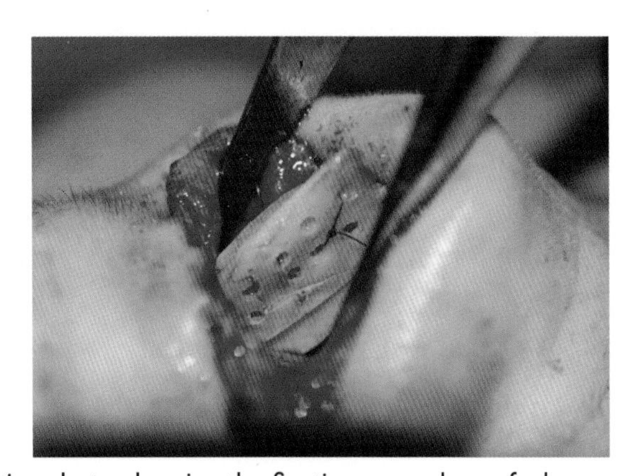

Figure 21 Intraoperative photo showing the fixation procedure of a bone graft to the caudal septum

The septal bone is thin and strong, which means that a stable caudal septum-strut complex can be made without affecting airway patency. Also, this surgical technique will avoid donor site morbidity caused by additional harvesting, and will not require foreign material. Using the bony septum will enable the surgeon to use more cartilage for tip grafting and augmentation. This surgical technique is suitable for patients having a small septal cartilage and wide bony septum with no deviation, patients with a history of septorhinoplasty, or in cases where the surgeons wants to avoid additional donor site morbidity.

(e) Resection of the Posterior Angle of the Septum

Caudal septal deviation in anteroposterior direction is caused by excessive nasal septal cartilage between the maxillary crest and the nasal roof. To straighten this, a small piece of septal cartilage from the junctional area between the anterior nasal spine can be removed, which will enable the caudal septum to become straight *(Figure 22)*. However, the cartilage needs to be reconnected to the anterior nasal spine and the maxillary crest, but it is difficult to reconstruct it with the same stability as before the removal. This reconstruction is difficult due to the three dimensional relationship between the cartilage and the bony shelf – the nasal spine and the maxillary crest is bent inwards in the nasal cavity. In cases where the posterior angle of the septal cartilage is dislocated from the anterior nasal spine, the excess portion of the dislocated caudal sepum should be excised, and the connection with the anterior nasal spine reestablished. When performing this maneuver, instantaneous straightening of the caudal septum can be verified, but could result in saddling due to the shortening of the caudal septum. Also, if the cartilage is very stiff and thick, incising the lower part will not ensure straightening. In these cases, additional placement of batten grafts is required. The most important part in correctly performing this fixation is to leave enough soft tissue around the spine during the dissection of the anterior nasal spine. If there is not enough soft tissue around the spine, holes need to be drilled in the bone to be able to fix it to the septal cartilage. However, not only is this surgical process technically difficult, it can also damage the stability of the nasal spine. If possible, leaving some soft tissue around the posterior septal angle and connecting it with the soft tissue around the anterior nasal spine will ensure stability of the caudal septum.

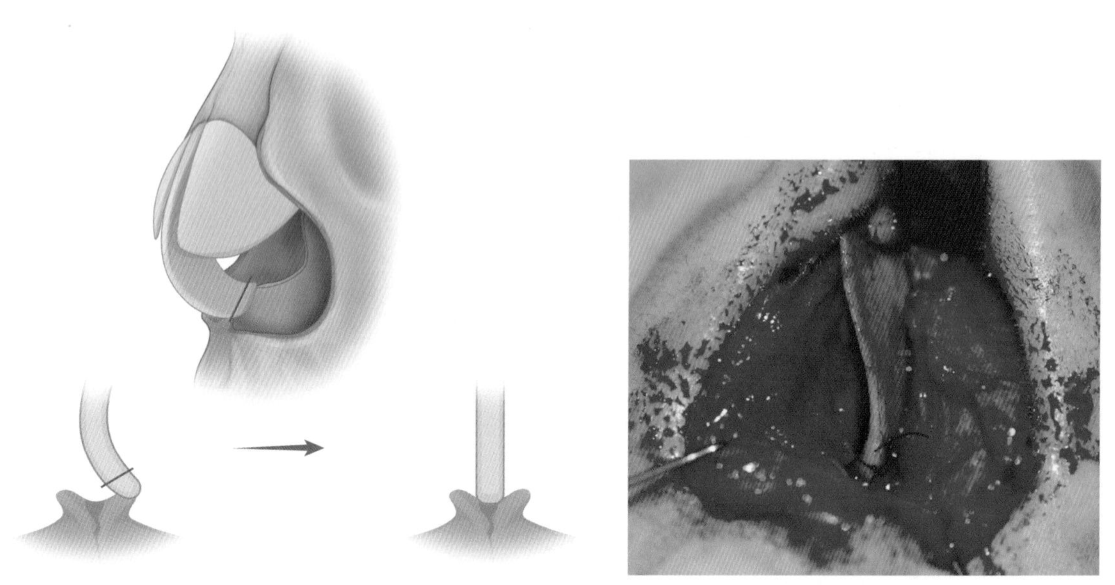

Figure 22 To straighten the deviated caudal septum, a small piece of septal cartilage from the junction between the anterior nasal spine can be removed, which will enable the caudal septum to become straight.

(f) Cutting and Suture Technique of the Caudal Septum

In cases of caudal septal deviation in the anteroposterior direction, a C-shaped convexity or acute angulations can be observed occasionally. To correct these deformities, the convex most part of the caudal L-strut septum can be incised and repaired with overlapping sutures. After the incision is made, the upper part is medialized and overlapped with lower part using three to four stitches using 5-0 PDS. When cutting and overlapping sutures are applied, immediate correction of the cartilage is identifiable *(Figure 23)*. When overlapping the cut cartilages, the surgeon must be cautious not to make the new height of the caudal septum shorter than its original height. If the stability of the newly built caudal septum is in question, a septal batten graft made from the central part of the cartilage or bone should be placed on the concave side for additional support *(Figure 24)*. If an increase in tip projection is needed, a septal extension graft should be applied. This will appropriately correct severely the bent caudal septum.

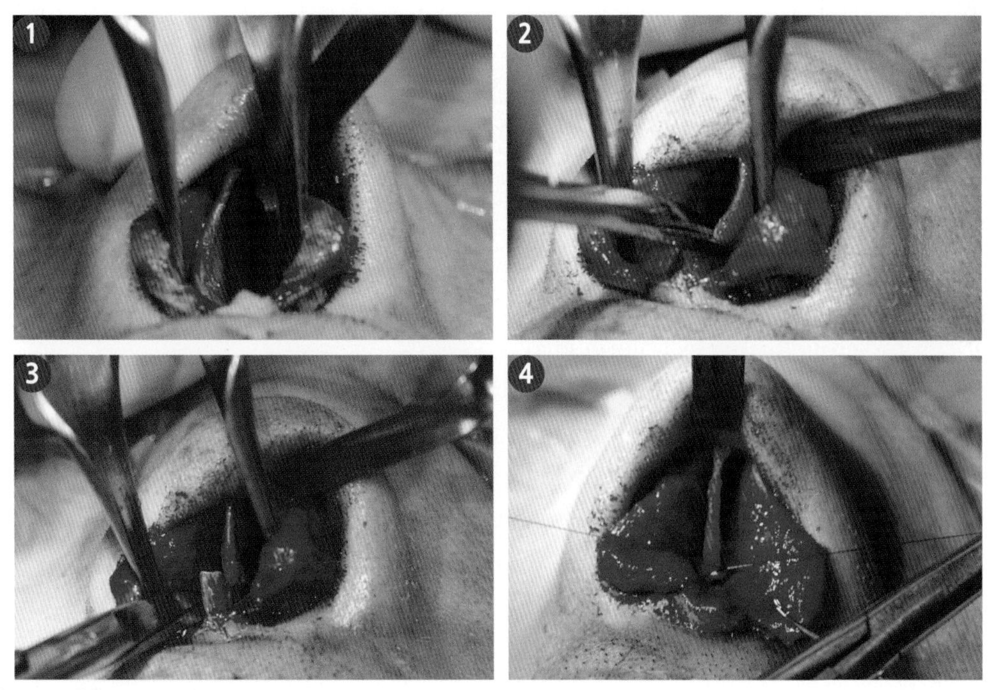

Figure 23 Intraoperative photo of cutting and suture technique to correct caudal septal deviation.

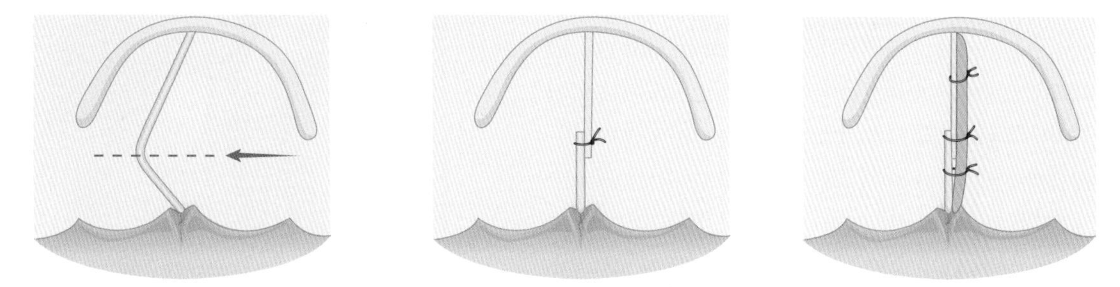

Figure 24 Illustration of caudal septum cutting and suture technique. Placement of a batten graft on the concave side of the septum can compensate for weakening of the caudal septum by this technique.

(g) Caudal Septal Relocation Suture

In cases of linear deviation where the nose appears to be deviated to one side, the caudal septum needs to be separated from the anterior nasal spine and then relocated to the opposite side – making the connection between the anterior nasal spine in a side-to-side manner *(Figure 25)*. If there is enough soft tissue around the anterior nasal spine, suturing will suffice for the procedure.

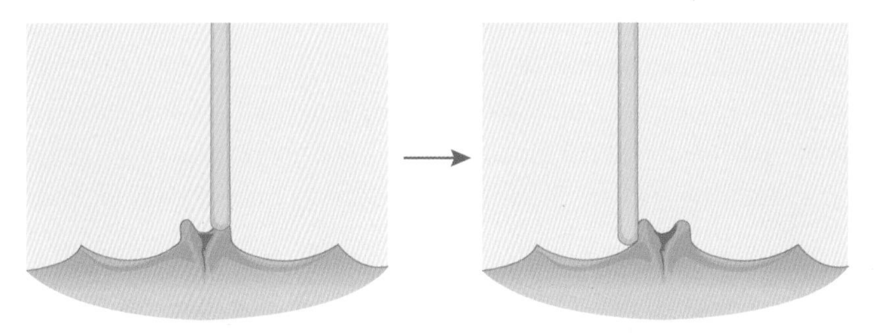

Figure 25 Caudal septal relocation suture.

(h) Paired Batten Grafts

If the caudal septum is weakened and shows an S-shaped deviation, the paired batten graft technique can be applied. This technique involves placing batten grafts on both sides of the caudal strut. This can be done if enough cartilage was harvested from the central compartment. The paired batten graft technique is useful in straightening and strengthening the caudal septum. However, using thick cartilage for this procedure could induce airway narrowing *(Figure 26)*.

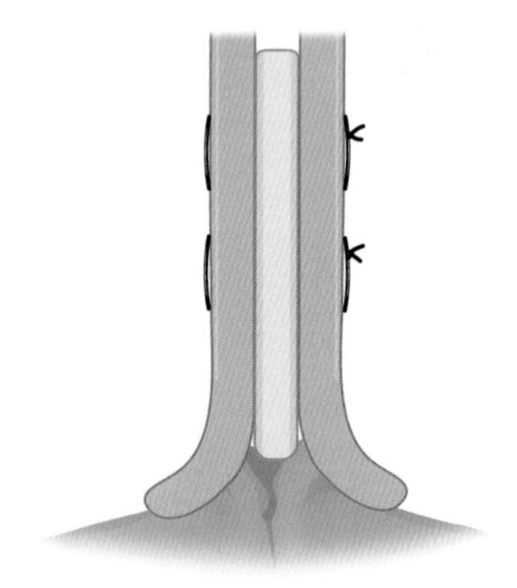

Figure 26 Paired batten grafts.

(i) Correction of Cephalo-Caudal Deviation

The caudal septum could only show deviation towards the anterior posterior direction, but could also show severe deviation in the cephalo-caudal direction *(Figure 27)*. In many cases of cephalo-caudal deviation, overly developed cartilages are seen in the caudal part. In these situations, the author first cuts off the overly developed excess cartilage in the caudal part perpendicularly. Then the removed cartilage is used as caudal septal

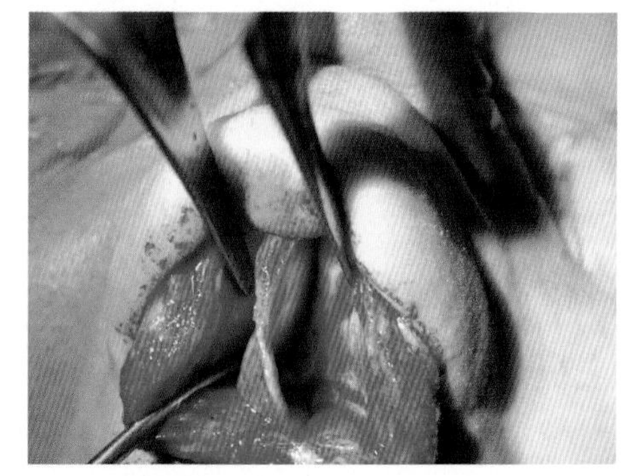

Figure 27 Intraoperative photo of caudal septal deviation in the cephalo-caudal direction.

extension graft placed on the wider nasal cavity to correct the deviation. This maneuver can compensate for the shortening of the caudal septum caused by the excision of cartilage *(Figure 28)*. Doing a wedge excision on the lower part of the caudal septum is another surgical option, which enables the surgeon to mobilize and fix the caudal septum in desired direction and location *(Figure 29)*.

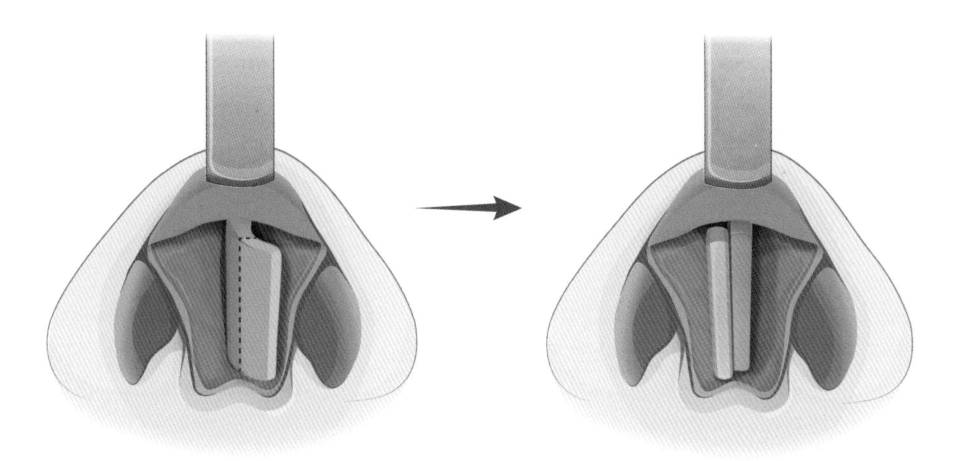

Figure 28 Excision of the deviated caudal septum and using the excised segment as caudal septal extension graft.

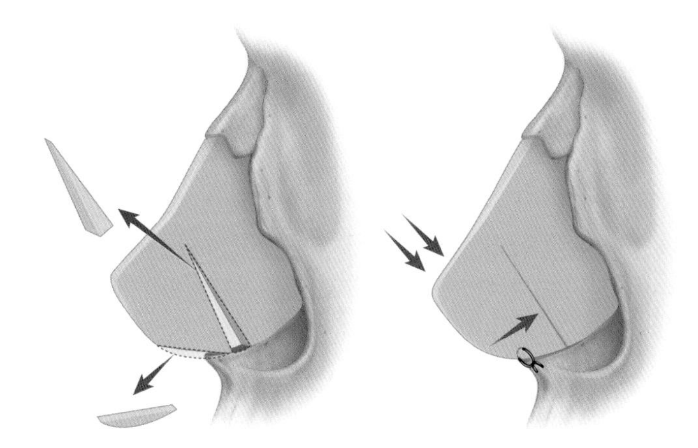

Figure 29 Wedge excision of caudal septum to correct a cephalo-caudal deviation

B) Extracorporeal Septoplasty

If the deviation of the nasal septum is too severe to be corrected with the aforementioned in situ techniques, extracorporeal septoplasty can be utilized. This method involves removing the near total part of the nasal septum from its location, and reimplanting it into position after reshaping it extracorporeally *(Figure 30)*. Extracorporeal septoplasty is a highly effective method in correcting severe deviations, but risks weakening the septal cartilage (especially the keystone area and the anterior nasal spine area) and is technically challenging. The following are various methods for stabilizing the reimplanted cartilage graft in extracorporeal septoplasty.

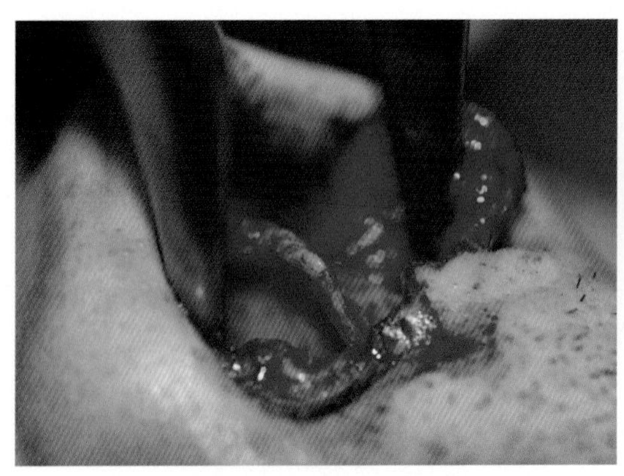
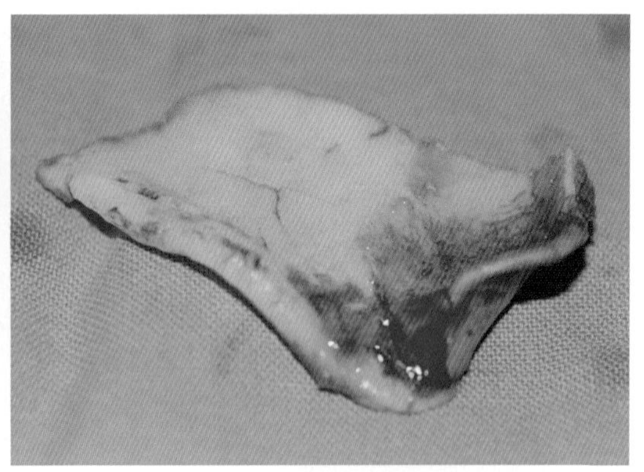

Figure 30 Severely deviated septal cartilage is taken out for extracorporeal septoplasty

- Suture fixation with the medial crura of the alar cartilage
- Utilizing U-shaped suturing between the upper lateral cartilage for fixation
- Anchoring by transseptal multiple mattress sutures
- Suturing through surgically made holes in the anterior nasal spine

The author prefers to perform his modification of the extracorporeal septoplasty technique. First, the osseocartilaginous skeleton needs to be exposed through an external rhinoplasty approach. Then the septal mucoperichondrial flaps are elevated. The septum is freed from the extrinsic forces of the deformed upper and lower lateral cartilages. Septal cartilage is removed except for the remaining few millimeters of the dorsal strip at the keystone area. Multiple techniques including scoring, wedge excision, and cartilage splinting are performed in order to straighten the removed cartilage. A straight and strong new L-strut is then formed extracorporeally *(Figure 31)*. The dorsal aspect of the new L-strut is fashioned into a "Y" shape by suturing one cartilage strip to the existing L-strut. The preserved cartilage tail at the keystone area is placed in the middle of the arms of the Y-shaped cartilage and then fixed using 4-0 PDS sutures. Caudal septum stability is obtained by suturing the newly shaped septal cartilage to the soft tissue around the anterior nasal spine using 5-0 PDS such that the anterior nasal spine is positioned in the middle and the arms of the new septum, which creates an inverted "Y" *(Figure 32)*. After fixing the new L-strut, the dorsal aspect of the septal cartilage is reconnected to the upper lateral cartilages using 4-0 PDS to provide additional stability. If necessary, septal bone or conchal cartilage can be harvested for spreader grafts or batten grafts for additional support. To ensure a successful surgery, it is important to leave less than 1 cm of the dorsal tip in removing the nasal septal cartilage. Leaving a sufficient amount of soft tissue around the anterior nasal spine is also important. If the anterior nasal spine is deviated towards one side, the new septum should be sutured with the soft tissue of the contralateral side. If the keystone itself is deviated, after the fixation of the graft, a wedge-shaped cartilage can be inserted to get a straight dorsal septum.

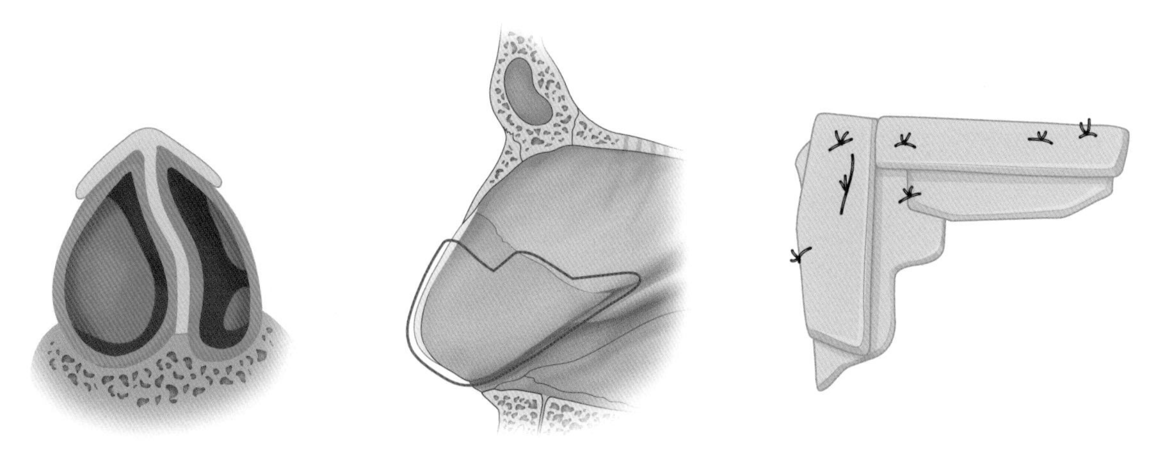

Figure 31 For extracorporeal septoplasty, septal cartilage is removed except for the remaining few millimeters of the dorsal strip at the keystone area. A straight and strong new L-strut which is formed extracorporeally and ready to be re-implanted.

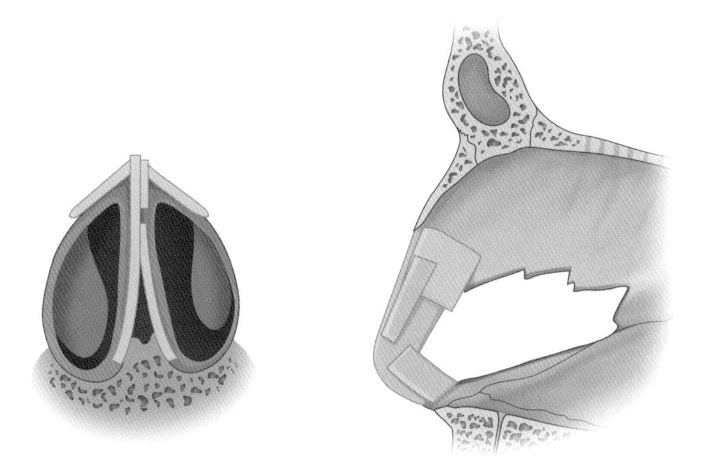

Figure 32 Newly formed L-stut is reconnected with the cartilage tail at the keystone area, and with the soft tissue around the anterior nasal spine.

(2) Correction of the Anterior Nasal Spine

The location and the direction of the nasal spine needs to be verified by sight during surgery. If there is a deviation in the nasal spine, a greenstick fracture needs to be made with an osteotome or a gouge. A complete fracture of the nasal spine must be avoided. A safer and easier way is to separate the septal cartilage, and then fix it on one side – letting it connect to the anterior nasal spine in a side-to-side manner. Overly protruding bone should be drilled out.

(3) Correction of the Upper Lateral Cartilaginous Deformity

Because the deformity of the upper lateral cartilage is usually a secondary deformity due to a deformed dorsal septum, the deviation of the upper lateral cartilage can basically be solved by straightening the septum, followed by placements of spreader grafts. Once the surgeon fixes all the components, the deviation will most likely be corrected. However, this method might leave some concavity or convexity on certain areas. If so, placing an onlay graft made from cartilage or Gore-Tex on the concave side will correct the deformity *(Figure 33)*.

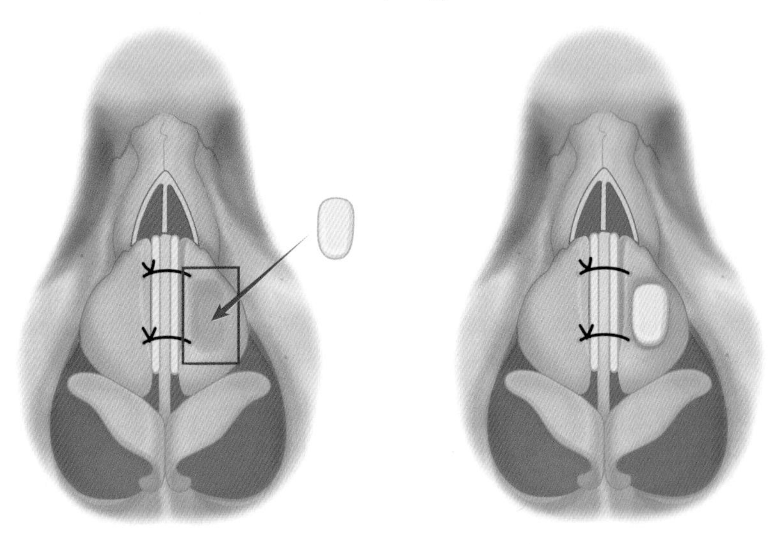

Figure 33 Deviation of the upper lateral cartilage can be corrected by straightening the septum, then placing spreader grafts. The remaining concavity is corrected by placing an onlay graft.

(4) Correction of the Lower Lateral Cartilage

In most cases, external nose deviation is caused by either bony deviation or the deformity of the cartilaginous dorsum constituted by the upper lateral cartilages and the septal cartilage. However, with some patients, the lateral crura of the lower lateral cartilages are too big and points towards the medial direction, deforming the lower third of the nose. To these patients, the asymmetry or deformity of the lateral crura as shown on the frontal view is responsible for the deviated nasal appearance *(Figure 34)*. This can be seen in patients with lateral crura that are concave on one side and convex on the other. These deformities can be corrected by flipping the lateral crus upside down (flip-flop technique), cephalic resection, lateral crural onlay, or lateral crural strut graft *(Figure 35)*.

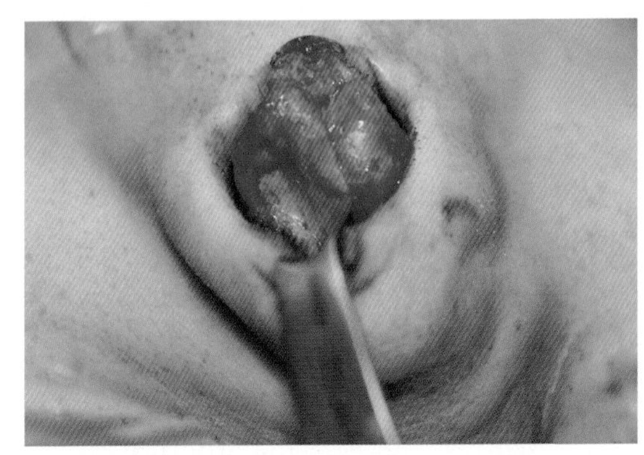

Figure 34 Intraoperative photo of a patient whose deviated nasal appearance was due to malformed and asymmetric lower lateral cartilages.

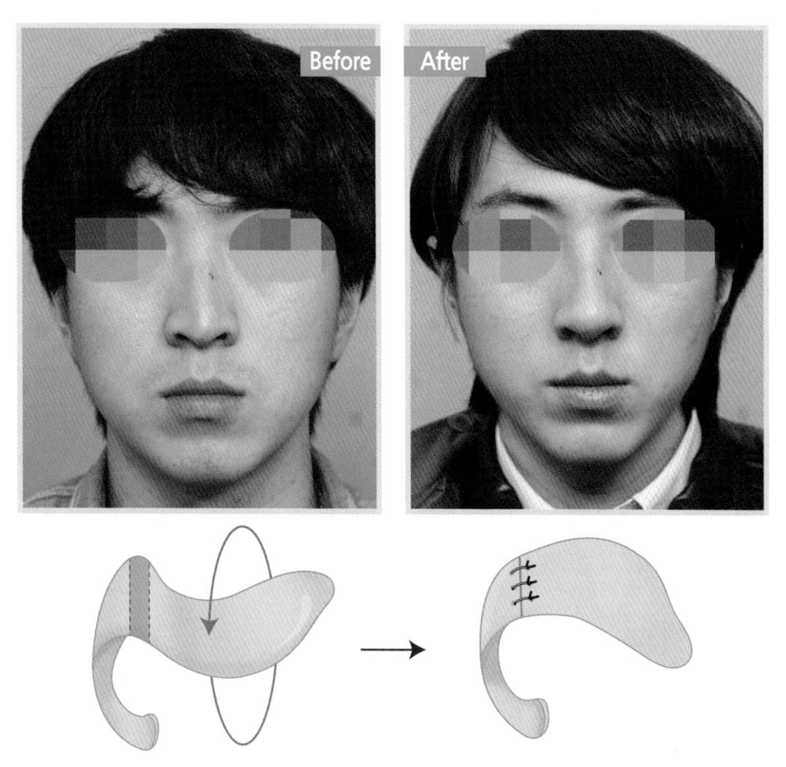

Figure 35 Concave lateral crus responsible for the deviated nose in this patient was corrected using flip flop technique.

Nostril asymmetry is commonly found in deviated nose patients *(Figure 36)*. These asymmetries could be derived from the deviation of the cartilaginous middle vault extending to the tip, or the lower lateral cartilage itself being deformed. Therefore, the deviation in the lower lateral cartilages should be first treated by correcting the deformities in the septum, and then be reevaluated after

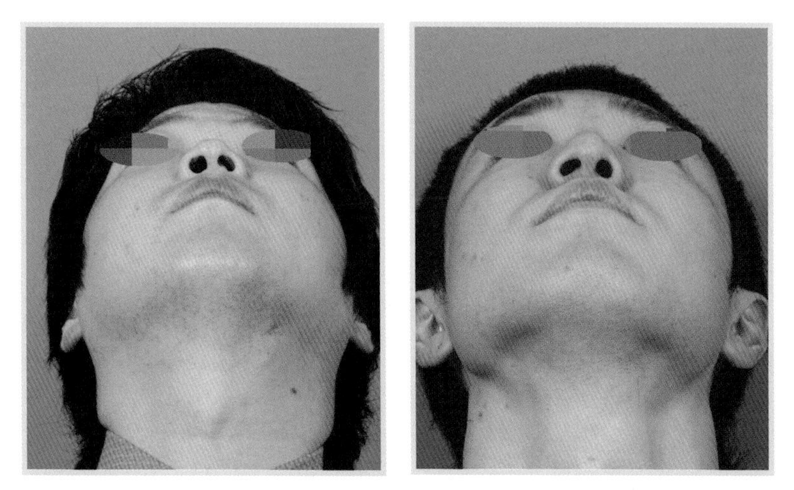

Figure 36 Nostril asymmetry is commonly found in patients with deviated noses. Correction of the nostril deformity should also be considered during rhinoplasty.

disconnecting the lower lateral cartilages from the upper lateral cartilages. If the lower lateral cartilages itself are deformed, various methods for tip surgery should be correctly applied to correct tip asymmetry. Such methods include cephalic trim, columellar strut, lateral crural overlay, interdomal suture, or various grafting methods.

4. Significance of Dorsal Augmentation in Deviated Noses

Dorsal augmentation is one of the last steps in correcting deviated noses. Through this procedure, the patient's bony and cartilaginous dorsum is restored to their aesthetic and functional balance. Commonly used procedures such as osteotomies or spreader grafting require suturing, and can cause dorsum irregularities in patients with thin skin. Also, unpredictable situations such as the inadvertent collapse of the keystone area can take place. In these situations, the need for dorsal augmentation arises. Deviated nose patients also show contraction of the tissue and the soft tissue where their deviation was originally. Appropriate dorsal augmentation prevents soft tissue deformities that cause deviation. Also, dorsal augmentation itself will make the nose appear longer and narrower. Implant materials for augmentation should be small in volume and soft. Because the correction of deviation requires extensive dissection and may weaken the underlying structures due to osteotomy and septal correction, dorsal augmentation with solid material such as silicone or costal cartilage can easily be displaced or can deform the underlying nasal skeleton. It is therefore recommended to use with soft implant materials such as Gore-Tex, fascia, conchal cartilage, crushed septal cartilage, diced cartilage, and fascia wrapped diced cartilage for dorsal augmentation.

5. Alar Base Modification

Some patients with deviated noses show asymmetry of the alar base, which means that one of their alar soft tissue is hypertrophic and their nostrils differ in size. For these patients, either unilateral alar base resection or asymmetric alar base resection cand be performed *(Figure 37)*. Failure in noticing and correcting this problem will cause dissatisfaction in patients.

6. Turbinoplasty

For patients who complain of nasal obstruction prior to surgery, decreasing the volume of the inferior turbinate or the middle turbinate needs to be performed. However, patients that do not have nasal obstruction might still have severely hypertrohied turbinates. Even if their septum is corrected, the hypertrophied turbinate could put pressure on the septum. This can cause relapse of the septal deviation, eventually causing nasal deviation. Therefore, properly addressing the turbinate using various methods described in the chapter "Turbinate Surgery" contributes in successfully correcting the deviated nose.

VI. Prognosis and Complications of Surgery

Surgical correction of deviated noses is considered to be one of the most difficult surgeries

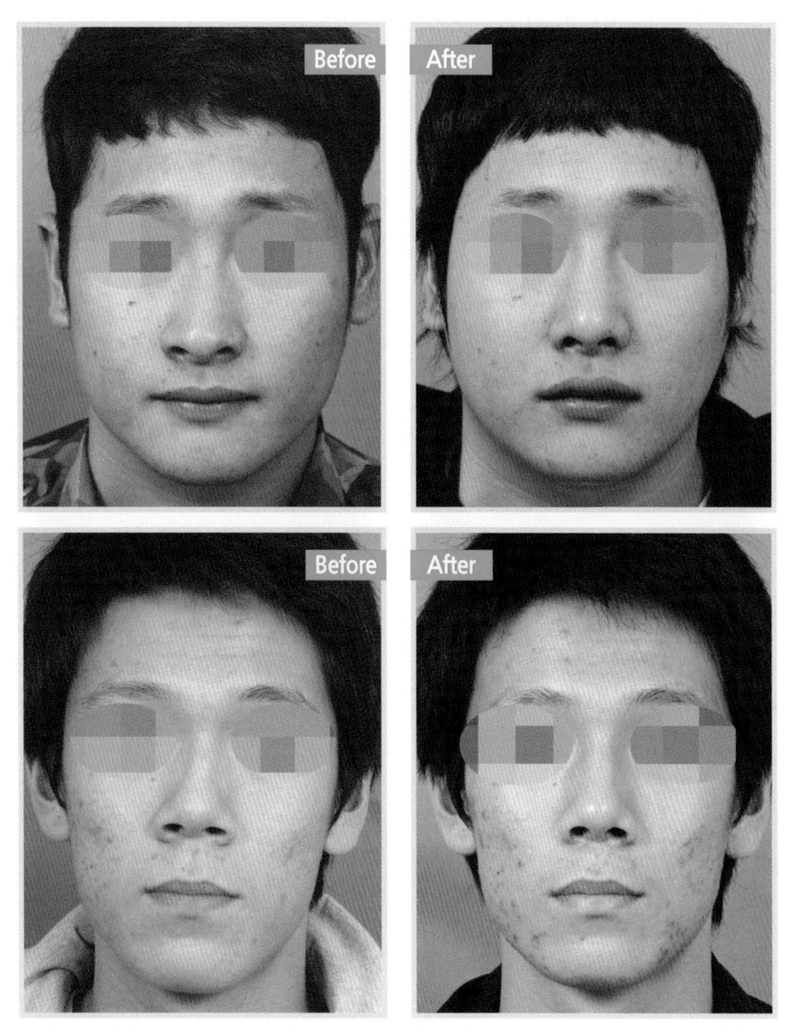

Figure 37 Alar base deformities are commonly associated with deviated nose. This problem must be addressed for the aesthetic success of rhinoplasty.

in rhinoplasty. The reason being is that there are various forms of deformities that are very complicated. Each patient will require different methods of surgery, and chances of relapses are high. The reason why relapses are common is because cartilaginous deformities have a huge impact on deviation, and their elasticity will keep on inducing them to return to their original shape prior to surgery. Excising out the deviated area of the cartilage is of course the most certain way of correcting it, but it could cause more structural instability. With patients with more severe deviations, their septal cartilage, upper lateral cartilages, and lower lateral cartilage will be deformed more severely. Surgical results will not always be satisfactory even if the surgeon performs all the right things. Structural weakening, inevitably following aggressive corrective procedures also hamper the acquiring a good surgical outcome. Especially, if preoperative planning is done poorly, or if there is a lack of thorough understanding of the dynamics of cartilages, the surgery itself and the results will not be successful. The following are the complications of surgery.

1. Incomplete Correction and Relapse of Deviation *(Figure 38)*

The probable causes of incomplete correction or recurrence of deviation are

- Secondary deformity of the bony vault as a result of osteotomy
- Failure to overcome the intrinsic memory of deformed cartilage
- Weakened cartilaginous supporting structure due to various surgical maneuvers
- Displacement or deformation of the dorsal implant material

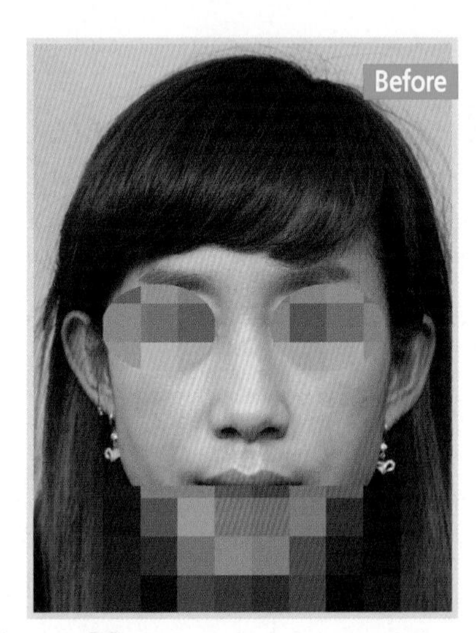

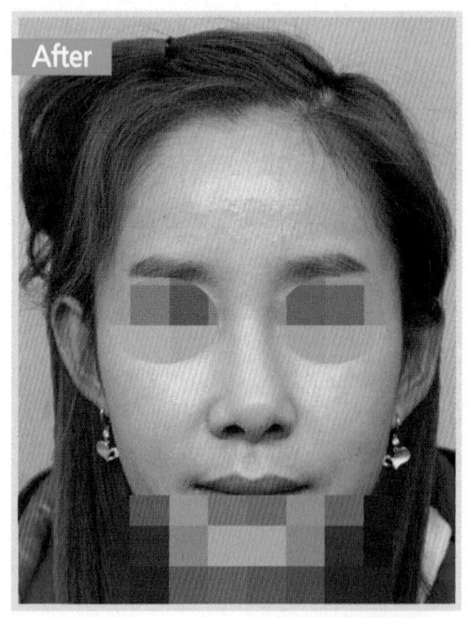

Figure 38 Patient showing incomplete correction of deviation after rhinoplasty.

2. Nasal Tip Deprojection due to Weakened Supporting Structure after Surgery

3. Short Nose Deformity *(Figure 39)*

This deformity may occur due to following reasons:

- Skin contraction due to immune or tissue reaction to the dorsally implanted material
- Loss of cartilaginous supporting power
- Resorption of the tip graft or septal extension graft

4. Saddle Nose Deformity *(Figure 40)*

Saddle deformities can occur with the similar etiologies that cause short nose deformities. Resorption the of dorsal implant can also be an important factor.

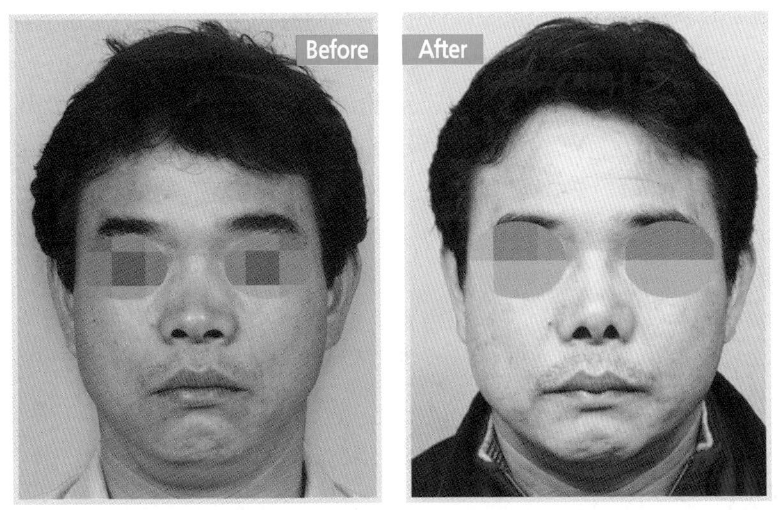

Figure 39 Patient showing a short nose deformity after rhinoplasty for correction of a deviated nose.

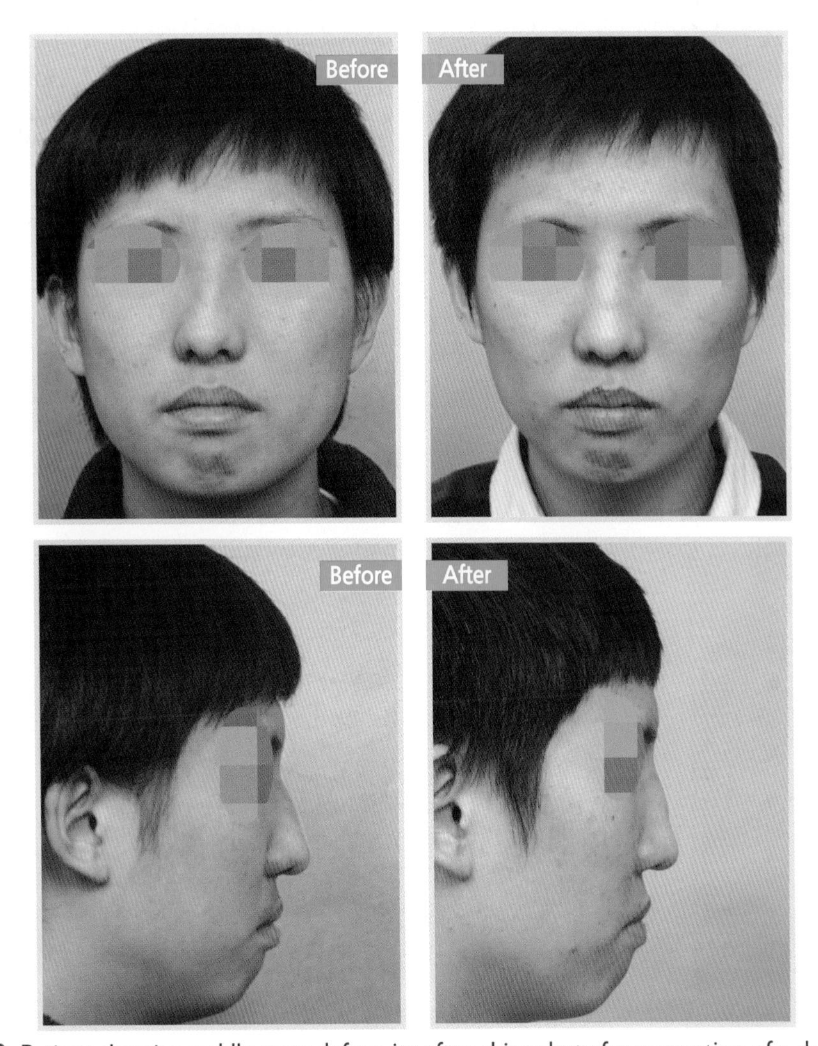

Figure 40 Patient showing saddle nose deformity after rhinoplasty for correction of a deviated nose.

5. Incomplete Correction of the Nasal Obstruction or Newly Developed Nasal Obstruction as a Result of Surgery

Causes of disturbed nasal breathing function are:

- Incomplete correction of the septal deviation
- Inadequate treatment for turbinate hypertrophy
- Stenosis, or dynamic collapse of the external valve or internal valve
- Collapsed bony dorsum as a result of osteotomy

In the author's experience, failed correction of the caudal septal deviation was the most common reason for functional dissatisfaction after rhinoplasty for correction of the deviated nose. Other than the aforementioned complications, several other complications might take place. The dilemma in treating deviated noses is that for perfect correction, the cartilages and the bones that form a nose need to be opened and disconnected, but such an aggressive method will damage the stability of the nose over a long period of time – causing a recurrence of the deviation, saddle nose, short nose, and other deformities. The author's own revision in rhinoplasty for deviated nose patients is about 7%, but overall dissatisfaction rate in this patient group was up to 20% in his series. Especially in cases of Type V patients, the correction of linear deviation was the most dissatisfactory in surgical outcome.

References

1. Boccieri A, Pascali M. Septal crossbar graft for correction of the crooked nose. Plast Reconst Surg 2003; 111: 629-38.
2. Bracaglia R, Fortunato R, Gentileschi S. Double lateral osteotomy in aesthetic rhinoplasty. Br J Plast Surg 2004; 57: 156-9.
3. Byrd HS, Salomon J, Flood J. Correction of the crooked nose. Plast Reconstr Surg 1998; 102: 2148-57.
4. Cho GS, Jang YJ. Deviated nose correction: different outcomes according to the deviation type. Laryngosocpe 2013, in press
5. Crestinu J. New data in the correction of twisted nose. Aesthet plast Surg 1986; 10: 231-4.
6. Ellis DAF, Gilert RW. Analysis and correction of the crooked nose. J Otolaryngol 1991; 20: 14-8.
7. Gilbert SE. Overlay grafting for lateral nasal wall concavities. Otolaryngol Head Neck Surg 1998; 119: 385-8.
8. Guyuron B, Behmend RA. Caudal nasal deviation. Plast Reconstr Surg. 2003; 111: 2449-60.
9. Guyruon B, Uzzo CD, Scull H. A practical classification of septo nasal deviation and an effective guide to septal surgery. Plast Reconstr Surg 1999; 104: 2202-9.
10. Hwang P, Mass CS. Correction of the twisted nose deformity: a surgical algorithm using the external rhinoplasty approach. Am J Rhinol 1998; 12; 213-20.
11. Jang YJ, Kwon MS. Modified extracorporeal septoplasty technique in rhinoplasty for severely deviated noses. Ann Otol Rhinol Laryngol 2010; 119: 331-5.
12. Jang YJ, Yeo NK, Wang JH. Cutting and suture technique of the caudal septal cartilage for the management of caudal septal deviation. Arch Otolaryngol Head Neck Surg 2009; 135: 1256-60.
13. Jang YJ, Kim JM, Yeo NK. Use of nasal septal bone to straighten deviated septal cartilage in correction of deviated nose. Ann Otol Rhino Laryngol 2009; 118: 488-94.
14. Jang YJ, Wang JH, Lee BJ. Classification of the deviated nose and its treatment. Arch Otolaryngol Head Neck Surg 2008; 134: 311-5.
15. Jang YJ, Sinha V. Spreader graft in septo-rhinoplasty. Indian J Otolaryngol Head Neck Surg 2007; 59: 100-2.
16. Jang YJ, Wang JH, Sinha V, Lee BJ. Percutaneous root osteotomy for correction of deviated nose. Am J Rhinol 2007; 21: 515-9.
17. Kim DW, Toriumi DM. Management of posttraumatic nasal deformities: the crooked nose and the saddle nose. Facial Plast Surg Clin N Am 2004; 12: 111-2.
18. Rohrich RJ. Gunter JP, Deuber MA, Adam WP. The deviated nose: optimizing results using a simplified classification and algorithmic approach. Plast Reconstr Surg 2002; 110: 1509-23.
19. Song HM, Kim JS, Lee BJ, Jang YJ. Deviated nose cartilaginous dorsum correction using a dorsal L-Strut cutting and suture technique. Laryngoscope 2008; 118: 981-6.
20. Stuker FJ. Management of the scoliotic nose. Laryngoscope 1982; 92: 128-34.
21. TerKonda R, Sykes JM. Repairing the twisted nose. Otolaryngol Clin North Am 1999; 32: 53-64.
22. Vuyk HD. A review of practical guidelines for correction of the deviated, asymmetric nose. Rhinoloy 2000; 38: 72-8.
23. Yeo NK, Jang YJ. Rhinoplasty to correct nasal deformities in post septoplasty patients. Am J Rhinol Allergy 2009; 23: 540-5.

Case 1

A 34-year-old male visited for a deviated nose after closed reduction surgery for nasal bone fracture 2 years ago.

Analysis Frontal: Tilted bony dorsum, curved cartilaginous dorsum (Type II deviation)
Basal: Nostril asymmetry, underprojected tip
Lateral and Oblique: Saddle-like dorsal concavity

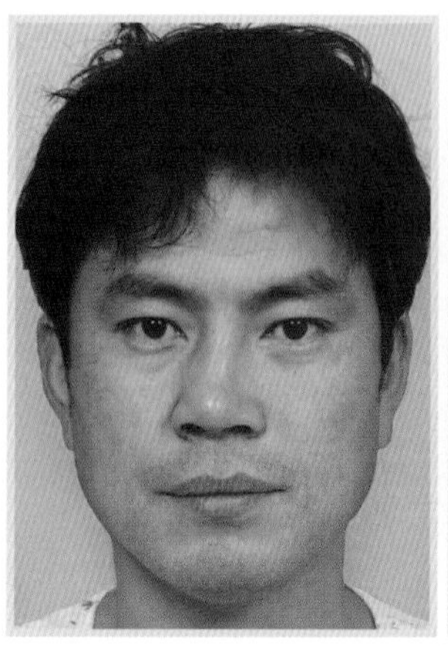
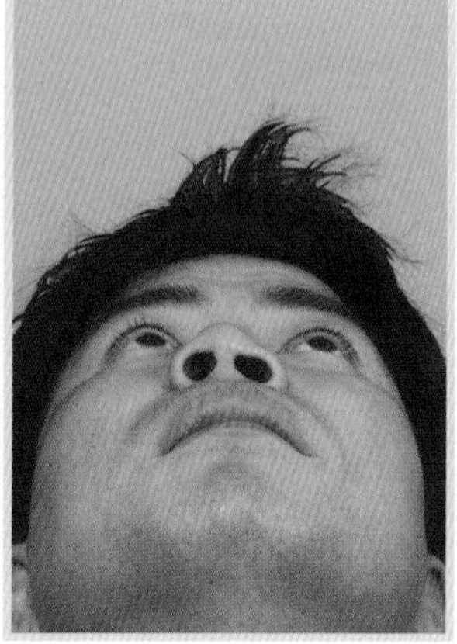
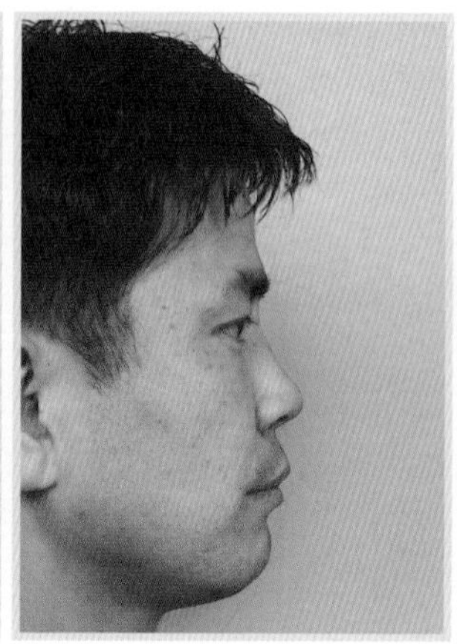
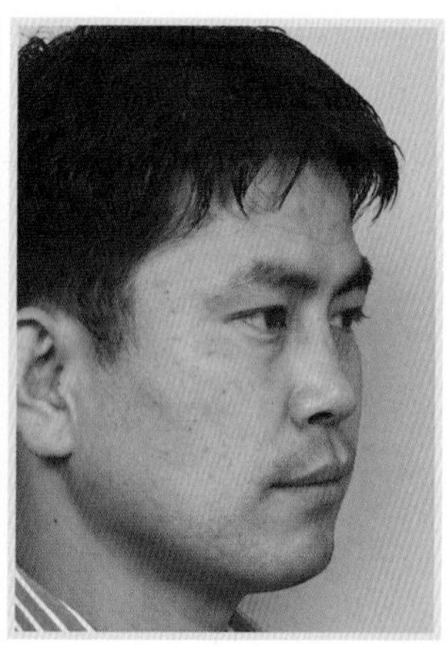

Operative Procedures

Open rhinoplasty approach
Septoplasty and harvest of septal cartilage and bone
Cutting and suture of the caudal septum
Medial and lateral osteotomies
Caudal septal extension grafting (left)
Modified vertical dome division technique with shield grafting
Dorsal augmentation using fascia and crushed cartilage
Tip graft camouflaging using fascia

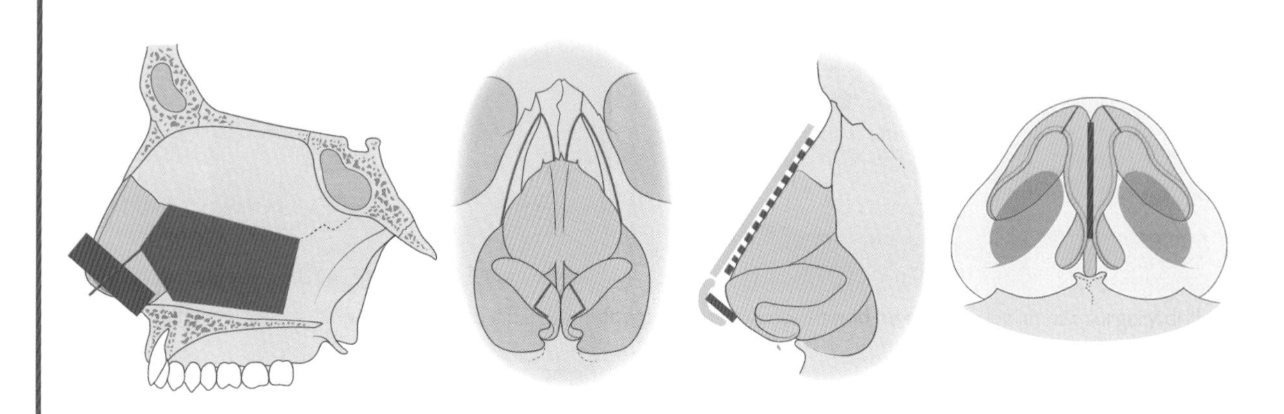

Postoperative Changes

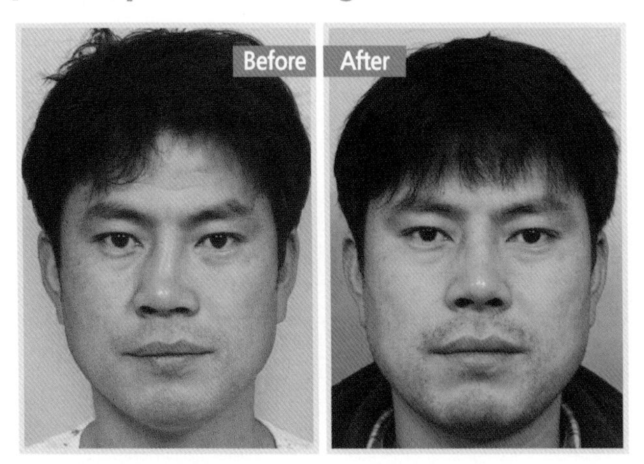

Frontal: Deviated nose was corrected successfully.

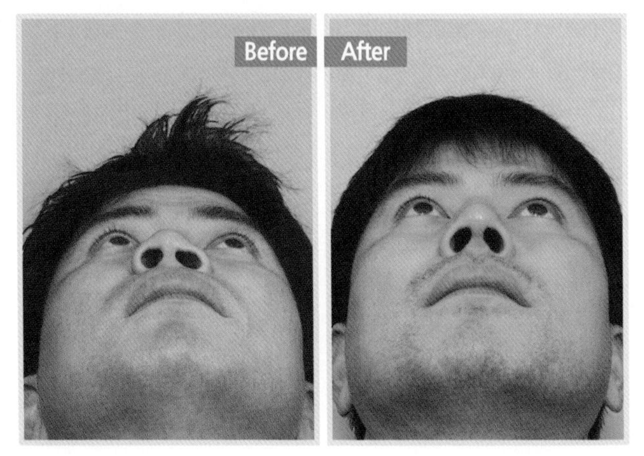

Basal: Nostril asymmetry was improved and tip projection was increased.

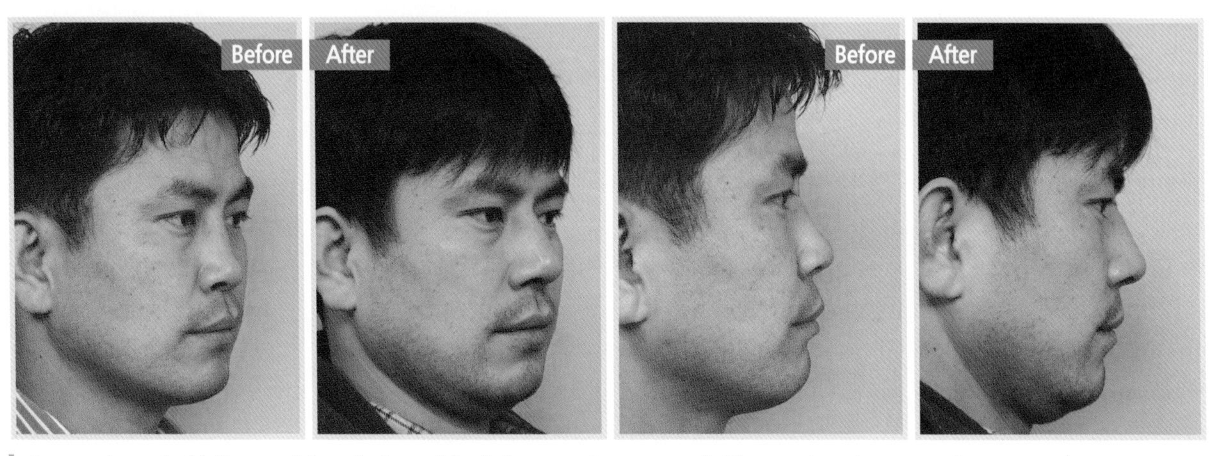

Lateral and Oblique: Nasal dorsal height was increased. Tip projection was improved.

Case 2

A 50-year-old male visited for a deviated nose with nasal obstruction.

Analysis

Frontal: Deviated nose, ptotic tip (Type I deviation)
Basal: Mild nostril asymmetry
Lateral and Oblique: Acute nasolabial angle, mildly convex nasal dorsum

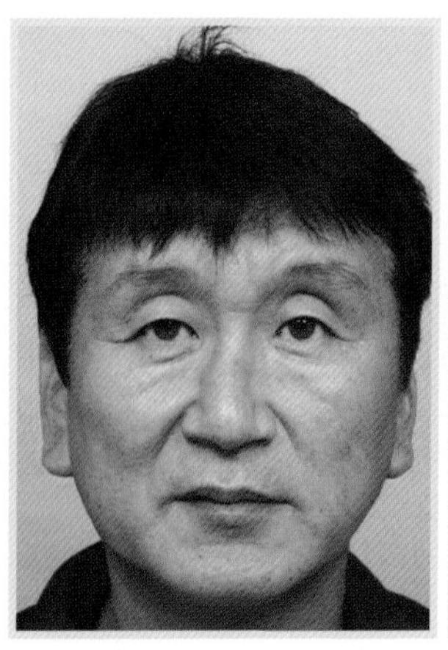
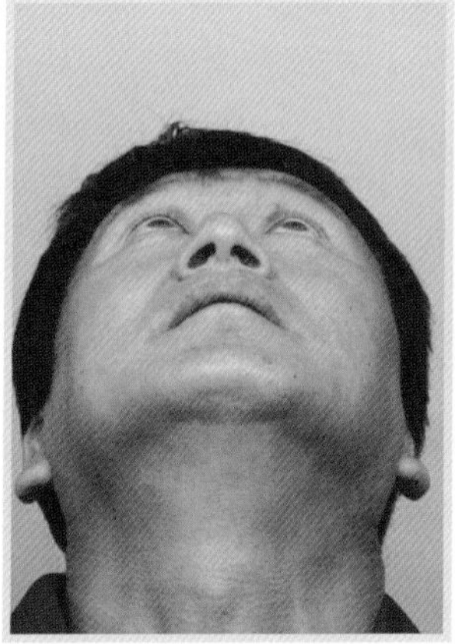
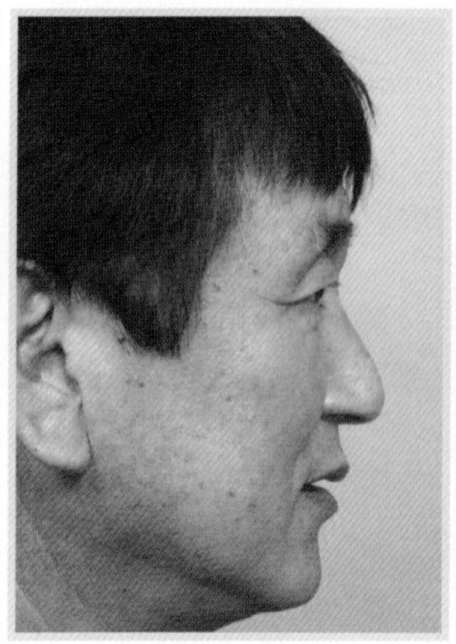
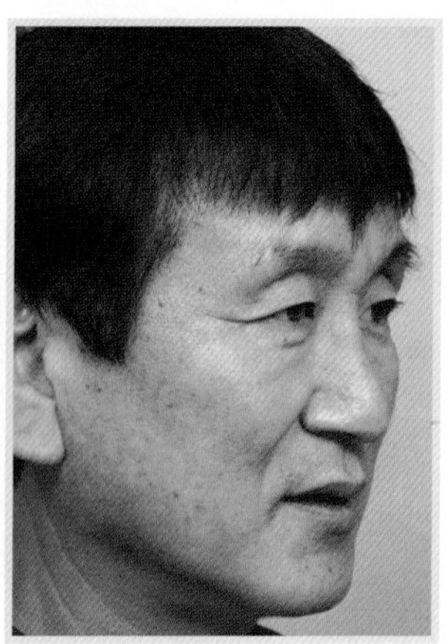

Operative Procedures

Open rhinoplasty approach
Medial and lateral osteotomies
Extracorporeal septoplasty
Reinforcement of the neo-septum with a spreader graft (left)
Dorsal augmentation using fascia lata

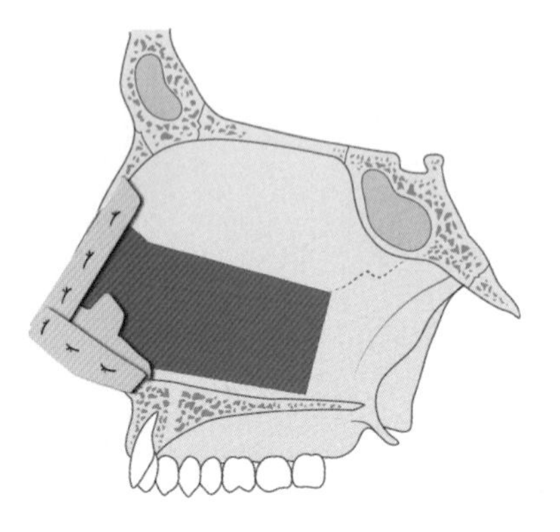
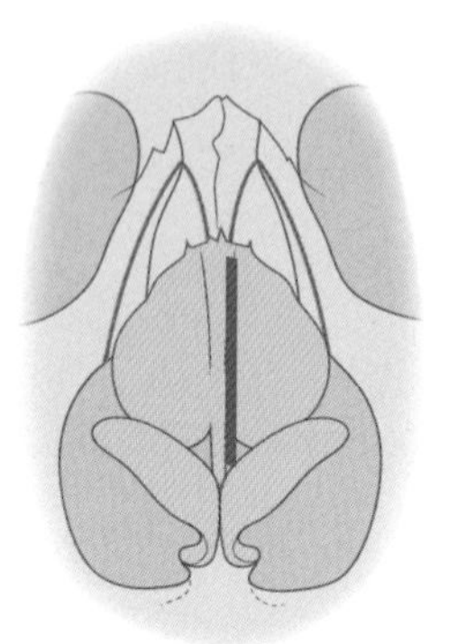
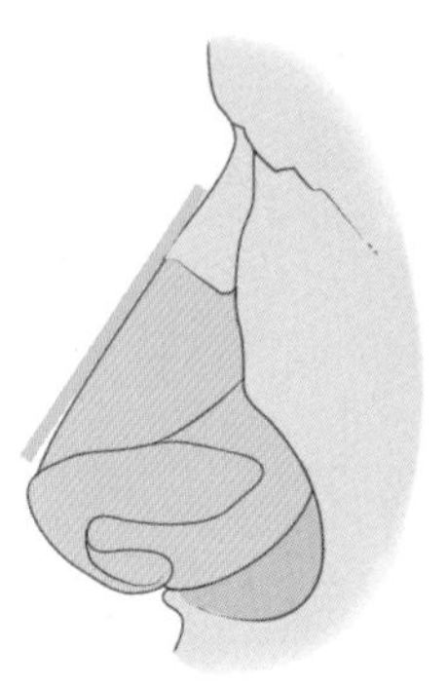

Postoperative Changes

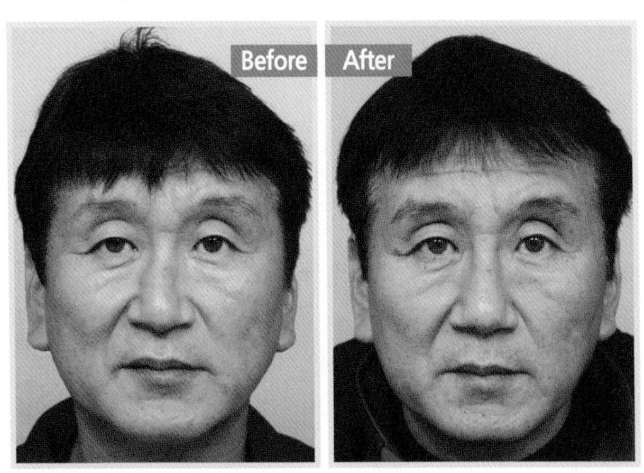

Frontal: Natural looking dorsal aesthetic lines were formed by the correction of the deviated nose. Ptotic tip was improved.

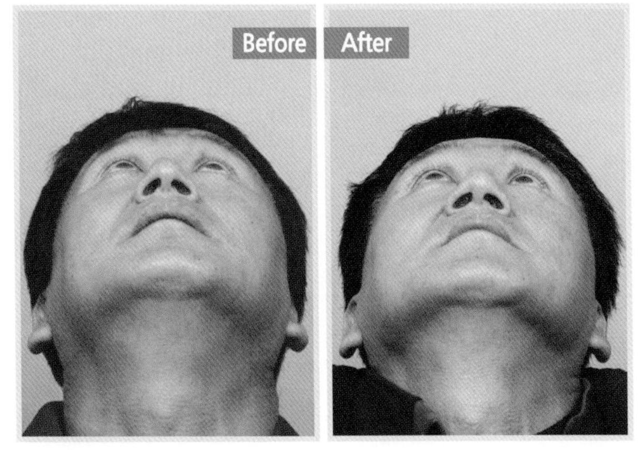

Basal: No definite change was observed.

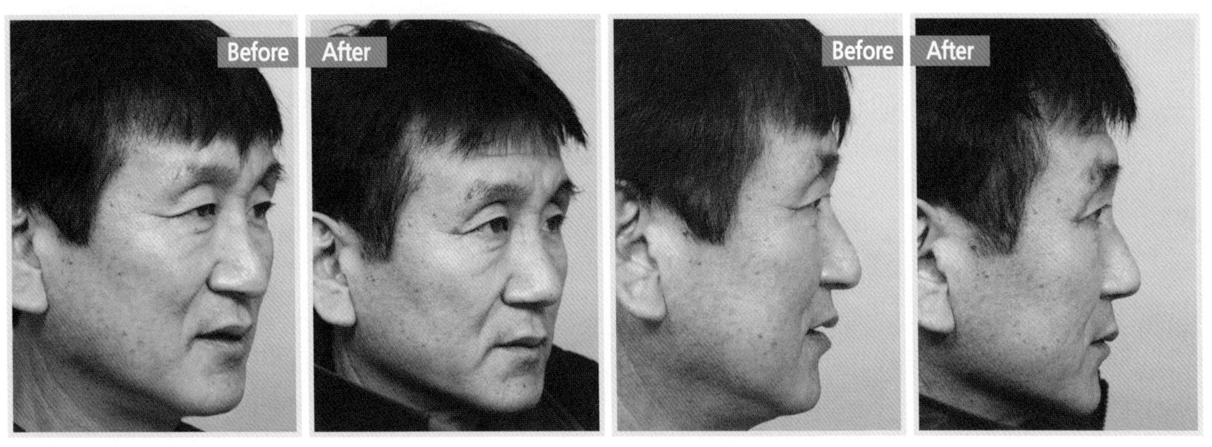

Lateral and Oblique: Ptotic tip was improved. Dorsal convexity was improved. Nasolabial angle was widened.

Case 3

A 22-year-old male visited for a deviated nose with nasal obstruction.

Analysis

Frontal: Deviated nose (Type III deviation), left nasal base located lower level than the right

Basal: Alar flaring, poor tip projection

Lateral and Oblique: Low nasal dorsum

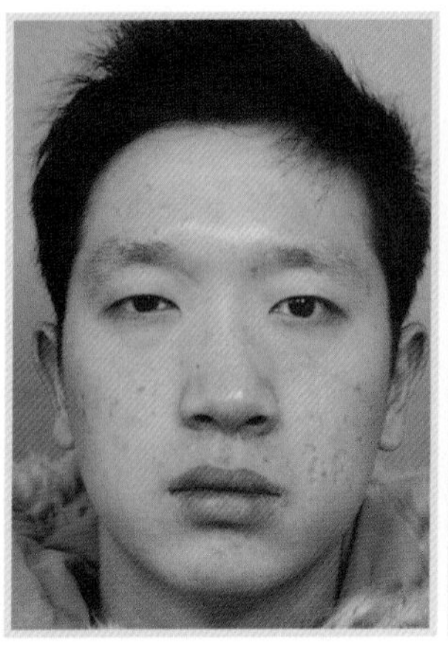

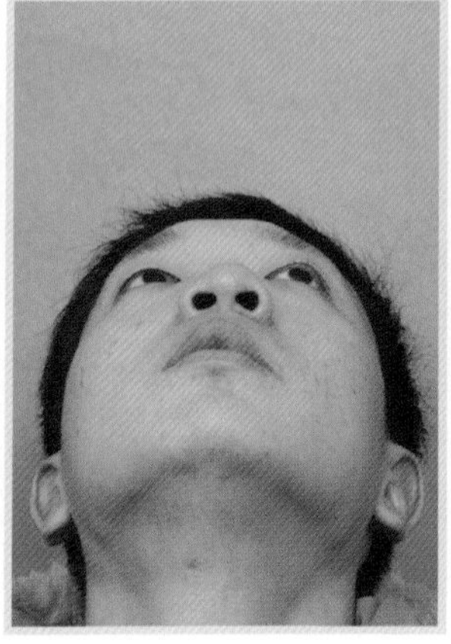

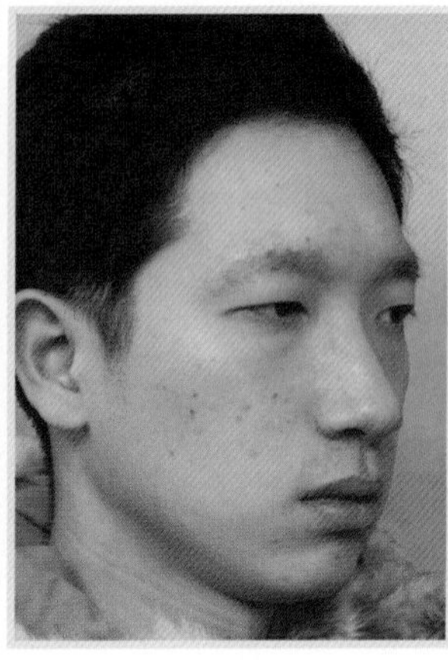

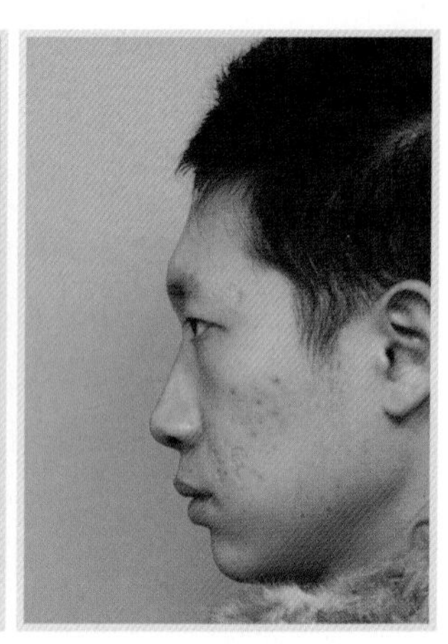

Operative Procedures

Open rhinoplasty approach

Septoplasty and harvest of septal cartilage and bone

Caudal septum repositioning

Medial, lateral, and percutaneous root osteotomies

Caudal septal extension grafting using septal cartilage (bilateral)

Spreader grafting using septal cartilage (right)

Tip graft camouflaging using processed fascia lata

Dorsal augmentation using processed fascia lata

Hanging ala correction by vestibular skin excision (left)

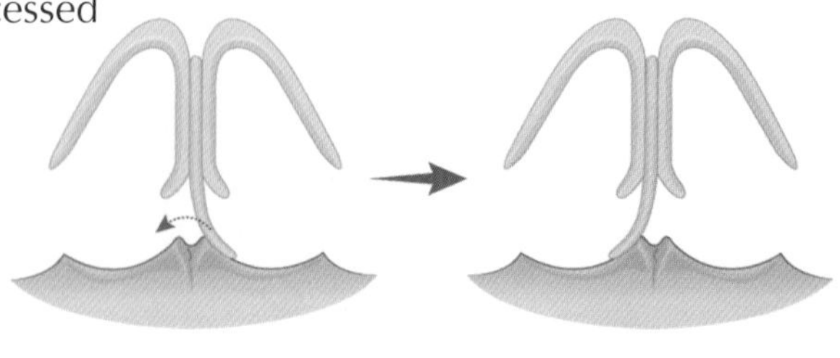

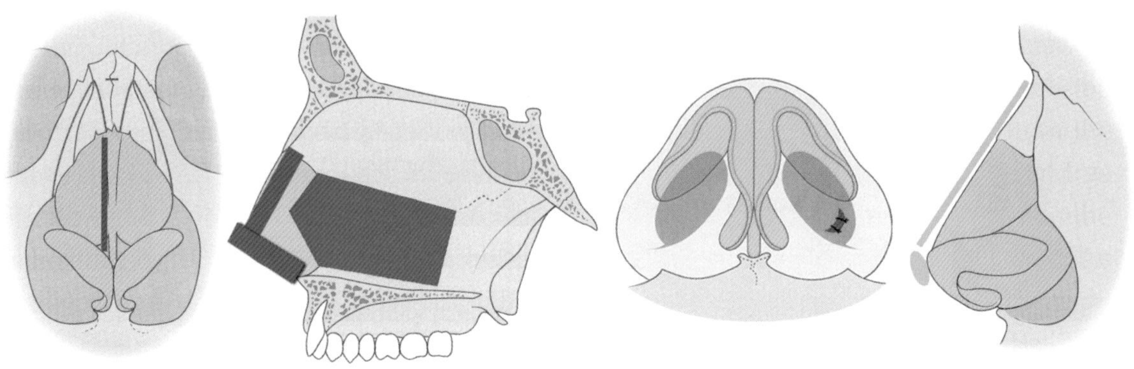

Postoperative Changes

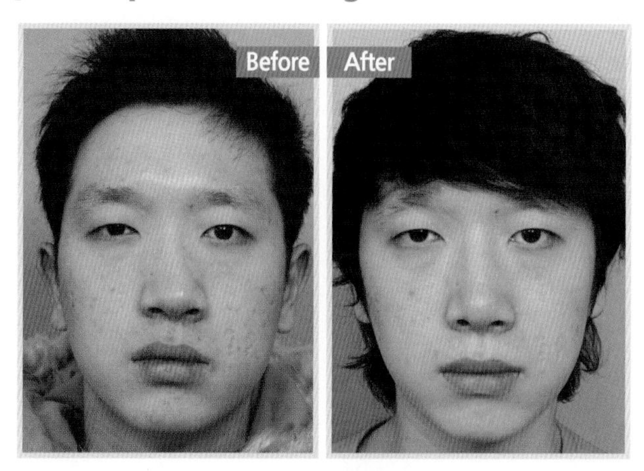

Frontal: Deviation was corrected.

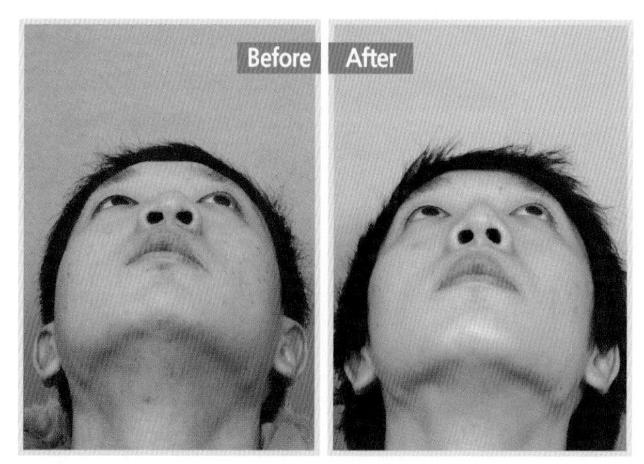

Basal: Tip projection and alar flaring were improved.

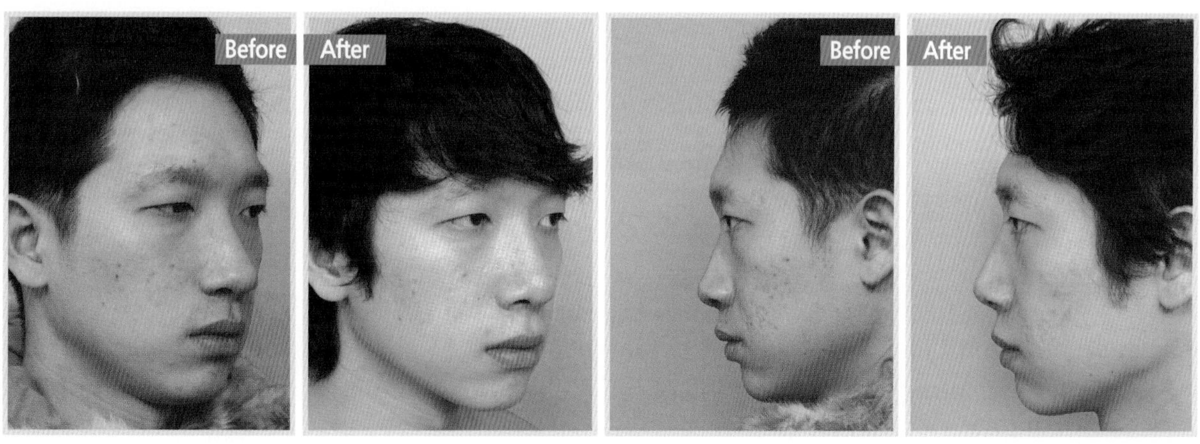

Lateral and Oblique: Dorsal height and tip projection were increased. Dorsal irregularity was improved.

Case 4

A 30-year-old female visited for a deviated nose with nasal obstruction.

Analysis

Frontal: Deviated nose (Type IV deviation)
Basal: Columella lobule ratio of 1:1
Lateral: Mildly convex dorsum with a polly beak shape

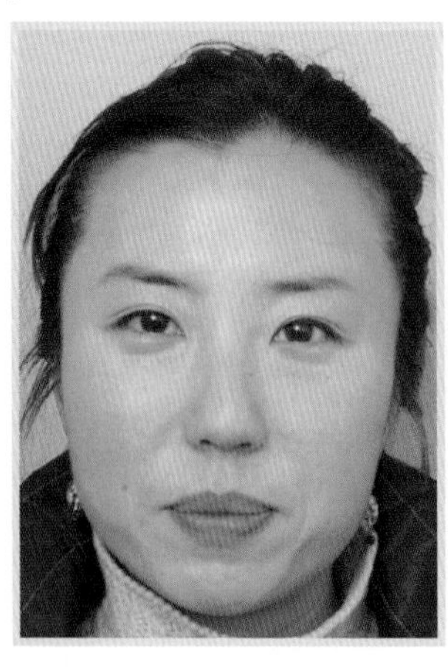

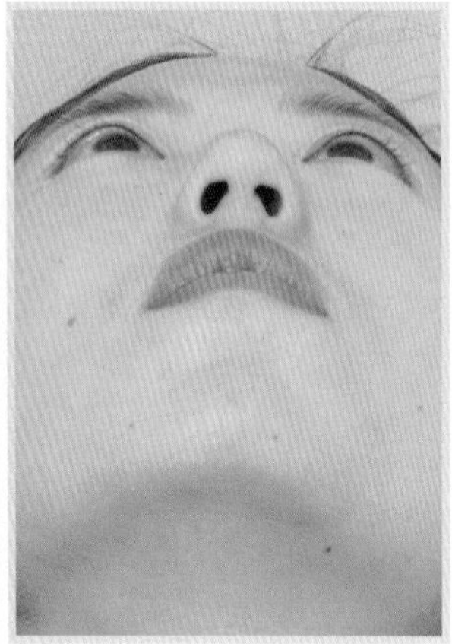

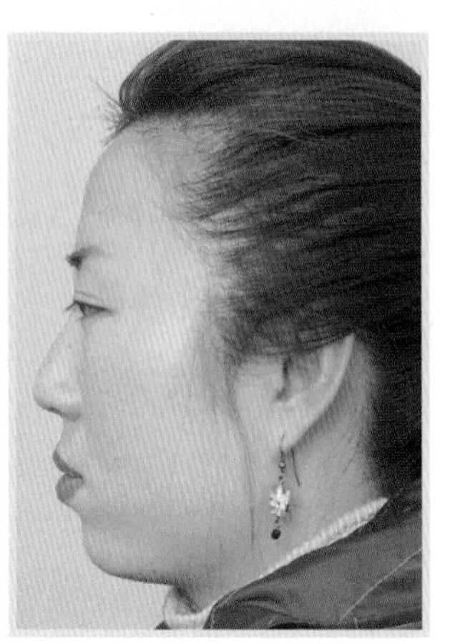

Operative Procedures

Open rhinoplasty approach
Septoplasty and harvest of septal cartilage and bone
Spreader grafting using septal cartilage (bilateral)
Cephalic resection (bilateral)
Transdomal suturing (bilateral)
Columellar strut application
Shield grafting using septal cartilage
Dorsal augmentation using silicone
Crushed cartilage grafting on surpatip

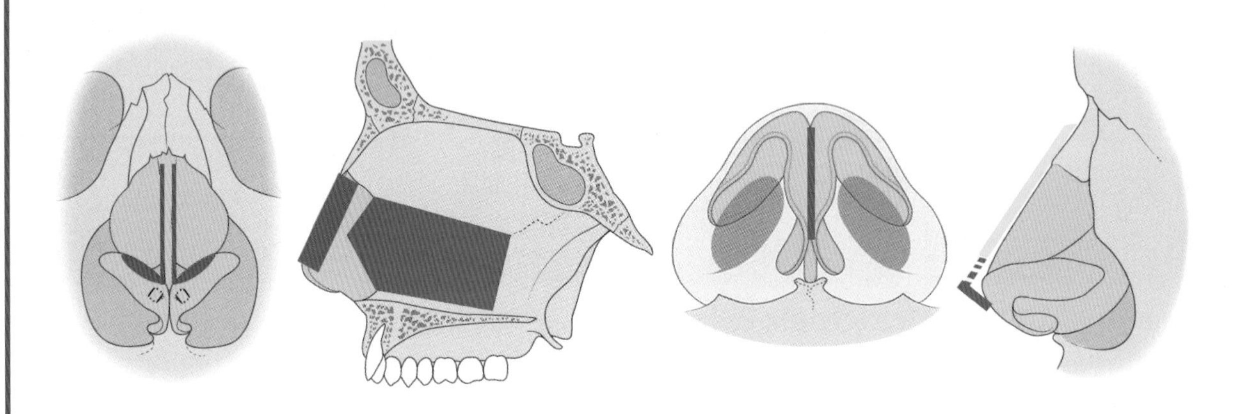

Postoperative Changes

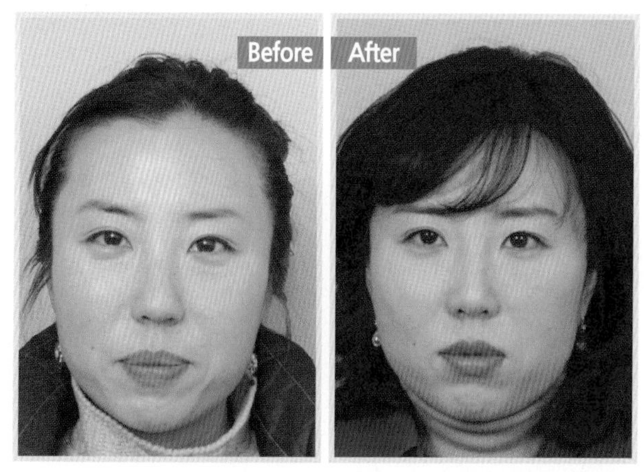

Frontal: Deviation was corrected. Aesthetic line was improved as well as the tip definition.

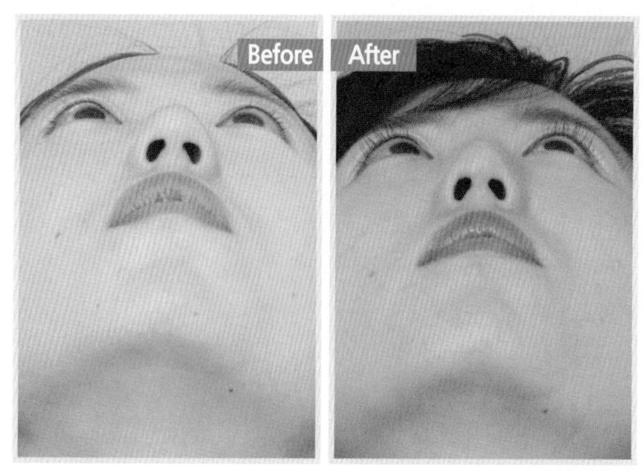

Basal: Tip projection was improved. Nasal base became the appropriate triangular shape.

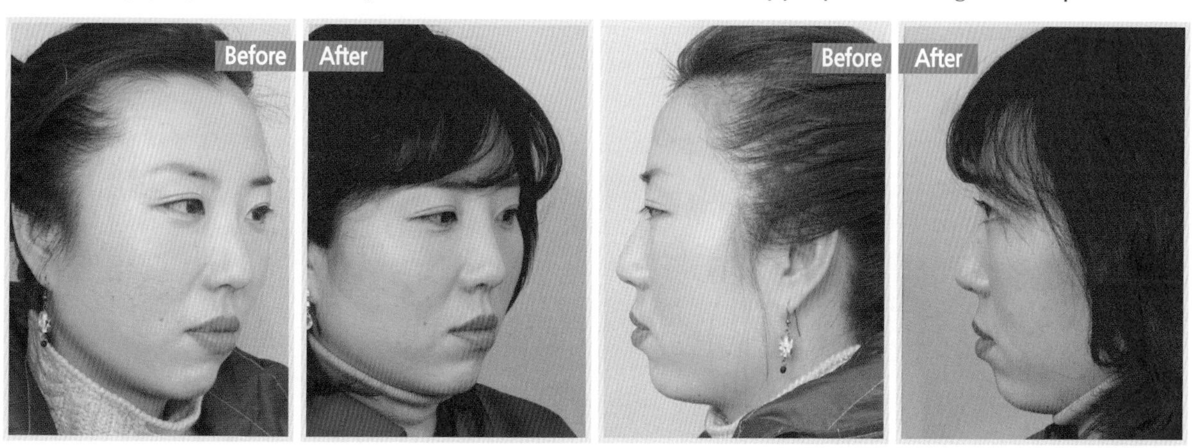

Lateral and Oblique: Slightly masculine dorsal shape was inadvertently created by the highly located radix. Dorsal convexity of cartilaginous portion was partially improved.

Case 5

A 27-year-old male visited for a nasal deviation with nasal obstruction.

Analysis

Frontal: Deviated nose (Type I deviation)
Basal: Poorly projected tip, lobule is longer than the columella
Lateral and Oblique: Mildly convex dorsum

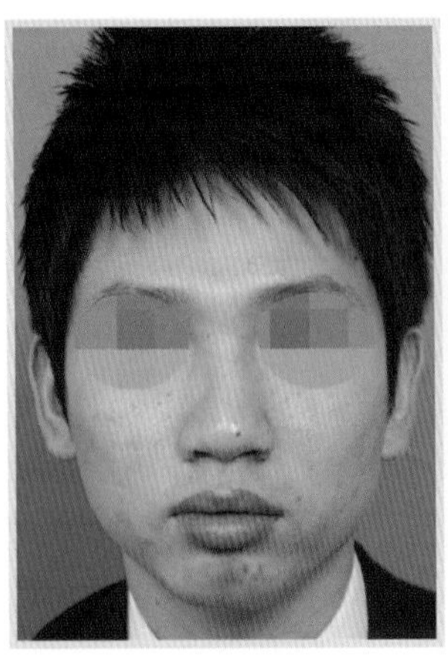
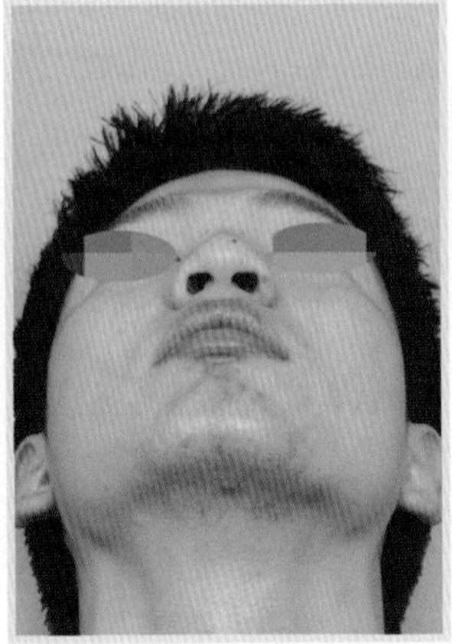
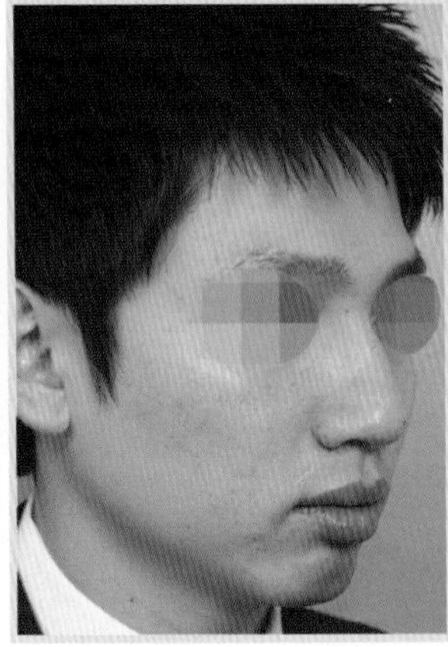
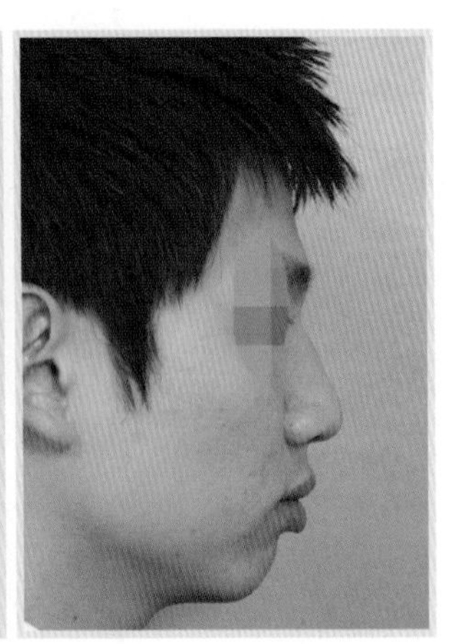

Operative Procedures

Open rhinoplasty approach
Septoplasty and harvest of septal cartilage and bone
Medial, lateral, and percutaneous root osteotomies
Spreader grafting using septal cartilage (bilateral)
Caudal septal extension grafting (left)
Multilayer tip grafting using septal cartilage
Dorsal augmentation using Gore-Tex

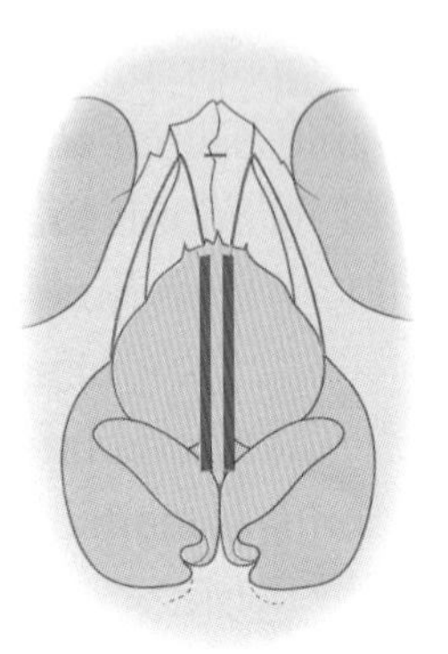
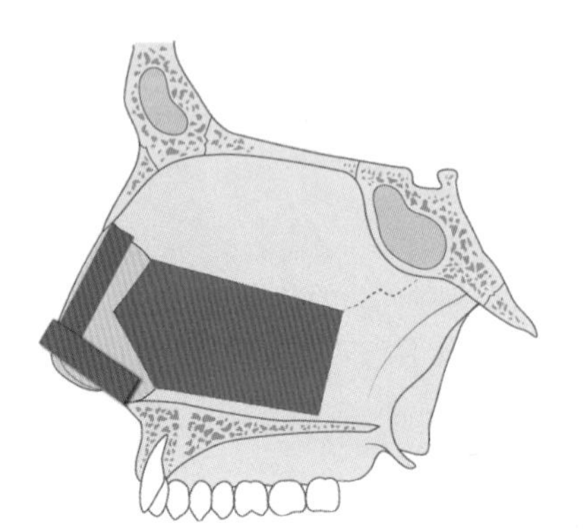
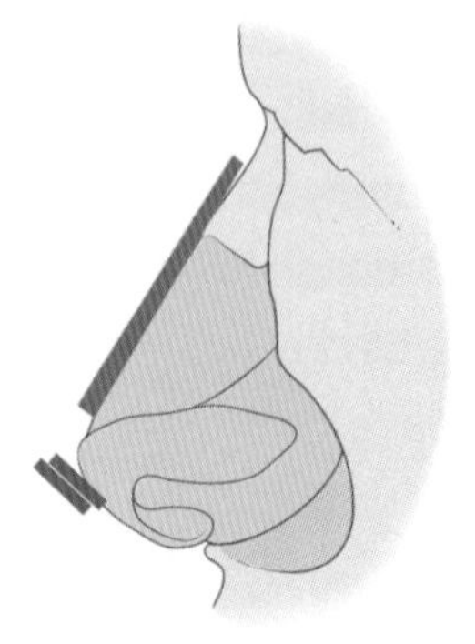

Postoperative Changes

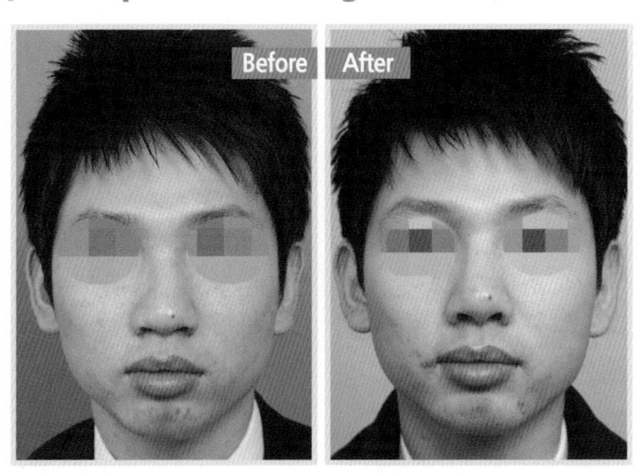

Frontal: Deviation was corrected. Natural and symmetric dorsal aesthetic lines were created. Nostril show was slightly increased.

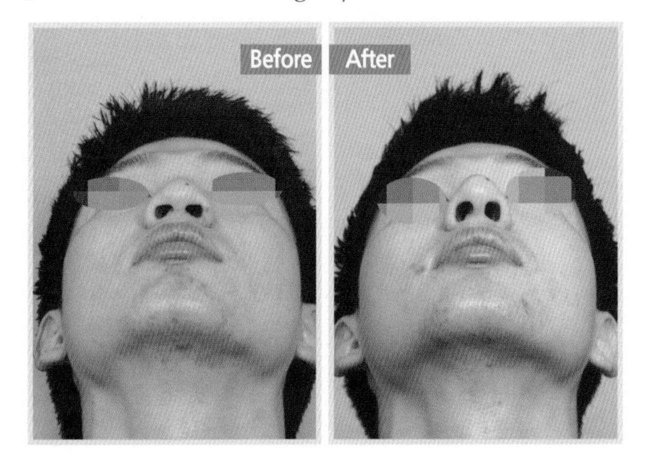

Basal: Tip projection was increased. Nostril shape and lobule-columella ratio were improved.

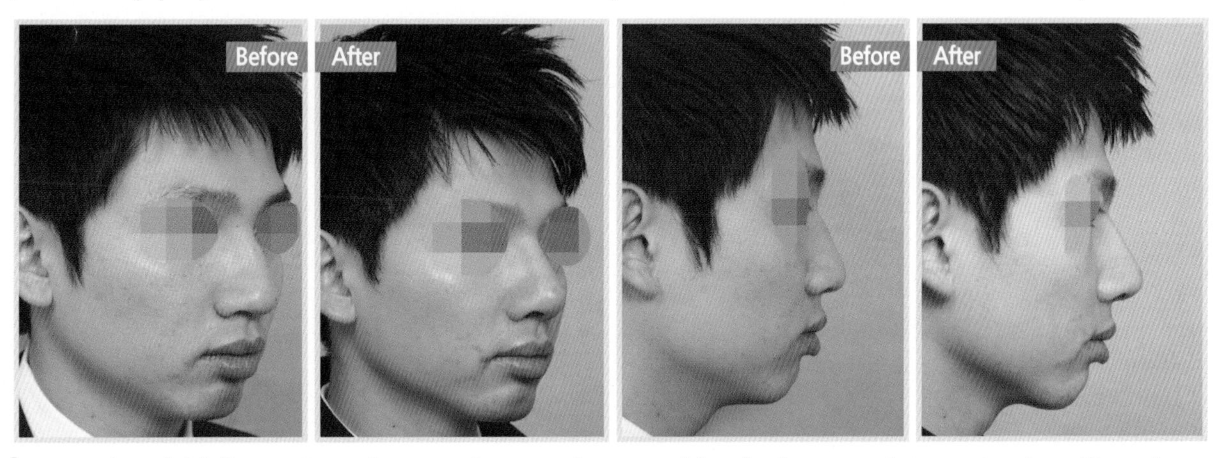

Lateral and Oblique: Dorsal convexity was decreased by the increased tip projection. Dorsal height was slightly increased.

Case 6

A 19-year-old female visited for a deviated nose.

Analysis

Frontal: Deviated nose (Type V deviation)
Basal: Underprojected tip, symmetric nostrils
Lateral: No gross abnormality

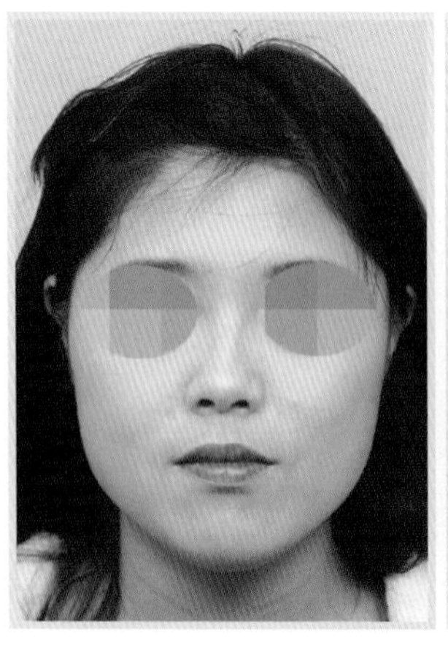
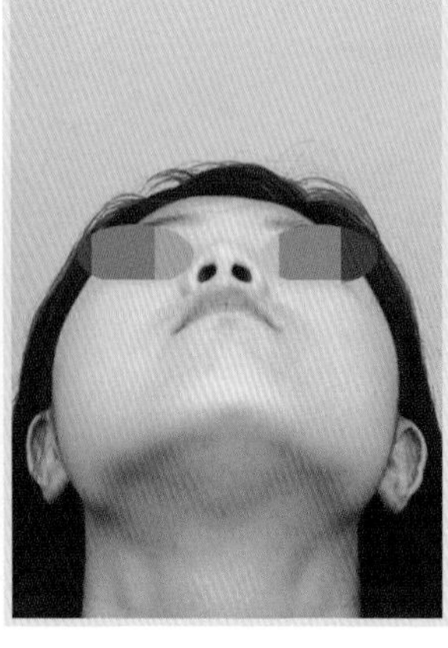
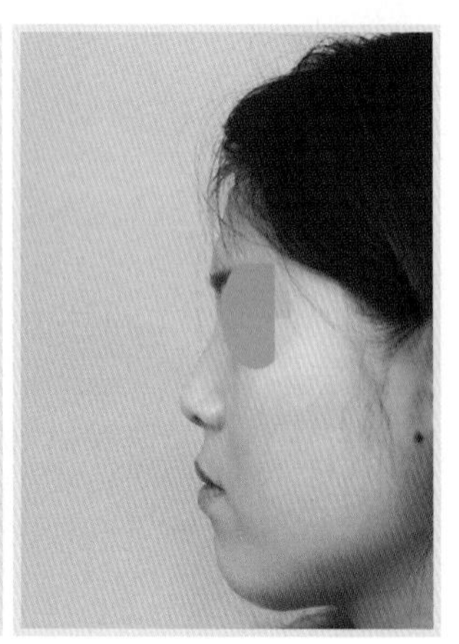

Operative Procedures

Open rhinoplasty approach
Septoplasty and harvest of septal cartilage and bone
Spreader grafting using septal cartilage (left)
Caudal septal extension grafting (bilateral)
Caudal septal relocation suture (right to left)
Medial, lateral and percutaneous root osteotomies
Multilayer tip grafting
Dorsal augmentation using fascia lata

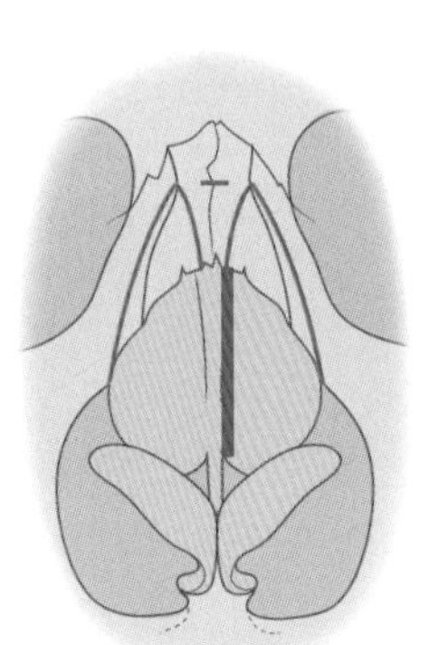
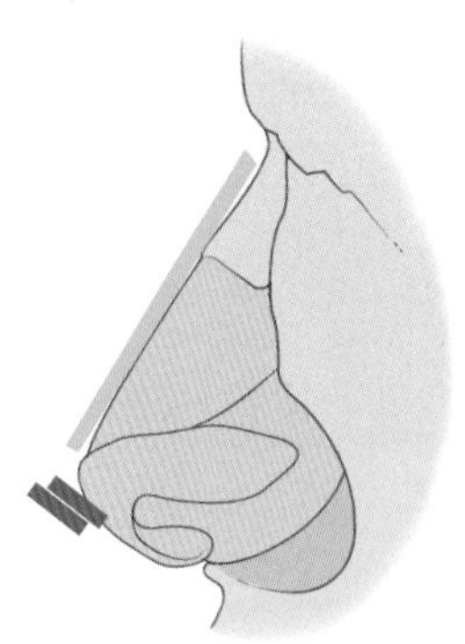
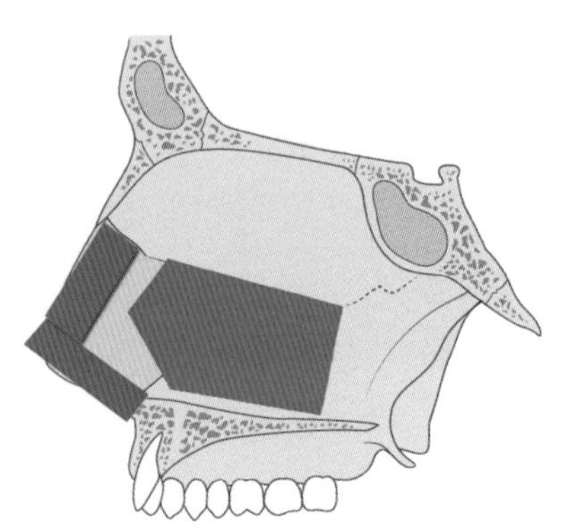

Postoperative Changes

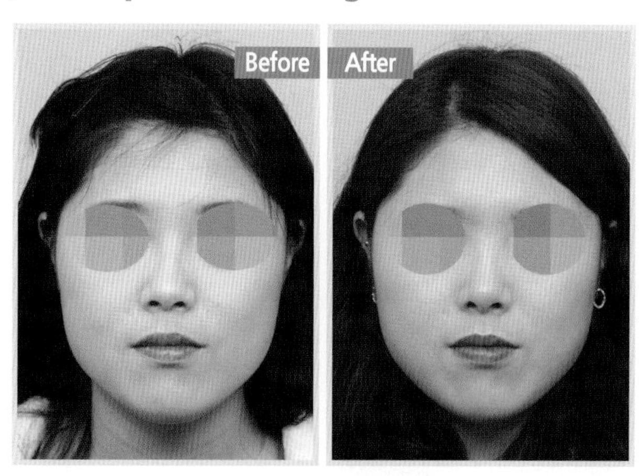

Frontal: Deviation was improved.

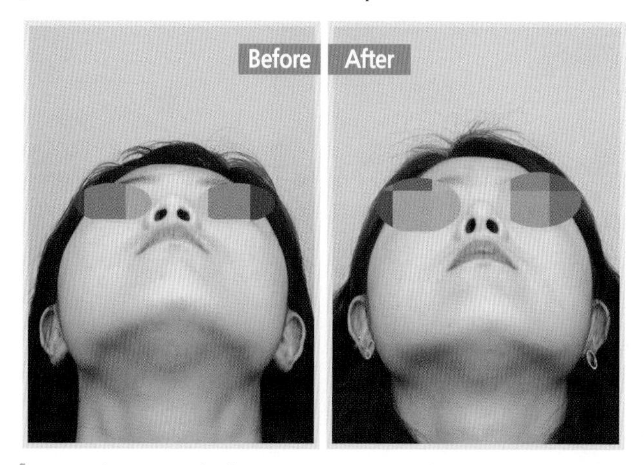

Basal: Nostril shape re-oriented more vertically. Right nostril apex located higher than the left. Tip projection was improved.

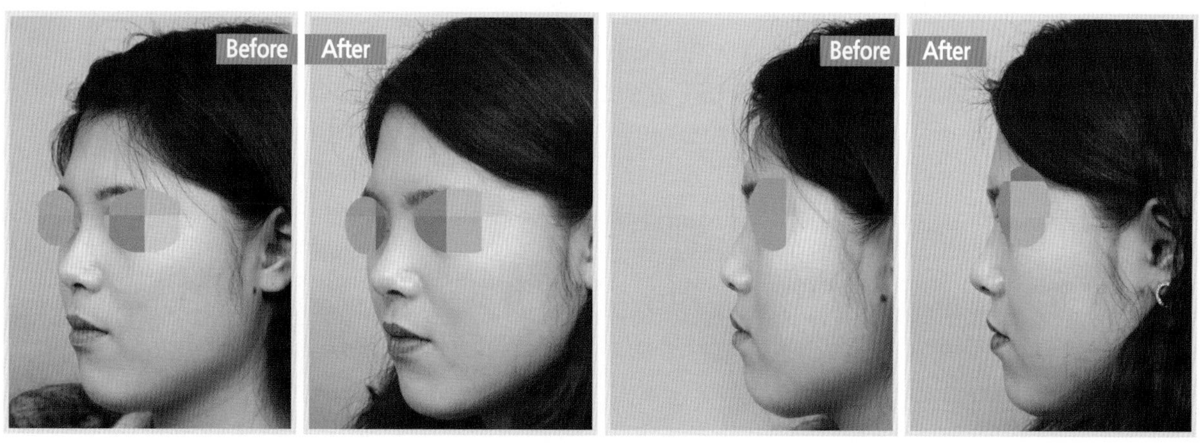

Lateral and Oblique: Slightly concave dorsal line was achieved by tip projection without dorsal height change.

Case 7

A 33-year-old female visited for a deviated nose with nasal obstruction following closed reduction for nasal fracture 4 months ago.

Analysis Frontal: Bony deviation to the right, cartilaginous deviation to the left (Type I deviation)
Basal: Non-specific
Lateral and Oblique: Isolated hump

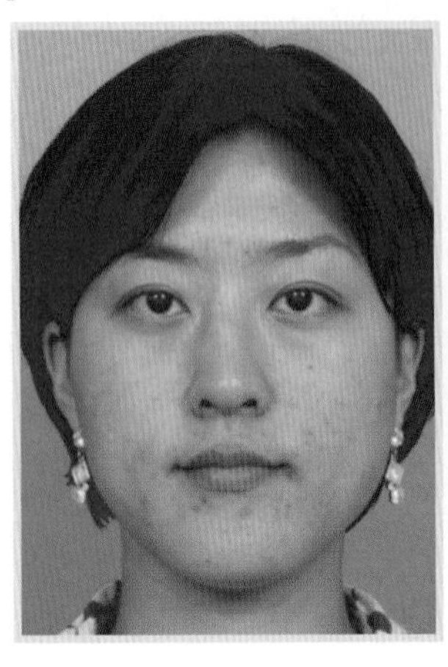
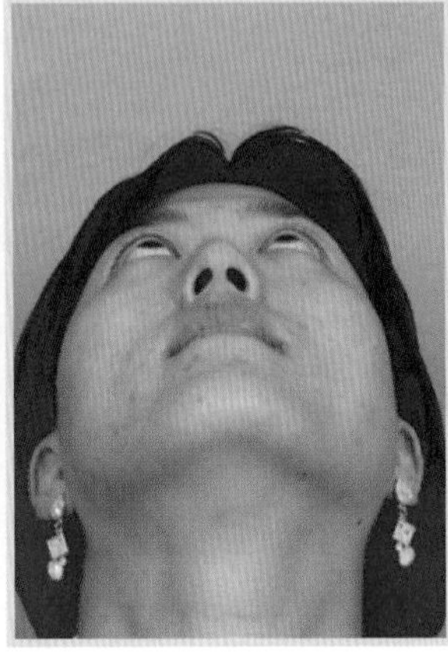
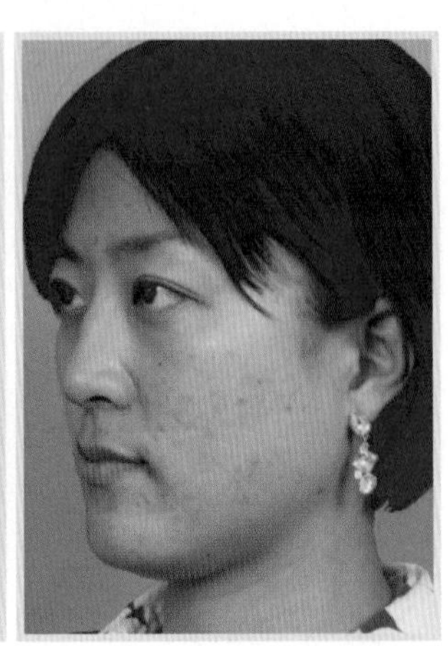

Operative Procedures

Open rhinoplasty approach
Septoplasty and harvest of septal cartilage and bone
Hump rasping
Spreader grafting using septal cartilage (right)
Caudal septal extension grafting using septal cartilage (right)
Batten grafting using septal bone (left)
Multilayer tip grafting using conchal cartilage
Dorsal augmentation using fascia lata

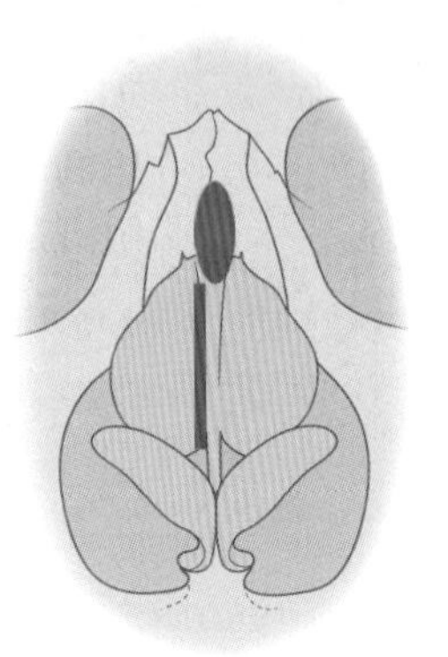
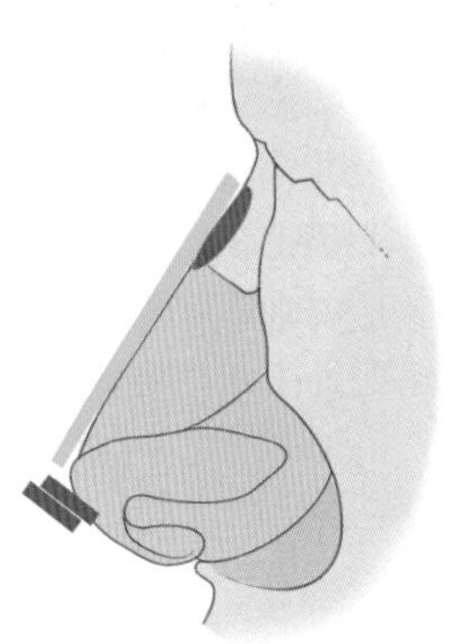
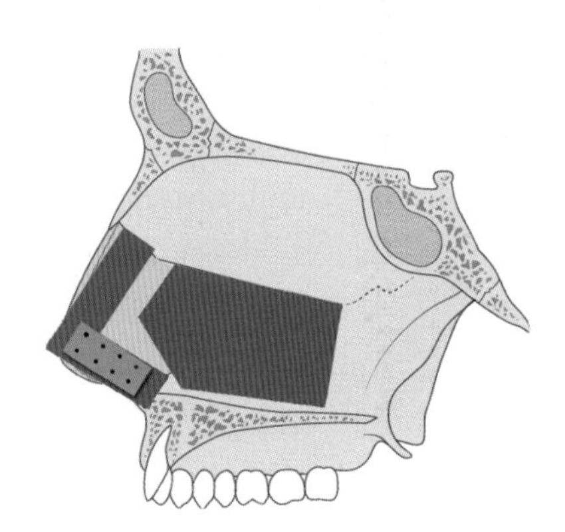

Postoperative Changes

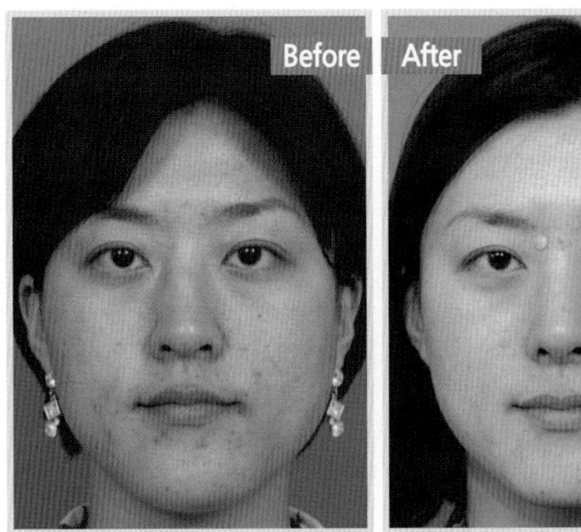

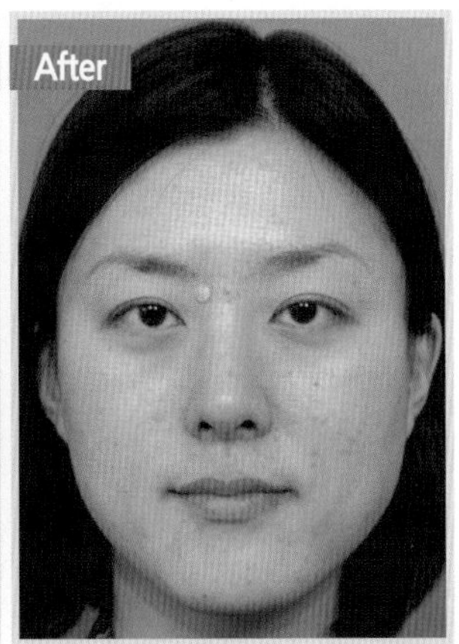

Frontal: Deviation was corrected. Dorsum was slightly widened.

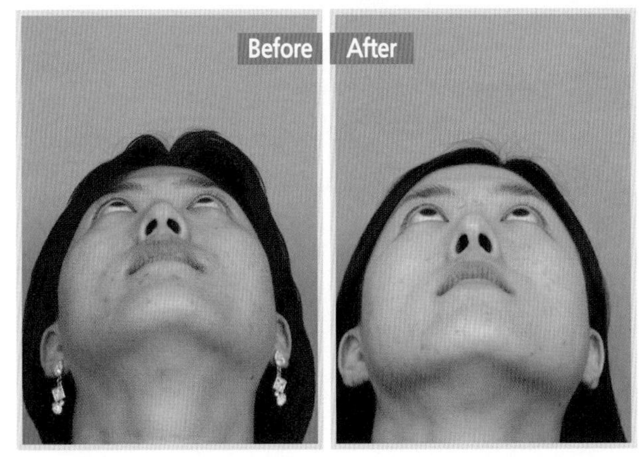

Basal: Tip projection was slightly increased.

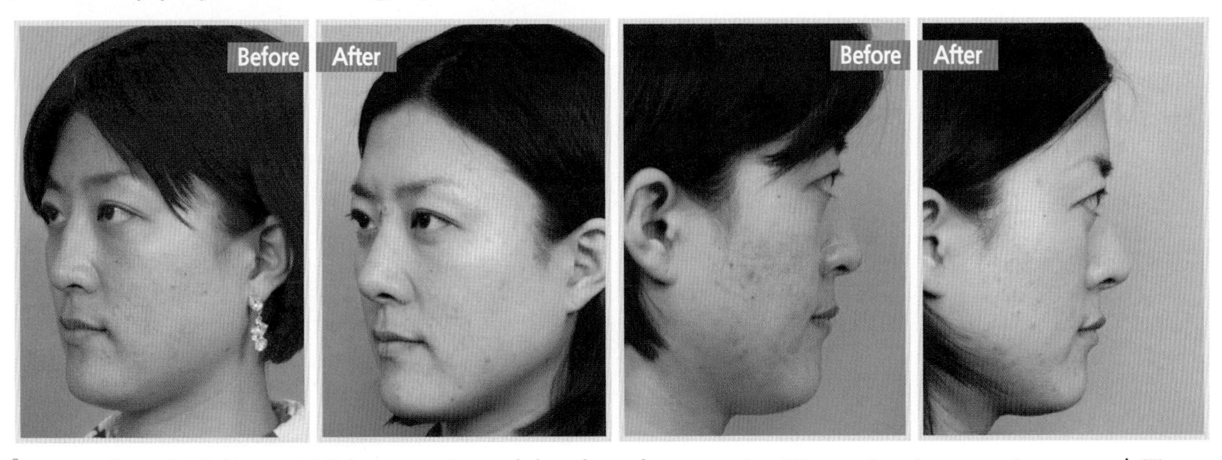

Lateral and Oblique: Mild correction of the dorsal convexity. Tip projection was increased. Tip definition was improved.

Case 8

A 17-year-old male visited for a deviated nose with nasal obstruction.

Analysis Frontal: Deviated bony dorsum, curved cartilaginous dorsum (Type II deviation), amorphous tip

Basal: Nostril asymmetry

Lateral and Oblique: Poor tip projection, low dorsal height

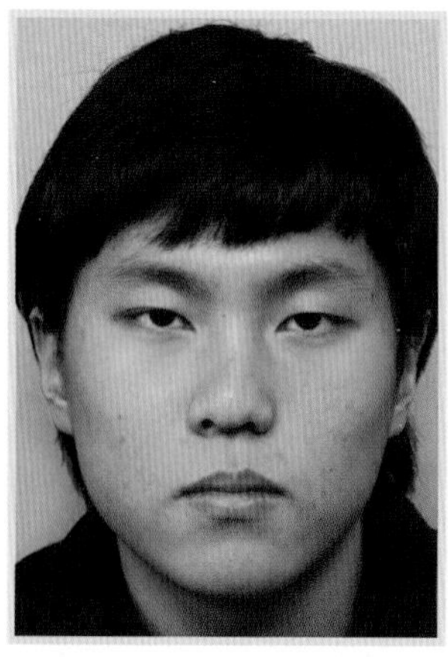
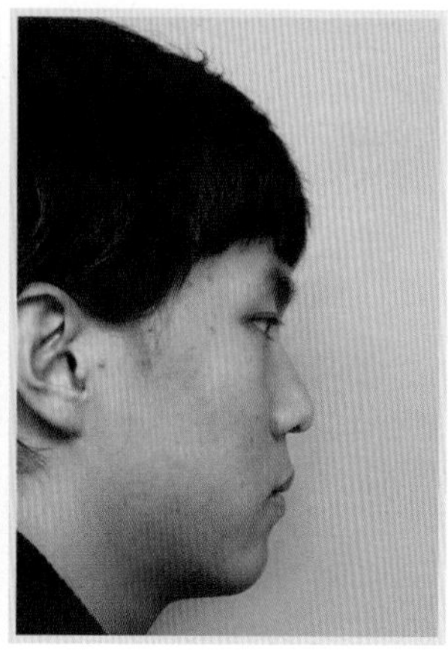
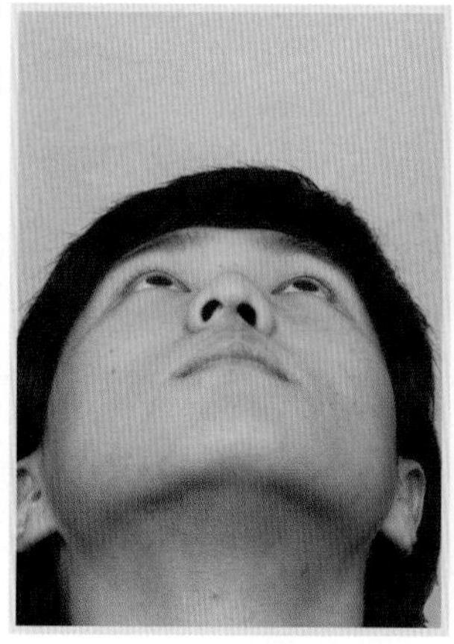
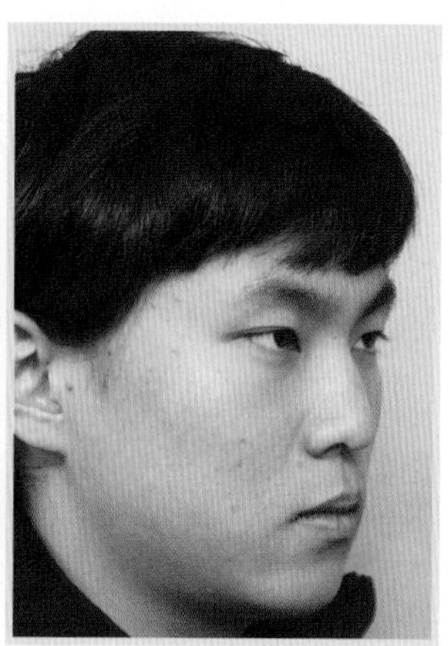

Operative Procedures

Open rhinoplasty approach

Medial, lateral, and percutaneous root osteotomies

Extracorporeal septoplasty

Shield grafting with backstop using septal cartilage

Dorsal augmentation using crushed cartilage and processed fascia lata

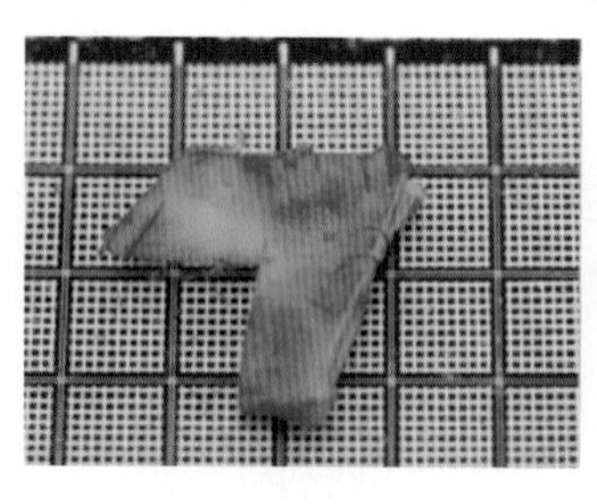
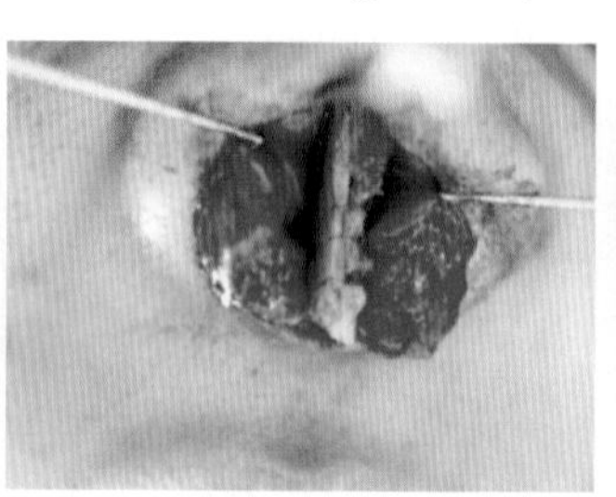
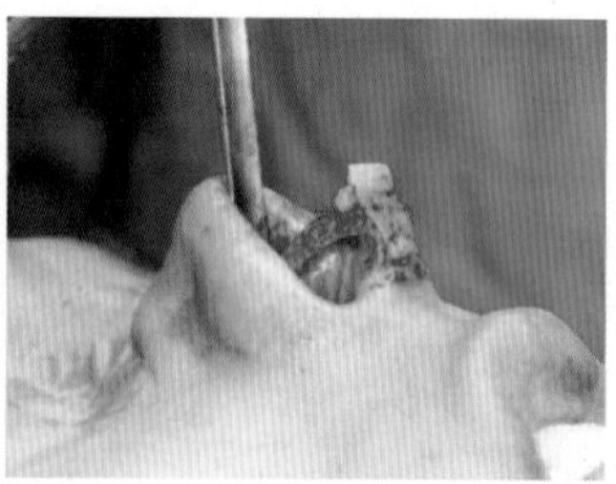
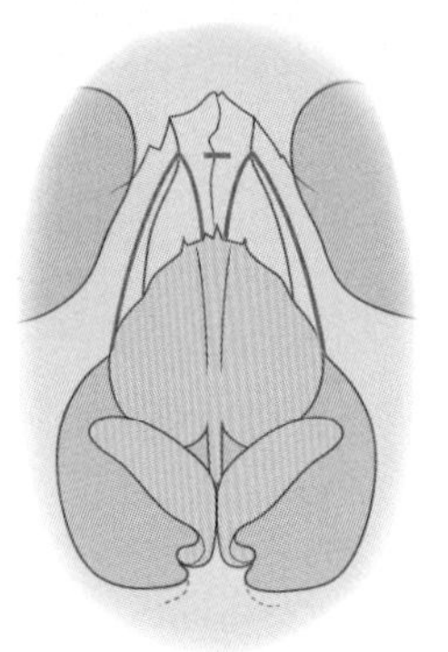
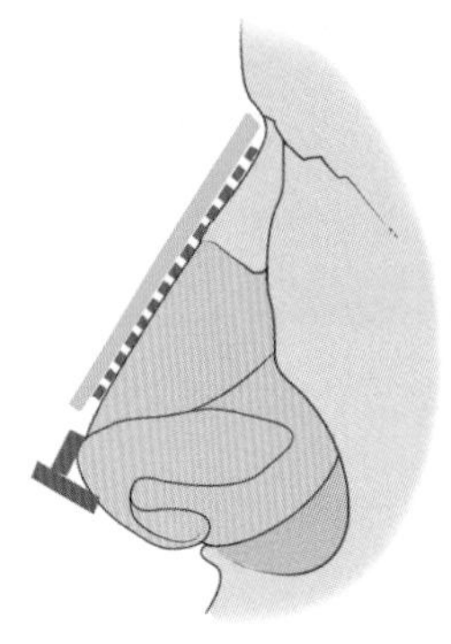
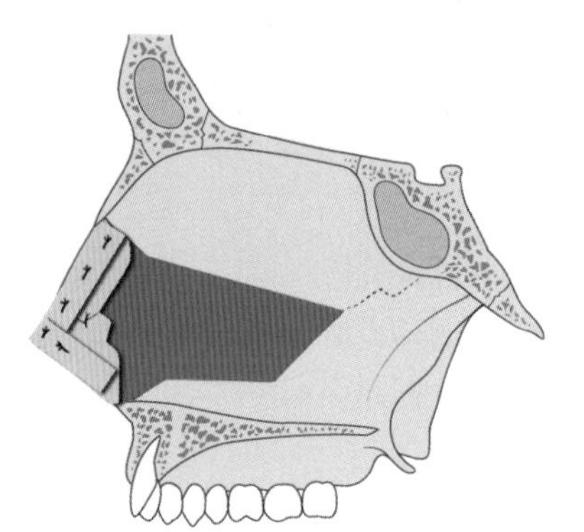

Postoperative Changes

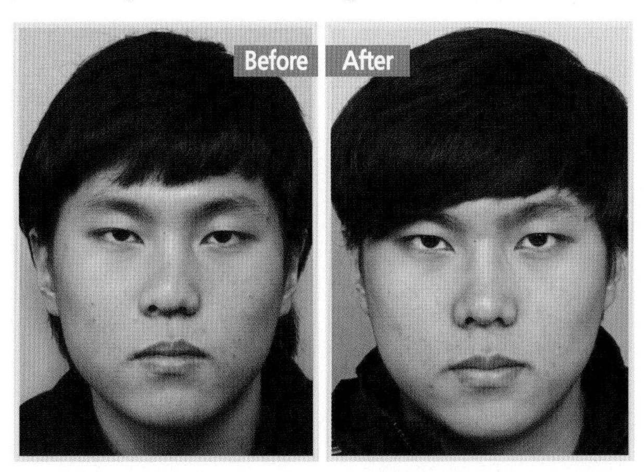

Frontal: Dorsal deviation and tip definition were improved.

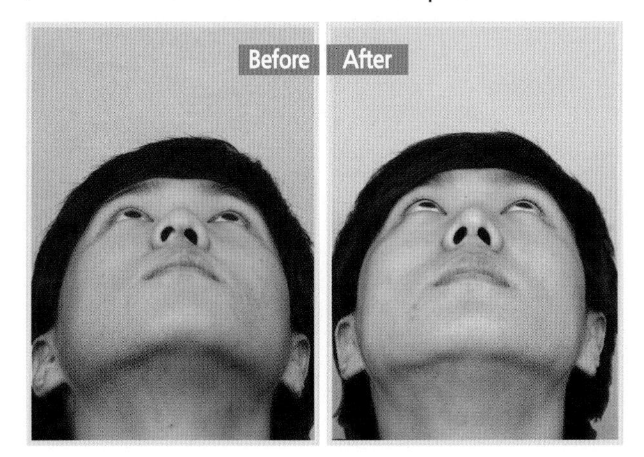

Basal: Nostril deformity was improved. Lobule-columella ratio was improved. Tip projection was increased.

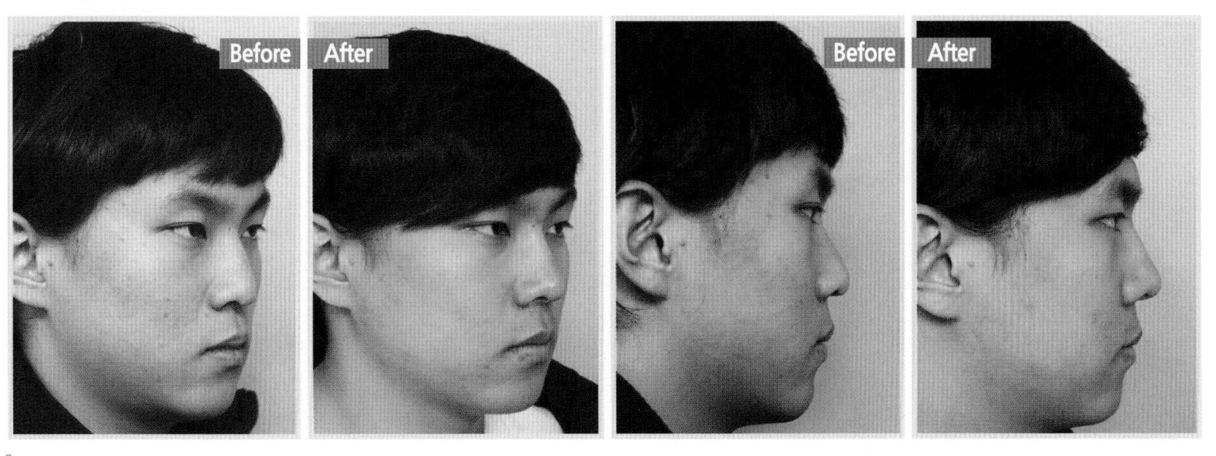

Lateral and Oblique: Tip projection and dorsal height were increased.

Case 9

A 47-year-old female visited for a deviated nose with nasal obstruction.

Analysis

Frontal: Tilted bony dorsum, curved cartilaginous dorsum (Type II deviation)
Basal: Nostril asymmetry, concave alar lobule (right)
Lateral: Good tip-dorsum relationship

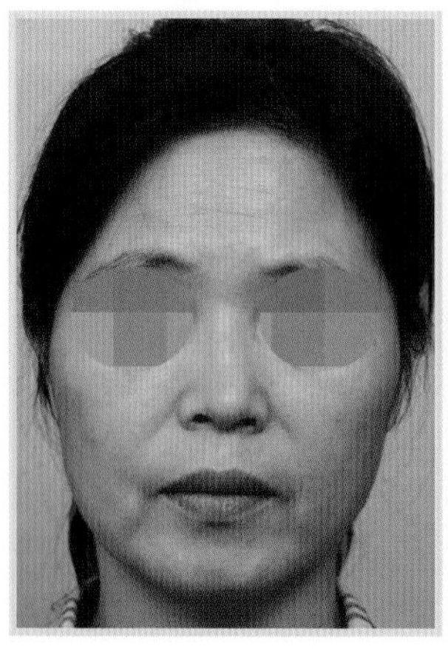
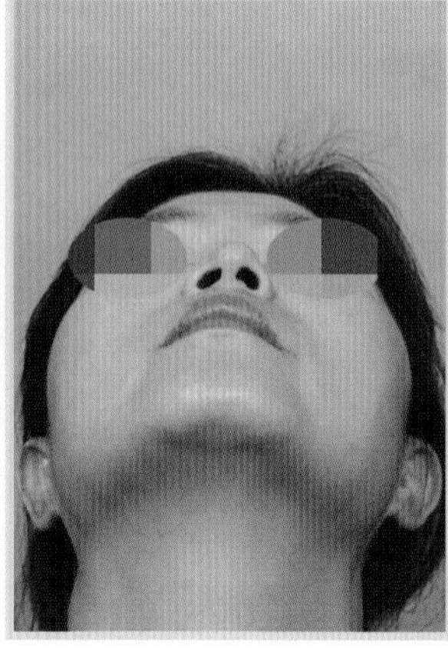
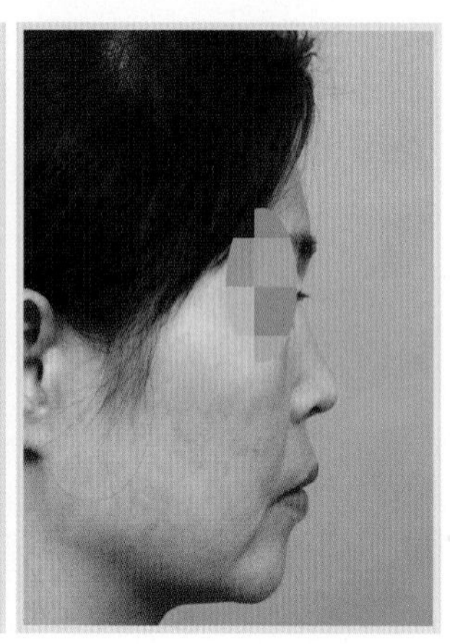

Operative Procedures

Open rhinoplasty approach
Caudal septum relocation suture
Spreader grafting (bilateral) using processed costal cartilage: homologous costal cartilage was used since the septal cartilage was too weak
Lateral crural onlay grafting using septal cartilage (right)
Septal extension grafting using processed costal cartilage
Dorsal augmentation using processed fascia lata

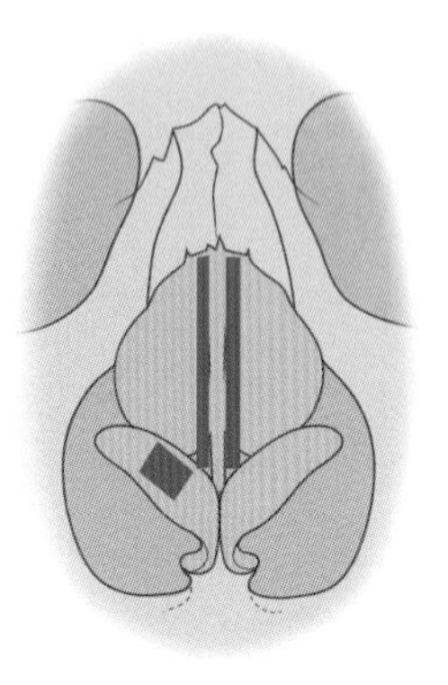
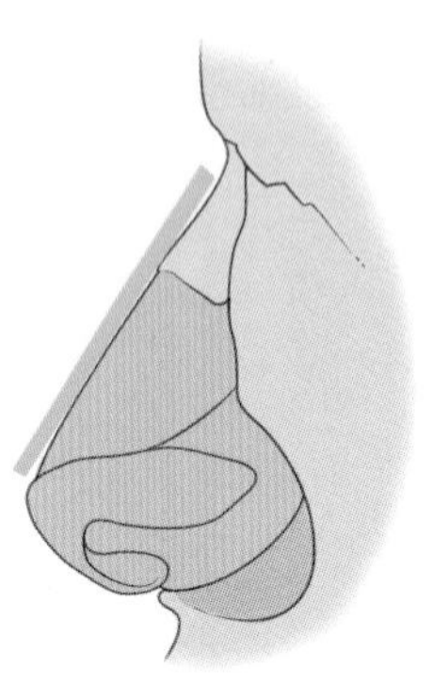
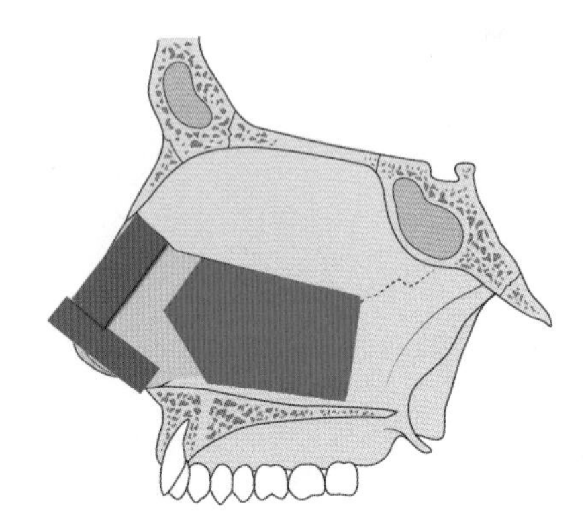

Postoperative Changes

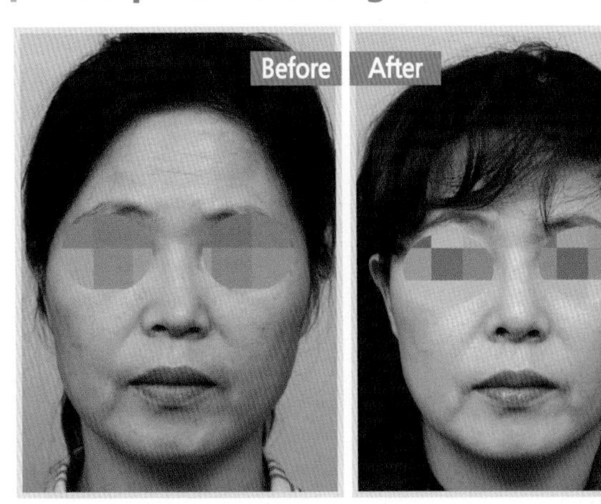

Frontal: Deviated nose was corrected and cartilaginous dorsum was slightly widened.

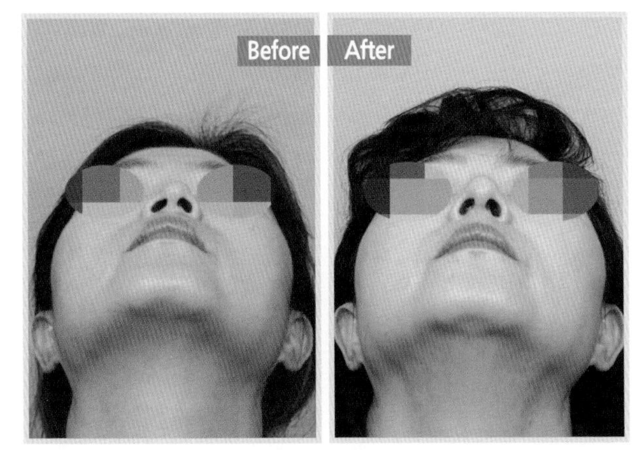

Basal: Right alar concavity was slightly corrected. Nostril asymmetry was improved. Tip projection was increased.

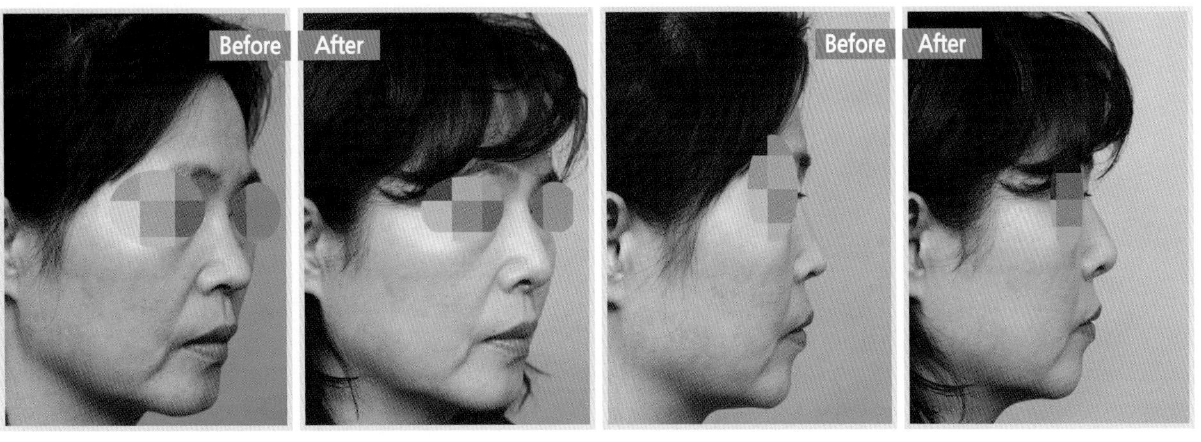

Lateral and Oblique: Slightly masculine dorsum was inadvertently created by the loss of dorsal concavity after dorsal augmentation.

Hump Nose (Convex Dorsum)

Yong Ju Jang

Dorsal hump reduction is a very common procedure among Caucasians. Generally the prevalence of a hump nose among Asians is low. However, more recently, as a result of complications related to external injury or developmental characteristics, there has been an increase in patients who are looking for surgical correction of their hump noses. Hump noses in Asians varies greatly in shape, and it would be more appropriate to describe the deformity as convex dorsum.

I. Anatomy

The skin of the nasal dorsum is thinnest at the rhinion, a little thicker at the cephalic region and thickest at the supratip and tip region *(Figure 1)*. Thus, the dorsum, which outwardly looks straight, in reality has a slight convexity around the rhinion. The dorsal line, which stretches out in a straight line, is composed of such a convex area and different levels of skin thickness in the dorsum.

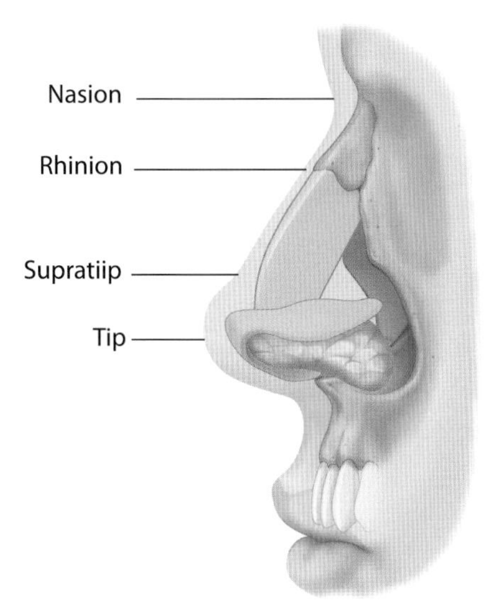

Figure 1 The skin of the nasal dorsum is thinnest at the rhinion and comparatively thinner at the cephalic to the rhinion and thicker at the supratip and the tip region.

II. Aesthetic Considerations

Observed from the front, the appearance of the dorsum is primarily determined by the dorsal aesthetic line. And such a line should be adequately created during the dorsal hump reduction. The dorsal aesthetic lines start from the supraorbital ridges, past the corrugators and meets at the medial canthal ligaments. Then, widening slightly at the keystone area, they go down parallel to each other until they reach the tip defining point. For males, it is desirable that the line connects to the tip without much disparity in the width, while for females, it is best if the line creates a gentle curve from the supraorbital ridge to the tip *(Figure 2)*. It is desirable that the dorsal line of a females should be located slightly lower than the line connecting the nasofrontal angle when it is observed from the side and the tip should take on a concave shape. For male subjects, to avoid looking feminine, the dorsal line should be slightly higher than that of a woman *(Figure 3)*. However, trying too hard to make the dorsal line concave can sometimes lead to excessive reduction of the dorsum and so special care must be exercised during this procedure. For proper management of convex dorsum, the surgeon needs to have a good understanding of the importance of radix augmentation. The radix is an area where the union of various nasal bones takes place. The soft-tissue of this area is made up of thick skin, a fatty layer, and muscle. To understand the exact location of the radix, one must understand what the nasion or radix stands for. The term nasion (sellion) is used to express the deepest part of the nasofrontal angle. And, with the nasion serving as the crux, the radix is an anatomical term that represents the region lying between the nasion all the way downwards to the lateral canthus and the corresponding distance upward.

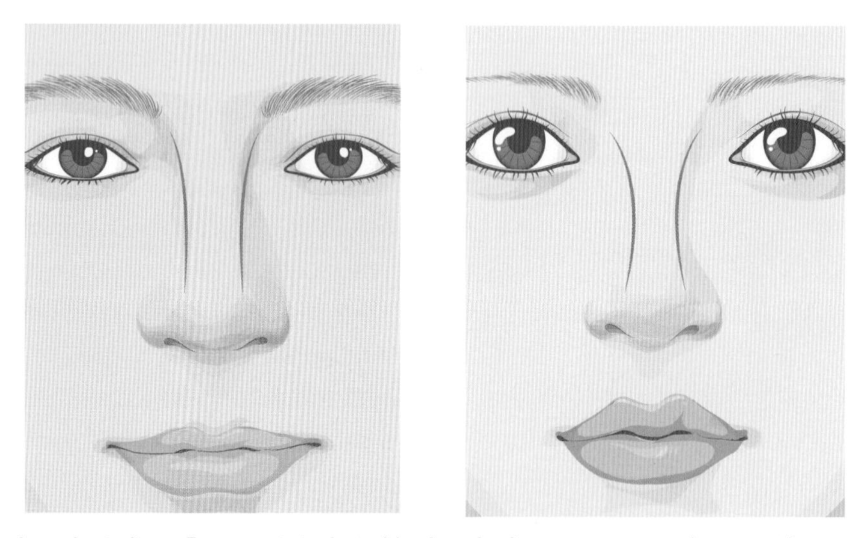

Figure 2 Dorsal aesthetic lines. For men, it is desirable that the line connects to the tip without much disparity in the width as shown in the left. For women, it is best if the line creates a gentle curve from the supraorbital ridge to the tip, as it appears in the right.

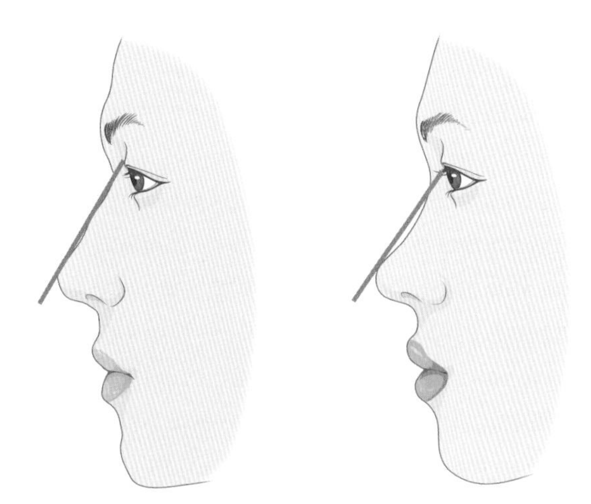

Figure 3 An ideal lateral view of the dorsal line. As shown in the left illustration, it is best when the line connecting the nasofrontal angle and the tip is slightly concave in female subjects. For the male patients, however, one must strive to acquire as straight a dorsal line as possible.

III. Classifications of the Convex Dorsum

Surgeons must be aware that the degree of deformity varies greatly among patients who visit seeking treatment for their dorsal humps. Different types of humps require distinct therapeutic plans. For the sake of convenience in treatment, the author suggests the following classification of the convex dorsum *(Figure 4)*.

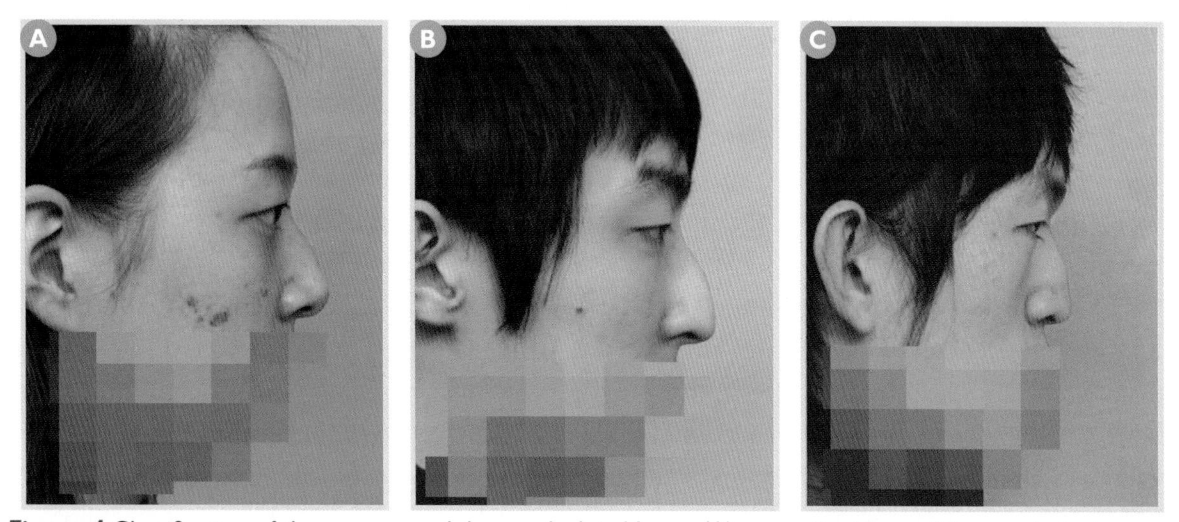

Figure 4 Classification of the convex nasal dorsum. Isolated hump (A), generalized hump (B), and relative hump with low tip (C).

- Isolated hump
- Generalized hump
- Relative hump with low tip

An isolated hump represents instances of an abrupt protrusion of a small hump in a triangular shape at the dorsal line. Isolated humps occur frequently in patients with a history of external nasal trauma. The total length of the hump is short and, when they are exposed during surgery; most of the hump can be found located around the rhinion. As proportional hump length over 45% of nasal length is defined as a generalized hump, a hump length below 45% of the nasal length is considered to be an isolated hump. The curvature of a generalized hump begins from the bony vault and goes all the way down to the cartilaginous dorsum in the form of a gentle curve. In many cases, patients showing generalized humps are without a history of external trauma and they are deemed to be the result of an inherited developmental problem. In treating such a deformity, there is a greater chance of success when the surgeon pays greater attention to the cartilaginous dorsum rather than the bony dorsum. In patients with relative hump with low tip, their dorsal convexity is due to the under projected tip. In the author's classification, when the tip projection with respect to nasal length is below 30%, the deformity is classified as a relative hump with low tip. Proper execution of tip augmentation is the most important determining factor for surgical success. In the author's patient series, generalized humps were the most common deformity. The second most common deformity was the isolated hump. Generally, the surgical outcome is the best in the isolated hump cases compared with other types of convex dorsum.

IV. Surgical Technique

1. Endonasal Approach *(Figure 5)*

The endonasal approach usually makes use of a marginal incision or an intercartilaginous incision. Meticulous dissection of the supraperichondrial and subperiosteal planes should be performed after incision. After dissecting the soft-tissue covering of the dorsum of the cartilaginous area, an incision at the periosteum of the caudal end of the nasal bone is made. The soft-tissue covering the bony vault is then dissected. During this procedure, it is not necessary to raise the periosteum excessively laterally, and must be limited to the area surrounding the hump planned for resection. Next, a retractor is inserted to raise the skin and, using a #15 blade, excise the cartilaginous vault along the intended incision line. To remove the bony part of the hump, insert a hump osteotome into the cartilaginous resection area and remove the osseocartilaginous hump in one lump. Then, using a rasp, polish the remaining bony until smooth. Should there be an isolated hump, a more simple method to treat this problem is to shave the cartilaginous hump with a blade and then, using a rasp instead of an osteotome, reduce the bony dorsum. If a distinct open roof deformity occurs following this procedure, use the osteotomy technique to correct this problem *(Figure 6)*.

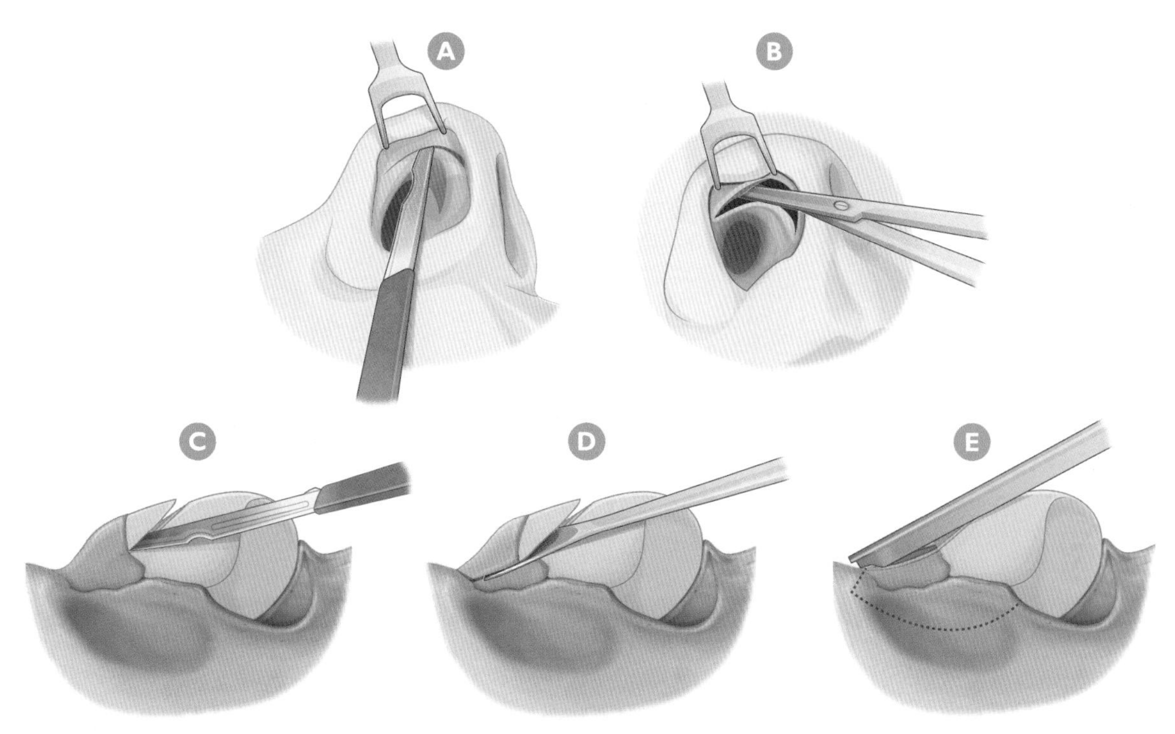

Figure 5 Surgical sequence in hump reduction via a closed approach

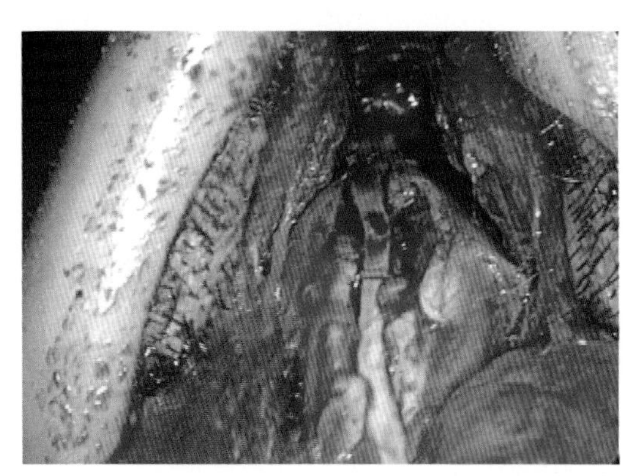

Figure 6 Open roof deformity of the nasal dorsum following hump removal

2. Open Approach

1) En-bloc Removal of Hump

The author usually uses the open approach on patients displaying characteristic features of a generalized hump. In particular, this method is recommended for relative beginners because of its good surgical view and the ease with which the intended operation can be performed. The skin flap is elevated using marginal and transcolumellar incisions. The dorsum is exposed by dissecting as close to the perichondrium as possible. During the dissection of the bony vault, when the periosteum is exposed, an incision is done on the periosteum using a blade followed by dissection towards the subperiosteal plane above the bony vault. As in the previously described endonasal approach, the cartilaginous and bony portions of the osseocartilaginous hump can be removed in an en-bloc manner *(Figure 7)*.

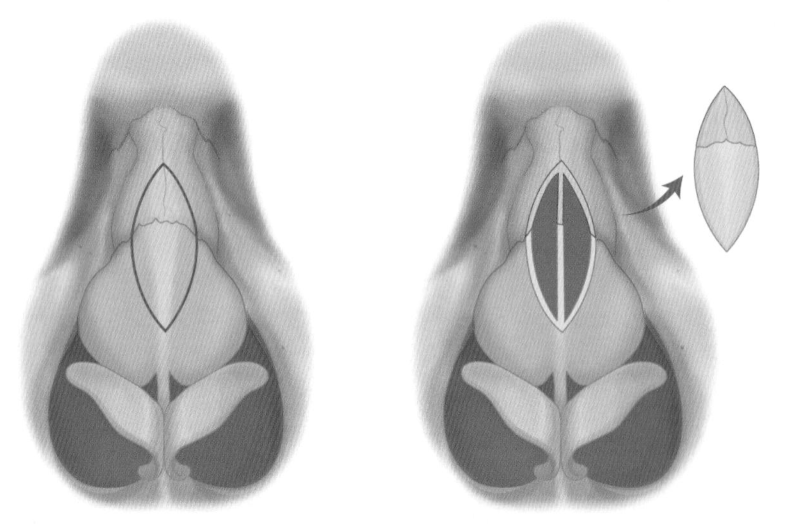

Figure 7 En bloc removal of hump.

2) Component Hump Reduction

This method involves separating the crural cartilage on both sides and, when the caudal portion of the septum has been exposed, subperichondrial tunnels are created followed by separation of the septal cartilage and upper lateral cartilages. In carrying out a component hump reduction, first, perform resection of the hump of the septum, which is separated and exposed in the midline. Next, using an osteotome, remove the nasal bone attached to the cephalic region together with the septal cartilage in one lump. In the next stage, using a rasp, remove the remaining bony hump. When performing rasping on the bony hump, it needs to be carried out in a slightly oblique direction to prevent the upper lateral cartilage becoming separated from the nasal bone. The bony dorsum needs to be rasped along the left and right dorsal aesthetic lines, and a hump reduction needs to be carried out in the middle while being supported with the thumb and the index finger of the other hand. In between rasping, the rasp needs to be shaken in water or cleaned with a brush to remove the bone fragments caught on the rasp. Then, re-drape the skin and observe the lateral dorsal line that has taken shape following the hump reduction. At this point, there is a high probability that the septum of the caudal region wherein the hump is excised will display a form of protrusion in the shape of a polly beak. Thus, the septal cartilage needs to be carefully excised in incremental fashion

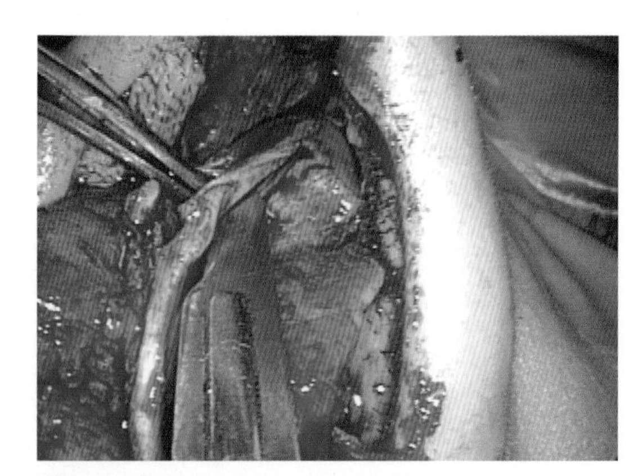

Figure 8 Resection of the dorsal septum during the component hump reduction procedure.

to attain the desired shape, covering the skin in between several times to confirm that the desired dorsal line is taking shape *(Figure 8)*. As a next step, reduction of the upper lateral cartilages can be performed if necessary. When the upper lateral cartilage are excessively excised, it can either result in the narrowing of the internal nasal valve or create a risk of the dorsal surface becoming uneven. Therefore, the author prefers to reduce the upper lateral cartilage as minimally as possible.

3) Hump Reduction without Osteotomy

Typical hump reduction techniques consisting of cartilaginous hump resection, hump osteotomy, and osteotomy is effective but may result in instability of the whole nose because of the aggressive nature of an osteotomy. An osteotomy is quite effective in reducing a hump and closing the open roof deformity, but carries the risk of destabilizing the whole nose in the long-run. It is therefore recommended to avoid the use of osteotomy if possible for the sake of securing a long lasting stable nose. In that regard, in mild convex dorsum or in a patient with small nasal bone, hump reduction can be done without osteotomy. The surgical technique starts with resection of the cartilaginous hump. What remains is a bony prominence immediately cephalic to the resected cartilaginous hump *(Figure 9)*. This bony hump is then gradually rasped to match the height of cartilaginous dorsum using a manual or powered rasp, not performing an osteotomy *(Figure 10)*.

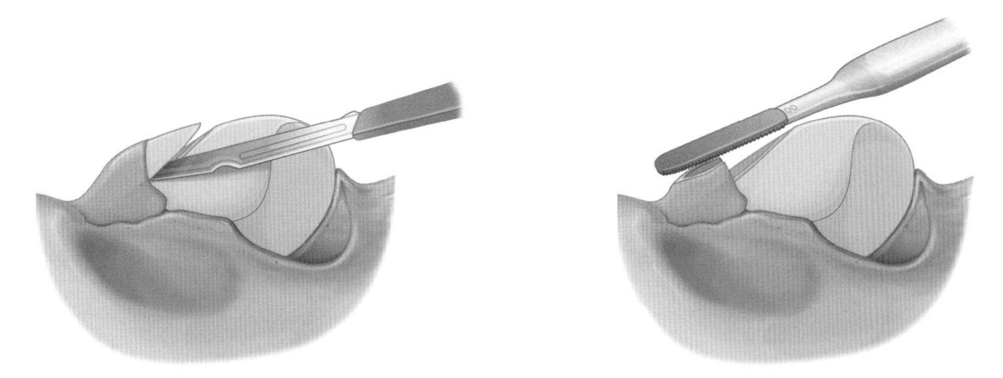

Figure 9 In hump reduction without osteotomy, the bony hump is reduced only by using a rasp.

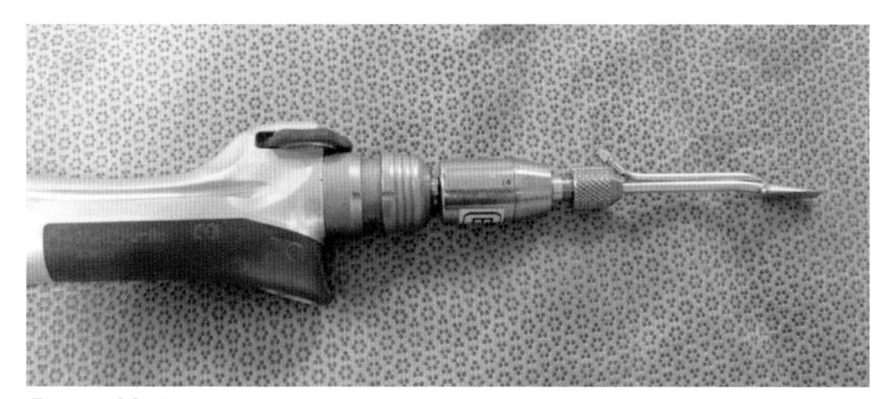

Figure 10 Powered rasp can ease the rasping procedure during hump reduction.

4) Osteotomy

Removing the hump during a dorsal hump reduction can lead to an open roof deformity and an osteotomy is needed to correct this problem *(Figure 11)*. A medial osteotomy is performed to induce a back-fracture at a proper level. This is necessary when the amount of hump removed is small or when the sidewall of the nose is thick and strong. Because an extensive gap is created between the nasal bone and the septum when a large hump is removed, a medial osteotomy may not be necessary.

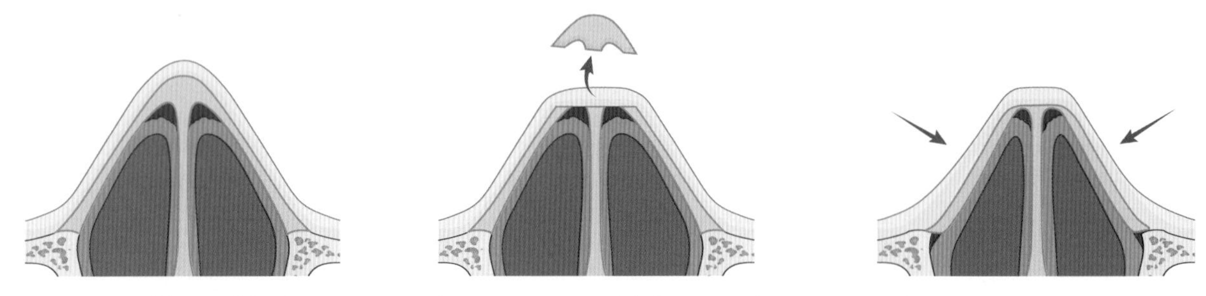

Figure 11 Osteotomy to close an open roof deformity subsequent to a hump resection.

5) Reconstruction of the Dorsum after Hump Reduction

Dorsal hump reduction can result in structural loss or weakening of the nasal dorsum, thus requiring proper reconstruction. Irregularities on the bony dorsum can be corrected by osteotomy and camouflage grafts. Reconstruction of the cartilaginous dorsum is usually performed by spreader grafting. The most important reason for performing the spreader graft procedure is the risk of middle vault collapse over time. Applying the spreader grafts properly can be helpful in the maintenance and reconstruction of the dorsal nasal roof and the internal nasal valve, as well as the reconstruction of the dorsal aesthetic lines. The spreader grafts can be inserted parallel to the septum in one or both sides of the nose. The grafts are fixed to the septum by means of horizontal mattress sutures using 5-0 PDS. Then, using 4-0 PDS, the upper lateral cartilages and spreader graft/septal complex are sutured and made immobile. The cartilage grafts for spreader grafts need to have reasonable thickness and strength in order for it to be effective. However, too thick a graft can widen the nasal dorsum excessively. It is therefore important to use grafts of adequate thickness. There is also a possibility of deviated nose formation as a result of poorly placed spreader grafting. If the resected part of the cartilaginous dorsum is limited only to the mid to cephalic portion of the cartilaginous dorsum, with preservation of normal anatomic relationship between the nasal septum and upper lateral cartilages, placement of spreader grafts may not be necessary. When performing component hump reduction, if there are well developed upper lateral cartilages, they need not be resected, instead, can be used as autospreader flap by rolling in the upper margin of the cartilages medially to function as spreader grafts *(Figure 12)*.

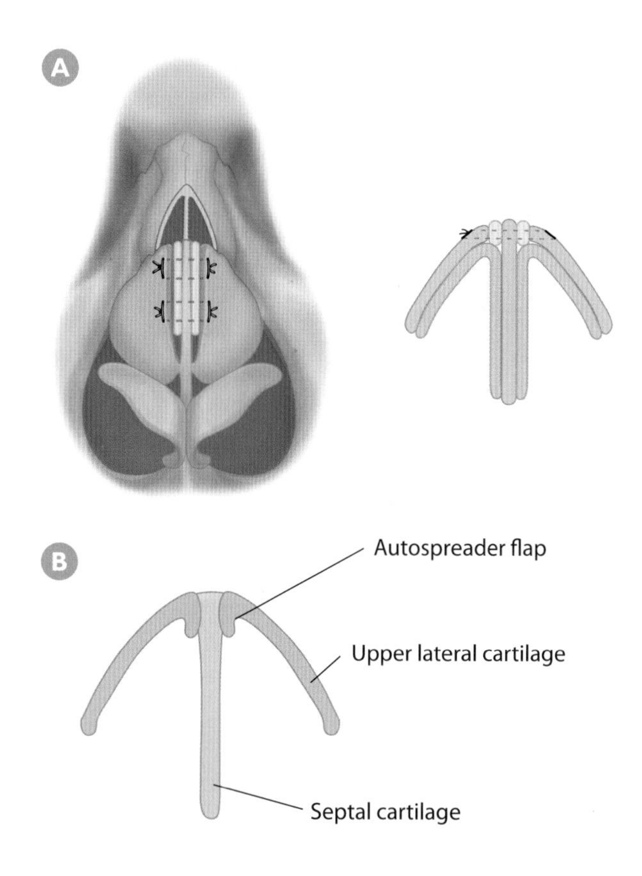

Figure 12 Spreader graft (A) and autospreader flap (B), aimed to prevent middle vault collapse after hump removal.

6) Tip Surgery in Dorsal Hump Reduction

Because dorsal hump reduction is a surgery to reduce the partial or general elevation of the dorsum, inexperienced surgeons may hope to achieve a successful surgical outcome with just a simple reduction. However, in clinical situations, things aren't that simple. Among hump nose patients who visit for surgical correction, there are many instances of an accompanying underprojected tip. If a simple hump reduction is performed on such patients, their nose will generally look smaller and flatter, making it very likely that the nose will look worse than before surgery. Thus, when performing dorsal hump reduction on patients with an underprojected tip and weak support, in most cases, surgery to improve the tip projection and support must be added. In the management of the convex dorsum, the author prefers to use tip surgery techniques that include shield grafts, multilayer tip grafts, and septal extension grafts, alone or in combination.

7) Radix and Dorsal Augmentation

In patients with convex dorsum, their radix normally looks relatively low, thus requiring augmentation to get a natural looking dorsum. Properly performed radix grafting combined with tip augmentation can soften the hump and can create an illusion of a straight dorsum *(Figure 13)* Radix augmentation should be performed in careful manner in patients who have a flat and low forehead. It is because radix grafting can make the nasion indistinct. In addition to radix augmentation, a full-length dorsal augmentation may be required in some patients. This is particularly useful in thin-skinned individuals to create the ideal dorsal aesthetic line and to cover dorsal irregularities following hump reduction. As for the material for dorsal augmentation in convex dorsum patient, it is advisable to use a material with a soft texture. When cartilage is selected for dorsal augmentation, the margin should be carefully beveled or crushed in order to avoid visible graft contour. Fascia can create initial good results, but may induce aesthetic problems later because of resorption. If silicone is selected for dorsal augmentation, it should be as thin and soft as possible. Gore-Tex can also be an excellent choice for radix or full-length dorsal augmentation. An aesthetically desirable surgical result can only be obtained when suitable augmentation is performed to match the elevation of the tip. Ultimately, it may be necessary to approach the treatments of dorsal hump reduction among patients in Asia not as a simple resection surgery, but a surgery for realigning and redistributing the height of the dorsum.

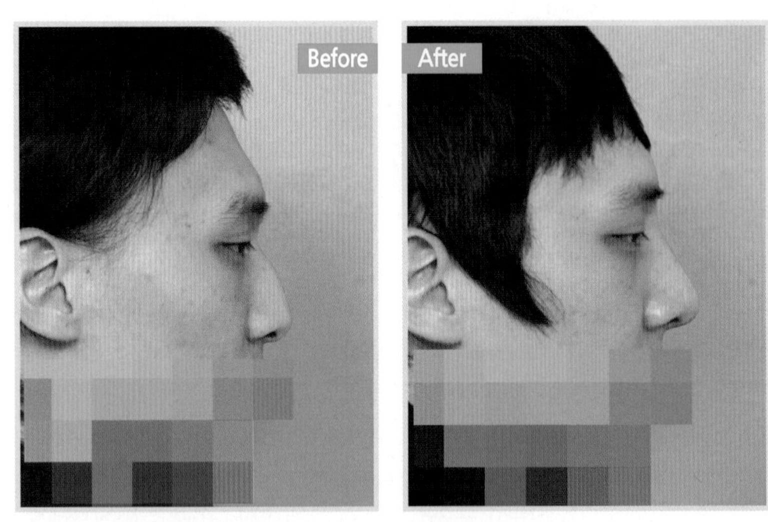

Figure 13 In order to get an aesthetically pleasing dorsal line in management of convex dorsum, a radix graft and tip augmentation should be performed together with hump reduction.

V. Complications

1. Undercorrection

This is the most common complication resulting in a polly beak deformity *(Figure 14)*.

The reasons for this phenomenon are:

- Underresection of hump
- Inadequate tip augmentation
- Inadequate radix augmenation

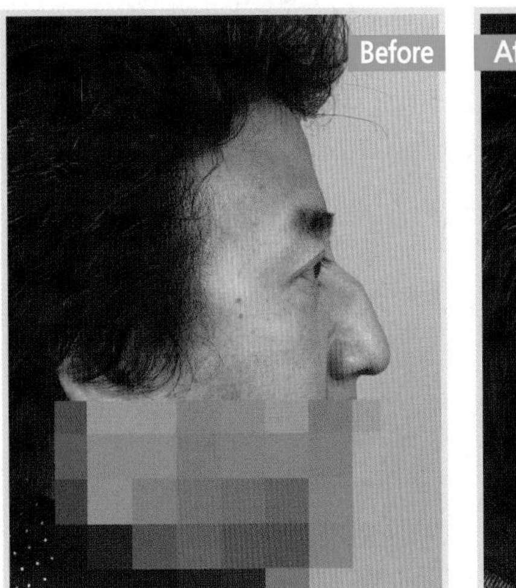

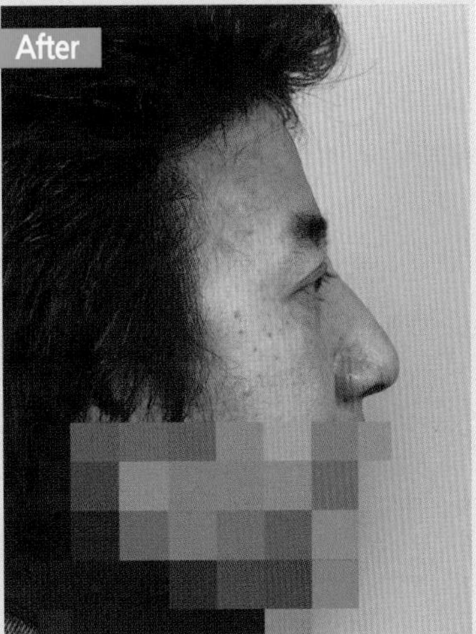

Figure 14 Undercorrection of the severe convex dorsum

2. Dorsal Irregularity

After surgery, a slight unevenness on the surface of the dorsum can be felt by palpation as well as seen visually *(Figure 15)*. Such unevenness must be prevented by meticulous shaving of the nasal dorsum or by careful camouflaging using thin implant materials such as Gore-Tex, temporalis fascia, and homologous fascia. If it is found in postoperative period, such techniques can be applied through an endonasal or open approach.

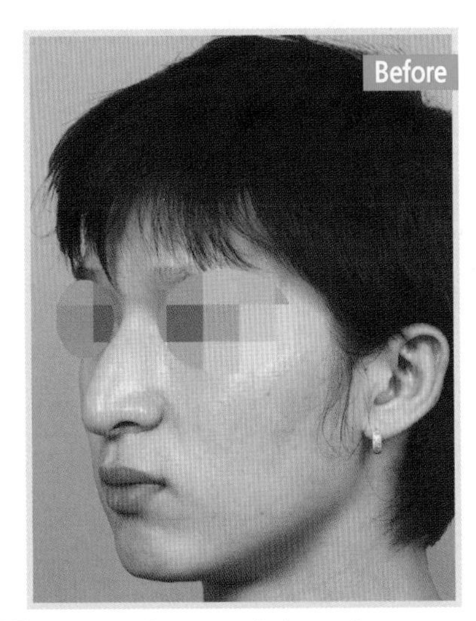

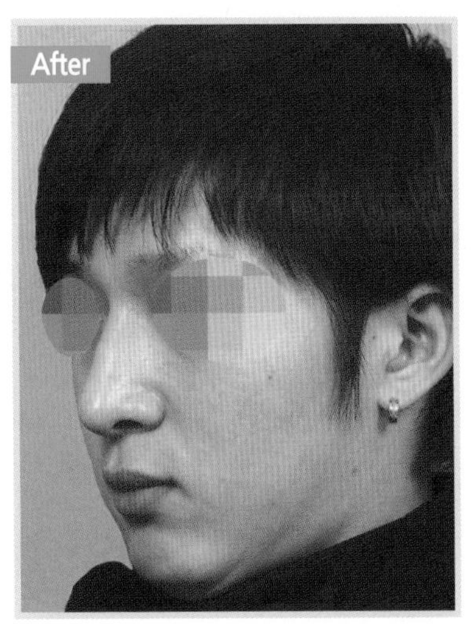

Figure 15 Patient showing slight undercorrection and dorsal irregularity after hump reduction.

3. Overcorrection

Overcorrection of the hump is commonly associated with an inverted-V deformity or saddle nose due to middle vault collapse *(Figure 16)*. This complication occurs when there is disjunction between the nasal bone and the upper lateral cartilages, brought about by severe resection of the hump, and by an improper lateral osteotomy which failed to properly medialize the bony segments. To prevent this complication, the surgeon must take care that the nasal bone and the upper lateral cartilage are not separated while performing rasping and the dorsum must be restored using a spreader graft. Surgical management of overcorrected dorsum should include dorsal augmentation with or without osteotomy.

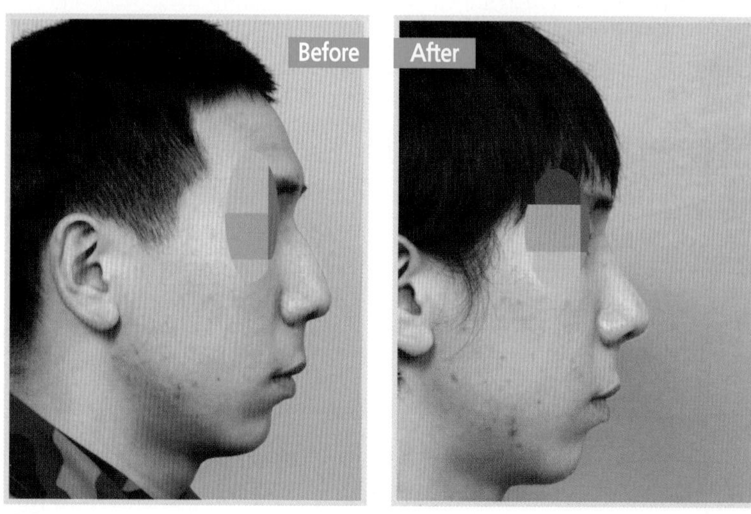

Figure 16 Saddle nose deformity following rhinoplasty to correct convex nasal dorsum.

4. Deviated Nose

This complication is caused by an osteotomy that heals in an unexpected way, poorly executed spreader grafting, and secondary deformity and weakening of the septal cartilage following hump reduction. To prevent this, the osteotomy should be performed very precisely and symmetrically. In addition, the strength and straightness of the cartilaginous dorsum must be adequately restored at the end of surgery. Surgical correction of the deviated nose after hump reduction is done using various surgical techniques applicable in correcting deviated noses in revision cases.

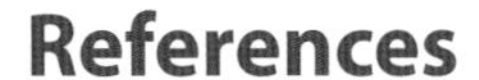

References

1. Camirand A, Doucet J, Harris J. Nose surgery: how to prevent a middle vault collapse-a review of 50 patients 3 to 21 years after surgery. Plast Reconstr Surg 2004; 114: 527-34.
2. Hall JA, Peters MD, Hilger PA. Modification of the Skoog dorsal reduction for preservation of the middle nasal vault. Arch Facial Plast Surg 2004; 6: 105-10.
3. Ishida J, Ishida LC, Ishida LH, Vieera JC, Ferreira MC. Treatment of the nasal hump with preservation of the cartilaginous framework. Plast Reconstr Surg 1999; 103: 1729-33.
4. Jang YJ, Kim JH. Classification of convex nasal dorsum deformities in Asian patients and treatment outcomes. J Plast Reconstr Aesthet Surg 2011; 64: 301-6.
5. Johnson CM, Toriumi DM. The upper two-thirds of the nose. In Open structure rhinoplasty. WB Saunders, 1990; 179-87.
6. Rohrich RJ, Muzaffar AR, Janis JE. Component dorsal hump reduction: the importance of maintaining dorsal aesthetic lines in rhinoplasty. Plast Reconstr Surg 2004; 114: 1298-308.
7. Romo T, Swartout BG. Reduction structured rhinoplasty. Dermatol Clin 2005; 23: 529-40.
8. Sheen, JH. Spreader grafts: A method of reconstructing the roof of the middle nasal vault following rhinoplasty. Plast Reconstr Surg 1984; 73: 230.

A 23-year-old male visited for a convex dorsum with nasal obstruction.

Analysis

Frontal: Mild deviation of the cartilaginous dorsum
Basal: Mildly asymmetric nostrils
Lateral: Deep radix, dorsal convexity

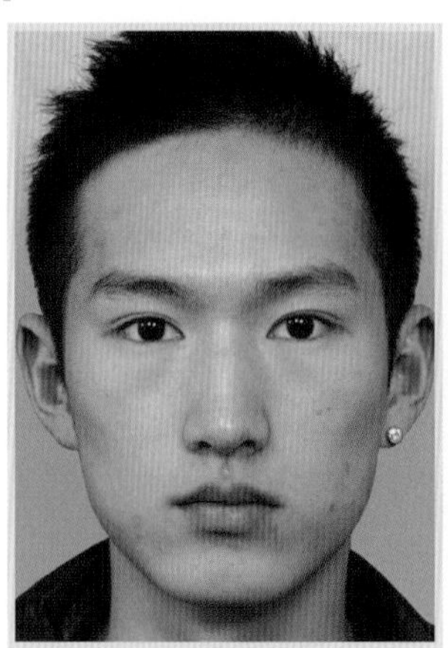
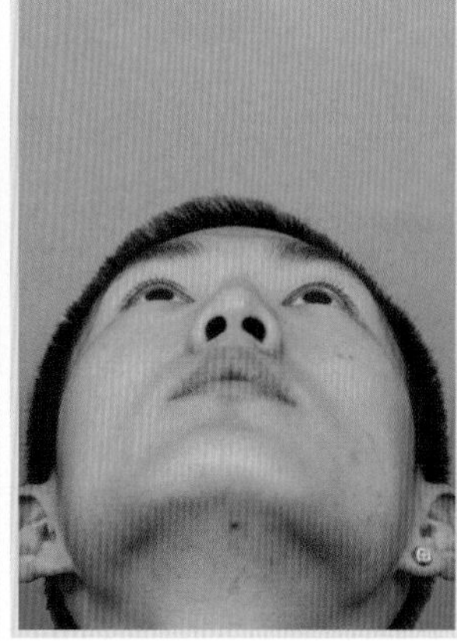
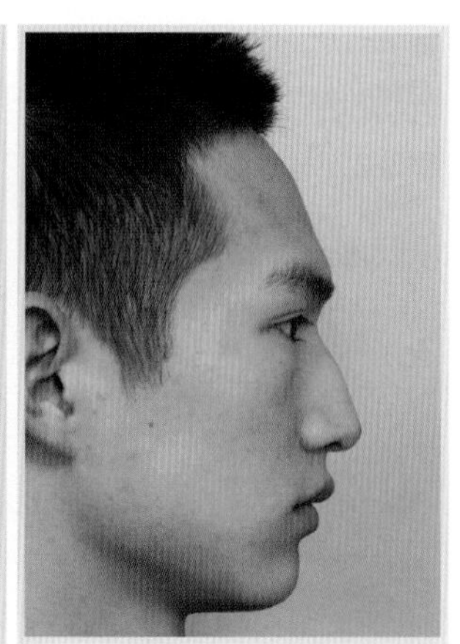

Operative Procedures

Open rhinoplasty approach
Septoplasty and harvest of septal cartilage and bone
Humpectomy and rasping
Multilayer tip grafting with backstop using septal cartilage
Columellar strut
Dorsum and radix augmentation using processed fascia lata

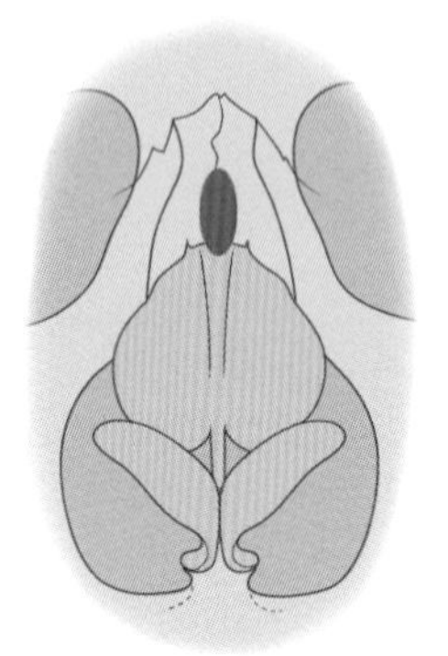
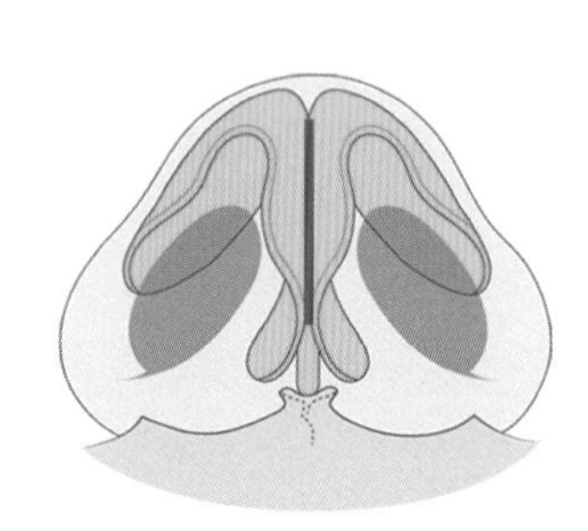
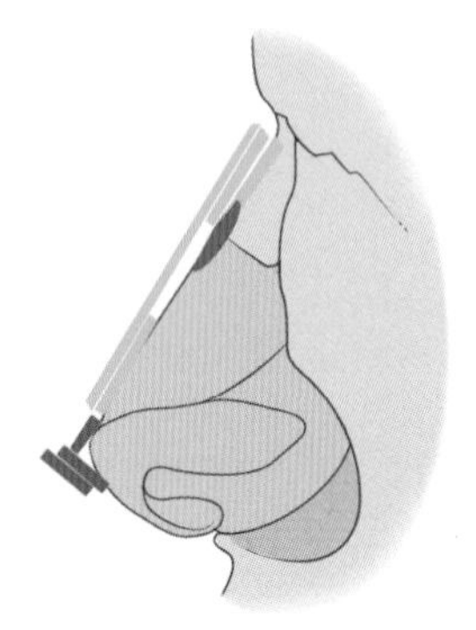

Postoperative Changes

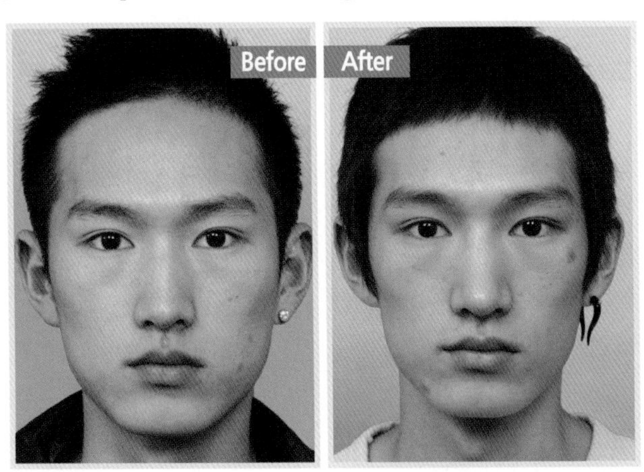

Frontal: Dorsal deviation was corrected. Nasal lengthening was achieved as a result of radix augmentation.

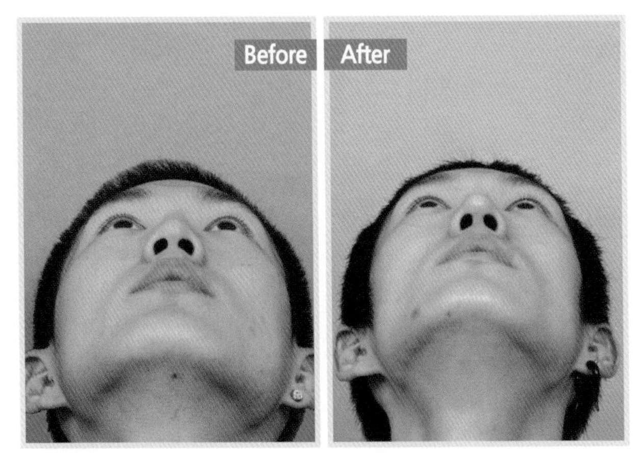

Basal: Tip projection was improved.

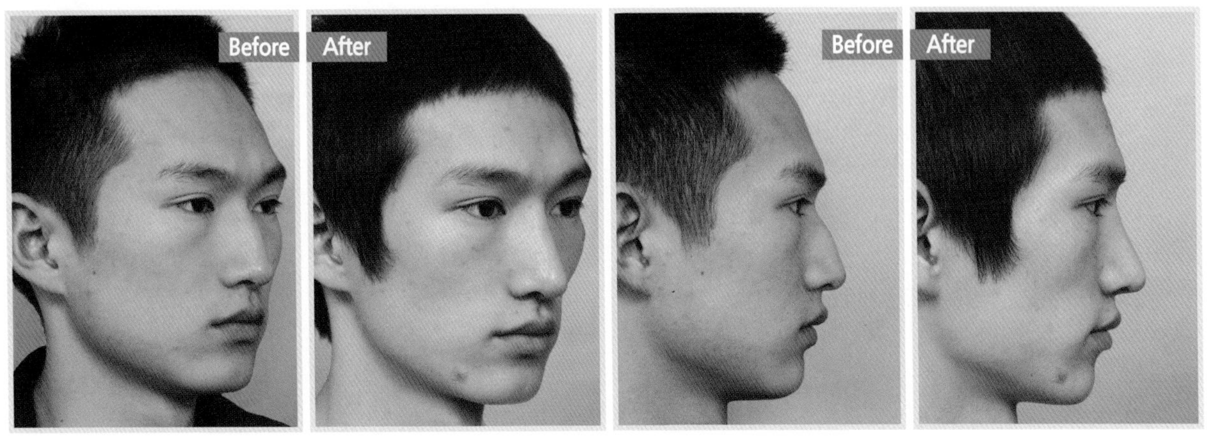

Lateral and Oblique: Radix height was augmented. Masculine dorsal aesthetic line was made by humpectomy and tip projection.

Case 2

A 19-year-old female visited for a convex dorsum with nasal obstruction.

Analysis

- Convex dorsum
- Bulbous tip
- Wide dorsum
- Septal deviation

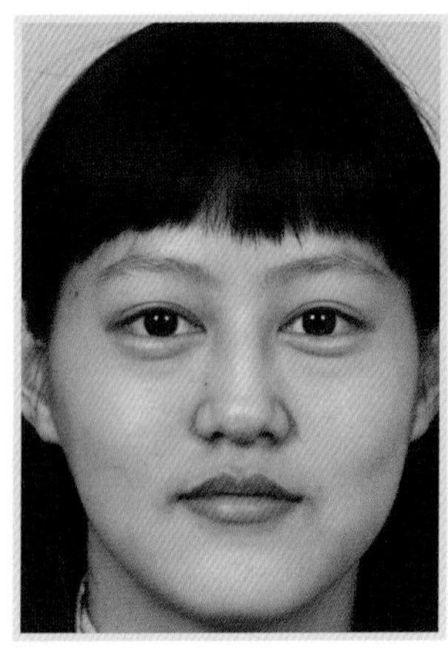
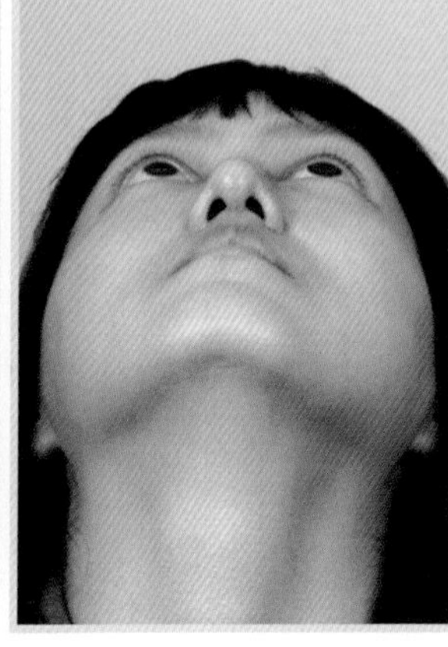
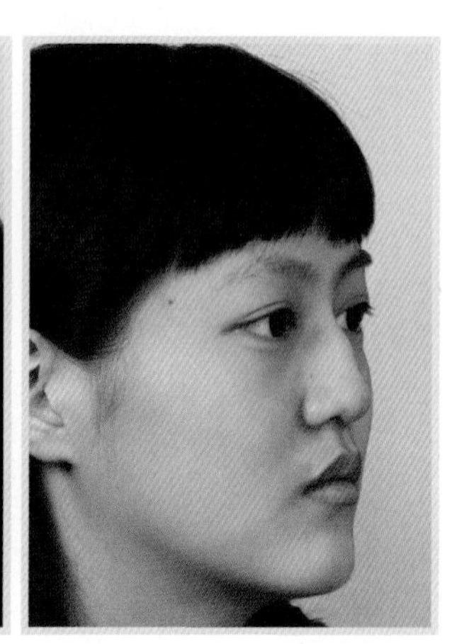

Operative Procedures

- Open rhinoplasty approach
- Humpectomy and rasping
- Lateral osteotomy
- Caudal septal extension grafting using septal cartilage (left)
- Spreader grafting using septal cartilage (bilateral)
- Conchal cartilage harvest
- Tip soft tissue defatting
- Shield grafting using conchal cartilage
- Radix augmentation using crushed conchal cartilage

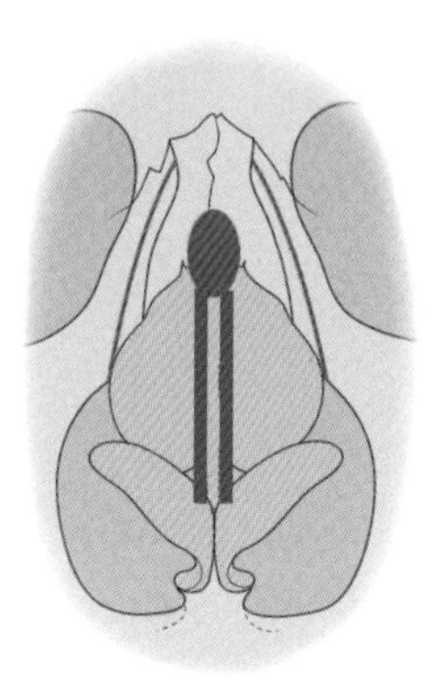
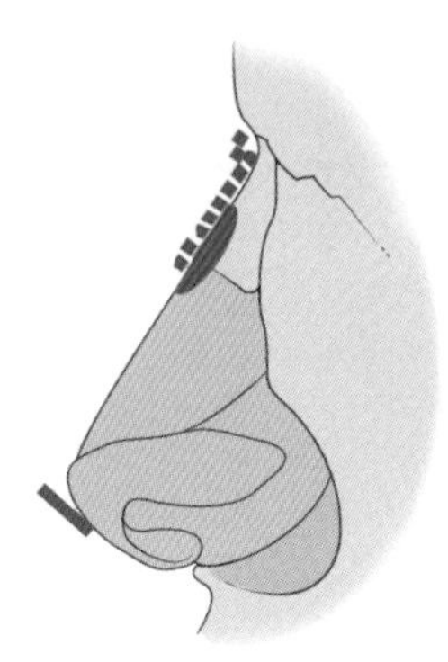
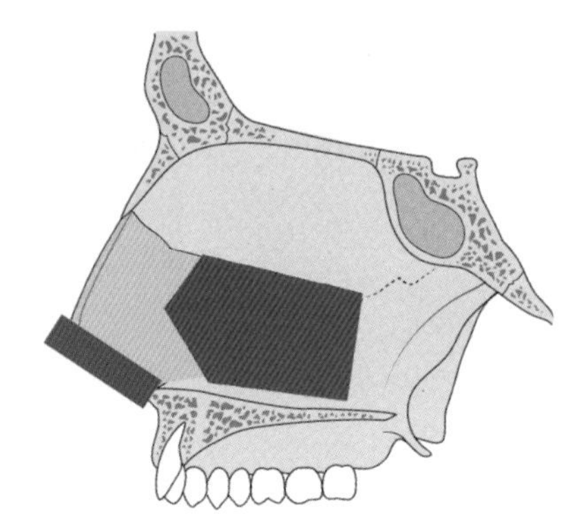

Postoperative Changes

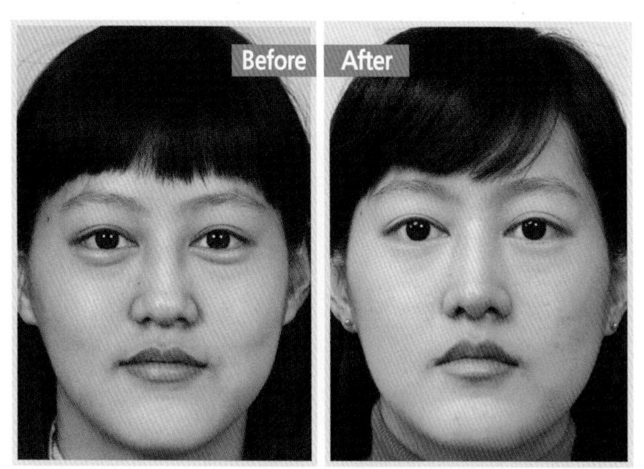

Frontal: Irregular surface of dorsum and tip bulbosity were improved.

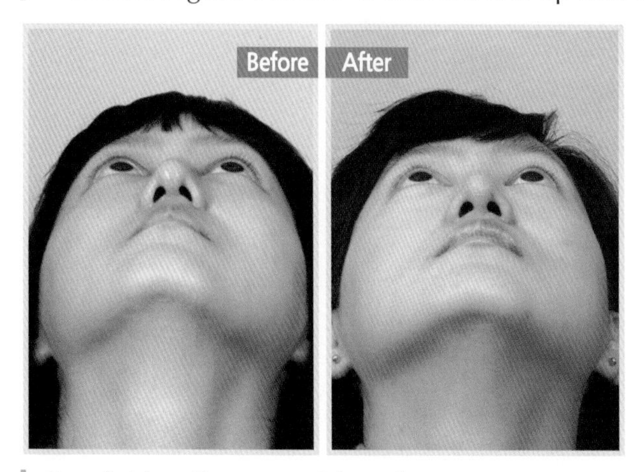

Basal: Nostrils were widened.

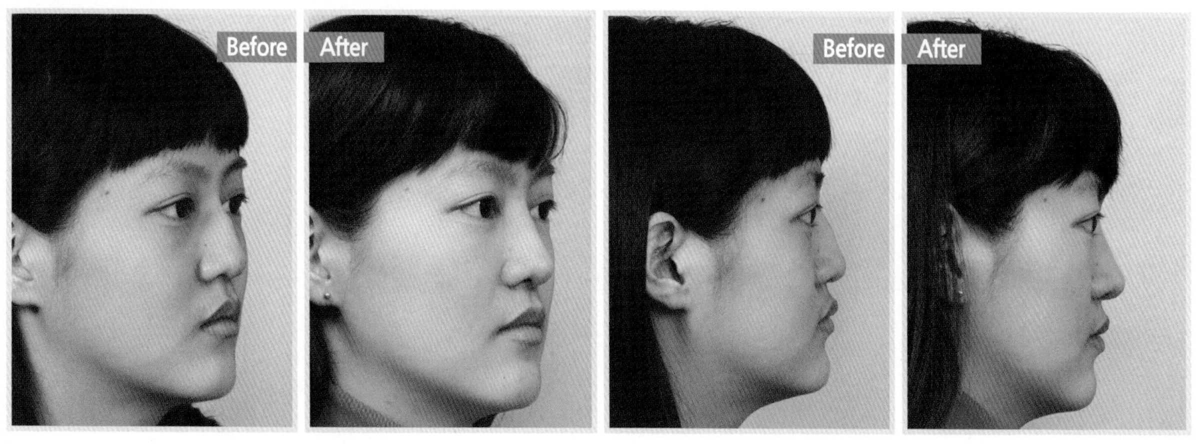

Lateral and Oblique: Appropriate dorsal aesthetic lines were created through hump reduction and tip projection.

Case 3

A 19-year-old female visited for a deviated nose and convex dorsum with nasal obstruction.

Analysis

Frontal: Deviated nose (Type I deviation)
Basal: Deviated columella, long infratip lobule
Lateral: Isolated hump

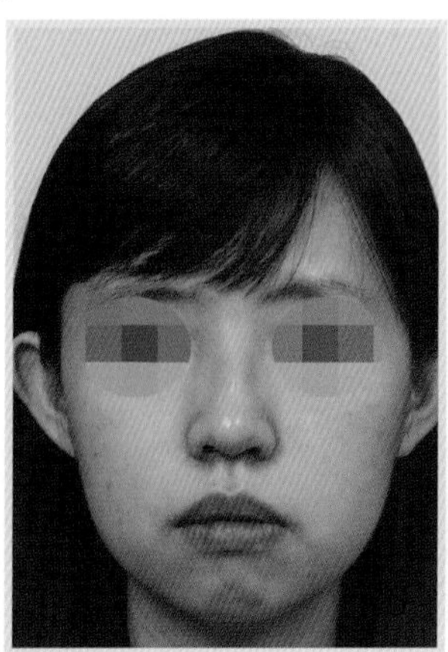
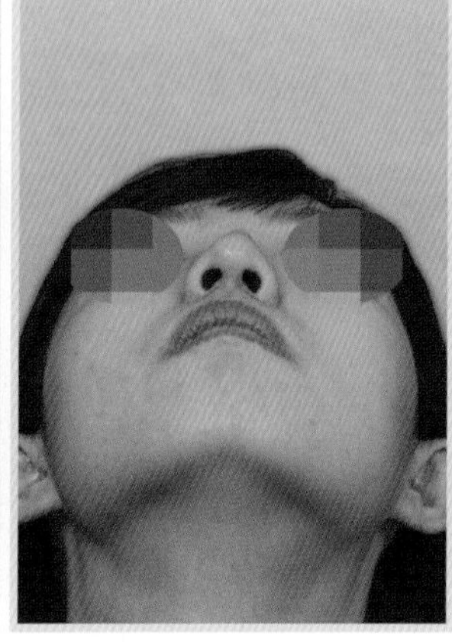
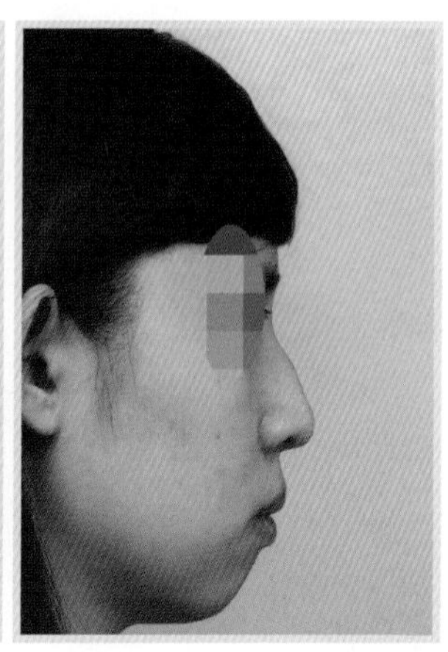

Operative Procedures

Open rhinoplasty approach
Medial, lateral, and percutaneous root osteotomies
Humpectomy and rasping
Caudal septum cutting and suture
Spreader grafting using septal cartilage (bilateral)
Batten grafting using septal cartilage (left)
Lateral crural onlay grafting using conchal cartilage (right)
Multilayer tip grafting with backstop using conchal cartilage
Tip graft camouflaging using processed fascia lata
Dorsal augmentation using processed fascia lata

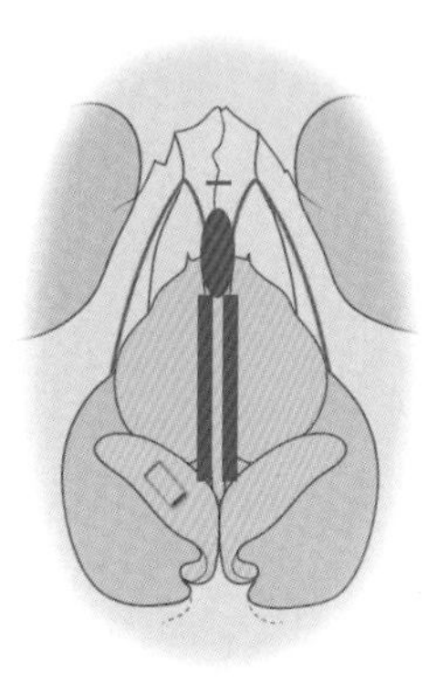
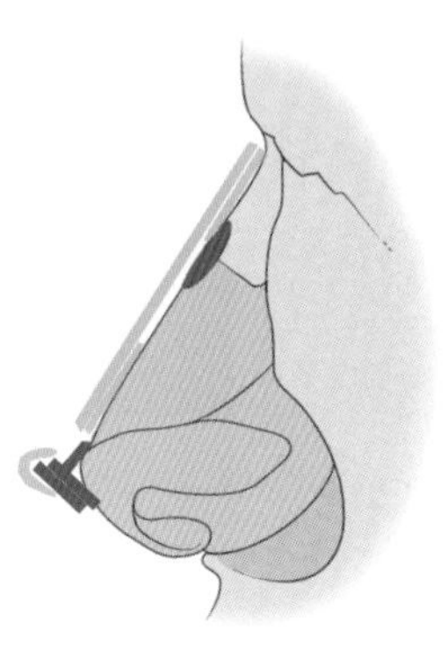
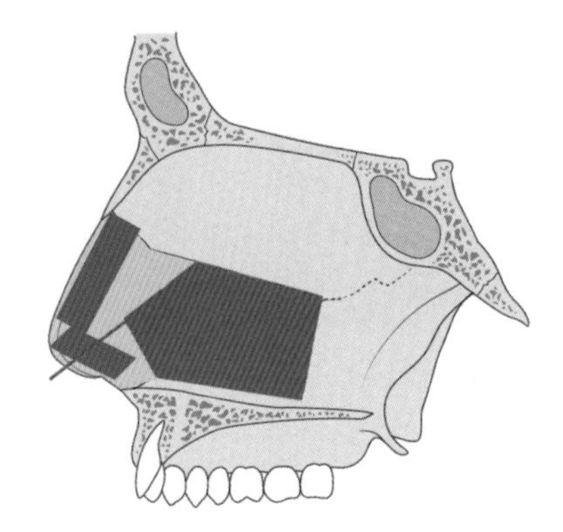

Postoperative Changes

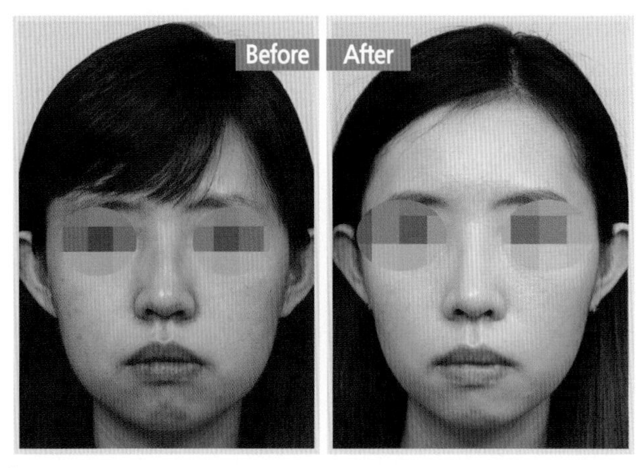

Frontal: Dorsal deviation was corrected.

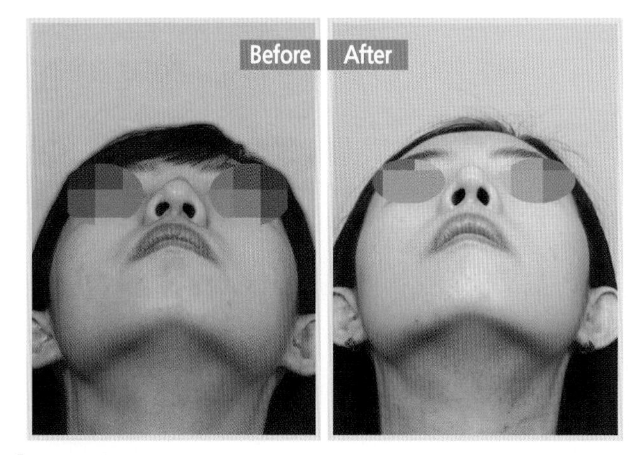

Basal: Tip projection was increased. Nostrils were given a more vertical orientation.

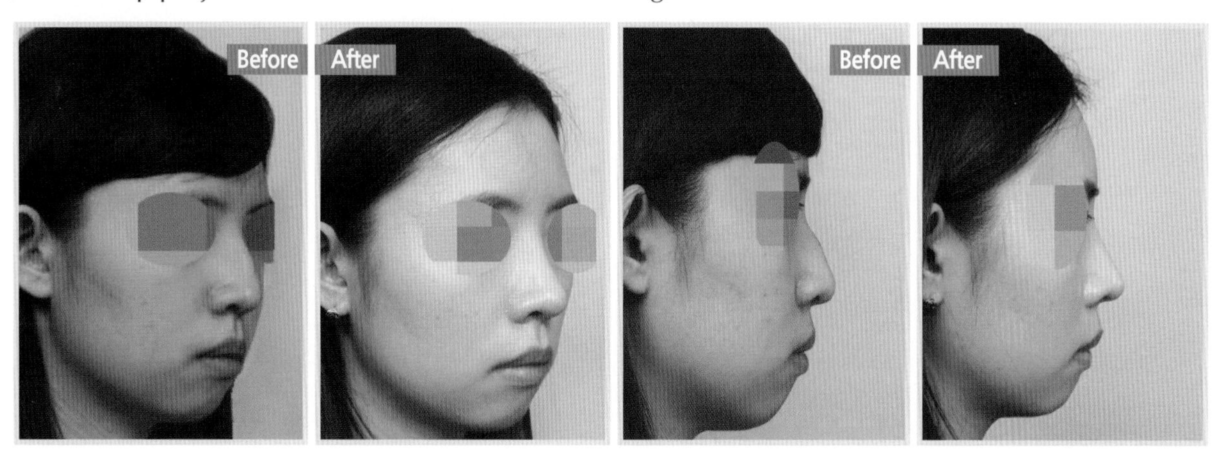

Lateral and Oblique: Smoothened dorsal concavity was made by hump rasping and tip projection.

Saddle Nose

Yong Ju Jang · Sang Min Hyun

A saddle nose deformity is characterized by an externally visible loss of dorsal height. This deformity results from the disruption of the bony or cartilaginous nasal supports. It not only has aesthetic defect but also causes functional problems for nasal breathing. So it remains one of the most challenging deformities to treat. Rhinoplasty surgeons must be fully aware of the pathophysiology and treatment strategies for saddle nose deformity.

I. Cause and Pathophysiology

Causes of saddle nose deformities include nasal trauma, excessive resection of septal cartilage during septoplasty, postoperative infection (perichondritis), excessive resection of the nasal dorsum during rhinoplasty, etc. *(Figure 1)*. It can also occur due to secondary chondritis following cautery of the septal mucosa to treat epistaxis. It may also be associated with certain conditions such as Wegener's granulomatosis, sarcoidosis, Crohn's disease, relapsing polychondritis, and long-term use of vasoconstrictors such as cocaine and oxymetazoline. Infectious diseases like syphilis, leprosy, septal abscess also can cause a saddle nose deformity *(Table 1)*.

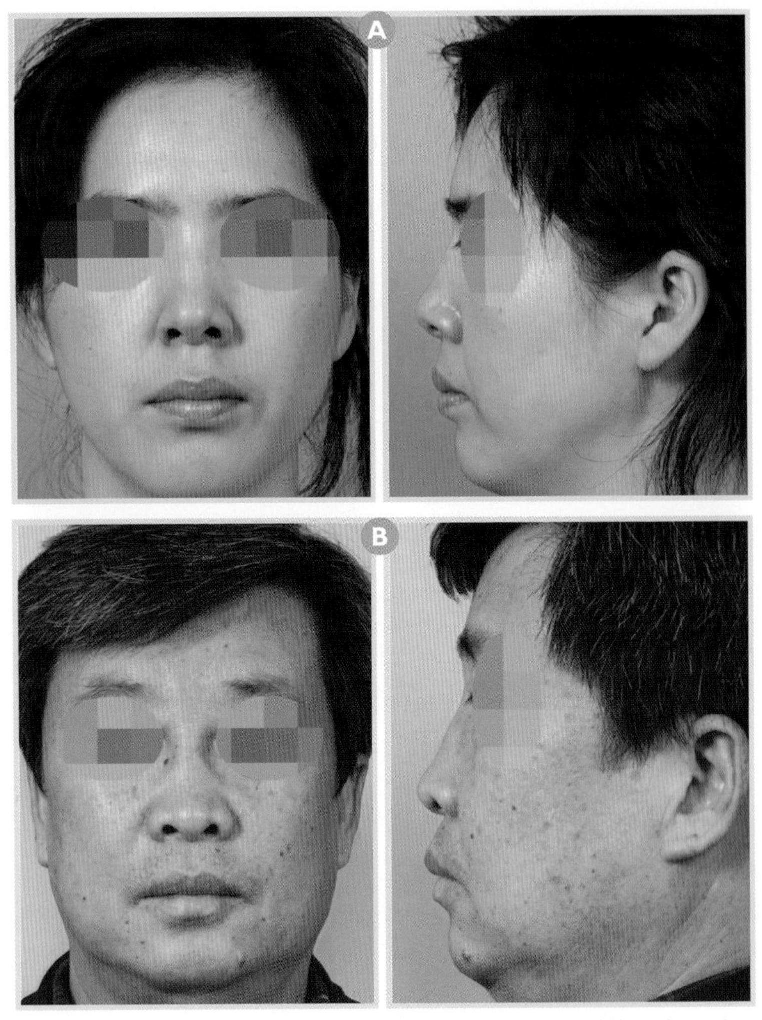

Figure I Saddle nose deformity caused by previous septoplasty (A) and nasal trauma (B).

Table I Causes of Saddle Nose Deformity

Nasal trauma
Septoplasty complication
Hematoma and abscess
Infection
Lost caudal support
Excessive resection of septal cartilage
Injury on keystone area
Overresected dorsum during rhinoplasty
Cauterization
Cocaine abuse
Medical diseases
Wegener's granulomatosis
Sarcoidosis
Relapsing polychondritis
Syphilis
Leprosy

As we can see in listed causes, most saddle nose deformities are associated with pathology of the septal cartilage. The septal cartilage is the key structure for nasal support as it supports the weight of soft tissue envelope of nose. Iatrogenic factors that lead to a saddle nose after septoplasty are dislocation of the caudal septum from nasal spine, excessive resection of the caudal portion of the L-strut, weakened nasal support due to not leaving enough L-strut, and disjunction of the bony-cartilaginous junction at the keystone area *(Figure 2)*.

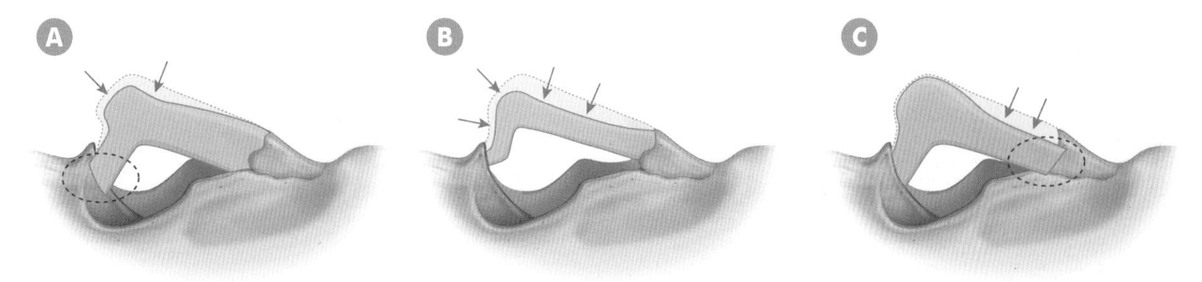

Figure 2 A saddle nose can occur due to dislocation of the caudal septum from the anterior nasal spine (A), excessive resection of the caudal portion of the L-strut, weak nasal support due to sparing not enough L-strut (B), and disconnection of the bony-cartilaginous junction in the keystone area (C).

According to our study, the most common causes of saddle nose deformity after septoplasty were shortening, weakening, and dislocation of the caudal septum. It is easily understood that shortening of the caudal septum can cause a saddle nose deformity, but dislocation of the caudal septum can also cause this deformity. Mobilization of the caudal septum during septoplasty can cause an abnormal rotation of septal cartilage at the keystone area, thus resulting in a saddle deformity *(Figure 3)*.

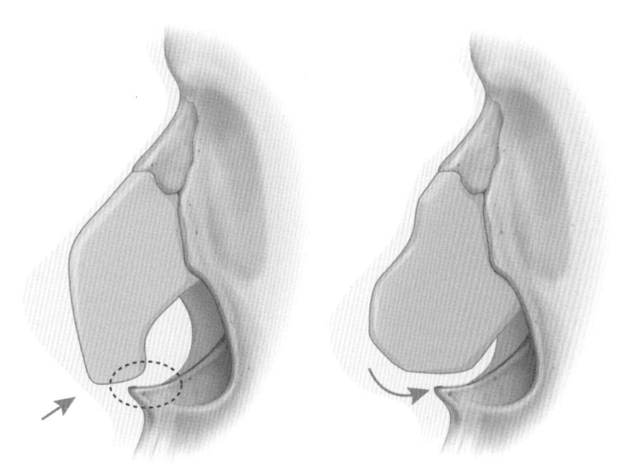

Figure 3 Rotation of the caudal septum from the anterior nasal spine caused by excessive resection of the caudal strut is a common cause for saddle nose deformity.

Derangements of the supporting structure of the quadrangular cartilage decrease dorsal and caudal height. Secondary to the lost septal support, the columella will collapse and the alar base will widen. The distance between the lower lateral cartilage and columella will decrease, which leads to lower lateral cartilage collapse during inspiration. The loss of nasal support decreases only the height of cartilaginous portion while height of bony portion remains intact, which leads to many deformities including a visible saddle deformity on the nasal dorsum. The saddle nose deformity not only causes middle vault and dorsal depression, but also loss of tip support and definition, columellar retraction, overrotation of the tip, and deprojection *(Figure 4)*.

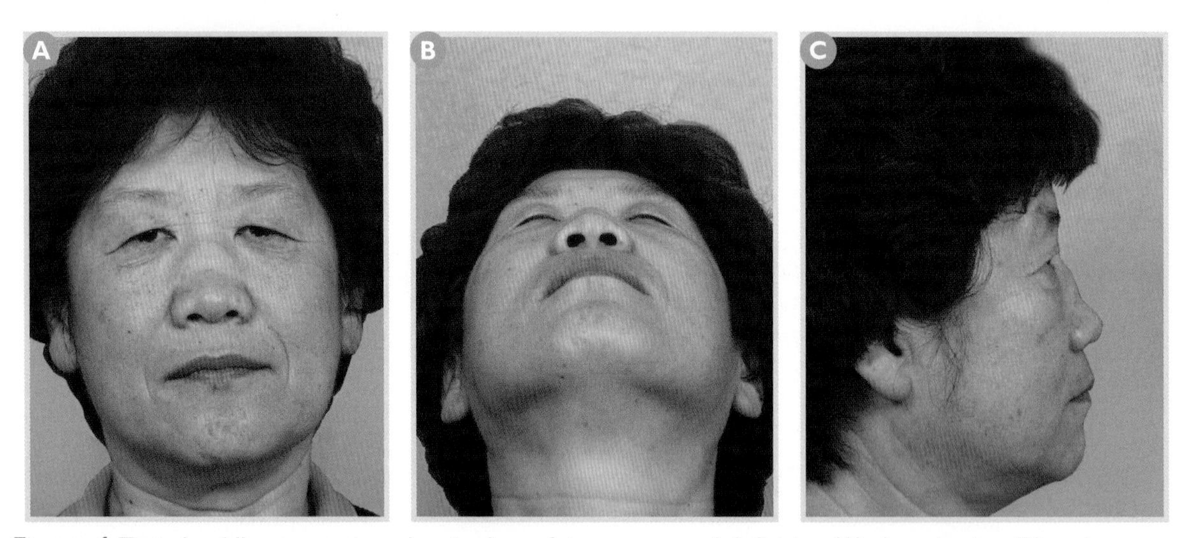

Figure 4 Typical saddle nose patient showing loss of tip support and definition (A), deprojection (B), and columellar retraction and tip overrotation (C).

II. Classification for Saddle Nose Deformities

The authors classify saddle nose deformities as follows *(Figure 5)*:

Type I: Minor supratip or dorsal nasal depression
Type II: Moderate to severe dorsal depression
Type III: Pan-nasal defect with severe dorsal deficiency in combination with lower third deficits
Type IV: Pan-nasal defect, relatively prominent tip projection only by the lower lateral cartilage

1. Type I Saddle Nose: Minor Supratip or Dorsal Nasal Depression

A Type I saddle nose has a slight depression of the nasal dorsum and columellar retraction with intact septal support *(Figure 6)*. Because the major mechanism for this deformity is weakness of the septal support, reinforcement of septal support is important during surgery. But if the septal framework is relatively intact and progressive aggravation is not expected, the aesthetic deformity can be corrected by performing only dorsal augmentation without reinforcement of the septal framework.

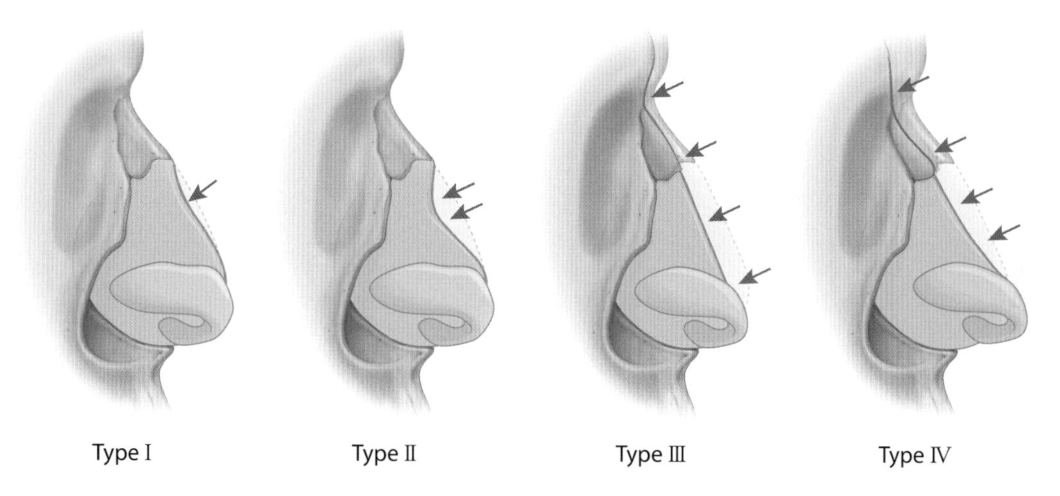

Figure 5 Classification of saddle noses.

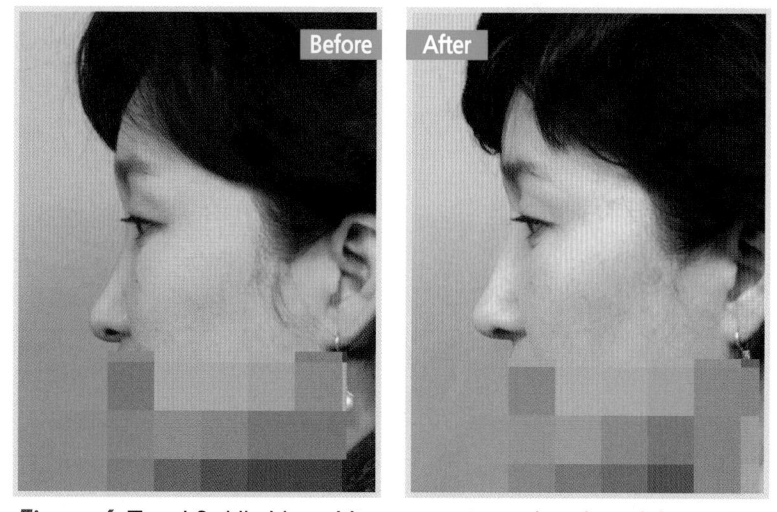

Figure 6 Type I Saddle Nose. Minor supratip or dorsal nasal depression.

2. Type II Saddle Nose: Moderate to Severe Dorsal Depression

Type II saddle noses show depression of the cartilaginous portion, columellar retraction and loss of tip support along with a more severe destruction of septal support than a Type I saddle nose *(Figure 7)*. Surgeons must improve the septal support during the surgery.

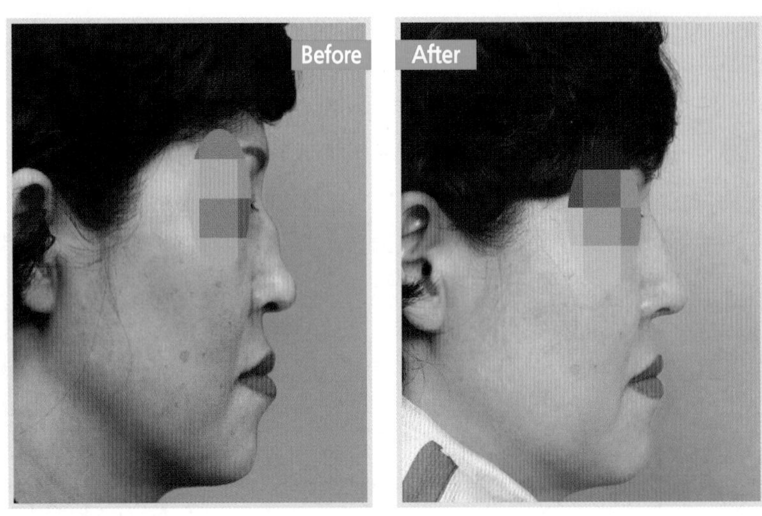

Figure 7 Type II Saddle Nose: Moderate to severe dorsal depression.

3. Type III Saddle Nose: Pan-Nasal Defect with Severe Dorsal Deficiency in combination with Lower Third Deficits

Type III saddle noses show the final stage of septal collapse *(Figure 8)*. It is a combination of bony dorsal deficiency with contraction of the nasal cavity lining. Sometimes it is accompanied by large septal perforation. In this type, patients may have an intact septal mucosa, but with no cartilage underneath once exposed during surgery. For the correction of the Type III saddle nose, a large amount of cartilage is required for septal reconstruction. And for raising the dorsal height, abundant augmentation material is required as well.

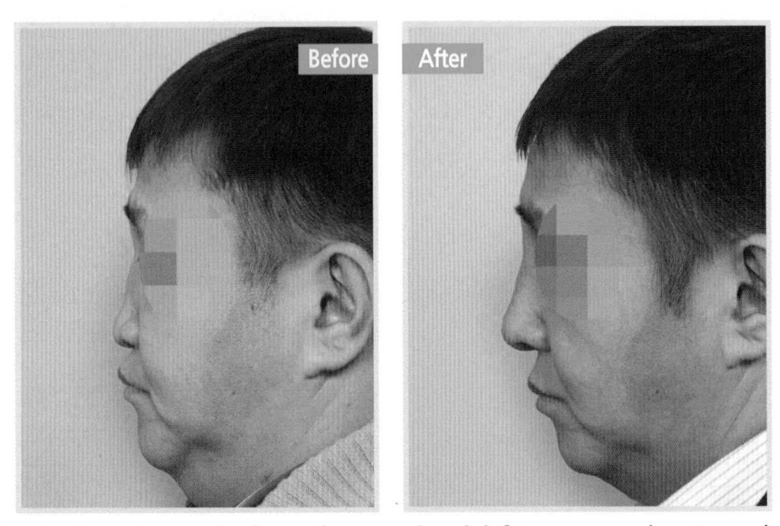

Figure 8 Type III Saddle Nose: Pan-nasal defect with severe dorsal deficiency in combination with lower third deficits.

4. Type IV Saddle Nose: Pan-Nasal Defect, Relatively Prominent Tip Projection only by the Lower Lateral Cartilage

Type IV saddle noses are usually associated with septal trauma at an early age *(Figure 9)*. Patients, who have had septal injury due to intranasal button battery or septal infection in childhood, have normal growth of the lower lateral cartilages but their dorsal height cannot grow normally show this deformity. The treatment strategy for Type IV saddle noses is same with the approach to a Type III saddle nose.

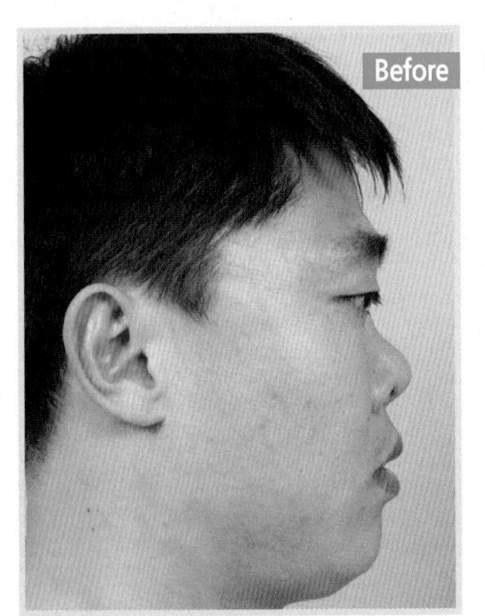

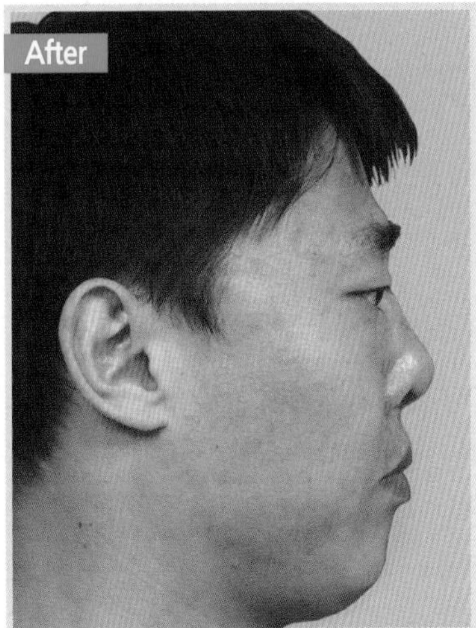

Figure 9 Type IV Saddle Nose: Pan-nasal defect showing relatively prominent tip projection by the lower lateral cartilage.

III. Surgical Treatment for the Saddle Nose

For improving the dorsal height, dorsal augmentation is necessary. In cases of correction of minor dorsal depressions, dorsal augmentation can be performed via an endonasal rhinoplasty approach using a marginal incision or an intercartilaginous incision. But for more than a moderate degree of saddle nose deformity requiring septal reconstruction, an external rhinoplasty approach is preferred. Treatment strategies for saddle nose deformities are the following:

1. Augmentation using Dorsal Onlay Grafts

If the tip support is relatively intact indicating a relatively healthy caudal septal support, a saddle nose can be corrected using only a dorsal onlay graft *(Figure 10)*. This method is aimed to augment the depressed dorsum without addressing the septal framework. This can be performed by

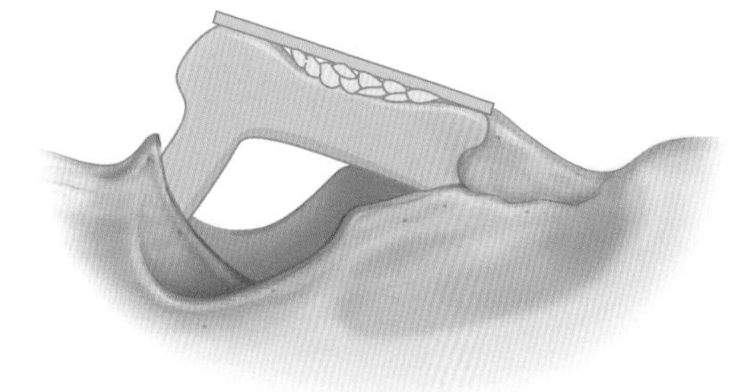

Figure 10 Dorsal onlay graft for saddle nose correction.

both endonasal and external approaches. Gore-Tex, fascia, fascia with crushed cartilage, diced conchal cartilage, and fascia-wrapped diced cartilage can be used to fill the depressed portion. For correction of the partially depressed dorsum like in Type I or Type II saddle nose deformities, the emphasis of treatment is the augmentation of cartilaginous dorsum. However the Type III or IV saddle nosed require full-length dorsal augmentation from the radix to nasal tip. In such cases, one can use costal cartilage, fascia-wrapped diced cartilage, Gore-Tex, silicone, etc. For dorsal augmentation, the use of soft materials is desirable. For saddle noses that have only a dorsal depression in the cartilaginous portion, fascia-wrapped diced cartilage laid on the depressed portion is a very useful for dorsal augmentation technique. In making fascia-wrapped diced cartilage, conchal cartilage is the preferred cartilage, and the temporalis fascia, fascia lata, or homologous fascia lata can be used for wrapping. Costal cartilage can be used on the dorsum as a mono-block graft after careful carving or a laminated graft of several cartilage strips.

2. Cartilage Framework Reconstruction

In cases of Types II, III, and IV saddle noses, the weakened septal framework should be reinforced or reconstructed. Evaluation of septal support can be easily done through inspection and palpation – observing a flat, deprojected tip and an easily collapsible lower third of nose by finger pressure. Reconstruction of the septal cartilage framework is one of most difficult procedures for rhinoplasty surgeons. In most cases, there is not enough septal cartilage for reconstruction purposes. The surgeon must be prepared to harvest cartilage such as conchal or costal cartilage to be able to enhance septal support. The method for septal reconstruction depends on the amount of septal cartilage remaining. If there is a very weak and thin L-strut remaining, reinforcement of the caudal and dorsal strut can be done using strong and thick cartilage. The authors prefer to use three different methods for septal reinforcement:

- One extended spreader graft is sutured to one side of the existing L-strut, and one caudal batten graft is placed contralaterally *(Figure 11A)*.
- Bilateral spreader grafts and bilateral batten grafts are placed on both sides of the existing L-strut. In this method, batten grafts should be relatively short, and spreader graft should fully cover the entire surface of dorsal L-strut *(Figure 11B)*.
- Bilateral extended spreader grafts are placed on both sides of the existing L-strut, and one caudal septal extension graft is sandwiched in between. In this method, the base of this graft is fixed to anterior nasal spine by drilling holes in the nasal spine, and suturing to the caudal septum in an end-to-end manner that will effectively lengthen the nose *(Figure 11C)*.

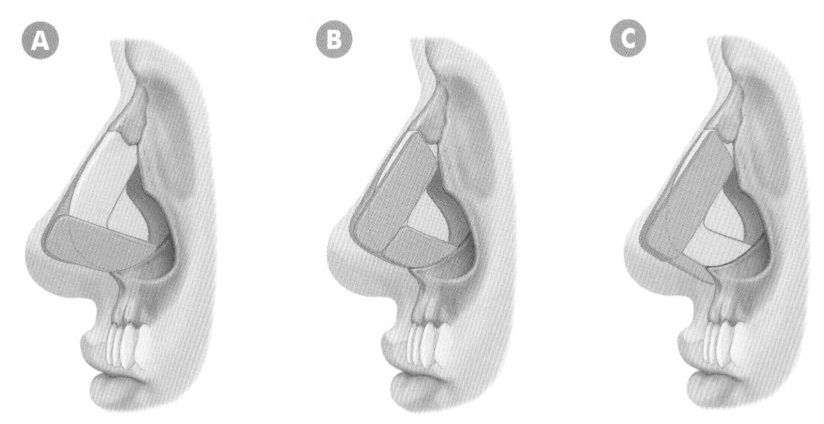

Figure 11 One extended spreader graft is sutured on one side of the existing L-strut, and one caudal septal extension graft is placed contralaterally (A). Bilateral spreader grafts and two batten grafts are sutured on the both sides of the existing L-strut (B). Bilateral extended spreader grafts are placed on both sides of the existing L-strut, and one caudal septal extension graft is sandwiched between them (C).

Some patients with saddle nose deformities have almost no septal cartilage left underneath the septal mucoperichondrium. In this scenario, both sides of mucoperichondrium should be fully elevated and a newly created septum using the costal cartilage inserted. For creating the neo-septal cartilage, using costal cartilage, one can insert an L-strut or a large quadrangular piece of cartilage mimicking the missing septal cartilage *(Figure 12)*.

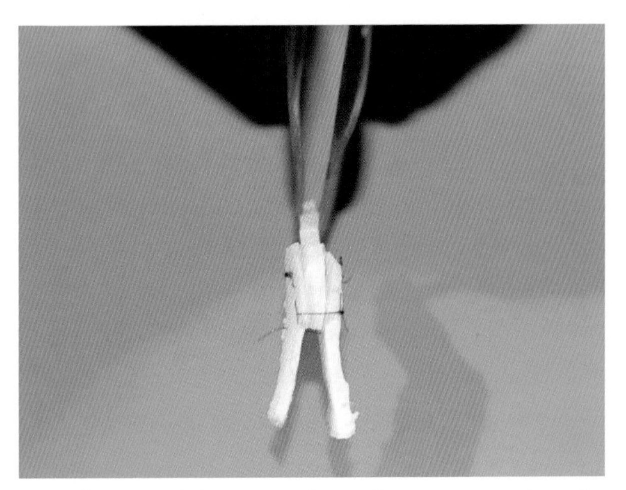

Figure 12 In cases of severe saddle nose deformities where almost no septal cartilage is left, one can build new L-strut using costal cartilage.

In cases of a totally absent septal cartilage, it is necessary to carve the cephalic portion of dorsal strut into an L-shape to fit on to the caudal margin of nasal bone. *(Figure 13)*. Securing a strong alignment between the new L-strut and nasal bone using wiring or suturing is extremely difficult. The L-shape carving of the dorsal strut can serve as an easier option despite its slight protrusion over the nasal bone, which can be sometimes beneficial for saddle nose correction.

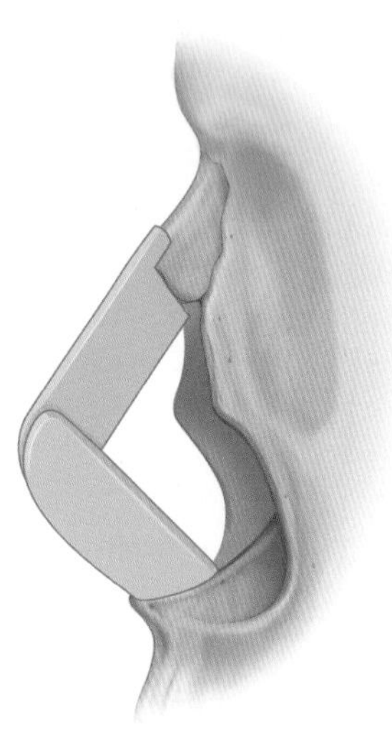

Figure 13 In cases of a totally absent septal cartilage, it is necessary to carve the cephalic portion of dorsal strut into an L-shape to fit on to the caudal margin of nasal bone.

The most difficult cases for septal reconstruction are the ones with septal perforations. If the patient does not suffer from perforation-related problems such as frequent epistaxis, crusting or nasal obstruction, rhinoplasty combined with septal reconstruction should be conducted first, addressing the septal perforation at a later time. In these cases, dissection of mucoperichondrium on caudal and dorsal part, not reaching to the perforation margin, should be performed very carefully. Septal reconstruction can be performed by placing cartilage grafts into the mucosal pocket above and front of the perforation margin. Simultaneous septal perforation correction and septal reconstruction is technically challenging and is not desirable because of the risk of ascending infection through the violated septal mucoperichondrial integrity.

3. Tip Surgery

After septal reconstruction has been performed, the lower lateral cartilages are secured by buried sutures to the newly formed anterior septal angle for proper support. If the tip projection is insufficient after this, one can additionally add a columellar strut, shield grafts and onlay grafts to achieve the desired tip projection. Before selecting the specific surgical techniques to be employed, the surgeon must consider patient's individual anatomy, available implants and grafts to reach the surgical goal.

IV. Complications after Saddle Nose Correction

Saddle nose correction can easily be associated with complications. Possible complications include:

1. Incomplete Correction and Recurrence

This is the most common complication. We have analyzed outcomes of saddle nose corrections and concluded that rate of incomplete correction and recurrence was up to 20-30%. The probable reasons for recurrence might be the reduction of implant volume, absorption of cartilages or fascia used for dorsal augmentation or for septal reconstruction, and loosening of the suture materials, with resultant weakening of the newly constructed septum *(Figure 14)*.

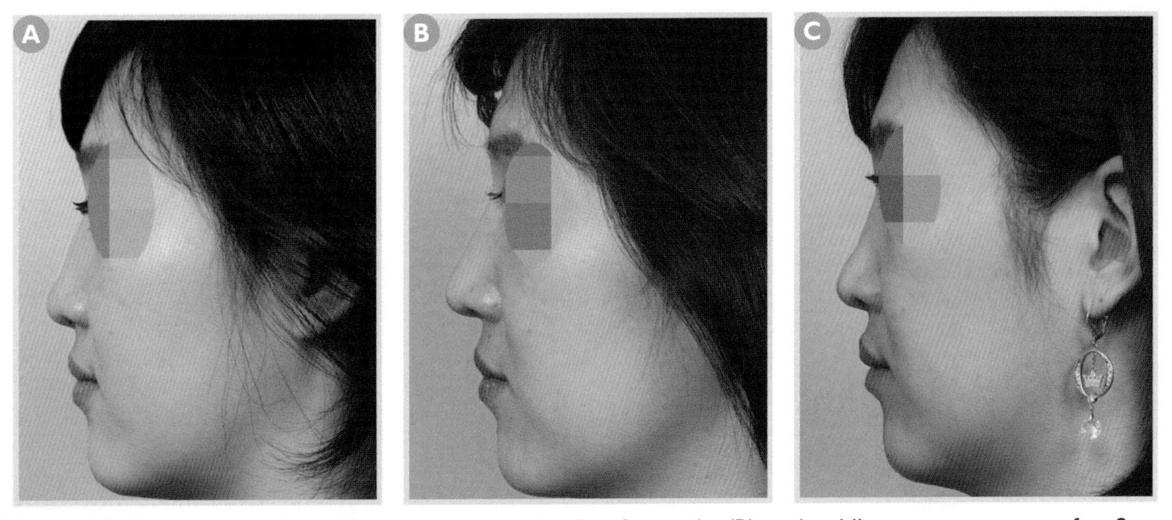

Figure 14 Preoperative view (A), satisfactory result after 2 months (B), and saddle nose recurrence after 2 years (C).

2. Scar on the Transcolumellar Incision Scar

Putting too much graft into the nose may increase the tension over the transcolumellar incision, increasing the risk of forming unsightly scar *(Figure 15)*.

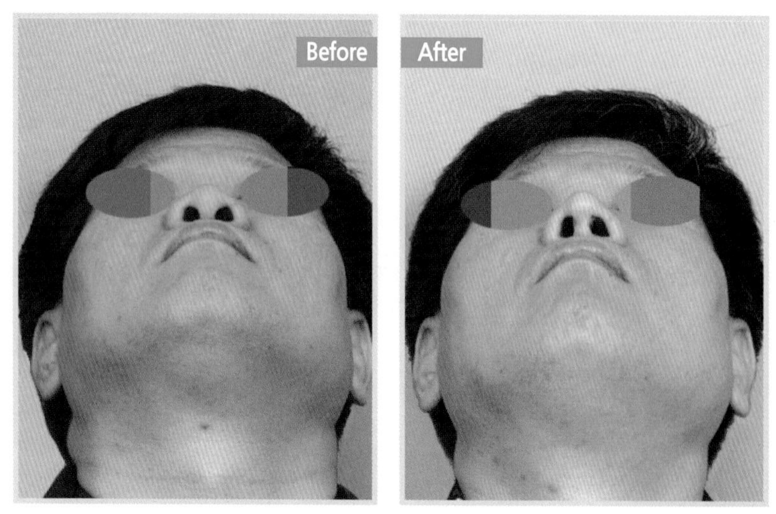

Figure 15 The patient had a visible transcolumellar incision scar after correction of saddle nose deformity using costal cartilage.

3. Secondary Nasal Deformity

When costal cartilage is used as dorsal augmentation material, warping and unnatural contours, and a toothbrush handle deformity can occur *(Figure 16)*.

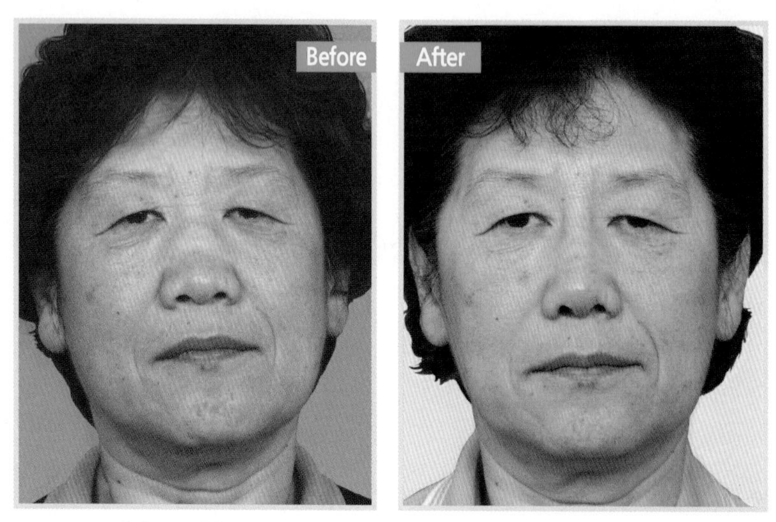

Figure 16 After correction of the saddle nose deformity using costal cartilage, the patient had an unnatural costal cartilage outline called the toothbrush handle deformity.

4. Nasal Obstruction

Nasal obstruction can occur when too thick a costal cartilage is used for septal reconstruction and protrudes to one side of the nose, or when septal reconstruction was not satisfactory, especially at the depressed portion.

References

1. Burget G. Aesthetic restoration of the nose. Clin Plast Surg 1985; 12: 463.
2. Christophel JJ, Hilger PA. Osseocartilaginous rib graft rhinoplasty: a stable, predictable technique for major dorsal reconstruction. Arch Facial Plast Surg 2011; 13: 78-83.
3. Daniel RK, Brenner KA. Saddle nose deformity: A new classification and treatment. Facial Plast Surg Clin North Am 2006; 14: 301-12.
4. Daniel RK. Rhinoplasty: septal saddle nose deformity and composite reconstruction. Plast Reconstr Surg 2007; 119: 1029-43.
5. Hyun SM, Jang YJ. Treatment outcome of saddle nose correction. JAMA Facial Plast Surg 2013, in press
6. Kim DW, Toriumi DM. Management of posttraumatic nasal deformities: the crooked nose and saddle nose. Facial Plast Surg Clin North Am 2004; 12: 111-32.
7. Kelly MH, Bulstrode NW, Waterhouse N. Versatility of diced cartilage-fascia grafts in dorsal nasal augmentation. Plast Reconstr Surg 2007; 120: 1654-9.
8. Pribitkin EA, Ezzat WH. Classification and treatment of the saddle nose deformity. Otolaryngol Clin North Am 2009; 42: 437-61.
9. Riechelmann H, Rettinger G. Three-step reconstruction of complex saddle nose deformities. Arch Otolaryngol Head Neck Surg 2004; 130: 334-8.
10. Tardy ME, Schwartz MS, Parras G. Saddle nose deformity: autogenous graft repair. Facial Plast Surg 1989; 6: 121.
11. Yeo NK, Jang YJ. Rhinoplasty to correct nasal deformities in post septoplasty patients. Am J Rhinol Allergy 2009; 23: 540-5.

Case 1

A 49-year-old male visited for a deformed nose with nasal obstruction. He had undergone septoplasty and closed reduction due to nasal bone fracture prior.

Analysis

Frontal: Deviated nose, flat nose, wide alar base

Basal: Poor tip projection, nostril asymmetry, tilted columella

Lateral and Oblique: Saddle nose (Type III), very low dorsal and tip height

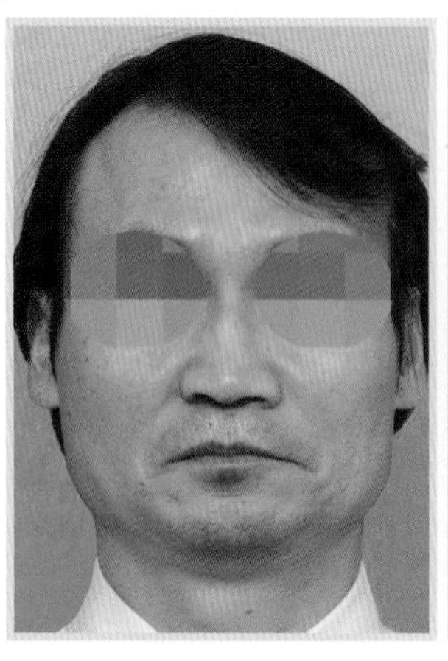

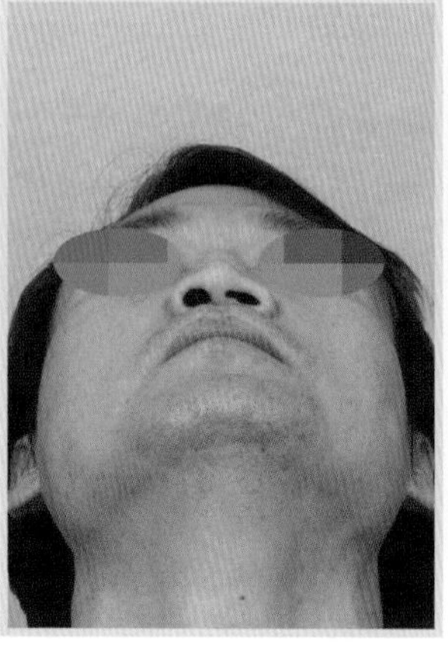

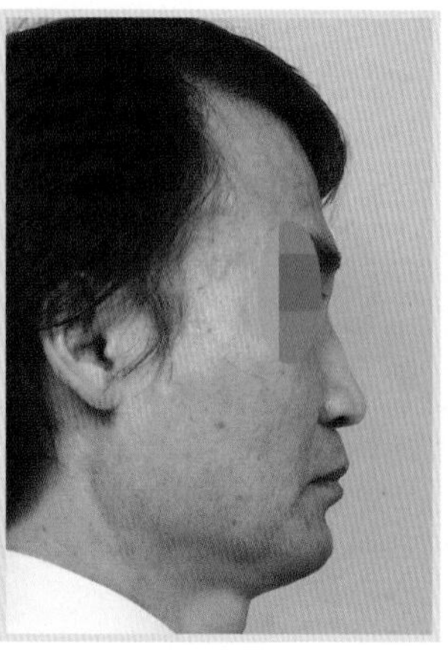

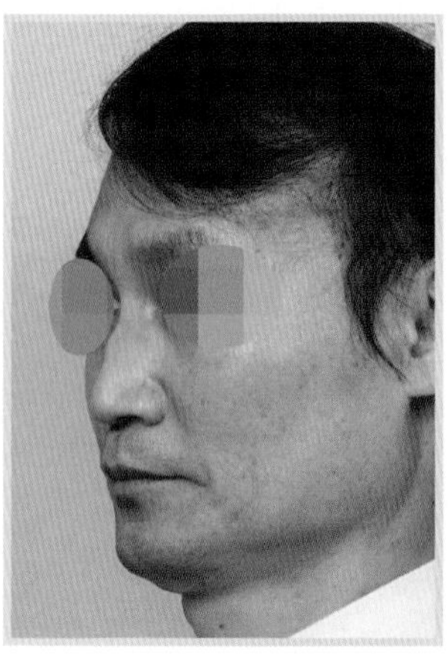

Operative Procedures

Open rhinoplasty approach

Costal cartilage harvest

Extracorporeal septoplasty using costal cartilage

Multilayer tip grafting using costal cartilage

Dorsal augmentation using processed fascia lata and crushed costal cartilage

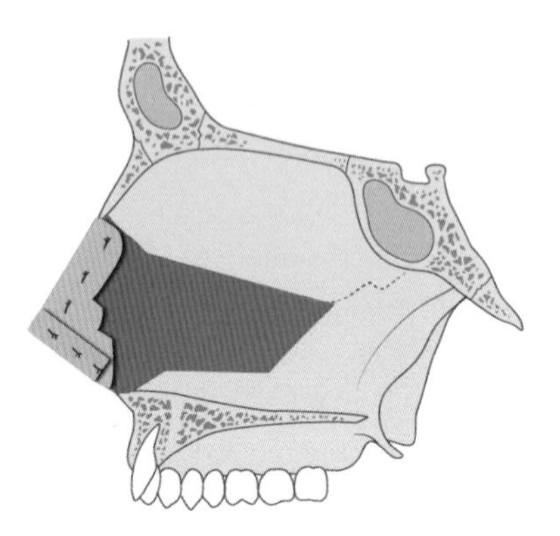

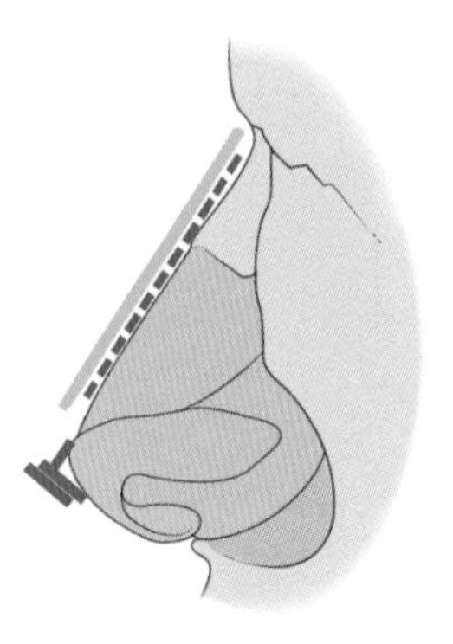

Postoperative Changes

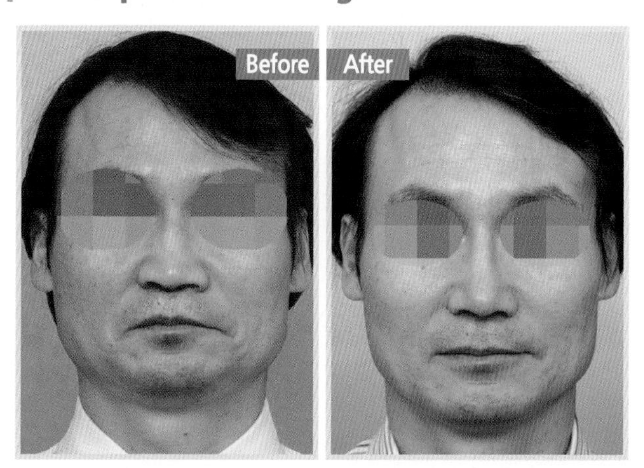

Frontal: Straightened dorsum with improved dorsal aesthetic lines were created

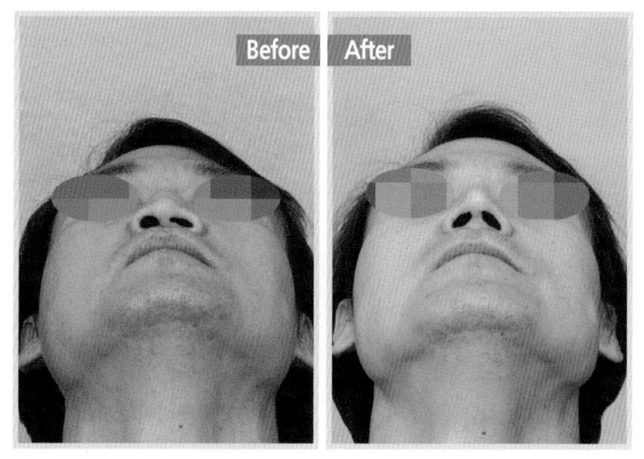

Basal: Tip projection was increased. Tilted columella was corrected. Nostril asymmetry was improved.

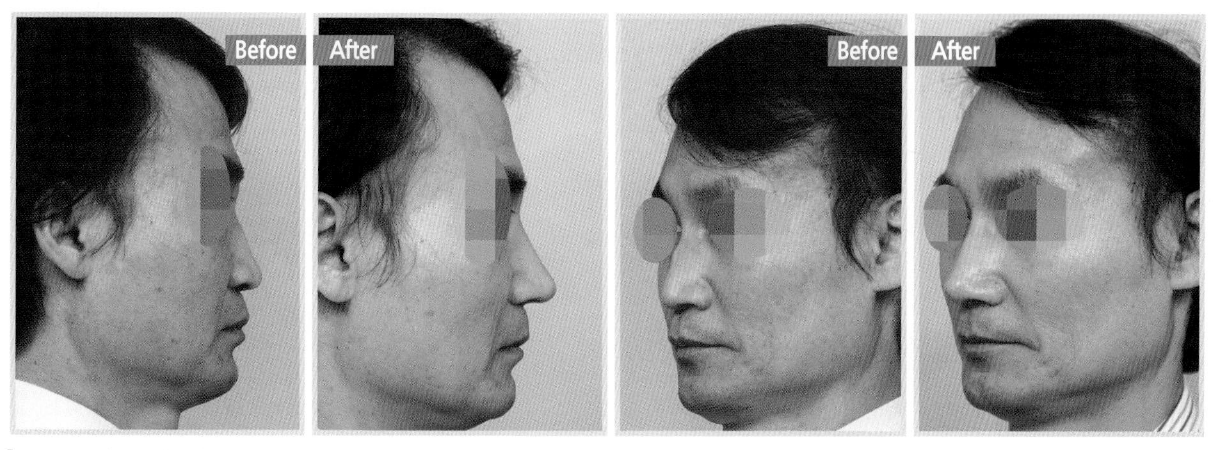

Lateral and Oblique: Dorsal irregularity was smoothened. Tip and dorsal heights were markedly increased.

Case 2

A 20-year-old female visited for a saddle nose deformity following nasal trauma 10 years ago.

Analysis

Frontal: Low dorsal height, bulbous and low tip
Basal: Nostril asymmetry, concave alar lobule
Lateral: Dorsal saddling (Type III), low tip

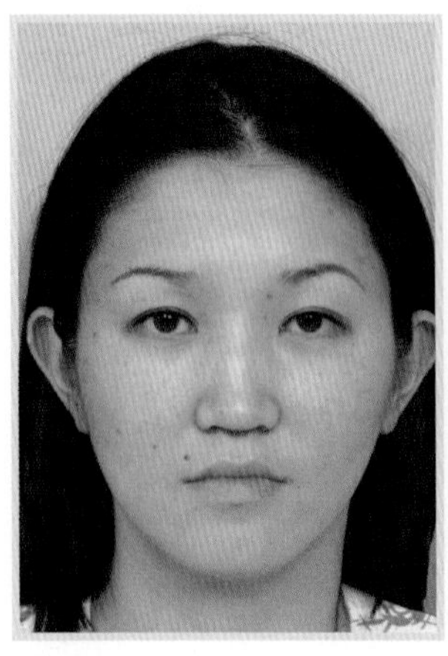
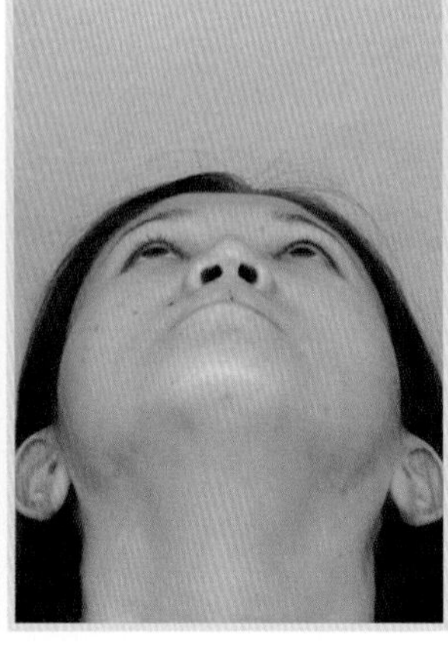
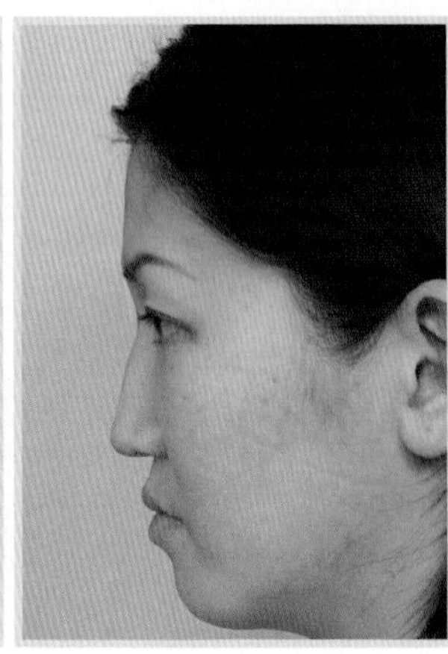

Operative Procedures

Open rhinoplasty approach
Costal cartilage harvest
Septoplasty
Batten grafting using costal cartilage (bilateral)
Spreader grafting using costal cartilage (bilateral)
Hump rasping
Multilayer tip grafting using costal cartilage
Lateral crural onlay grafting using septal cartilage (right)
Dorsal augmentation using fascia-wrapped diced cartilage

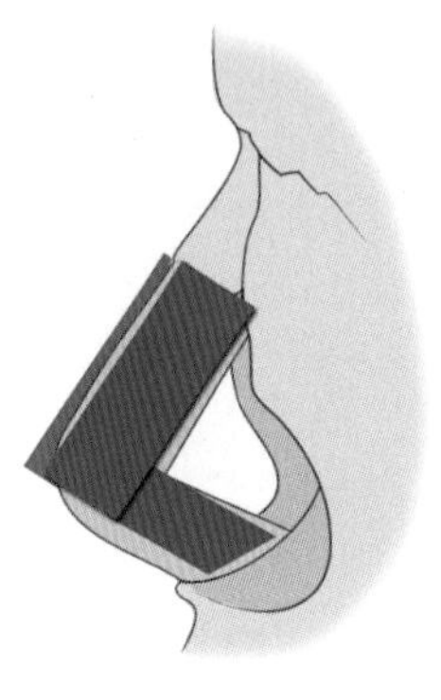
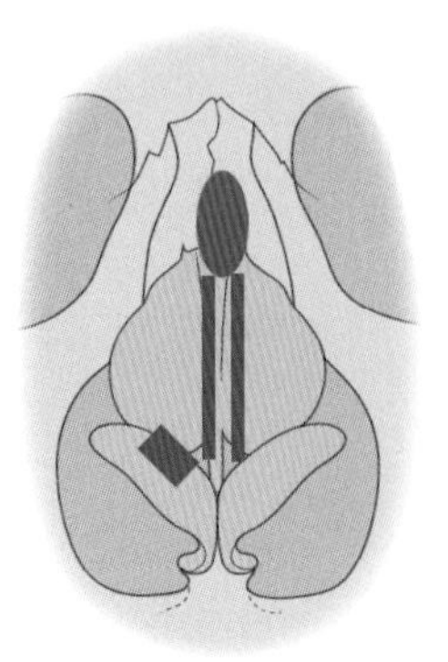
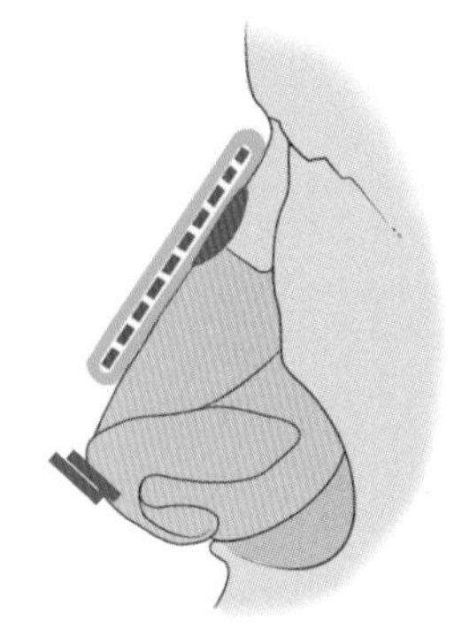

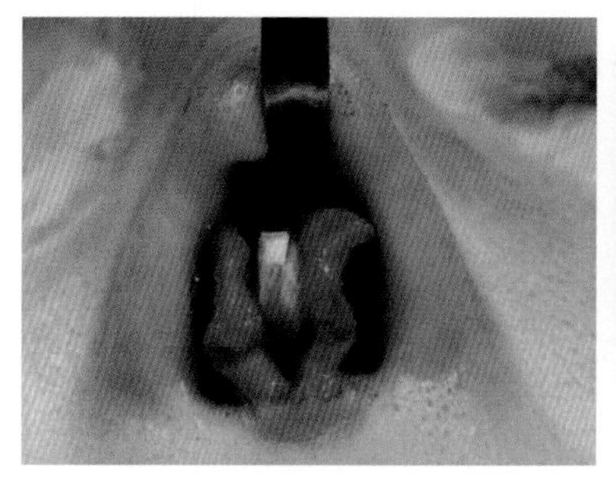

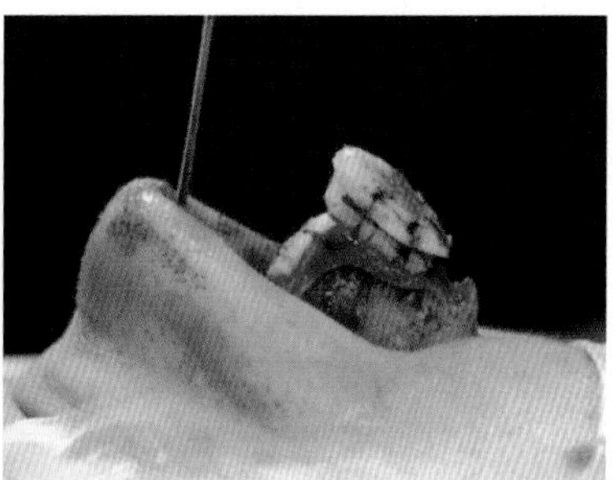

Postoperative Changes

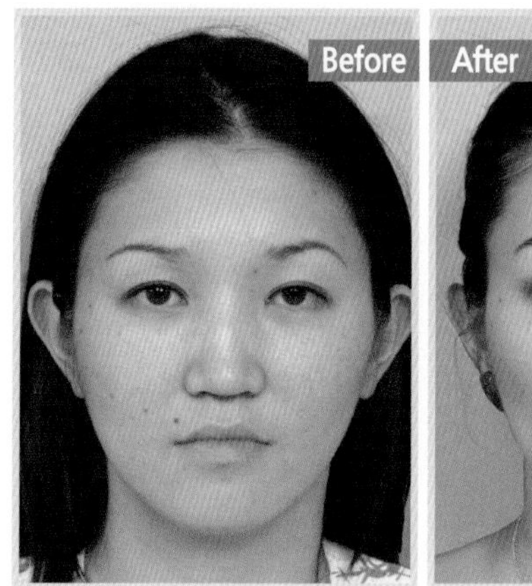

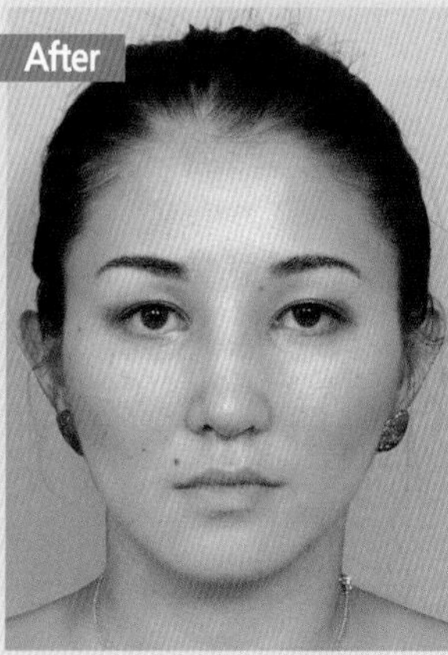

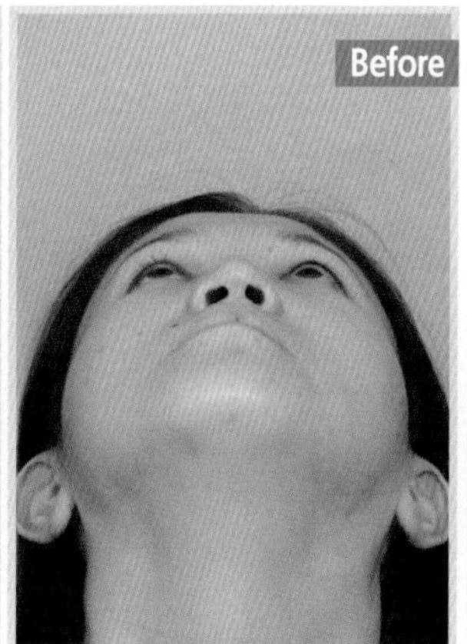

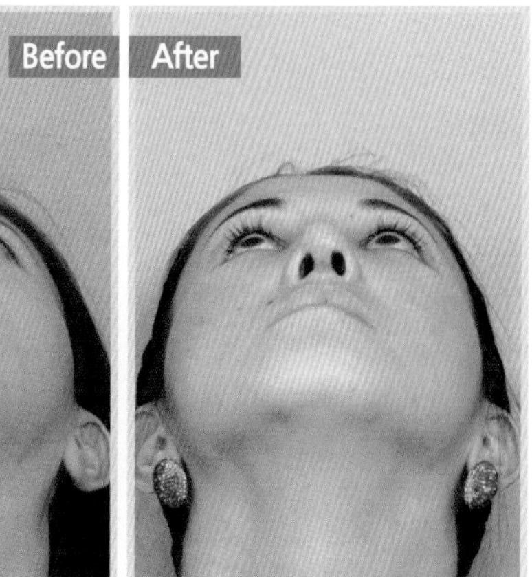

Frontal: Dorsal height was augmented. Tip projection was improved. Alar width narrowed.

Basal: Nostril asymmetry was improved. Tip projection was increased. Right alar concavity was corrected.

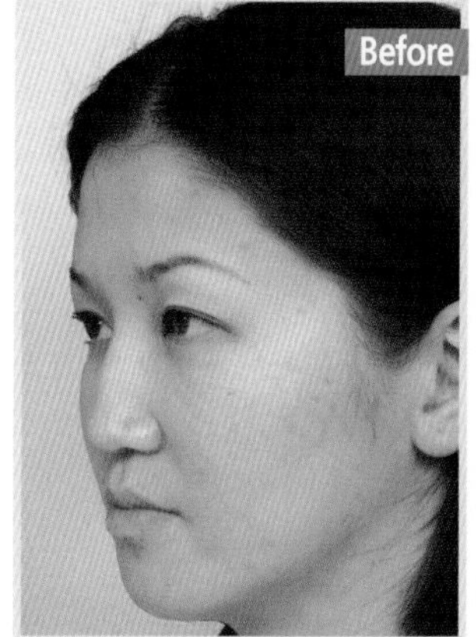

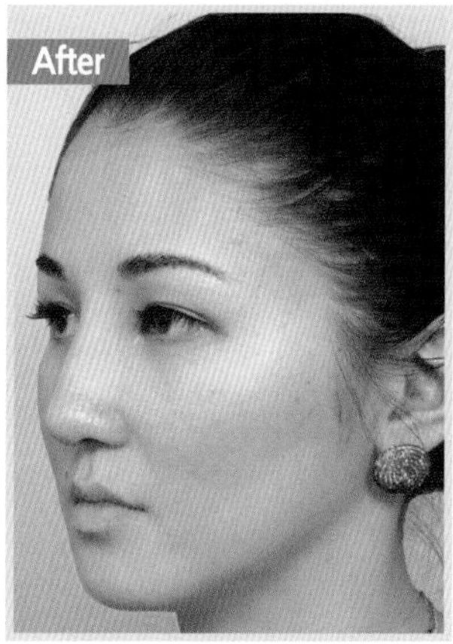

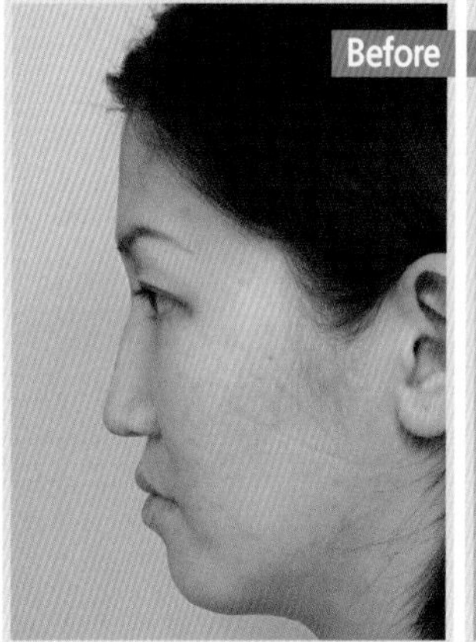

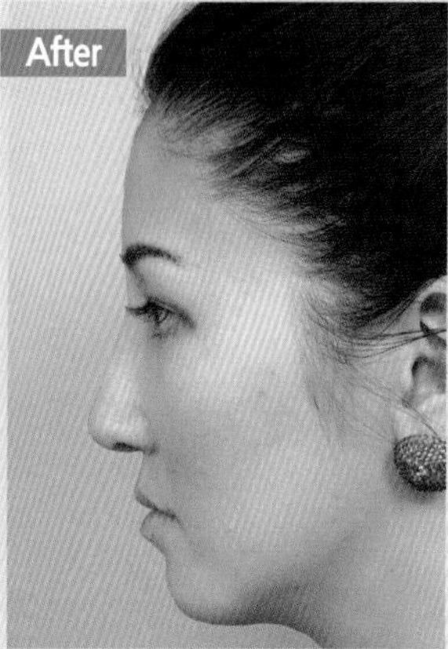

Lateral and Oblique: Tip projection was increased. Tip definition was improved. A natural looking dorsal line was created by correction of the saddle deformity.

Case 3

A 16-year-old female visited for a saddle nose deformity. She had history of insertion of mercury cell battery in nasal cavity when she was child.

Analysis

Frontal: Low dorsal height, wide alar base, retracted columella
Basal: Poor tip projection and definition, nostril asymmetry
Lateral and Oblique: Saddle nose (Type IV), pan-nasal defect, relatively prominent tip projection
Endoscopy: Large septal perforation

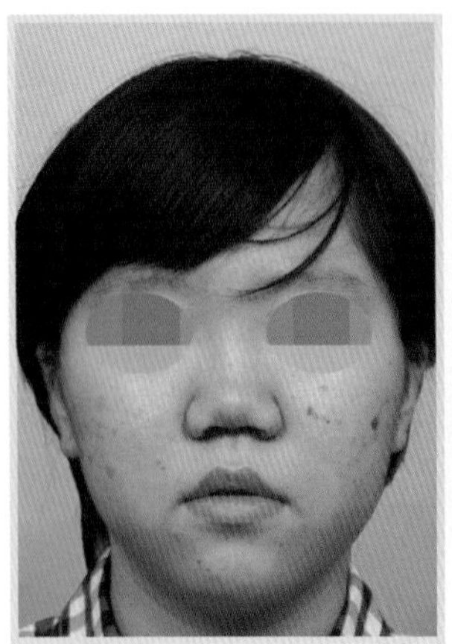
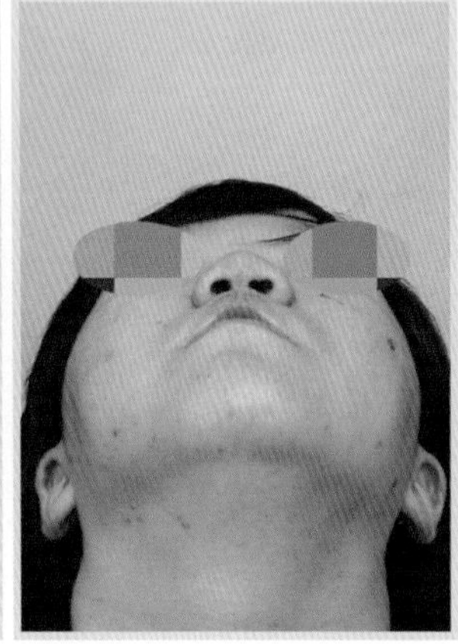
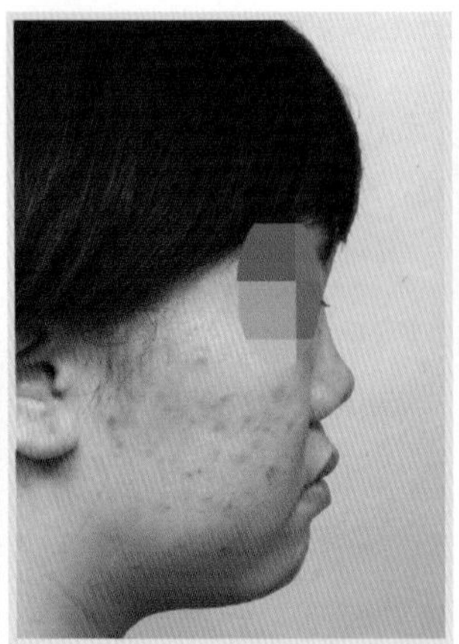
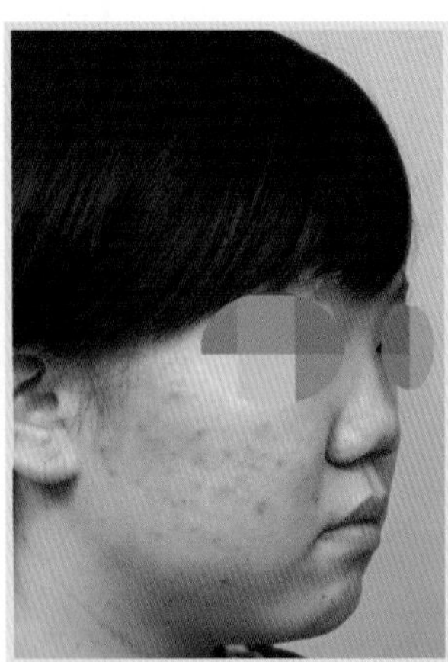

Operative Procedures

Open rhinoplasty approach
Costal cartilage harvest
Spreader grafting using costal cartilage (left)
Caudal septal extension grafting using costal cartilage (bilateral)
Multilayer tip grafting using costal cartilage
Dorsal augmentation using crushed costal cartilage and processed fascia lata
Alar base resection (bilateral)

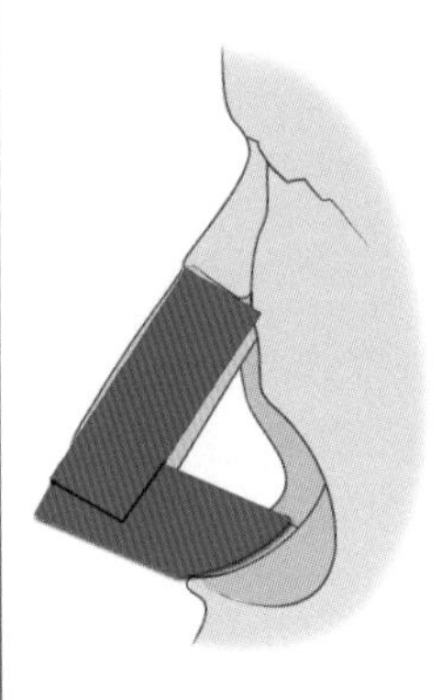
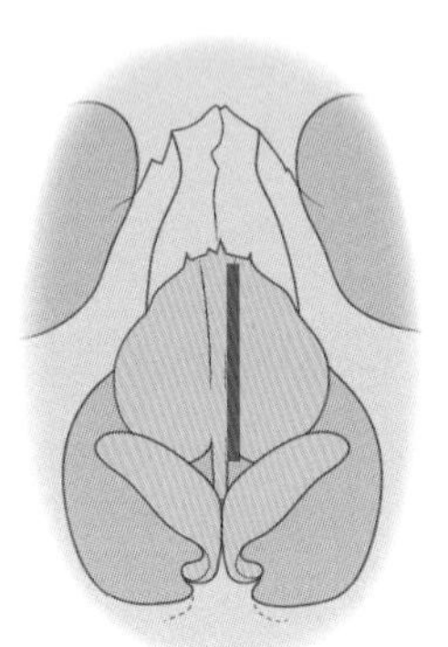
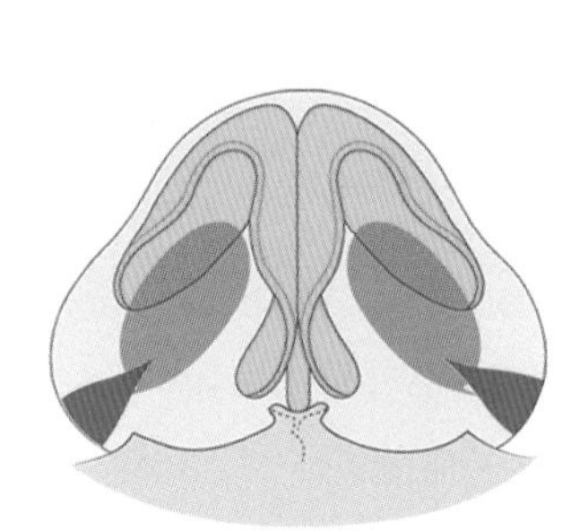
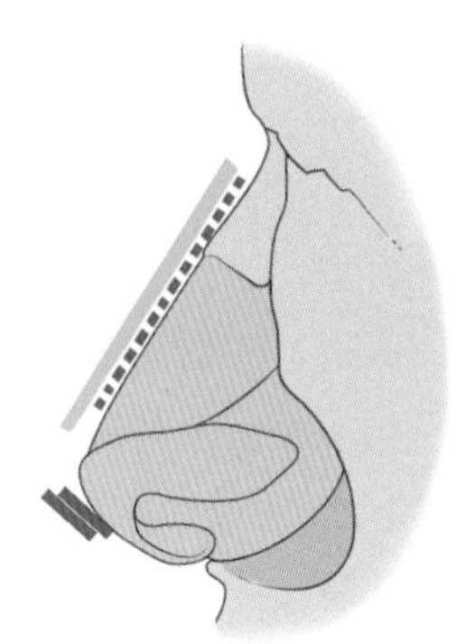

Postoperative Changes

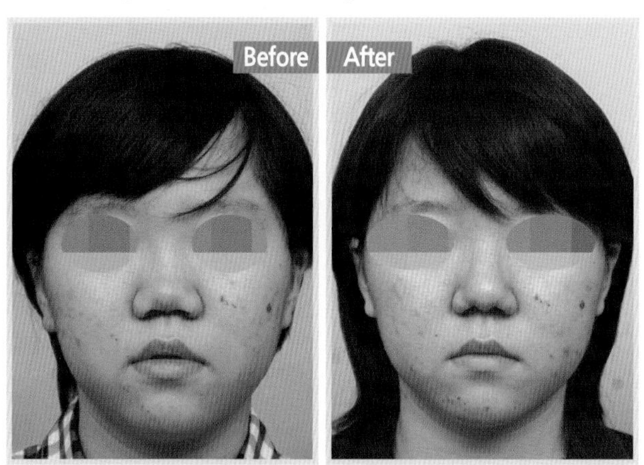

Frontal: Dorsal aesthetic lines were improved by the formation of a nasal bridge. Although the nasal dorsum is wide, the alar width was narrowed.

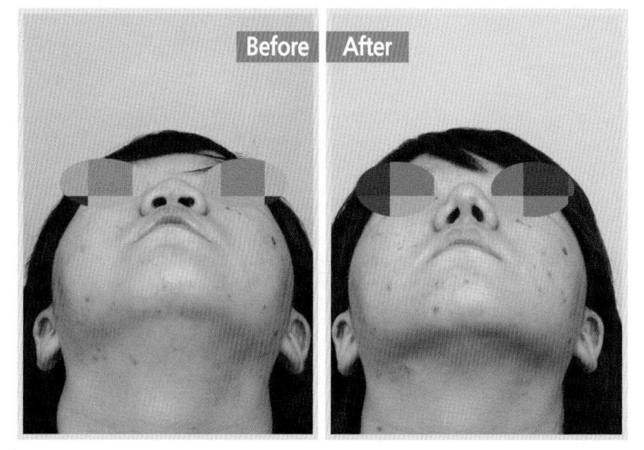

Basal: Tip projection was increased. Alar width was narrowed. Nostrils were given a more vertical orientation. However, a concavity on right alar lobule was formed.

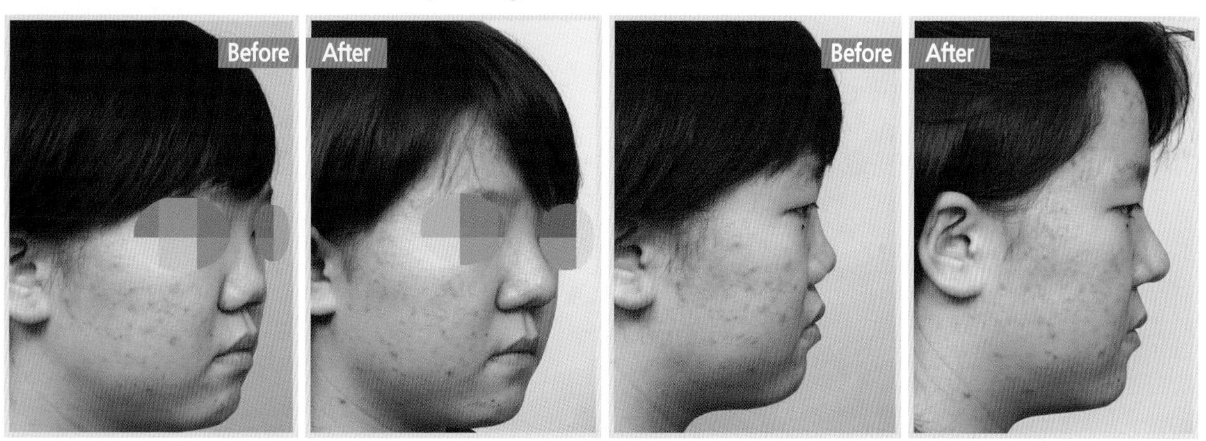

Lateral and Oblique: Nasal dorsal height was augmented. Nasal tip was derotated. Tip projection was increased and tip definition was improved. However, a masculine dorsal line was inadvertently created because of the highly located nasal starting point.

Short Nose

Yong Ju Jang

"Short nose" is a term that describes a nose characterized by excessive show of the nostrils in the frontal view and a wide nasolabial angle, giving the nose an upturned appearance. This deformity is also referred to as an "upturned nose". In some patients who have a small nose, a concave nasal dorsum, and a low nasion level, this deformity can easily be corrected simply by dorsal augmentation. However, the main problem in this group of patients is the upturned appearance of the tip. Therefore, proper derotation of the nasal tip is the most important step in surgical correction. Although cephalically rotating the nasal tip is an easy procedure, caudally rotating the tip, which is the main procedure involved in the correction of short nose, is a very difficult procedure. In clinical practice, short noses that develop as a complication of previous rhinoplasty is the most commonly encountered scenario, and this deformity is one of the most difficult to treat.

I. Classification and Etiology

Short noses can largely be classified into apparent short nose and absolute short nose, with no clear distinction between thee two entities. However, the patient who has a severely small or flat nose can be considered to have absolute short nose because the nasal starting point is distant from the forehead in these cases. The patient who has an upturned nose can be considered to have apparent short nose *(Figure 1)*.

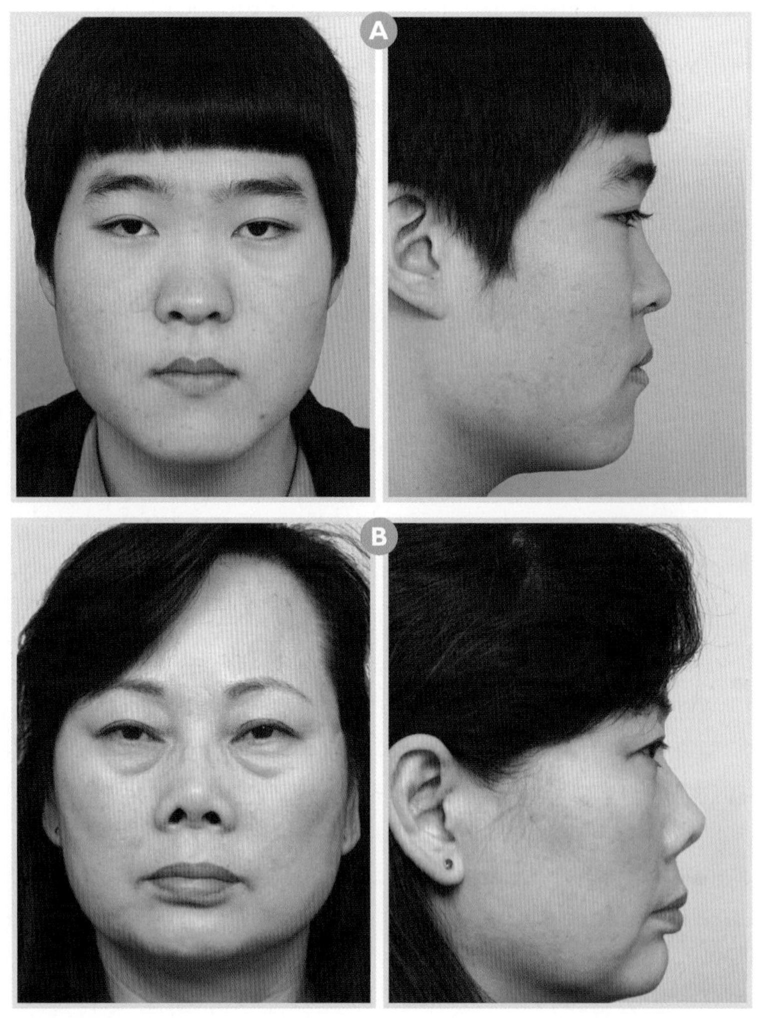

Figure 1 Absolute short nose (A), which exhibits the characteristics of a small nose, and apparent short nose (B), which has the appearance of upturned nose.

1. Facial Features Contributing to a Nose that Appears Short *(Figures 2, 3)*:

- Over-rotation of the nasal tip
- Concave nasal dorsum
- Deep and low radix
- Disproportionately high nasal tip relative to the nasal length
- Wide nasolabial angle
- Wide columellar-lobular angle
- Alar-columellar discrepancy due to alar retraction
- Long philtrum

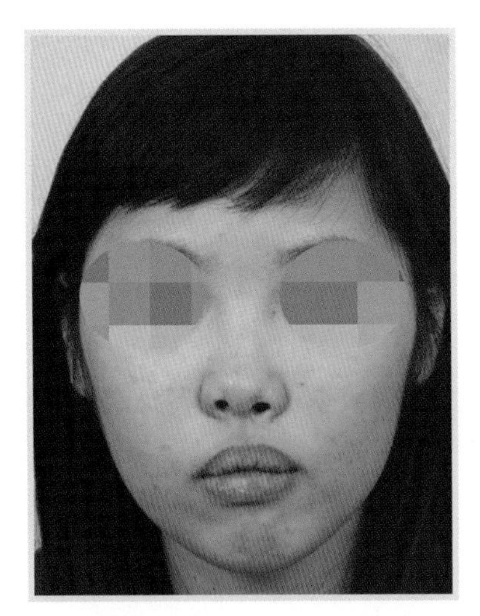
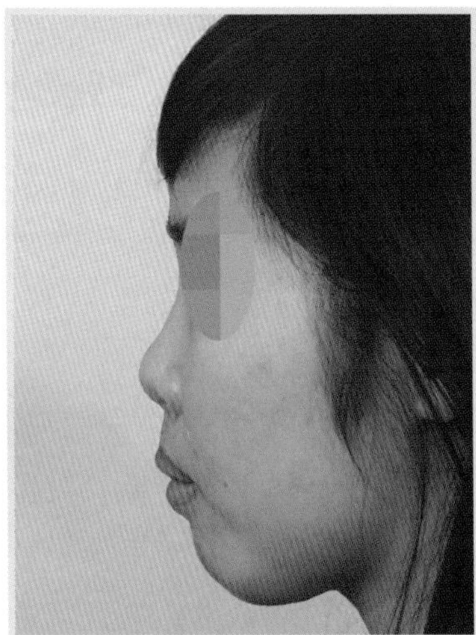

Figure 2 The congenital short nose. This is characterized by distinct nostril show on the frontal view, a concave dorsum on the lateral view, and a wide nasolabial angle.

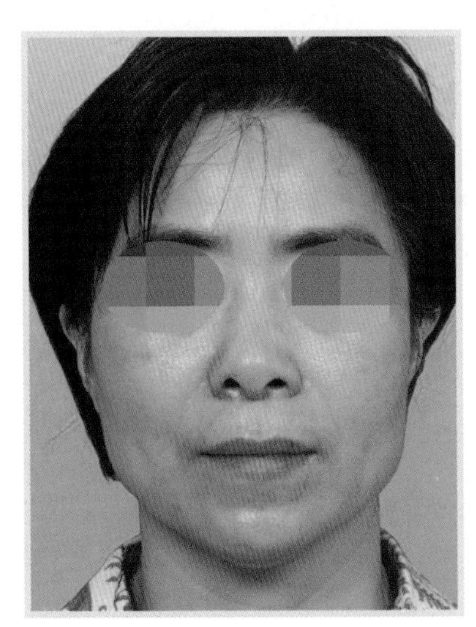
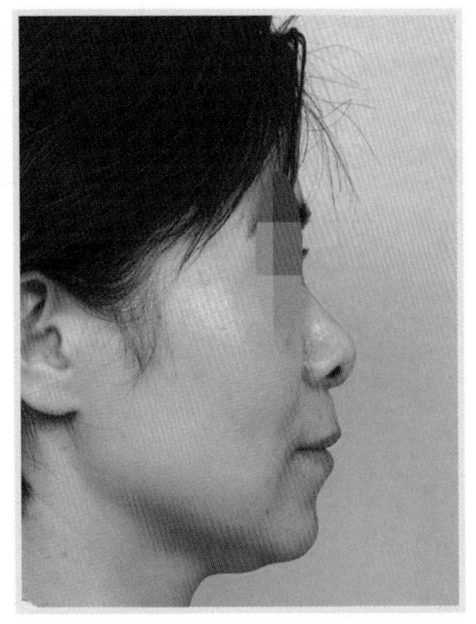

Figure 3 The congenital short nose. The nose appears to be short because the columellar-lobular angle seen on lateral view is very wide.

2. Etiologies of Short Noses:

- ☑ Trauma
- ☑ Postoperative complication (rhinoplasty, septoplasty, tumor surgery) *(Figure 4)*
- ☑ Infection and inflammation (septal abscess, hematoma)
- ☑ Developmental problem (Binder syndrome)

As described in the etiology, a short nose most commonly develops as sequelae of nasal surgery *(Figure 4)*. In order to avoid creating sequelae in the form of a short nose, the surgeon should be extremely careful not to perform over-resection of the dorsum, aggressive cephalic resection of the lateral crus, shortening of the caudal septum, wide resection of the dorsal septum, and aggressive defatting of the skin-soft tissue envelope. In particular, an aggressive rhinoplasty maneuver that includes excessive cartilage work is more likely to result in a short nose in the pediatric population compared to adults.

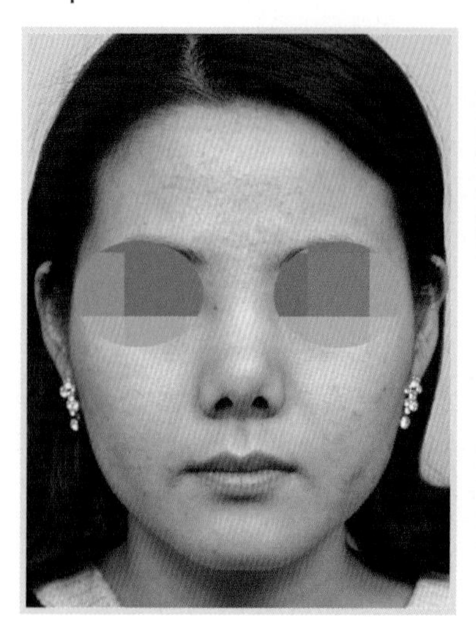
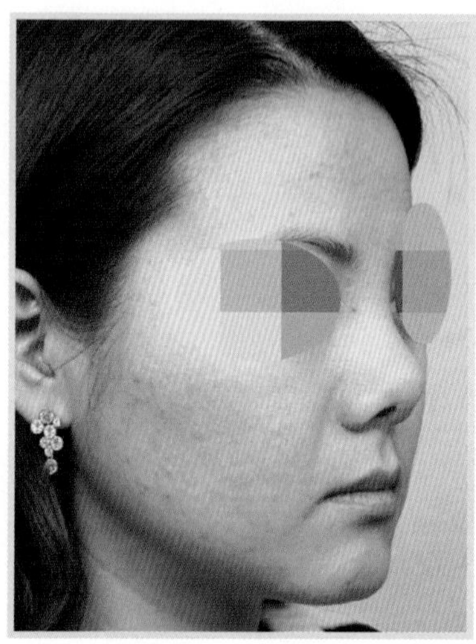
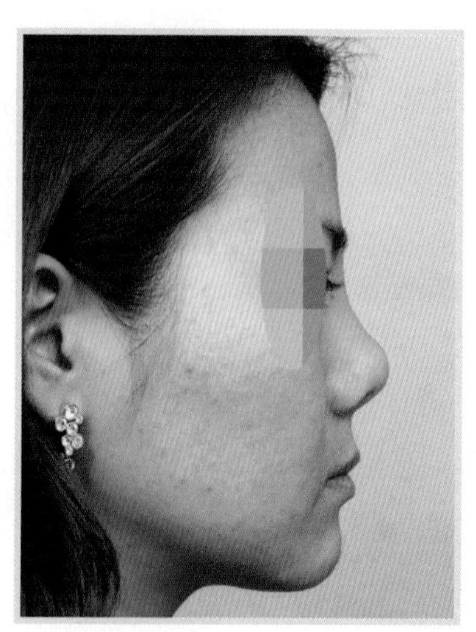

Figure 4 Short nose as a complication of a previously implanted silicone for dorsal augmentation.

II. Surgical Treatment

A short nose is one of the most difficult deformities to correct, and it requires the use of challenging surgical techniques for correction. Setting the proper goal of correction should depend on which of the factors described above make the nose appear shorter. The most important thing to consider aside from the morphology is the mobility and the characteristic of the skin-soft tissue envelope; therefore, this should be closely examined. When a short nose is due to complications of previously performed silicone rhinoplasty, the nasal soft tissue of these patients is often severely thickened and hardened. The skin-soft tissue envelope is likely to exhibit structural changes or injury due to scarring from the previous surgery during the healing period even in patients in whom primary rhinoplasty was performed without the use of silicone.

Most short nose patients have a concave dorsum, which is anatomically related to a short nose. Successful correction of a short nose is determined by the interaction between the internal cartilage framework and the external skin soft tissue; successful results can be obtained by extending the internal lining (internal framework) of the nasal cavity and the external soft tissue envelope.

The surgery must proceed with the actual extension of the length of the nose while simultaneously creating the visual illusion of a nose that appears to be longer. Short nose treatment must include taking into account the anatomical diversity of the short nose patient and the patients' expectations on the results of the surgery. In most cases, meeting both of these demands is difficult using only one surgical technique alone. Multitudes of surgical techniques are required to meet the demands.

1. Lengthening the Internal Framework

1) Lengthening of the Central Compartment

After the skin soft tissue envelope has been elevated, the exact shape of the central compartment should be evaluated. In particular, the issues of scar contracture of the skin soft tissue envelope and weakened nasal framework should be considered in the revision case.

The ultimate goal of the surgery is repositioning the central compartment and the nasal tip, as well as maintaining an adequate supporting structure to the tip. A strong internal framework is essential for achieving long-term predictable results; thus, the decision of which cartilage can be used to reconstruct the cartilage framework will affect the results. According to the author's experience, reconstruction of the nasal septum by using an autologous or homologous costal cartilage and the placement of an extended spreader graft produce superior results *(Figure 5)*.

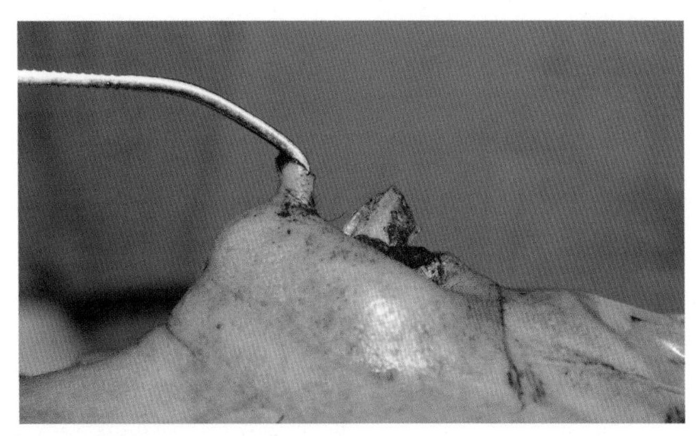

Figure 5 Surgical procedure to lengthen the central compartment by extended spreader graft using autologous costal cartilage.

The mid-portion of the quadrangular cartilage, not included in the L-strut, can be used appropriately for septal lengthening. However, in many patients, especially females, the cartilage is very thin and weak. This thin and weak cartilage cannot withstand the contractile force of the soft tissue during healing, thus may be deformed in the long run, which makes it not suitable for septal reconstruction and lengthening. Moreover, because short nose surgery is usually performed in revision cases, additional harvestable septal cartilage is not available in most situations. The length of the nose can be increased by using the extended spreader graft with conchal cartilage;

however, conchal cartilage is not suitable for lengthening the framework because this cartilage is not so strong and straight *(Figure 6)*. Despite concerns over the complications related with the use of alloplastic implants, Medpor can also be used for this purpose, and good surgical outcomes have been reported by some authors.

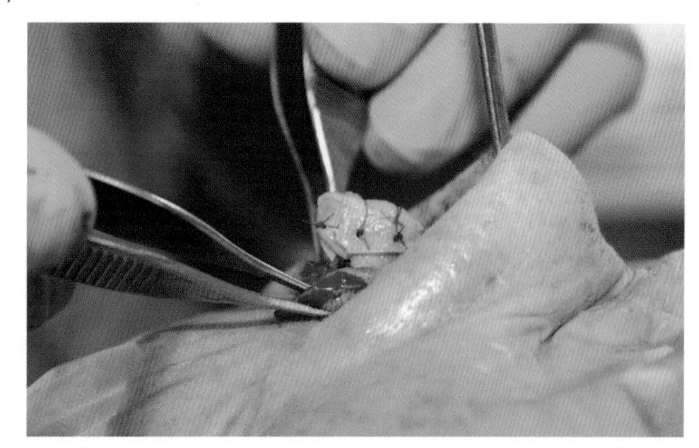

Figure 6 Central compartment lengthening using conchal cartilage.

A short nose is usually accompanied by overrotation of the tip. The septal extension graft, especially the extended spreader graft, is effective for lengthening short noses and counter rotating the nasal tip. The concept of septal cartilage framework reconstruction is the same for short noses as for saddle nose correction, except that greater attention should be paid to lengthening in the caudal direction in the former.

(1) When the Remaining Septal Cartilage is Strong and the Structure is not Defective

An extended spreader graft or caudal septal extension graft is placed *(Figure 7)*. Various forms of septal extension grafts are available, and the choice should be determined by the status of the septal cartilage and the amount of available cartilage. Sufficient lengthening of the nose can be achieved by a strong extended spreader graft. It is placed on both sides of the septum and in a direction that is 3-10 mm more caudal to the anterior septal angle. Strong septal cartilage is a prerequisite for a successful surgical outcome.

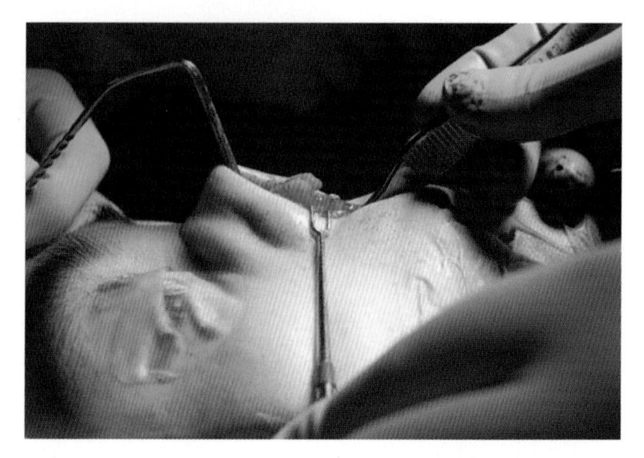

Figure 7 Application of extended spreader grafts by using septal cartilage. The grafts could be extended in the caudal direction from the anterior septal angle.

(2) When the L-strut Remains Thin and Weak

The caudal strut and dorsal strut should be reinforced by strong and thick cartilage with conservation of the remaining L-strut.

Several methods are available:

A) Place the extended spreader grafts on both sides of the dorsal strut and place the caudal extension graft between them. The caudal graft is sandwiched by the dorsal grafts and is placed in an end-to-end manner with the caudal septum. This graft is placed in the center of the nose framework; therefore, it is placed more caudally to the original caudal septum. The bottom portion of the graft is fixed to the anterior nasal spine by making drill holes, and secured to the caudal septum in an end-to-end fashion *(Figure 8)*.

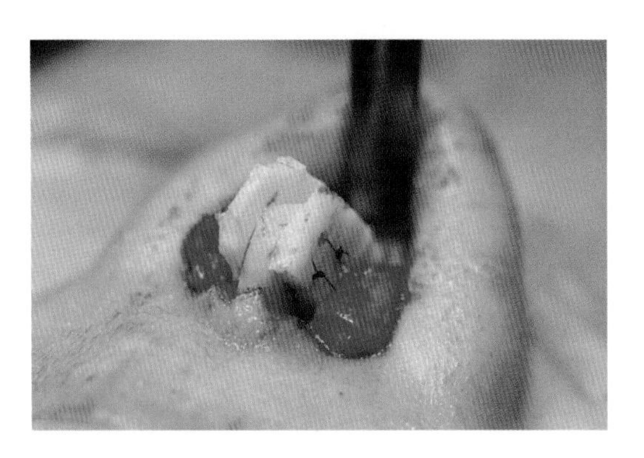

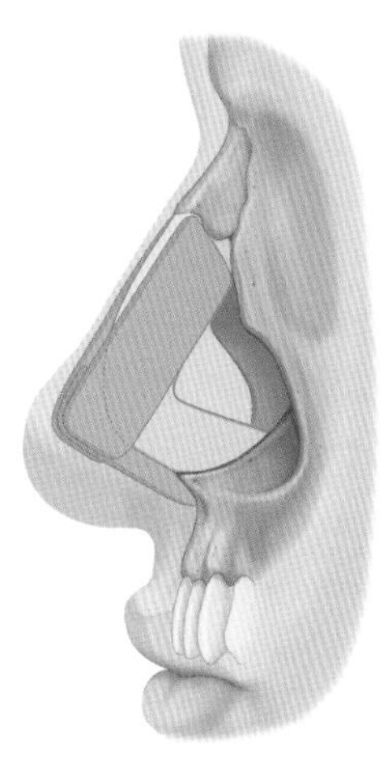

Figure 8 Extension of the internal framework using a caudal septal extension graft sandwiched on both sides by extended spreader grafts.

B) Place a batten graft on one side of the caudal strut and an extended spreader graft on the other side of the dorsal strut. The extended spreader graft is extended caudally when using this method *(Figure 9)*. In addition to this typical

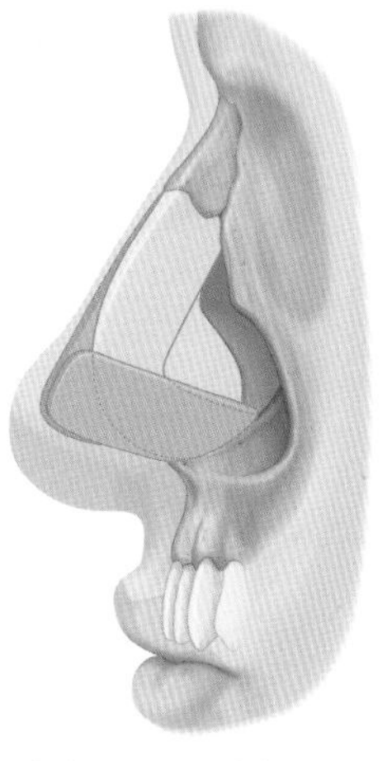

Figure 9 Extension of the internal framework with an extended spreader graft on one side and a batten graft on the other side.

method, a variety of modified techniques can be utilized *(Figure 10)*. The selection of the specific technique should be based on the quality and quantity of grafting cartilage and the condition of the remaining L-strut during surgery.

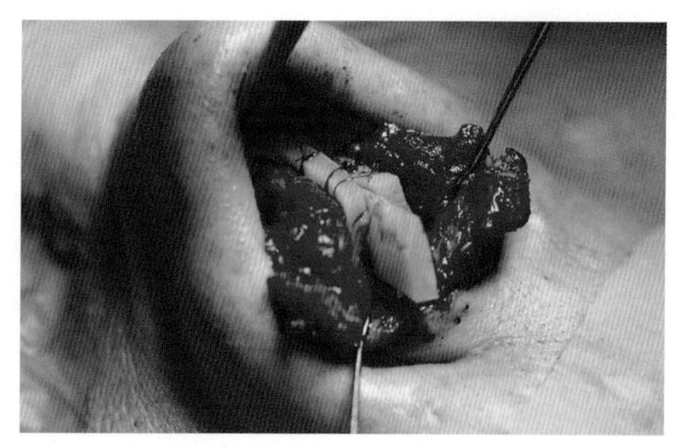

Figure 10 Surgical procedure to lengthen the central compartment by inserting a graft between the spreader grafts.

2) Correction of the Lateral Compartment

If lengthening of the central compartment is not combined with adequate lengthening of the lateral compartment, the nose may look pinched and unnatural. It is therefore important to address the lateral compartment of the nose accordingly to get an aesthetically harmonious surgical outcome. A number of techniques are useful in that regard.

(1) Alar Rim Graft

An alar rim graft can be applied by using septal, auricular, or costal cartilage *(Figure 11)*. The function of this graft is to prevent alar retraction that can occur after surgery and to rotate the alar rim caudally.

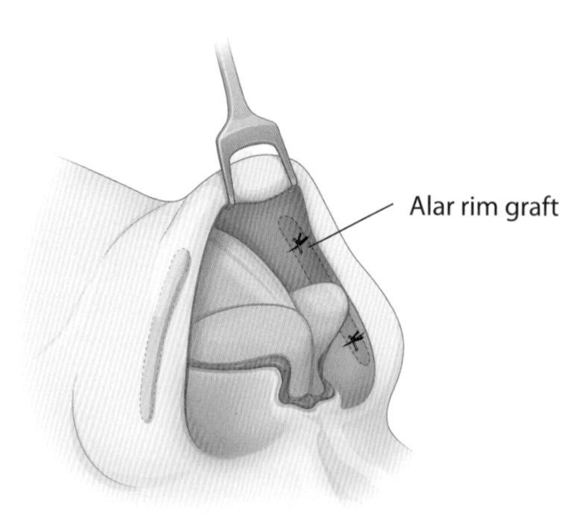

Figure 11 Alar rim graft.

(2) Auricular Composite Graft

The soft tissue of the internal alar surface is often insufficient when a short nose is associated with severe alar retraction. Inserting the graft to the alar lobule side and suturing a marginal incision after surgery is difficult in this situation. In such cases, satisfactory results may be achieved with an interposed composite graft, which is a harvested composite graft that includes cartilage and skin from the cymba concha or cavum concha *(Figure 12)*.

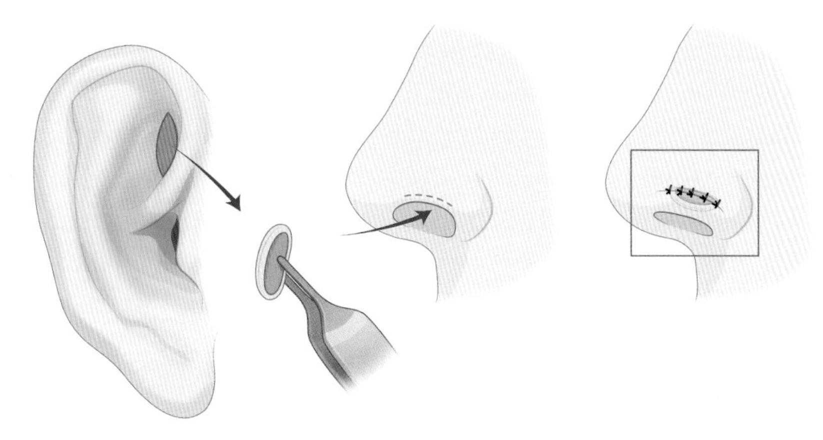

Figure 12 Correction of inner lining deficiency and retracted alar by using a composite ear cartilage graft.

(3) Lateral Crural Strut Graft

This is a graft placed underneath the lateral crus, which is freed off from the vestibular skin. The lateral crus and graft complex must be relocated to a caudally positioned pocket in order to correct the alar retraction in some patients. The lateral crura can maintain an adequate shape when it is fixed to the caudal position and it matches the caudal part of the central component *(Figure 13)*.

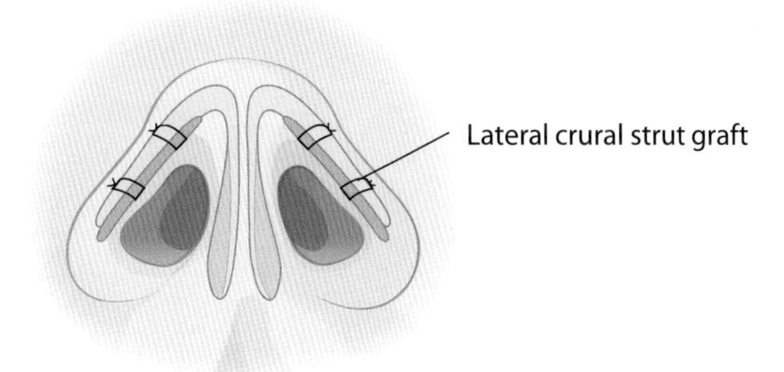

Figure 13 Lateral crural strut graft.

3) Dorsal Augmentation

The nose appears to be shorter when the dorsum looks concave. Dorsal augmentation is a very important surgical procedure because the nose appears longer after the correction of the concavity by dorsal augmentation in short noses. Concavity of the nasal dorsum looks more prominent when the nasion is located in much lower position than normal. When the nasal dorsum, especially the radix, is elevated, and a nasal starting point is subsequently created on the side that is closer to the forehead; the nose becomes longer in these patients *(Figure 14)*. The nasal dorsum must be elevated by using an implant, which surgeon feels comfortable in cases of primary rhinoplasty. However, sufficient augmentation is often impossible due to the limited ability to stretch the skin-soft tissue envelope adequately in revision rhinoplasty patients whose nasal skin is severely thickened, contacted, injured, or has lost its normal elasticity. Therefore, dorsal augmentation is performed within the range of the tension-free closure of transcolumellar incision. It must be understood that the division of the forehead and the nose becomes unclear in patients with poor forehead development if the increase in the height of the nasion is excessive. Since many patients have short noses resulting from complications of silicone, removal of the silicone and insertion of another implant material is necessary. For this purpose, the author prefers to use costal cartilage, processed fascia lata with cartilage, as the dorsal implant material. Gore-Tex can be used if the patient does not have a severe infection.

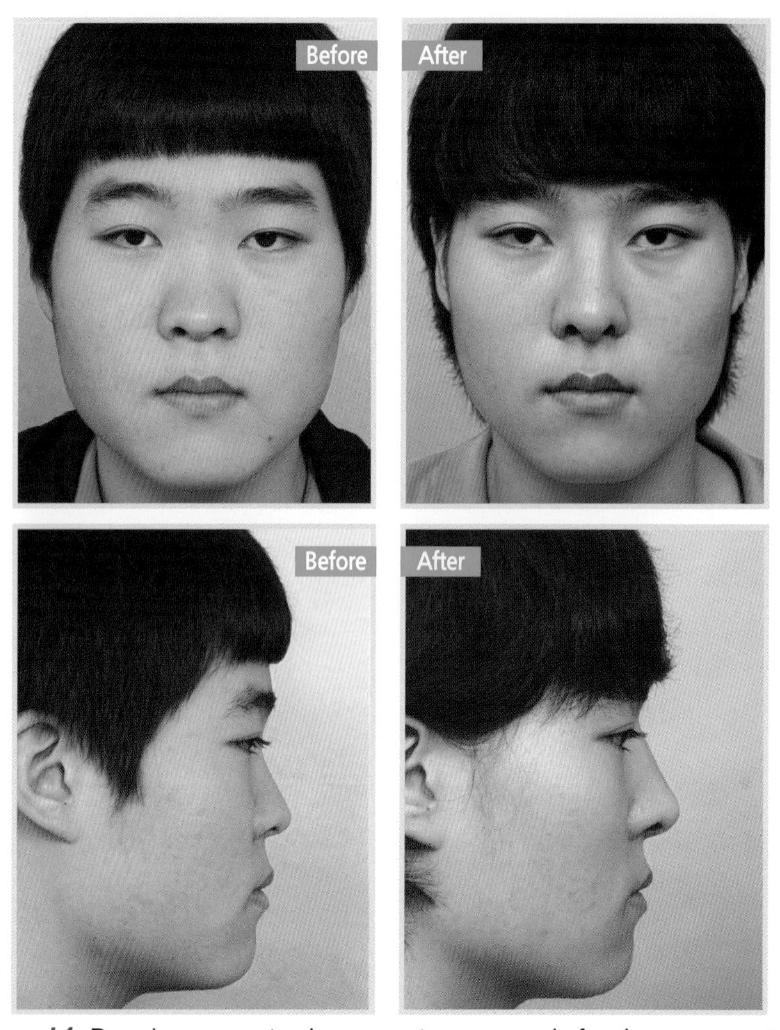

Figure 14 Dorsal augmentation has a very important role for short nose patients.

4) Nasal Tip Surgery

The nose also appears short if the nasal tip is cephalically rotated. If the columellar-lobular angle is particularly wide, the nose appears to be cephalically rotated. As such, caudal rotation of the nasal tip is necessary in order to make the nose appear longer. The best surgical technique for derotation of the nasal tip (caudal rotation) is the multilayer tip grafting technique *(Figure 15)*.

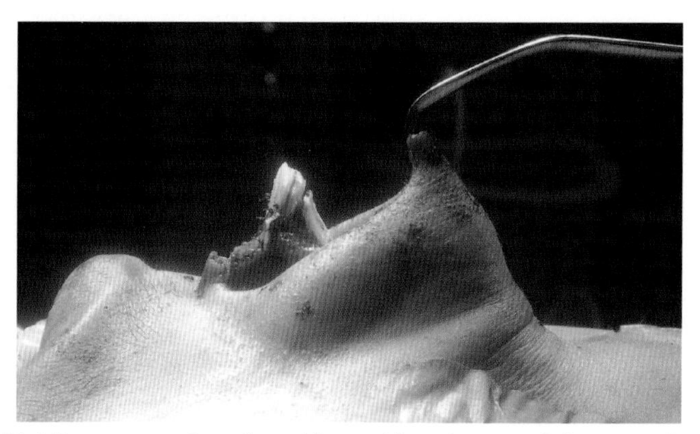

Figure 15 Multilayer tip grafting for additional lengthening of the central compartment.

When performing this type of tip grafting, it is necessary to focus more on increasing the length of the nose rather than on raising the height of the tip. Therefore, the multilayered tip graft should be placed caudally. Even if the caudal rotation of the tip is adequate, the nose appears short when the tip is greatly projected in patients with a short nose *(Figure 16)*.

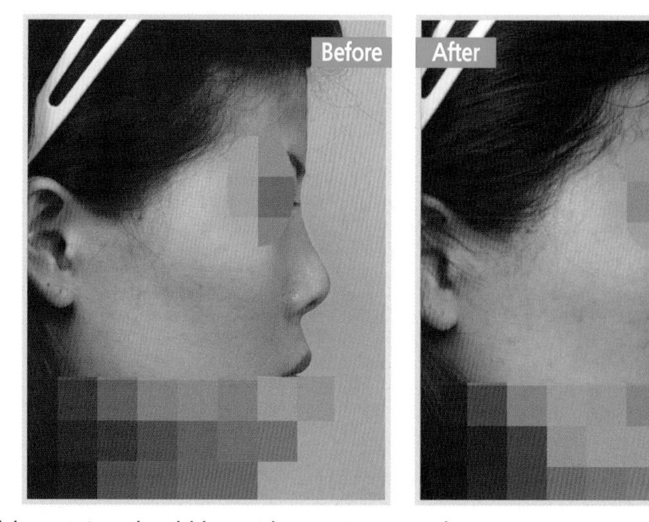

Figure 16 Careful attention should be paid to patients in whom tip projection is increased after surgery because this may exaggerate the appearance of a short nose.

Severe fibrosis and scarring are present in short nose patients. Therefore, the longer septum created by the septal extension graft is often not reached by both of the lower lateral cartilages in these patients. The mobility of the lower lateral cartilages must be ensured by sufficient dissection between the lower lateral cartilage and upper lateral cartilage and the lateral extension of a marginal incision. However, covering both sides of the already lengthened central compartment may be difficult even with these techniques. To overcome this, it is possible to cover the midline structures by application of the cartilage flap technique modified from the dome division technique, in which both sides of a medially based cartilage flap are developed by incising and dissecting the lateral crus of the lower lateral cartilage from the underlying vestibular skin, and rotated medially to cover the extended spreader graft *(Figures 17, 18)*. This method is very effective for correcting a short nose. The cartilage devoid area on the middle to lateral crus may appear after application of this technique. An additional lateral crural onlay graft can be placed at the cartilage-devoid portion if the defect is big enough to result in alar retraction.

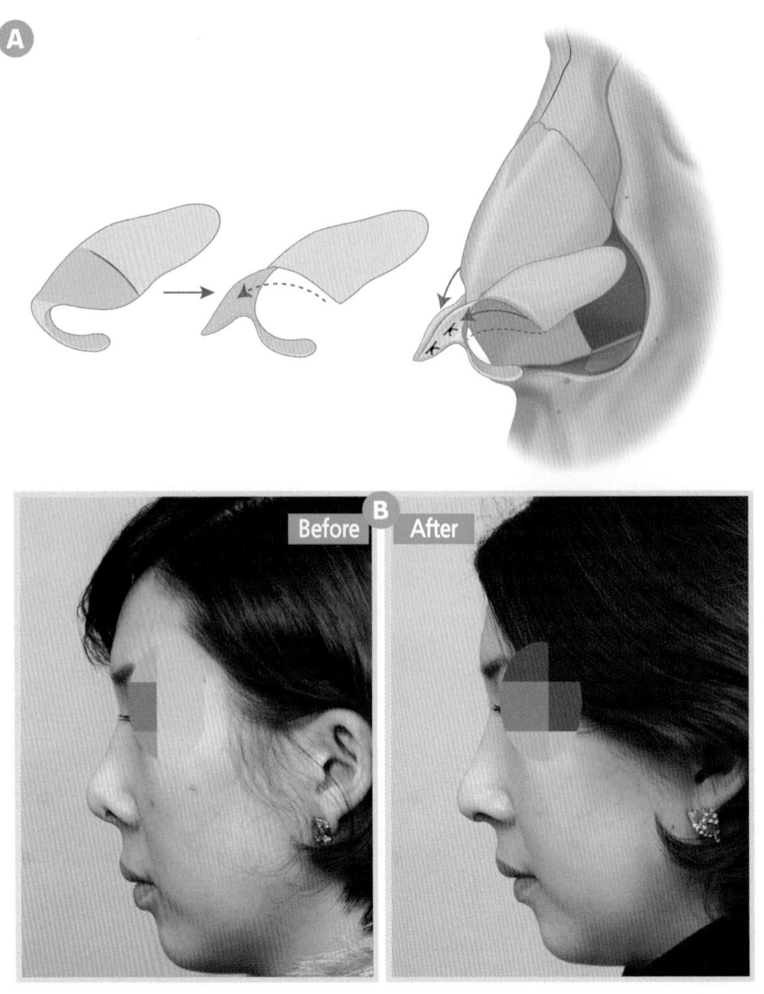

Figure 17 Additional central compartment lengthening can be facilitated when a cartilage flap technique is applied after using the dome division technique (A). Example of a patient treated with this method (B).

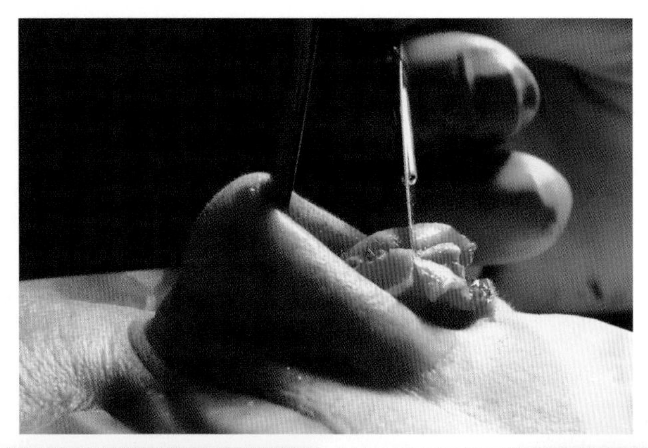

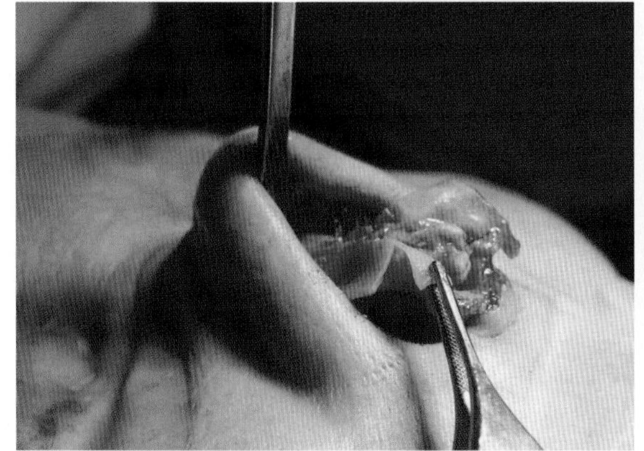

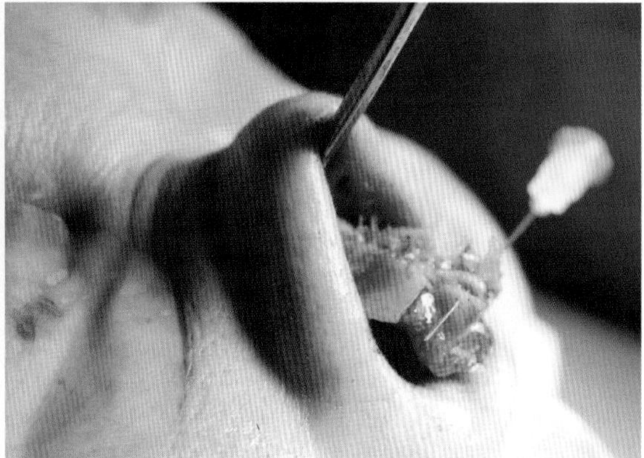

Figure 18 Cartilage flap technique.

5) Other Considerations

It should be noted that the soft tissue envelope of the skin covering the nasal skeleton must be widely dissected. Dorsal augmentation, various forms of tip grafting, and extension of the central compartment using septal extension grafts may exert excessive tension to the skin which should cover all of the grafts; thus, suturing the transcolumellar incision is often difficult at the final stage of surgery. Sufficiently wide dissection of both septal mucoperichondrium is necessary in order to solve this problem. In addition, wide dissection around the upper lateral cartilage and soft tissue around the alar cartilage is also important. In order to lengthen the internal mucosa more easily, one can make vertical incisions in the septal mucosa. The vertical incisions on both sides should not be made at the same location to prevent a mucosal defect. Making a few horizontal scoring incisions from the inner side of the skin flap reaching to the dermis is sometimes useful when the skin has thickened and hardened because of repeated inflammation *(Figure 19)*. Furthermore, closure of the transcolumelar suture can be made easier by creating a relaxing incision-which is an extension of the incision in the infero-lateral aspect of the lower flap of the transcolumellar incision *(Figure 20)*.

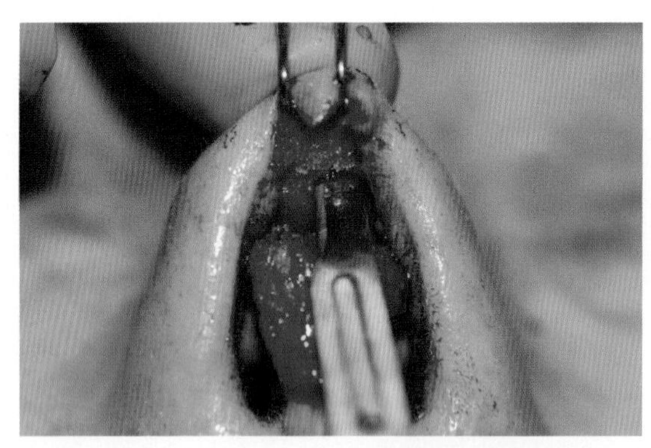

Figure 19 Horizontal scoring incisions can be made on the inner surface of the skin in order to facilitate the easier pulling of hard, thickened skin.

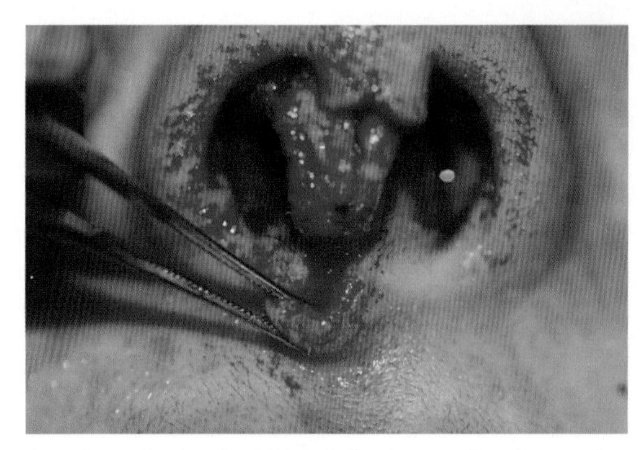

Figure 20 Relaxing incision placed on the both sides of the lower flap for easier closure of the trascolumellar incision.

In order to address the difficulty of covering and extending the skin of short nose patients, a method can be used in which the patients themselves pull the skin of the nose to increase the elasticity of the skin.

III. Complications and Difficulties of Treatment

Complications of surgery include complaints of insufficient length extension and caudal rotation, postoperative infection, and scar formation. One of the issues associated with short nose treatment is that complications appear more frequently in revision cases compared to congenital short noses. Performing revision rhinoplasty for patients with a short nose is very difficult for surgeons because the graft material is not sufficient in most of these patients and dissection is challenging because of the previous surgery. Furthermore, adequate lengthening of the nose is often difficult because of the fibrosis and contracture that has occurred in the dissected soft tissue. Multiple grafts must be inserted at the nasal tip to achieve the desired lengthening of the nose. In revision cases, because of the poor blood supply and difficulty in complete closure of the transcolumellar incision, there is an increased risk of infection of the grafted cartilages. Careful wound care is required and complete closure of all the incisions is mandatory with the use of skin grafting in extreme cases *(Figure 21)*.

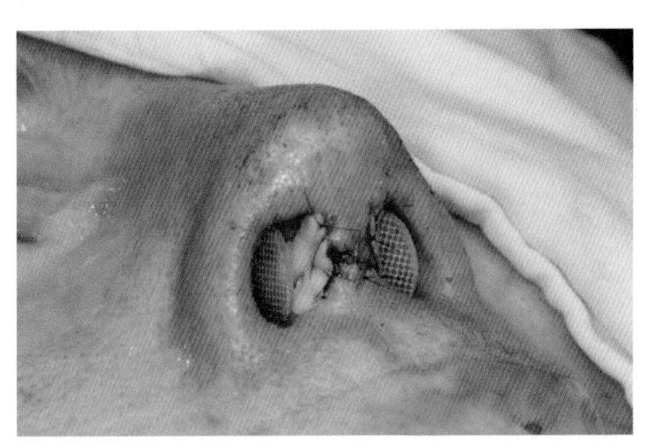

Figure 21 Postauricular skin graft applied to compensate the lack of skin at the marginal incision at the end of surgery.

Integrity of the columellar skin is the most precious part to be valued in managing these type of patients. When there is excessive wound tension detected during wound closure, a certain degree of extension must be relinquished. If this occurs, a portion of the central compartment should be shortened again and the incision resutured. When the color of the skin suture site after surgery is poor, hyperbaric oxygen therapy and frequent dressings are desirable for facilitating wound recovery. In our experience, infection after surgery occurs frequently when using costal cartilage for patients in whom the short nose is due to repeated rhinoplasty. If such a problem occurs, it must be treated with antibiotics and debridement by removing a portion of the inserted costal cartilage graft.

References

1. Guyuron B, Varghai A. Lengthening the nose with a tongue and groove technique. Plast Reconstr Surg 2003; 111: 1533.
2. Gruber RP. Surgical correction of the short nose. Aesthet Plast Surg 2002; 26: 6.
3. Naficy S, Baker SR. Lengthening the short nose. Arch Otolaryngol Head Neck Surg 1998; 124: 8091.
4. Palaci JM, Bravo FG, Zeky R, Schwarze H. Controlling nasal length with extended spreader grafts: a reliable technique in primary rhinoplasty. Aesthet Plast Surg 2007; 31: 645-50.
5. Sandel HD, Perkins SW. Management of the short nose deformity in revision rhinoplasty. Facial Plast Surg 2008; 24: 310-26.
6. Toriumi DM, Patel AB, DeRosa J. Correcting the short nose in revision rhinoplasty. Facial Plast Surg Clinic North Am 2006; 14: 343.

Case 1

A 47-year-old female visited for a short nose deformity. She had undergone open rhinoplasty 4 years ago.

Analysis

Frontal: Flat nose, marked nostril show

Basal: Slight nostril asymmetry

Lateral and Oblique: Low radix, short dorsal length, wide nasolabial angle

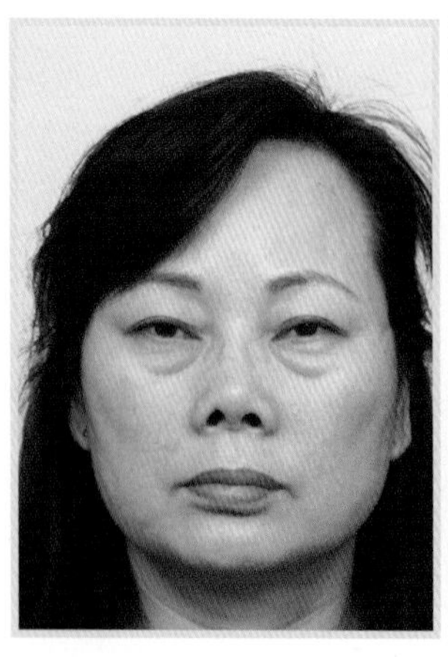
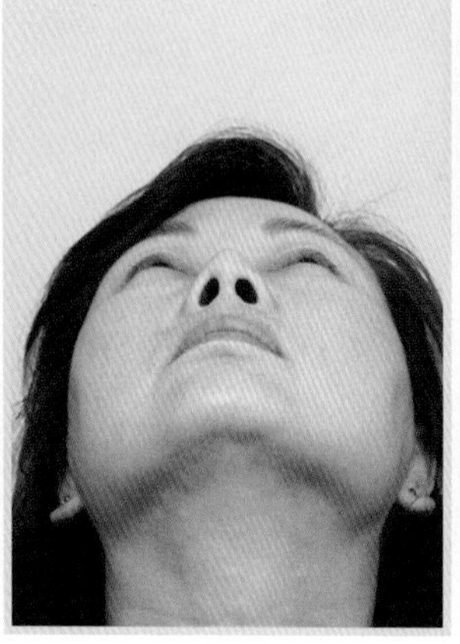
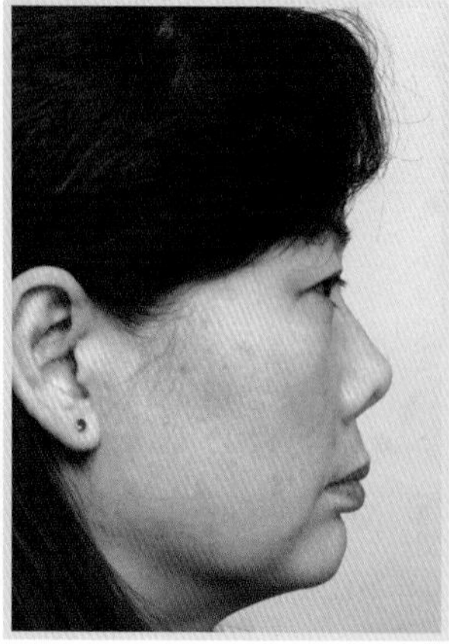
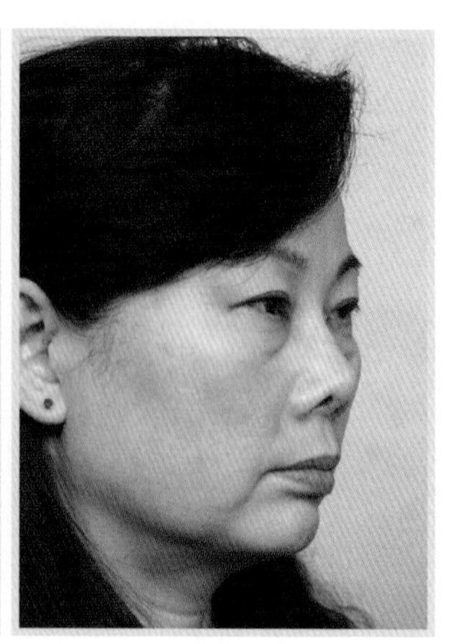

Operative Procedures

Open rhinoplasty approach

Costal cartilage harvest

Removal of previously inserted tip graft

Extended spreader grafting using costal cartilage (bilateral)

Caudal septal extension grafting using costal cartilage-sandwiched between two extended spreader grafts

Coverage of the lengthened midline cartilage framework using cartilage flap

Dorsal augmentation using crushed costal cartilage and Gore-Tex

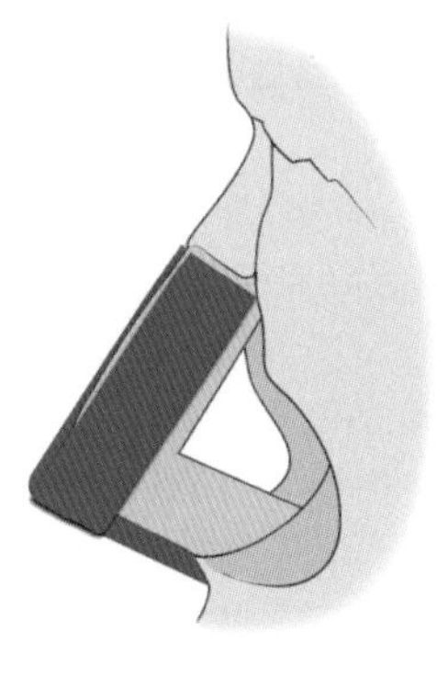
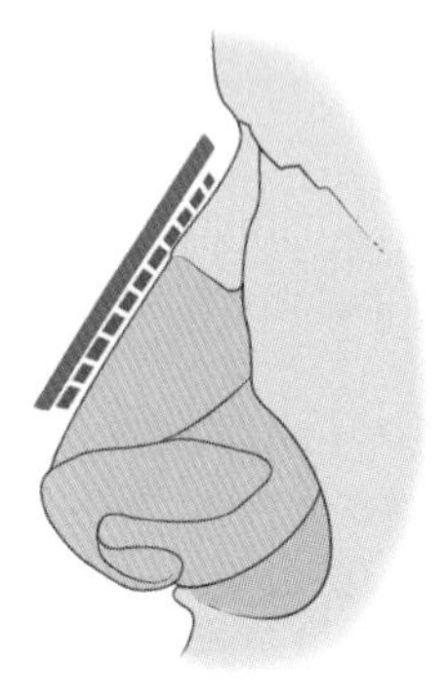
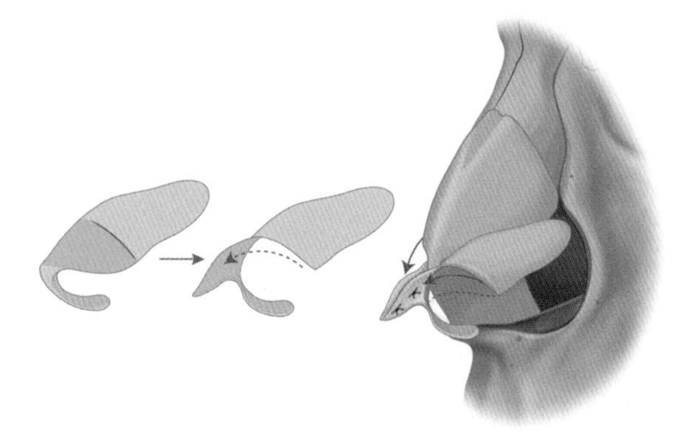

Postoperative Changes

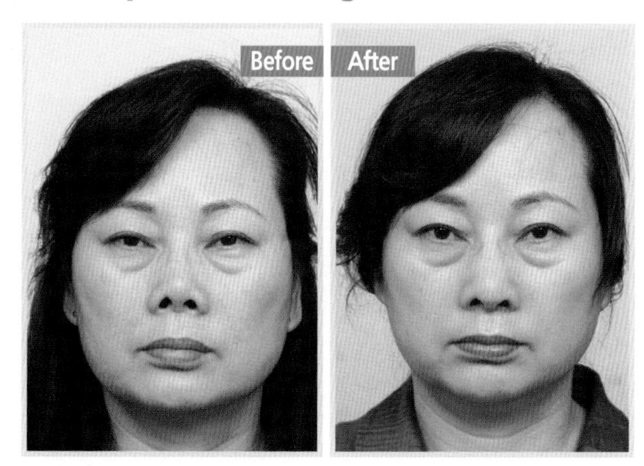

Frontal: Nostril show was improved. Dorsal aesthetic lines became natural looking.

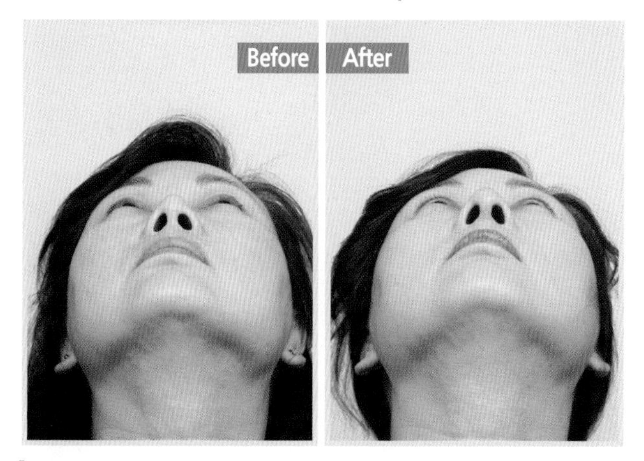

Basal: Nostrils became widened and tip projection showed no change.

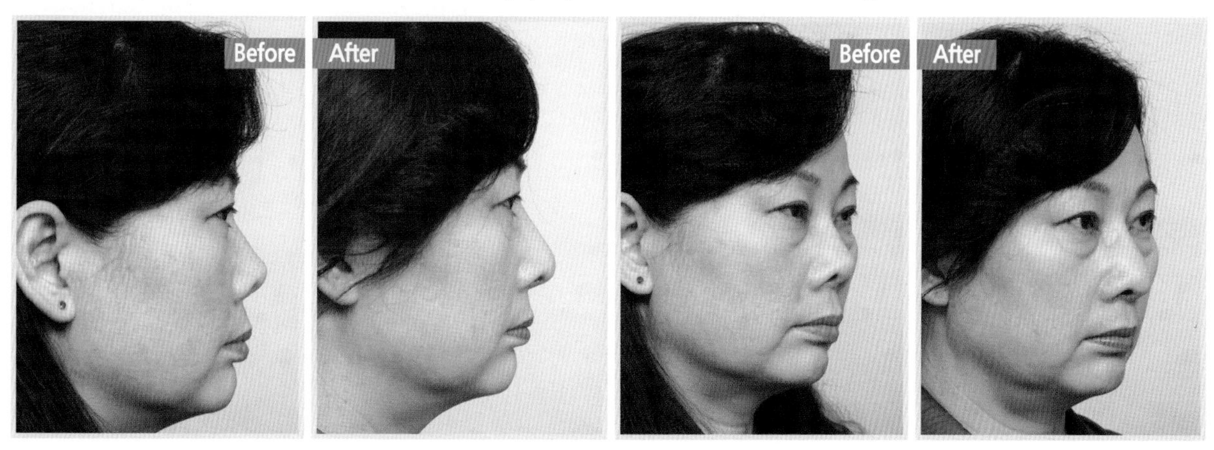

Lateral and Oblique: Dorsal height was augmented. Nasolabial angle was narrowed, and the nose looks less upturned.

Revision Rhinoseptoplasty

Yong Ju Jang

More than in any other surgery, rhinoplasty has the highest potential for revision surgery. The reasons for a secondary rhinoplasty include patient dissatisfaction over the cosmetic result of the first surgery and complications. Because surgical complications are usually accompanied by cosmetic failure, it is difficult to make a clear distinction between the two aspects. Rhinoplasty is performed with a clear cosmetic purpose in mind and whether the patient is satisfied with the aesthetic outcome determines the success or failure of the surgery. However, as this is strictly a subjective matter, it is inevitable that the level of satisfaction varies from person to person. This fact is a major reason behind the relatively high likelihood of revision surgery. In addition, it is quite common to see the use of an implant material during rhinoplasty, thus, surgical complications originating from the physical properties of the implant material leads to greater chances of revision surgery. Furthermore, changes in the supporting structure of the nose occurring as a consequence of surgery can over time affect the shape and function of the nose. This also is another factor that increases the likelihood of a revision surgery. Revision rhinoplasty is an extremely complex field of surgery that involves complicated problems and surgeons must be fully aware of the challenges of revision surgery.

I. Understanding the Psychological States of Patients Facing Revision Surgery

The main characteristics and problems related to the psychological state of patients requiring revision rhinoplasty are as follows:

- Patients seeking secondary surgery frequently tend to be more obsessed over minor facial details compared to those who do not seek revision surgery. In other words, they tend to have an obsessive personality wherein they become preoccupied with minor problems, which others often don't even realize.

- Patients who experience an unsuccessful primary surgery will suffer psychological pain as a result of that failure and this in turn will adversely affect their relationship with others.
- Most patients undergoing revision surgery experience difficulty in trusting their doctors. Thus, patients who elect to have revision surgery by a different doctor rather than the one who performed the primary surgery usually have much doubt on whether he/she chose the right surgeon for the job. Additionally, in cases where the doctor who is responsible for the failed surgery is entrusted with the secondary surgery, the patient frequently experience severe anxiety.

II. Anxiety Felt by Doctors Performing Revision Rhinoplasty

Besides the patient factor, an additional factor that weighs in on the surgery is the mental burden felt by the surgeon. When the same surgeon is performing the secondary surgery, it is difficult for the surgeon to be confident over the results of secondary surgery and he/she is liable to experience severe anxiety over the fear that the results of the secondary surgery will again be unsatisfactory. Furthermore, patients tend to be reluctant to pay for the secondary surgery and such a money-related factor can lead to an unpleasant situation. Overcoming it while carrying out the secondary surgery can be difficult. The anxiety felt when performing revision surgery can be lessened if the surgeon is different from the one responsible for the primary surgery. Nevertheless, the burden of anxiety felt from an unsuccessful primary surgery is heavy regardless of whoever performed the surgery.

III. Surgical Technique Related Problems of Revision Surgery

The technical difficulties related to revision surgery as compared to primary surgery are the following:

- Distorted normal anatomical structures due to the previous operation
- Difficulties in the dissection of the skin and cartilaginous tissue
- Heightened risk of infection due to compromised blood supply in the revision wound
- Higher probability of severe contraction of the wound during healing, compared to the primary surgery, thereby increasing the risk that the surgical result would be contrary to what is expected.
- An increase in difficulty in obtaining sufficient amounts of autologous grafts
- Damage to the nasal supporting structures caused by the primary surgery can be aggravated by the secondary surgery.

IV. The Importance of Preoperative Consultation in Preventing Unsatisfactory Surgical Outcomes

Dissatisfaction over rhinoplasty results is inevitable. The main task, therefore, for the surgeon is discovering their own ways to lower the dissatisfaction rate and finding proper steps to take care of the existing factors responsible for the dissatisfaction.

From such a perspective, the most important factor is probably a good doctor-patient relationship. Prevention is the best means to deal with discontent over surgical outcome. Thus, the process of rhinoplasty begins from the moment the surgeon meets the patient first as an outpatient. During preoperative consultation, adequate explanation must be provided concerning the possible changes by surgery, how the surgery is done, the cost, and possible complications. Good rapport with the patient based on mutual trust must be established during this discussion as well as an understanding of the patient's reaction pattern and character. Properly performed consultations with the patient prior to surgery will reduce the dissatisfaction rate. Most cases of litigation over patient dissatisfaction usually arise from breakdown in the basic doctor-patient relationship. Surgeons need to recognize if the patient has psychological problems during consultation. It would be best if patients be required to receive psychiatric consultation prior to surgery in order to discover any possible problems in advance. However, as most are not willing to undergo psychiatric consultation, this is extremely difficult to implement. Therefore, it is important to try and sort out patients who are suitable for surgery by means of careful consultation.

V. Prerequisites for Satisfactory Surgical Outcomes

Postoperative dissatisfaction does not have a direct correlation with how well the surgery is performed. The problem lies with how the patient views the result. In addition to consultation and proper understanding of the patient, the following matters need to be settled before proceeding with surgery:

- ☑ The patient must have a cosmetic problem that is both recognizable to others and correctable through surgery.
- ☑ The problem with the patient must be within the scope of the surgeon's technical skills.
- ☑ There must be a consensus between the patient and the surgeon regarding the anticipated result.
- ☑ The patient must be physically and psychologically fit to undergo surgery.
- ☑ The accompanying risks of surgery must be acceptable to both the patient and the surgeon.

In case these conditions are not met and it is deemed unreasonable to continue with the surgery, the surgeon must be able to politely, and without hurting the patient's pride, decline to perform the operation.

VI. Characteristics of Patients having a High Probability of Dissatisfaction

Recognizing in advance patients who have a high potential for postoperative problems is a very important element, and whether to perform or not the surgery on patients belonging to the following categories should be seriously reconsidered.

1. Patients with Unrealistic Expectation Towards the Surgery

Should the patient have a subconscious expectation that the surgery will be a great help in solving his personal, familial, and social problems, there is a high risk that he/she would be unhappy with the result of surgery. Also, a patient who has an unrealistically high expectation that is beyond what the surgery can deliver is likewise an unsuitable candidate for surgery. For example, a broad and gently sloping nose typical to an African cannot be transformed into a slender and high nose of a Caucasian with just a single surgery.

2. Patients Who Don't Have a Clear Understanding of His/Her Cosmetic Problem

There are cases where some patients, unable to clearly explain what their cosmetic problems are, display attitudes which can be summed up in the following dialogues: "Doctor, do what you think is necessary"; "Doctor, in your opinion, what is the problem with my nose?". As such patients tend to shift all responsibility on the doctor after the rhinoplasty, the doctor need to exercise caution on such patients.

3. Patients with Vague Motivation for Surgery

Patients who, without being aware of some definite problem, seek surgery for secondary reasons such as to improve the chances of employment or to please their spouse need to be persuaded to have a more definite motivation.

4. Patients Displaying Undependable and Exaggerated Attitudes

"Finally! I have found the doctor to cure all my problems. I will entrust everything to you." There is high possibility that patients displaying such exaggerated language of confidence or gratitude prior to surgery can easily undergo a sudden change in attitude and create a difficult situation. In addition, a patient who does not follow the hospital routine, seeking a personalized and special treatment also is very likely to create problems after surgery.

5. Patients with Communication Problems

In some cases, patients fail to grasp what is being explained to them by their doctors or are so engrossed in their own thoughts that it is difficult to reach a consensus during consultation. Such patients are very likely to deny having received most of the preoperative instructions that the doctor had painstakingly provided them before surgery.

6. Body Dysmorphic Disorder

Body dysmorphic disorder or dysmorphophobia denotes a condition wherein a patient is persistently distressed over a physical deformity that is imperceptible to others or over a normal physical form prompting him/her to resort to surgery to correct such conditions. This can be an expression of a latent psychosis. When a patient's anxiety or emotional response greatly exceeds what is deemed normal comparative to the level of deformity, it is called minimal defect syndrome and such patients have difficulty getting satisfaction from surgery.

7. Abnormal Psychological State

A patient who is taking medication for anxiety disorder or has a history of mental disorder should, with the patient's consent, receive psychological consultation. In some cases, patients display symptoms of excessive suspicion or aggressiveness during consultation in which case surgery must be avoided whenever possible. Also, for the sake of his/her health, it is best to delay surgery while a patient is experiencing major events such as the death of a spouse or a layoff.

8. Patients Who Have Difficulty being Satisfied with Previous Surgeries

If a patient displays an illogical discontent over a satisfactory surgical result of a primary surgery, there is a high probability he/she would be dissatisfied with all subsequent revision surgeries. Patients exhibiting a general distrust of doctors tend to belong to this category.

VII. Surgeon Factors Contributing to Postoperative Discontent

Cases wherein a doctor attempts difficult surgeries beyond the scope of his/her capabilities, leading to unsatisfactory surgical results, or failing to be fully focused and be at his/her best during surgery can lead to serious problems. In addition, if the doctor fails to provide adequate consultation prior to surgery and create a working doctor-patient relationship, or if the surgeon treats his/her patients brusquely or carelessly after surgery, the patient is liable to project such accumulated non-surgical discontent in the form of discontent over the surgical result. The reason for this is because patients have a tendency to judge the surgery not on its technical merits but on how fairly he/she has been treated throughout the whole process of surgery. From time to time, surgeons can misconstrue patient discontent as an expression of personal antipathy and react too defensively. This too can become a problem. Should this postoperative problem occur, although it can be troubling from the doctor's perspective, it is best to encourage the patient to express all the difficulties and indisposition involved, not to a third party but to the doctor who performed the surgery.

Ⅷ. How to Deal with Dissatisfaction

1. Solution for Dissatisfaction Caused by an Obviously Unsatisfactory Result

In this case, the surgeon must honestly acknowledge the fact that the operation has been unsatisfactory and show empathy towards the anguish felt by the patient. The surgeon must also be able to reassure the patient that the current problem can be improved over time. And, although it may be extremely difficult for the surgeon, it is important to encourage the patient to express his/her thoughts and feelings truthfully. During this process, getting into an argument or a fight with the patient must be avoided. Then, a secondary surgery should be suggested in the next 6-12 months. During this waiting period, the patient may become accustomed to his/her changed appearance and, in some cases, the patient may come to feel that the secondary surgery may not be necessary. By this time, the wound would have completely healed. Howerver, if the patient is too depressed with the surgical outcome, and cannot maintain normal daily activities, revision surgery can be performed much earlier than 6 months. Should the surgeon feel that the problem is beyond his/her ability to solve, or if the rapport with the patient is damaged beyond repair, recommending the patient to another surgeon can be a good alternative. In this case, every effort must be made to avoid giving the impression that the surgeon is attempting to dodge the problem irresponsibly.

2. When the Surgical Result was Deemed Satisfactory yet the Patient's Subjective Dissatisfaction is Causing Problems

When faced with such a problem, the surgeon should make an objective and calm determination of whether or not the doctor himself is subconsciously trying to shift the blame on the patient in order to deny the fact that the surgery was unsatisfactory. If such is not the case, the doctor should be assertive in helping the patient and being sympathetic to his/her suffering. Nevertheless, even when the doctor is confident that there isn't any problem with the surgical results, the patient can be persistent in his/her request for a secondary surgery. In such a situation, efforts should be made to help the patient overcome the obsession for a secondary surgery by providing the patient a detailed explanation of the risks associated with revision surgery. In dealing with these patients, it is necessary to maintain a sincere and patient attitude.

3. The Patient Complains Strongly about the Surgeon Who Performed the Previous Surgery

It is essential that the surgeon make a clear determination of the patient's problem and show a sympathetic attitude toward the patient's suffering. However, there are cases where the patient visiting for a secondary surgery complains continuously about the surgeon who performed the primary operation. To allow this is to happen is not appropriate. And, if the patient's relationship with the earlier surgeon is still workable, whenever possible, it is best to advise the patient to return to the first surgeon for consultation. In addition, it should be explained to the patient that even the best surgeon can occasionally have a bad result while an inexperienced surgeon can also at times obtain an excellent result. It is best not to proceed with a surgery for a patient while the patient is involved in a lawsuit with the primary surgeon.

4. The Patient is Satisfied but not the Doctor

It is usual for the doctor to be more critical about the result of surgery than the patient. Also, as it is difficult to be 100% sure about the measures taken to solve the various problems encountered during the surgery, it is understandable to have concerns during the postoperative recovery period. However, even though there may be aspects that are unsatisfactory from the surgeon's perspective, if the patient does not raise the issue first, it is not necessary to bring it to the patient's attention. This matter has nothing to do with a doctor's honesty. As the issue of being satisfied with a surgery is largely a subjective matter, it is inappropriate to show discontent by calling to attention to specific areas that the patient is not even aware of.

IX. Types of Problems Requiring Secondary Surgery and Methods of Treatment

Around 8-15% of patients who underwent primary rhinoplasty require revision surgery. Various problems, particularly tip deformities, are mentioned as major causes of revision surgery in overseas publications. However, in Korea, the most common cause of revision surgery are related to problems with the nasal dorsum. This is because, in Korea, unlike in western countries where complex tip surgery or reduction is frequently performed, the most common surgery being carried out is dorsal augmentation. In order to properly treat various deformities requiring revision, a multitude of rhinoplasty techniques should be used based on the surgeon's own experience. There are no standard treatment methods for each specific problem. The treatment strategy needs to be individualized

1. Unsatisfactory Surgical Result

To be dealt with according to the principles stated above.

2. Dosal Implants such as Silicone are Positioned Properly without Symptoms of Infection or Displacement yet the Patient is Anxious about the Possibility of Infection and Wishes to have the Implant Removed

If the existing implant is removed, the dorsum will again be lowered and it is common for these patients to have difficulty accepting this change after surgery. Thus, augmentation of the nose usually needs to be performed using a new material. However, such secondary surgery has a very high risk of complications. Therefore the most appropriate solution is to persuade the patient to go on living in their current condition.

3. Displacement, Malposition, Infection, and Extrusion of Implant

In this case, the implant should be removed using an endonasal or open approach. It is important to note that a capsule gets built up whenever a silicone is implanted and this capsule must be properly addressed. The microdebrider can effectively remove the thick, inflammed, and irregularly-shaped capsule attached to the nasal dorsum, which can affect the final shape of the revision dorsal augmentation. If the capsule is in good shape and condition, and not inflamed, it can be preserved, especially on the skin side because capsule removal might injure the skin-soft tissue envelope. Following the removal of the implant, if the dorsum becomes too low, an alternative dorsal augmentation material needs to be selected to replace the original material *(Figure 1)*. For this purpose, Gore-Tex, dermofat, alloderm, or fascia wrapped diced cartilage, or costal cartilage can be used. To manage an extrusion of silicone implant through the skin, the surgeon should remove the extruded implant and can perform immediate dorsal augmentation if there is no sign of frank infection. Regardless of whether the material of the implant is silicone or Gore-Tex, if there is a sign of active infection, the implant must be removed. The most difficult aspect when faced with such a problem is deciding on how to treat the deformity of the dorsum that appears after the removal of the implant. It is advisable to perform secondary rhinoplasty only after removing the implant followed by several months of healing, and when it has been determined that the infection has completely resolved *(Figure 2)*. However if after the removal of implant, there is excessive collapse and contraction of the nose which can impair normal daily activities, revision rhinoplasty can be done even after few weeks after implant removal.

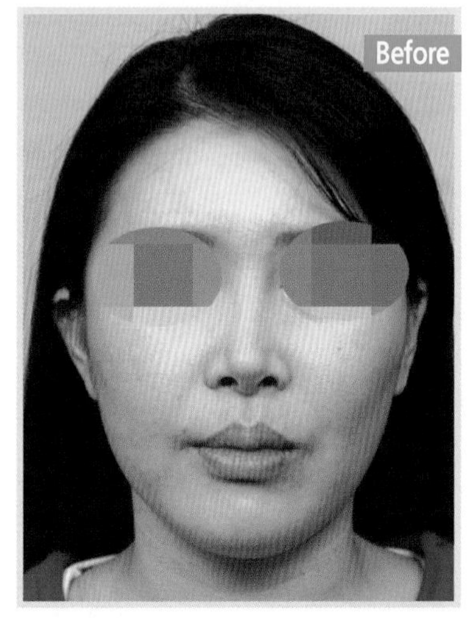

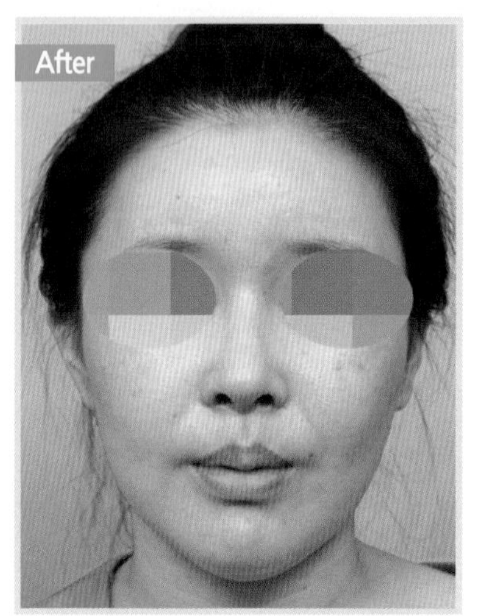

Figure 1 Silicone showing unnaturally obvious contour was removed and the dorsum was augmented using the combined use of processed fascia and crushed septal cartilage.

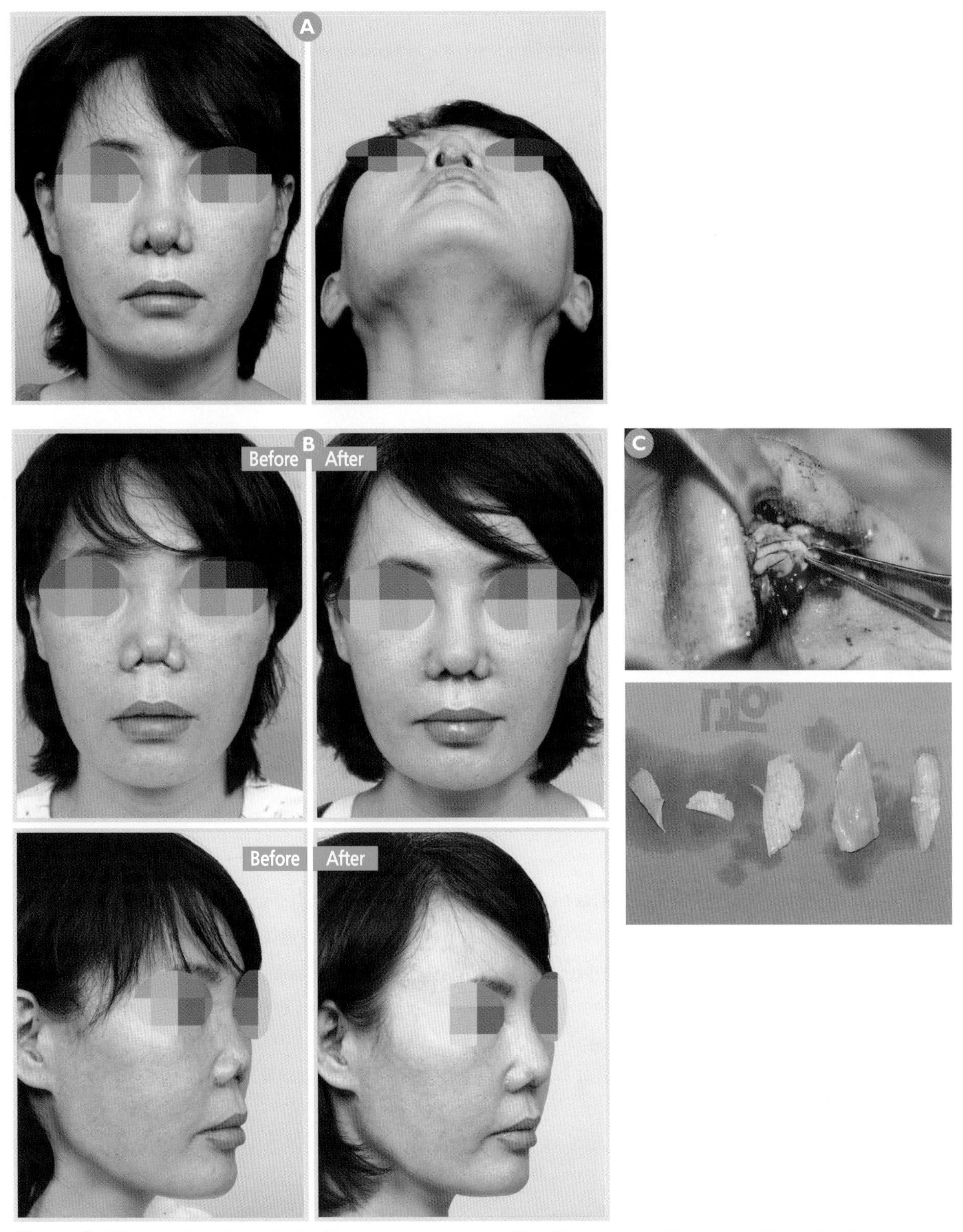

Figure 2 Silicone induced infection in this patient was corrected by silicone removal. Delayed revision rhinoplasty was performed using dorsal augmentation with costal cartilage, reconstruction of cartilaginous framework using costal cartilage, and repair of the inner lining defect using composite conchal cartilage graft. Before removal of the silicone implant (A). Before and after photos of revision rhinoplasty (B). Composite conchal cartilage graft and costal cartilage grafts used for revision (C).

4. Short Noses

This problem commonly happens as a long term complication of rhinoplasty using silicone implants or fascia grafts, or the destruction of nasal supporting structures due to aggressive septal work in primary rhinoplasty. This is one of the most difficult problems to deal with. Short noses should be corrected adhering to the surgical principles of lengthening the central and lateral segments, tip grafting with lengthening purpose, and dorsal augmentation. Elasticity and distensibility of the skin soft tissue envelope is a critically important determining factor on the success of surgery. After removal of the silicone implant, the dorsum is best reaugmented using biologic tissue implants *(Figure 3)*.

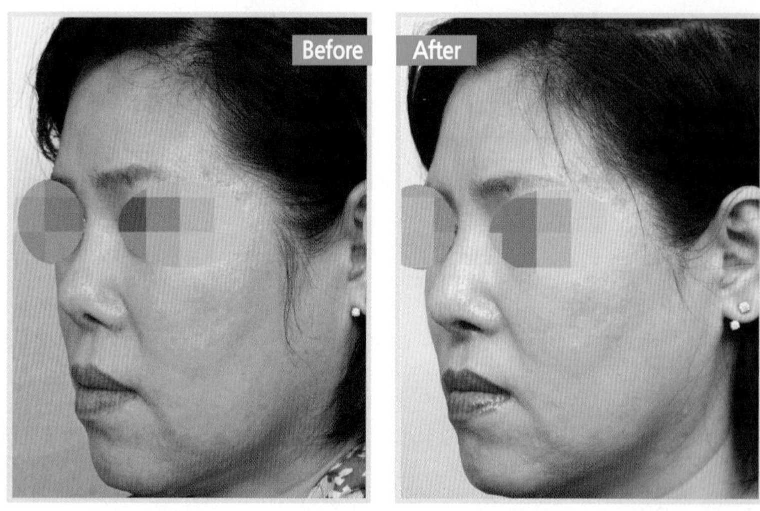

Figure 3 Short nose deformity in this multiply revised nose was corrected using costal cartilage

5. Warping and Visible Contour of the Costal Cartilage on the Nasal Dorsum

When there is warping or prominent contour of the costal cartilage implanted at the dorsum, it is first removed then re-sculptured, or turned into a generally crushed cartilage and then reimplanted in the dorsum. Using this method will render the dorsum a little lower than its original height but this procedure will help correct the warping while maintaining the dorsum at an acceptable height. If the patient dislikes the rigid feeling by the costal cartilage, or wants aesthetic perfection, the surgeon can use alloplastic implants such as Gore-Tex or silicone in revision *(Figure 4)*.

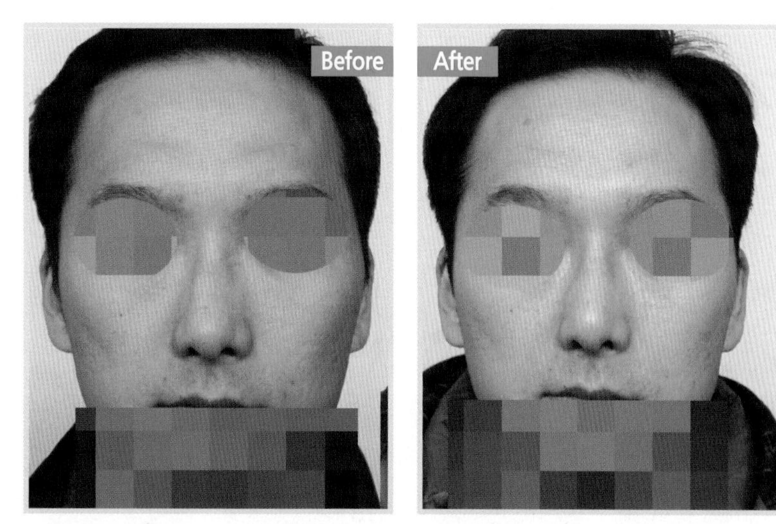

Figure 4 Costal cartilage on the dorsum showing visible graft contour was removed and replaced with Gore-Tex.

6. Contour Irregularity due to Resorption of Fascia or Cartilage on the Dorsum

The biologic grafts placed on the dorsum such as fascia, fascia wrapped diced cartilage, crushed cartilage, and dermofat can show decreased volume over time because of resorption, resulting in loss of dorsal height or contour irregularity. These kinds of aesthetic complications are managed by revision dorsal augmentation using alloplastic implants such as Gore-Tex or silicone which have less risk of long-term volume change than biologic tissue.

7. Residual Deviation and Recurrent Deviation Following Surgical Correction of the Deviated nose

The whole corrective procedure using an open rhinoplasty approach should be done under the assumption that it is a primary surgery. It is very important to make a correct diagnosis of the cause of recurrence; whether it is bony deviation or cartilaginous deviation or a combination of both. In most revision cases of deviated noses, it is common to have inadequate septal cartilage that can be used for structural reconstruction of the nose. Thus, the need for additional use of conchal cartilage, costal cartilage, or homologous cartilage increases *(Figure 5)*.

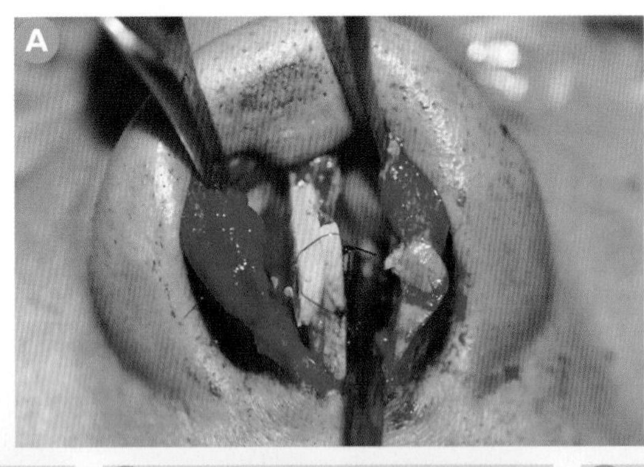

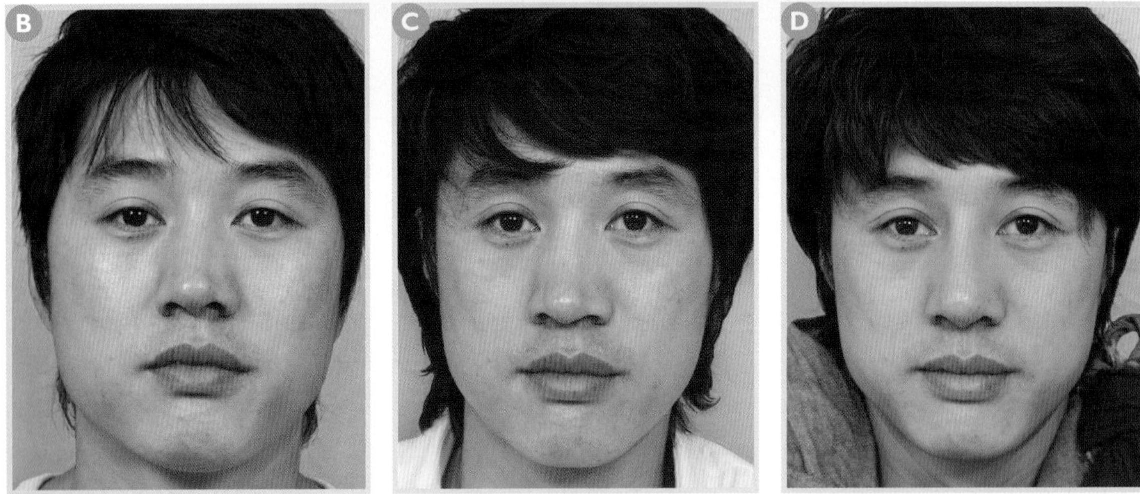

Figure 5 Intraoperative photo of septal reconstruction using costal cartilage for revision of the deviated nose (A). Before primary rhinoplasty (B), 1 year after first operation (C), and 6 months after revision rhinoplasty (D).

8. Minor Dorsal Saddle Deformity

After any kind of rhinoplasty procedure, occurrence of a saddle nose deformity or partial concavity on the nasal sidewall can commonly be encountered during long term follow up. If the degree of saddle is not so severe, the surgeon can correct this problem using simple camouflage or concealment procedures by using diced conchal cartilage, fascia-wrapped diced cartilage, or Gore-Tex.

9. Undercorrection of Convex Nasal Dorsum

Undercorrection of the dorsal convexity is the most common complication of hump reduction. A small prominence around the rhinion can be managed by rasping through an endonasal approach. However, a general convexity which is persisting or recurring after rhinoplasty should be managed by revision tip augmentation, hump reduction, and radix augmentation *(Figure 6)*.

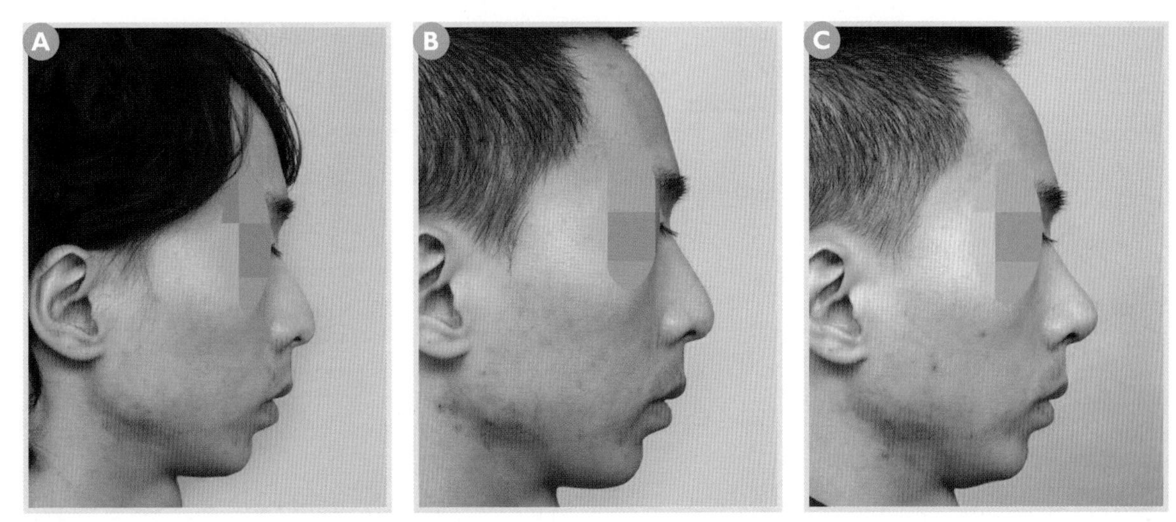

Figure 6 Residual convexity in this patient was corrected by additional hump reduction, tip augmentation, and radix grafting. Before surgery (A), 1 year after primary surgery (B), and 6 months after revision rhinoplasty (C).

10. Visible Tip Graft Contour, Over Projected Tip

Aggressive tip grafting in thin-skinned individuals may end up with visible contours of the tip graft causing aesthetic dissatisfaction. In addition, placement of too large or too much grafts on the tip may result in overprojection of the nasal tip. This problem can easily be managed through a limited marginal incision followed by trimming of the grafted cartilage. If the patient wants a smoother contour of the tip, the surgeon can interpose fat, dermis, or fascia between the skin and the grafted cartilage *(Figure 7)*.

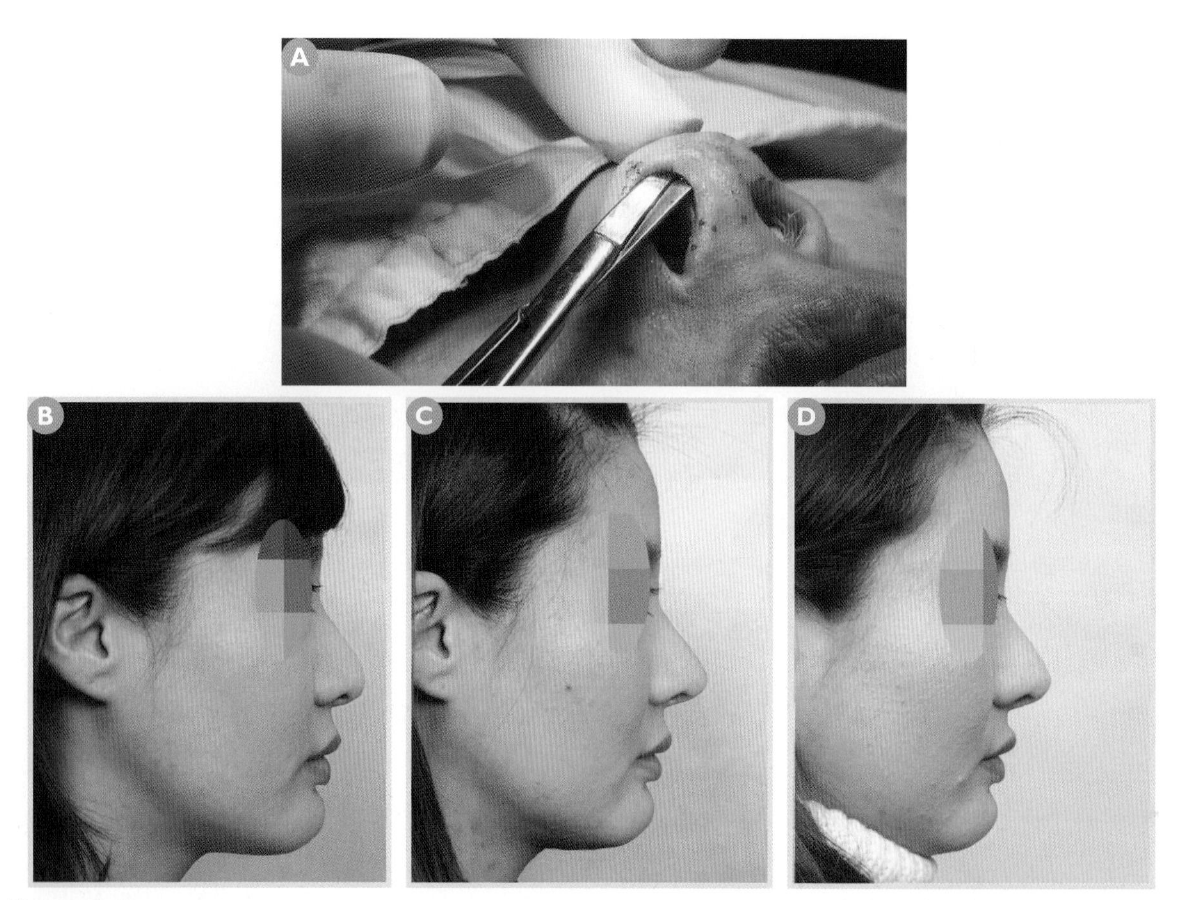

Figure 7 The overprojected tip in this patient was corrected by trimming of the tip graft via a limited marginal incision (A). Before surgery (B), 1 year after primary surgery (C), and 6 months after revision rhinoplasty (D).

11. Tip Graft Infection

Post-rhinoplasty infection is mainly due to dorsally implanted materials, or too much tip grafting on the nasal tip. Typical signs of infection are swelling, erythema, discharge, tenderness, and granulation tissue formation around the incision site *(Figure 8)*. In most cases, conservative

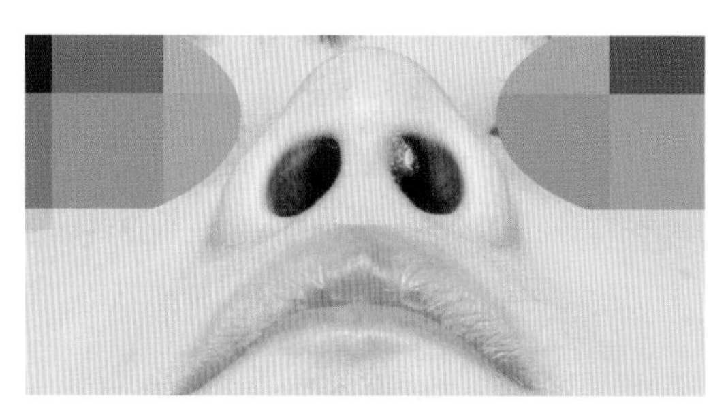

Figure 8 Granulation tissue formed at the incision, a telltale sign of implant-related infection.

management of such infections fail and may result in a permanent scar on the skin soft tissue envelope, or result in loss of the covering skin in the worst cases.

In order to prevent this scenario, once there is a salient sign of infection, the surgeon should not hesitate in removing the tip graft. Methicillin-resistant *Staphylococcus aureus* (MRSA) which is often isolated on these situations, cannot be controlled by using IV antibiotics only. Therefore any foreign body in the nose should be removed as promptly as possible. Removal of the implant or graft through an endonasal incision and irrigation of the wound usually brings about dramatic improvement of the infection *(Figures 9, 10)*.

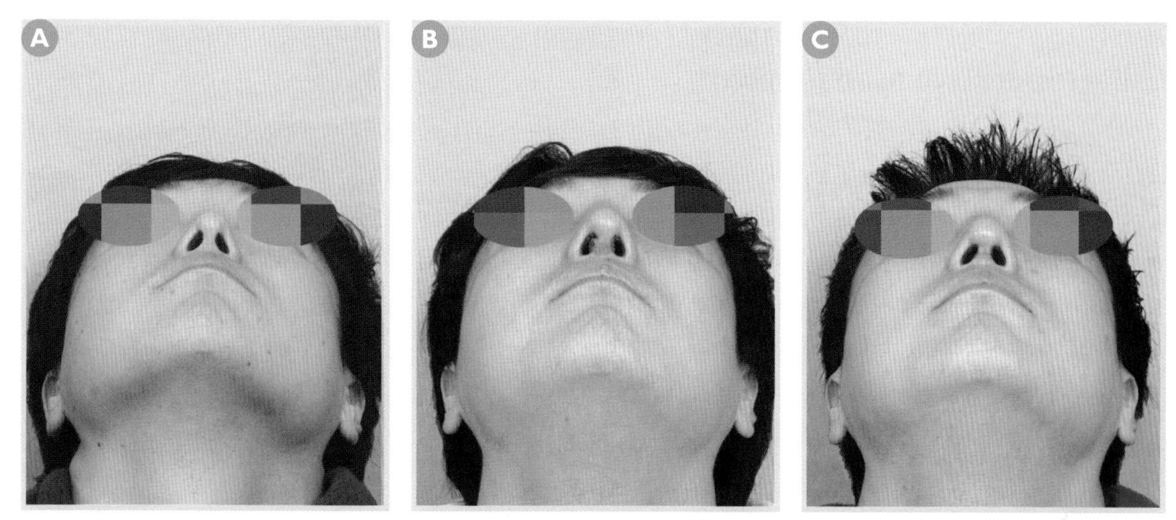

Figure 9 Tip graft infection was improved after removal of cartilage grafts. Before surgery (A), 2 weeks after primary surgery (B), and improved infection after removal of the grafts (C).

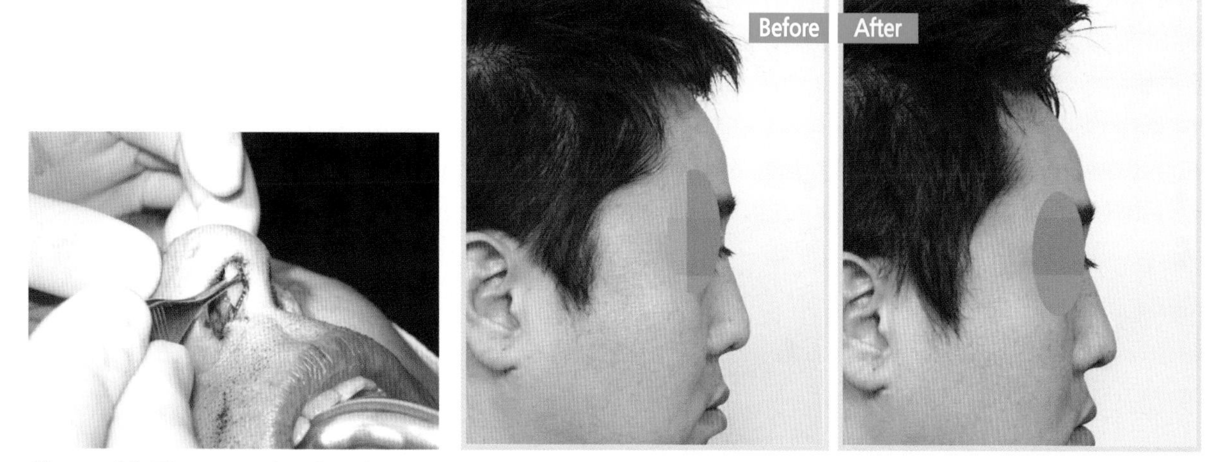

Figure 10 Three months after the removal of the tip graft to treat infection, revision tip augmentation was conducted via an endonasal incision. Profile view of patient showing improved tip projection after revision tip surgery.

12. Persisting Nasal Obstruction or Newly-Occurred Nasal Obstruction Following Rhinoplasty

In order to solve this perplexing problem, one should choose the most conservative treatment method first. For example, prescription of medications to treat rhinitis, and simple outpatient procedures to correct turbinate hypertrophy should be performed first. If there is persisting nasal septal deviation, septoturbinoplasty should be performed again. If there is an obvious problem with the internal valve, surgical procedures such as spreader grafts or alar batten grafts should be performed preferentially via an open approach. In the author's experience, caudal septal deviation was the most common reason for persisting or recurrent nasal obstruction.

X. Postoperative Management

The outpatient treatment for patients who underwent revision surgery must be carried out with greater care than those who underwent primary surgery. It should be assumed that the risk of postoperative infection is higher than that of the primary surgery, and antibiotics should be prescribed for the appropriate duration. Outpatient follow-up should also be performed more frequently. Finally, the patients should be educated to recognize the various signs that accompany infection and to visit the hospital at the first suspicion of infection.

XI. Conclusion

Revision rhinoplasty is an extremely difficult field of surgery. Even more difficult than the technical aspect of the surgery is having the surgeon maintain an attitude of calm, composure and sympathy for the patient's suffering. In addition, the patient must be made to feel that the surgeon is attempting to help the patient. The suffering of one patient caused by an unsatisfactory surgery is of such nature that it is more than enough to negate the happiness derived by ninety-nine other patients from their successful operations. Although it is possible to reduce the rate of unsatisfied patients or the occurrences of complications, it is not possible to completely eliminate them. Nevertheless, it is possible to reduce patient discontent resulting from the technical aspect of surgery through the efforts of the surgeon. Discontent coming from the doctor-patient relationship can likewise be reduced through perseverance. Therefore, the author would like to emphasize the fact that doing one's best at all times is the only means of reducing secondary surgery.

References

1. Adamson PA, Galli SK. Rhinoplasty approaches: current state of the art. Arch Facial Plast Surg 2005; 7: 32-7.
2. Bagal AA, Adamson PA. Revision rhinoplasty. Facial Plast Surg 2002; 18: 233-44.
3. Becker DG, Becker SS, Saad AA. Auricular cartilage in revision rhinoplasty. Facial Plast Surg 2003; 19: 41-52.
4. Bracaglia R, Fortunato R, Gentileschi S. Secondary rhinoplasty. Aesthet Plast Surg 2005; 29: 230-9.
5. Clark JM, Cook TA. Immediate reconstruction of extruded alloplastic nasal implants with irradiated homograft costal cartilage. Laryngoscope 2002; 112: 968-74.
6. Constantian MB. What motivates secondary rhinoplasty? A study of 150 consecutive patients. Plast Reconstr Surg 2012; 130: 667-78.
7. Daniel RK, Calvert JW. Diced cartilage grafts in rhinoplasty surgery. Plast Reconstr Surg 2004; 113: 2156-71.
8. Davis RE, Bublik M. Psychological considerations in the revision rhinoplasty patient. Facial Plast Surg 2012; 28: 374-9.
9. Foda HM. Rhinoplasty for the multiply revised nose. Am J Otolaryngol 2005; 26: 28-34.
10. Neaman KC, Boettcher AK, Do VH, Mulder C, Baca M, Renucci JD, Vander Woude DL. Cosmetic rhinoplasty: revision rates revisited. Aesthet Surg J 2013; 33: 31-7.

Case 1

A 23-year-old female visited for a saddle nose deformity. She had undergone endonasal rhinoseptoplasty 2 years ago using Gore-Tex.

Analysis Frontal: Wide dorsum, displacement of Gore-Tex implant

Basal: Poor tip projection, nostril asymmetry

Lateral and Oblique: Low dorsal height, concave dorsum

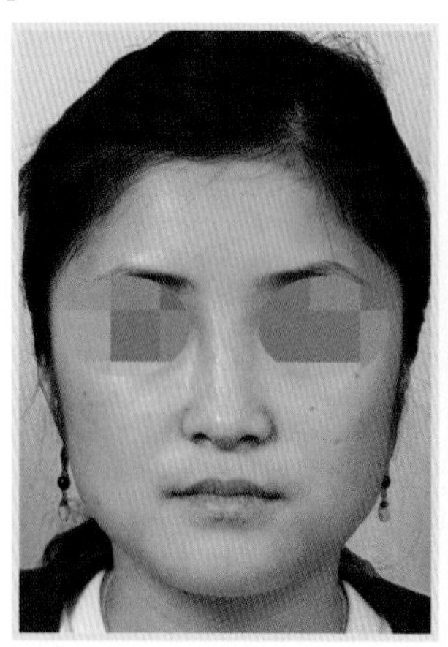
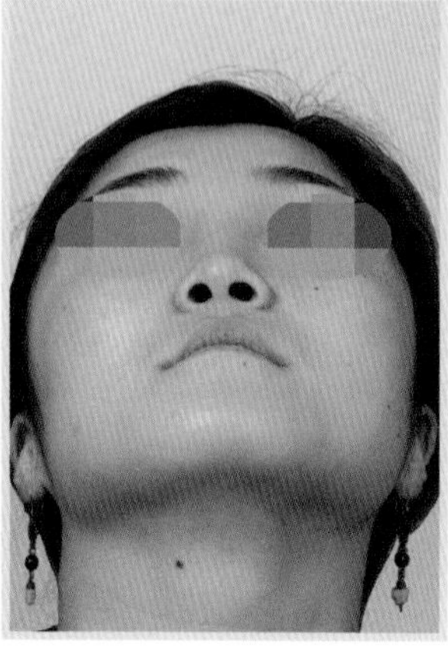
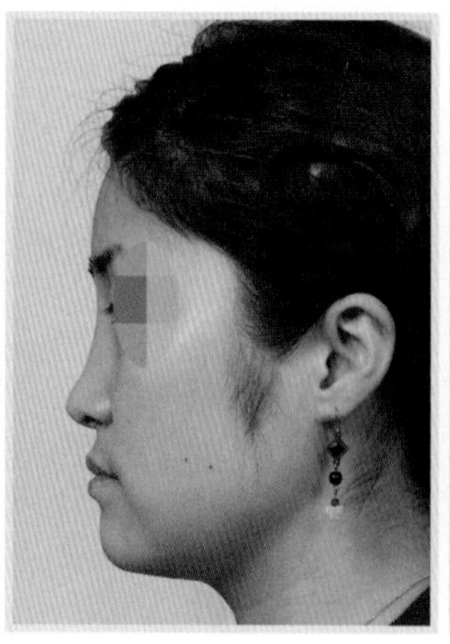
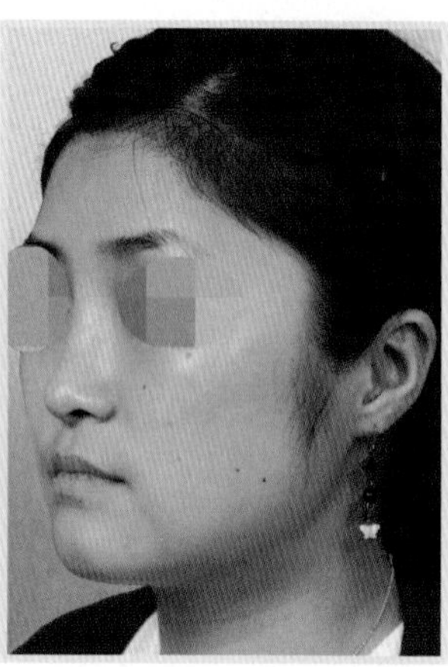

Operative Procedures

Open rhinoplasty approach

Implant removal

Costal cartilage harvest

Extracorporeal septoplasty reinforced with costal cartilage

Interdomal and intercrural suturing

Tip onlay grafting using crushed costal cartilage

Shield grafting using costal cartilage

Dorsal augmentation using crushed costal cartilage and processed fascia lata

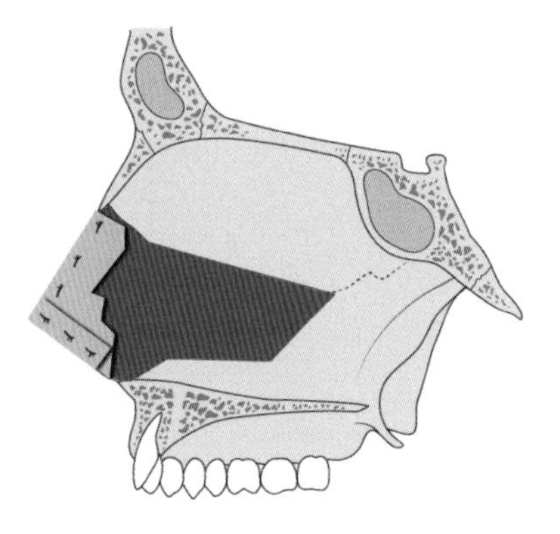
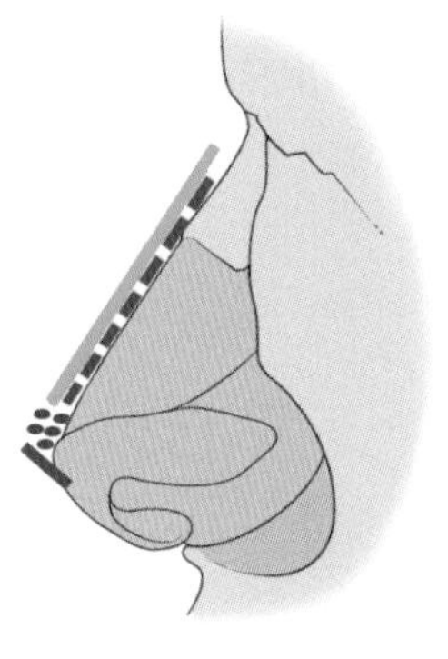
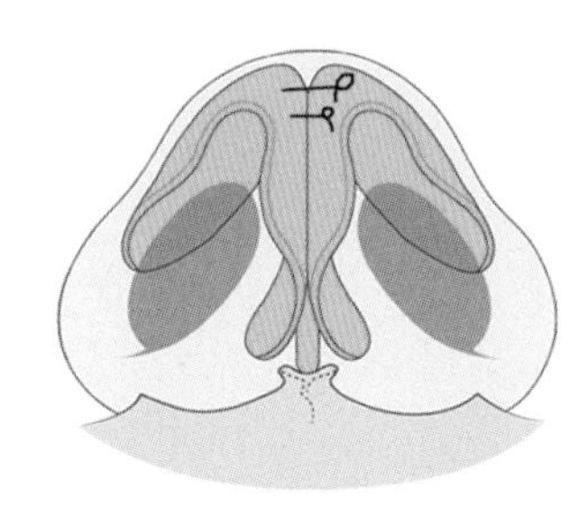

Postoperative Changes

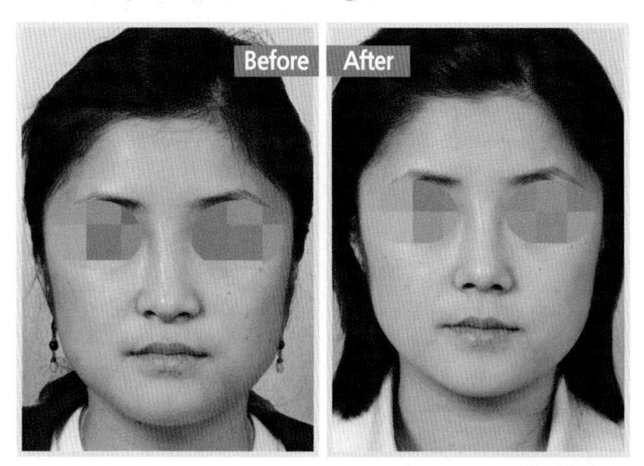

Frontal: Dorsal aesthetic lines were improved with the correction of the deviated nose.

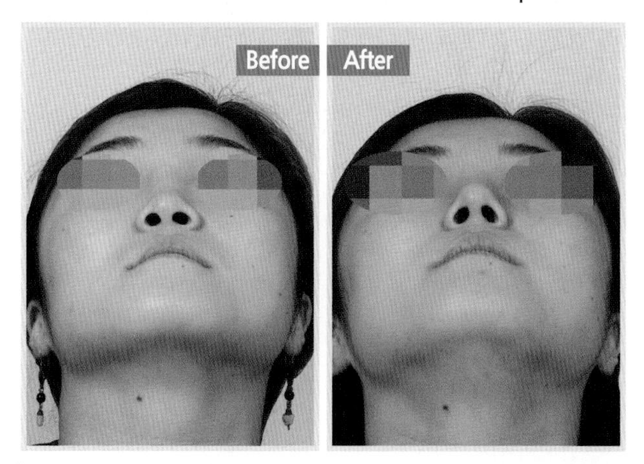

Basal: Tip projection was improved. Nostrils became symmetric.

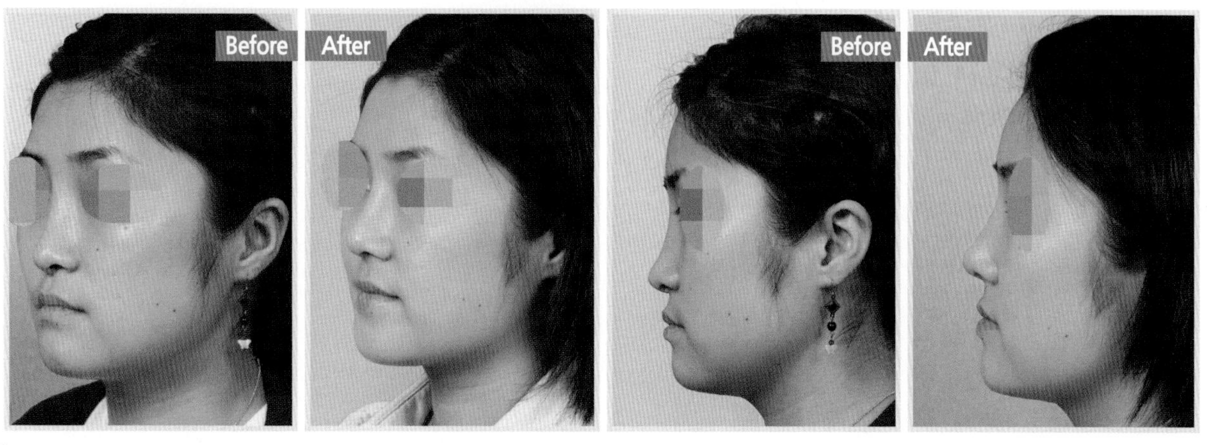

Lateral and Oblique: Dorsal height was augmented. Tip projection was increased. Nasolabial angle was widened.

Case 2

A 44-year-old female visited for an upturned nose deformity with continuous discharge from the right nasal cavity.

Analysis

Contracted nose
Upturned nose
Nostril asymmetry
Alar retraction (right)
Silicone extrusion through the right nasal cavity

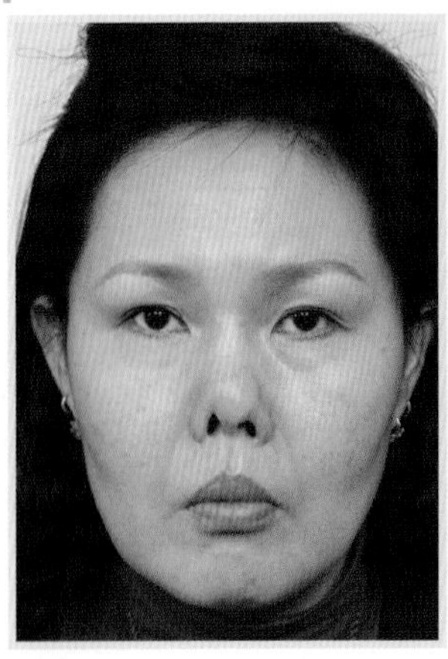
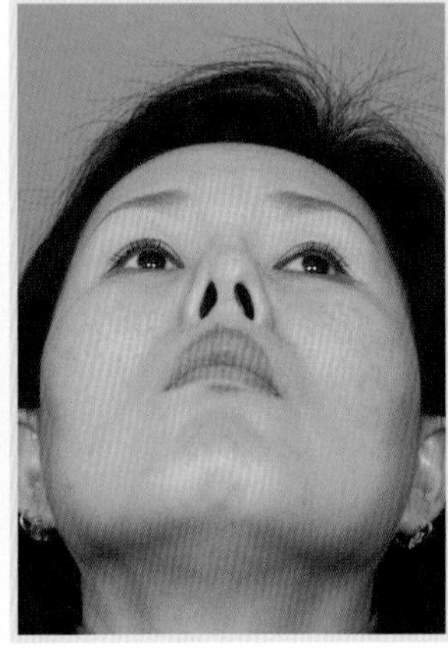
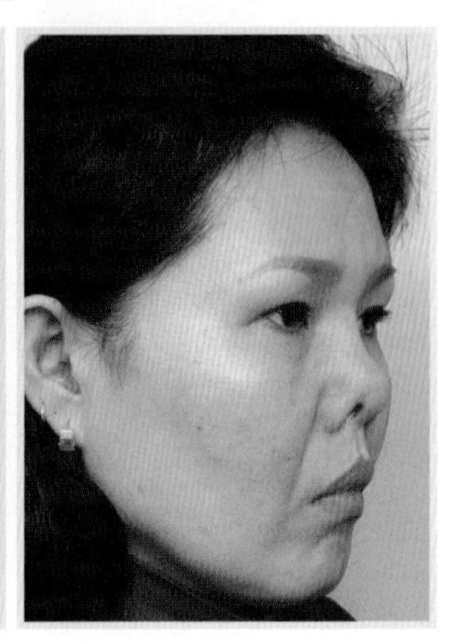

Operative Procedures

Open rhinoplasty approach
Extruded silicone implant removal
Costal cartilage harvest
Extended spreader grafting using costal cartilage (bilateral)
Caudal septal extension grafting using costal cartilage (left)
Lateral crural strut grafting using septal cartilage (right)
Cephalic resection (left)
Tip augmentation with shield grafting
Medial and lateral osteotomies
Dorsal augmentation using perichondrium and costal cartilage
Right nasal cavity mucosal defect repair using a conchal cartilage composite graft

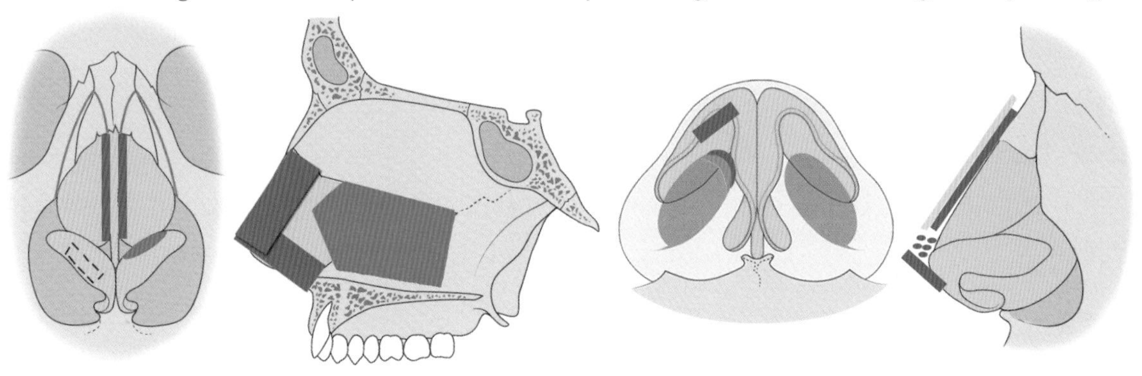

Postoperative Changes

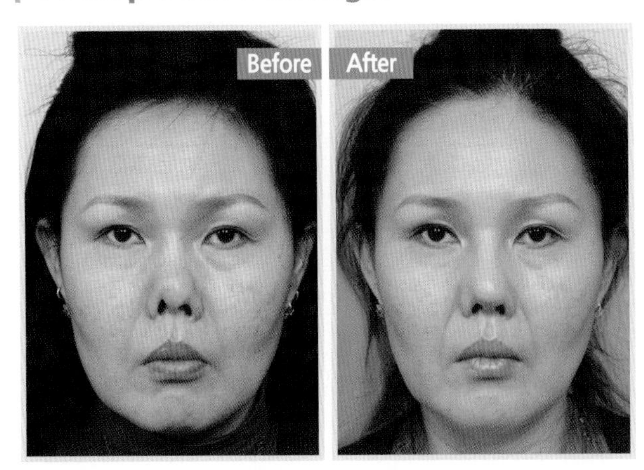

Frontal: Alar retraction was improved. Dorsal height was increased. Nostril show was decreased.

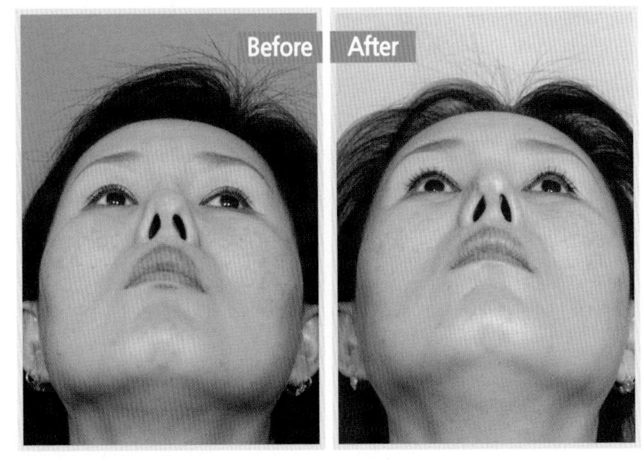

Basal: Nostrils were slightly narrowed. Hypertrophic scar was formed at the left marginal incision.

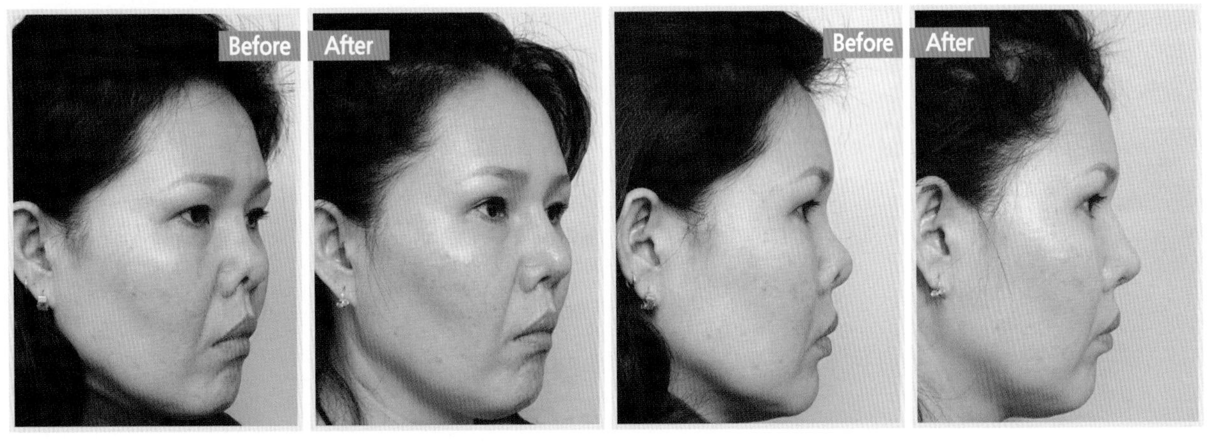

Lateral and Oblique: Nasal dorsal height was augmented. Right alar retraction was corrected. Tip definition and projection were improved.

Chapter 32

Nasal Bone Factures

Jae Hwan Kwon

I. Introduction

The nose is a relatively weak, protruding part of the face and is therefore frequently fractured in facial injuries. Nasal bone fractures can occur even with low impact, and are twice as likely to occur in men than in women. The most common causes of nasal bone fractures are traffic accidents, sports injuries, and interpersonal violence. Adequate treatment is important because without it, even small fractures can result in significant functional and cosmetic problems such as external nose deformities, nasal obstruction, septal perforation, and facial growth disturbances in children. Although guidelines and methods for the treatment of nasal bone fractures have been established, the optimal method for recovering the shape and function of the nose has not yet been determined. Rhinoplasty immediately after trauma must be considered carefully because both the soft and bony tissues are deformed after a nasal bone fracture and the nasal bone is small in Asians. Furthermore, revision septoplasty and rhinoplasty are frequently required in 40-62% of patients with nasal bone fractures because of residual deformation of the nose even after closed reduction. Adequate management and treatment of nasal bone fractures and nasal septal fractures have a significant effect on overall results.

II. Anatomy and Pathophysiology

1. Anatomy

The bony part of the nose consists of the frontal process of the maxilla and the nasal processes of the frontal, ethmoid, vomer, and nasal bones. The nasal bone is thin and caudally wide; therefore, fractures frequently occur at this site. The cartilaginous portion of the nose consists of the septal cartilage in the middle, two upper lateral cartilages, and two lower lateral cartilages. The upper lateral cartilage is attached to the caudal part of the nasal bone, which is supported by the quadrangular cartilage in the middle. The lower lateral cartilage plays an important role in the cosmetic appearance of the nasal tip and in absorbing the impact of an external force. Cartilage can generally be deflected without fracturing because of its ability to absorb the impact. It is possible to estimate the amount of force required to fracture the cartilage *(Figure 1)*.

The nasal septum is composed mainly of the quadrangular cartilage and vomer inferiorly, and the perpendicular plate of the ethmoid posteriorly and superiorly *(Figure 2)*. The damage caused by severe nasal septal injuries may affect the growth of the face because the nasal septum has a long growth period lasting up to 12-13 years.

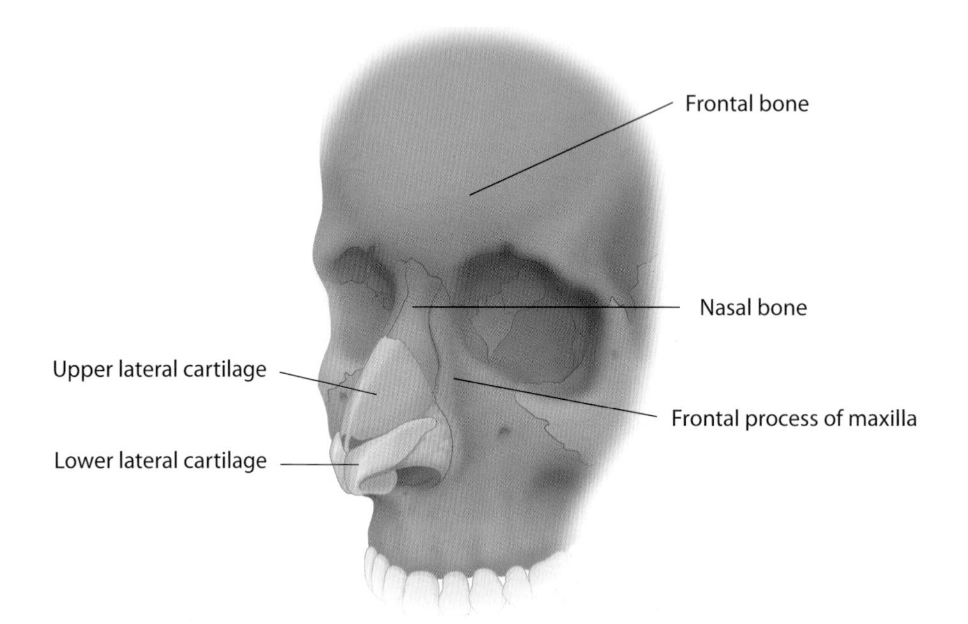

Figure 1 The nose is composed of cartilage and bone.

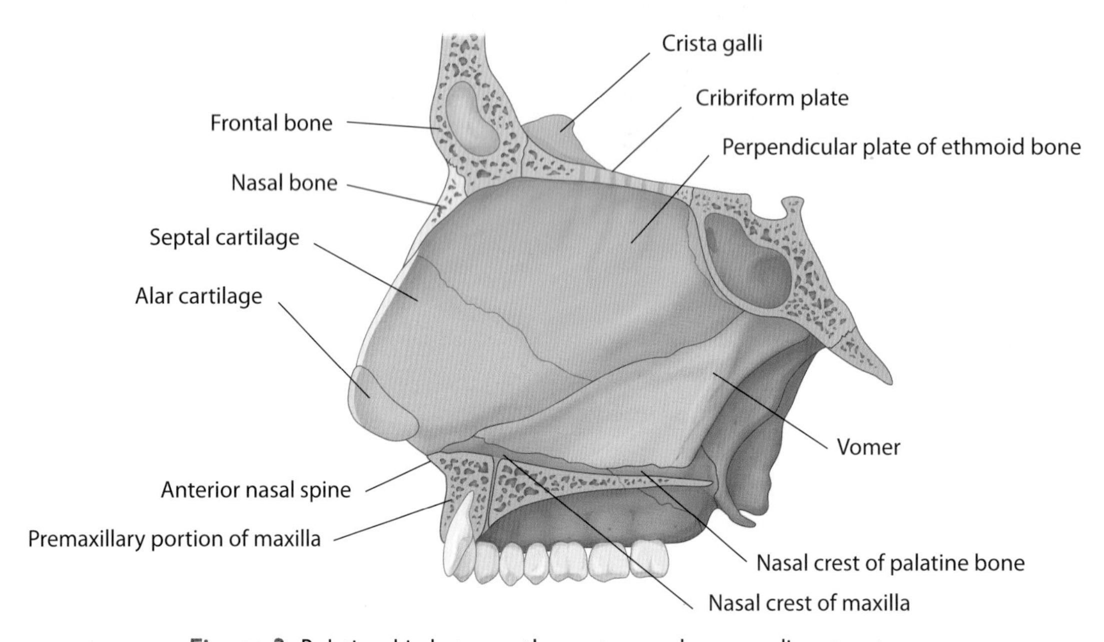

Figure 2 Relationship between the septum and surrounding structures.

2. Pathophysiology

A force applied laterally to the nose causes an infracture on the same side of the force and an outfracture on the opposite nasal bone. This results in deviation of the nasal axis with dislocation of the nasal septum *(Figure 3)*.

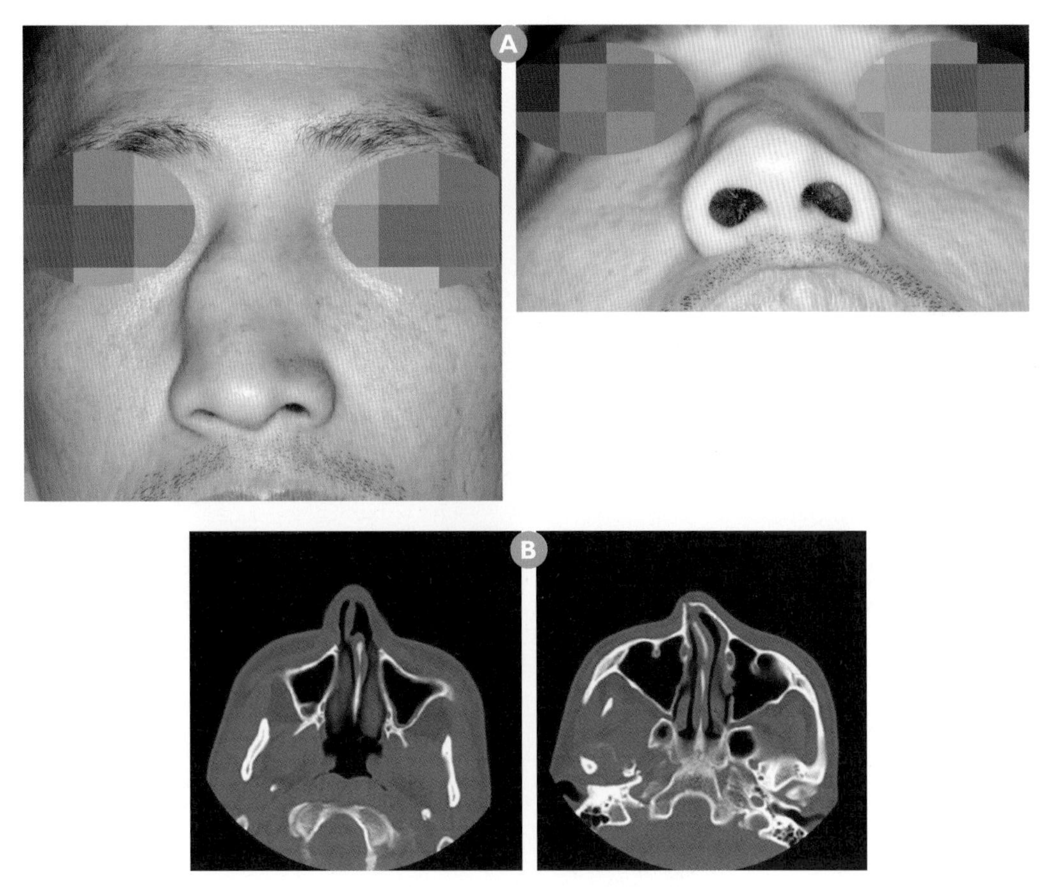

Figure 3 Infracture on the ipsilateral side caused by a force applied on that side and outfracture of the opposite nasal bone. Facial photographs of the patient (A) and CT findings (B).

Damage to the front of the face which can be the result of car accidents or fall, is often accompanied by a nasal bone fracture, fracture or dislocation of the caudal nasal septum, saddle deformity of the nasal dorsum, or cephalic rotation of the tip *(Figure 4)*. Young patients mostly present with large pieces of fractured nasal bone, whereas the elderly usually present with a comminuted fracture. Nasal bone fractures are less common in pediatric patients because of the high cartilage content of their noses and incomplete ossification of the nasal bone. However, when they do occur, they present as a greenstick fracture with cartilage damage. Decreased height of the nasal dorsum or tip and deviation of the nasal bony pyramid as a result of incomplete septal fracture reduction are common findings.

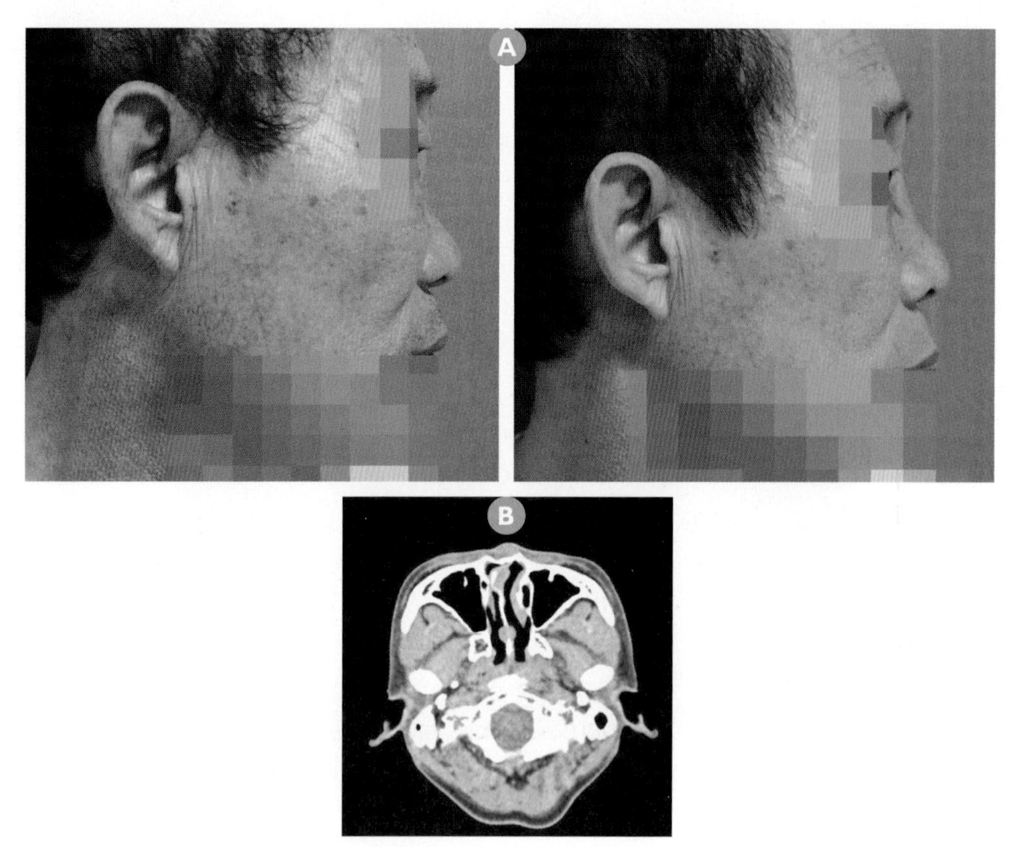

Figure 4 Injury caused by an anterior force. This type of injury is mainly sustained in falls or vehicular accidents and is accompanied by a saddle deformity and cephalic rotation of the tip because due to the nasal bone fracture and caudal septal fracture from the strong impact. Preoperative and postoperative facial photographs of the patient (A) and CT findings (B).

III. Diagnosis

A complete history in patients with nasal bone fractures should include the mechanism of injury, the time elapsed since the injury, any previous history of facial injury, and the presence of nasal bony or septal deformities. A detailed history of previous nasal surgery is important because trauma can cause nasal deformities. Determining the shape of the nose before the injury using previously taken photographs is also important because more than 50% of individuals without a history of nasal injury have nose deformities. Information on the shape of the nose may be more accurate when obtained from identification documents such as a driver's license or from previous CT images rather than from a direct interview with the patient. Symptoms of nasal obstruction, congestion, and sleep apnea should be assessed and a history of medications being taken such as nasal sprays or allergy medicines should be obtained before surgery. It is important to know how long after the injury the patient visited the clinic. If the patient presents to the clinic within a few hours of the injury without nasal swelling, a closed reduction can be performed because the nasal deformity can be precisely identified. Beyond a few hours, surgery has to be delayed for 7-14 days, after resolution of the nasal swelling, and rhinoplasty may be necessary when the patient presents after ossification of the fractured nasal bones. Assessment of nasal bone fractures must include external and internal examinations of the nose. Visual inspection of the external appearance of the nose is necessary to determine the presence of nose deformities. Pain and crepitus on palpation are important clues in making a diagnosis. A more accurate assessment is necessary to identify mobile bony or cartilaginous fragments if an open wound exists. A CT scan rather than plain X-ray film is necessary to visualize the nasomaxillary suture and nasociliary groove with a fracture line. Furthermore, soft tissue swelling can mask the fracture line in cases of a simple nasal bone fracture. Cerebrospinal fluid (CSF) rhinorrhea is suspected when clear discharge is drained from the nasal cavity, and may indicate cribriform plate injury as a result of nasal septal injury. In most cases, CSF rhinorrhea recovers spontaneously; however, head elevation with the patient in the supine position is recommended to minimize CSF leaks. If the CSF rhinorrhea does not improve after 10-14 days, lumbar drainage or surgical reconstruction should be considered. For nasal cavity exams, blood clots need to be removed and the nasal cavity is examined after administration of a vasoconstrictor. Damage to the nasal septum is suspected when mucosal injury is detected. Septal hematomas should be incised and drained immediately to prevent cartilage necrosis. If septal fractures are not properly corrected, complications such as a deviated nose and saddle nose are more likely to occur.

IV. Treatment of Nasal Bone Fractures

The ideal treatment of nasal bone fractures remains controversial, and several treatments are commonly used depending upon the surgeon's preference or the established treatment plan.

1. Timing of Surgery

Early reduction immediately after injury may not be sufficient for correction of the defect because of soft tissue swelling, whereas late reduction can be difficult because of the presence of fibrous connective tissue and osteogenesis of the fractured nasal bone. In most cases, conservative treatment including analgesics, antibiotics, ice packs, and head elevation should be instituted and a closed reduction should be performed within ten days of the fracture. However, in certain cases, a closed reduction is still possible three weeks after the injury. Early management is important in cases requiring an open reduction, and patients without edema within a few hours of injury can be treated immediately.

2. Anesthesia

The anesthetic method depends on the surgeon's preference. The patient's age, degree of cooperation, health status, and cost should be considered in choosing between local and general anesthetics. Local anesthetics can be classified into topical and infiltration preparations. Topical anesthesia can be achieved using gauze soaked with 4% lidocaine with oxymetazoline or phenylephrine hydrochloride (Neo-Synephrine®) placed in the nasal cavity for eight to ten minutes. This results in mucous membrane decongestion and the anesthesia acts on the anterior ethmoidal nerve at the dorsal aspect of the nasal septum, pterygopalatine ganglion at the middle turbinate, nasopalatine nerve at the nasal floor, and sphenopalatine artery. Infiltration anesthesia consists of a mixture of lidocaine and epinephrine that is administered at a dose of up to 500 mg (2% lidocaine, 25 mg) in adults. Injection of small volumes followed by massage is recommended to avoid deforming the nose after injection.

3. Closed vs. Open Reduction

Non-displaced simple fractures do not require any surgical intervention. Closed reduction is the optimal treatment for unilateral medially displaced fractures, whereas open reduction is required for severe nasal bone fractures. A septal fracture may be overlooked in a closed reduction *(Figure 5)*. Murray, et al. suggested that one of the causes of closed reduction failure is a poor understanding of the pathophysiology of fractures. In more than 50% of patients, the nasal bridge shows a combined C-shaped septal fracture, which should be treated by closed reduction with septoplasty, reserving closed reduction only in mild injuries. The disadvantages of open reduction are the relatively high cost and risk of complications. The indications for closed and open reductions are given below.

Indications for closed reduction

- ☑ Unilateral or bilateral nasal bone fracture
- ☑ Nasal bone fractures with a septal fracture
- ☑ Degree of deviation not exceeding half of the nasal width

Indications for open reduction

- Severe nasoseptal fracture
- Fractured bone displaced more than half of the nasal width
- Fracture and displacement of the caudal septum
- Open wound fracture
- Persistent external nose deformity after closed reduction

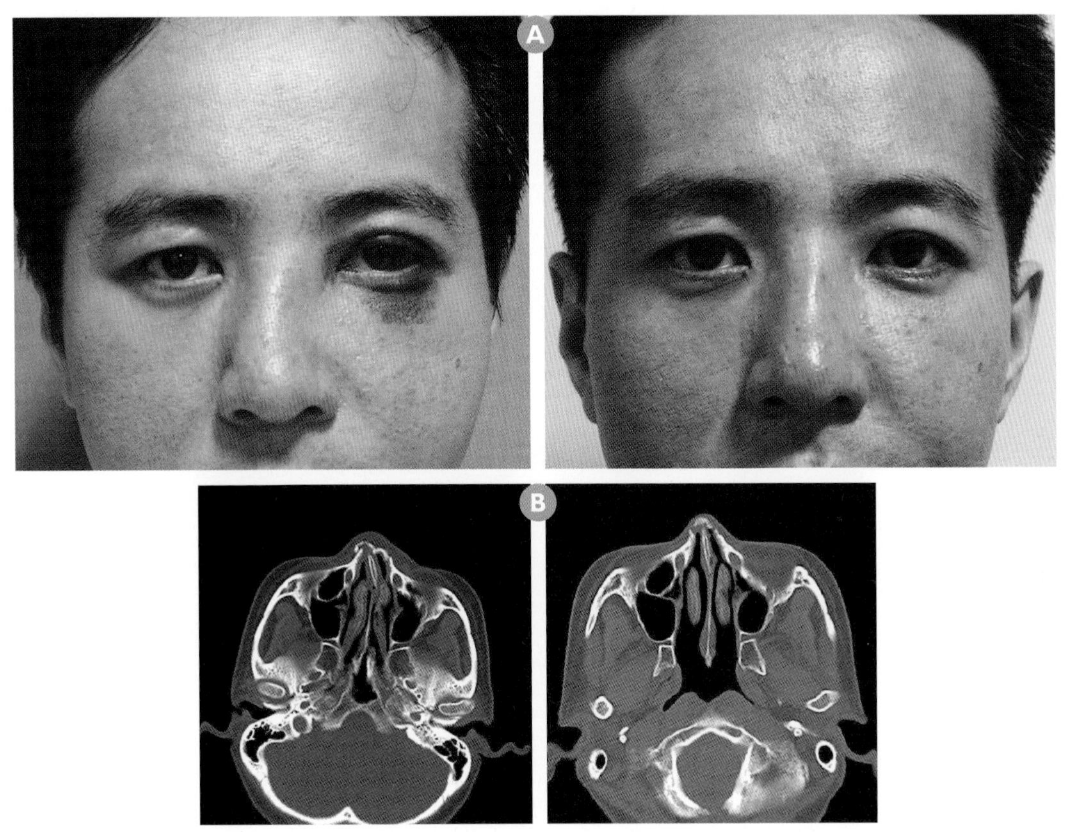

Figure 5 When the nasal bone fracture is accompanied by a septal fracture, it can be corrected by closed reduction (A) and preoperative and postoperative CT scans are obtained (B). A remaining deformity after treatment is observed with undercorrection of the fracture.

1) Closed Reduction

The principle of closed reduction is the application of force in the direction opposite that of the force that caused the injury, and centered alignment of the nasal bone and septum. An elevator is initially inserted into the nasal cavity and pressure is applied to the nasal bone in an upward and lateral direction, with pressure on the displaced bone using the thumb and index finger. The septum can be corrected using Asch forceps *(Figures 6, 7)*.

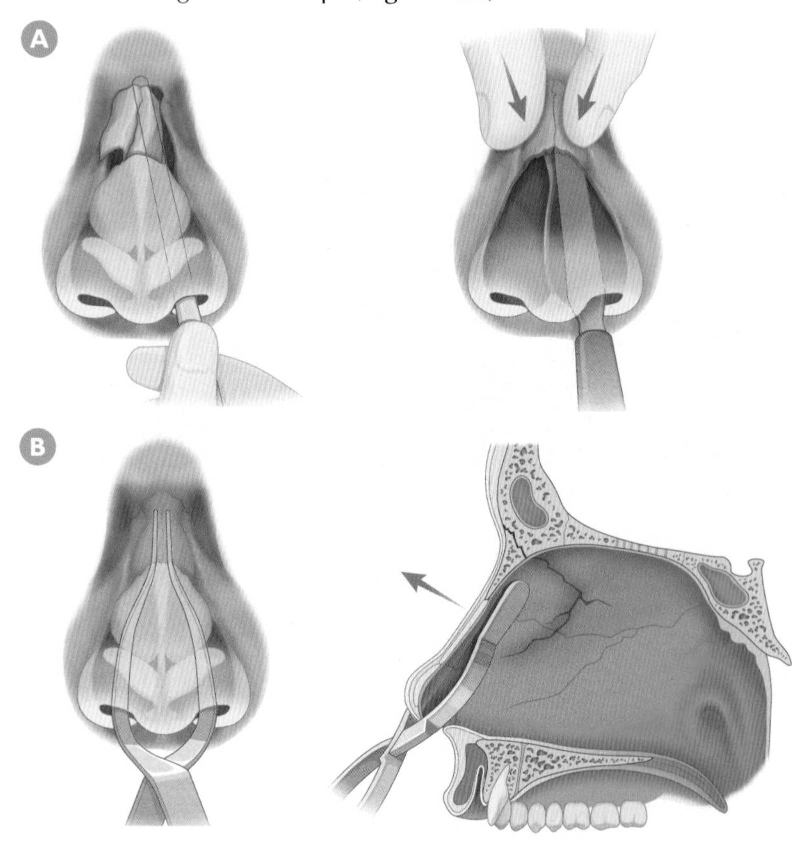

Figure 6 Schematic diagram of closed reduction. After elevator insertion into the nasal cavity, pressure is applied to the upper and lateral sides of the nasal bone. The fractured bone is returned to its original position with the thumb and index finger placed externally as support (A). The septal fracture is corrected using Asch forceps (B).

The elevator is inserted into the nasal cavity to a depth equal to the distance from the nostril to the displaced bony fragment without injuring the cribriform plate. An overlapped fractured bone chip can be corrected using Walsham forceps. In incomplete fractures, nasal packing is not always necessary, but an external splint is required to maintain the bony fragment in position after reduction. The patient should be informed prior to surgery that open reduction or rhinoplasty may be required at a later time.

2) Open Reduction

An open reduction is intended to restore a significantly displaced nasal bone through extensive

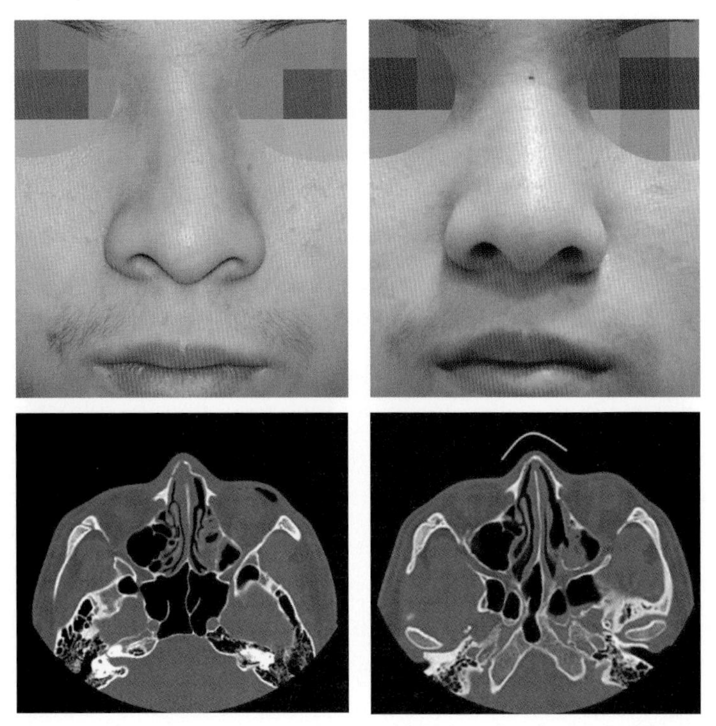

Figure 7 A left nasal bone fracture was corrected by closed reduction under local anesthesia.

surgical resection, reconstruction, and fixation. It is not commonly used in nasal bone fractures. It is recommended for comminuted fractures, nasoseptal fractures that cannot be corrected by closed reduction, and nasal bone fractures with soft tissue injury. Open reduction should be performed immediately after the initial swelling subsides, as it is more difficult to correct after four to six months because of the development of secondary deformities.

(1) Incisions and Exposure

The most appropriate approaches for the correction of a nasal bone fracture depend on the injured site and reconstruction type. The caudal end and the posterior half of the septal cartilage are exposed and fixed through a complete transfixation incision or hemitransfixation incision. The nasal dorsum is approached through an intercartilaginous or marginal incision. Occasionally, an open rhinoplasty approach is necessary. In rare cases, severe damage to the upper third of the nose can be accessed directly through a nasofrontal crease incision for nasoethmoid fractures. Under exceptional circumstances, severe cases can be approached through a lateral rhinotomy, bicoronal scalp incision, or midfacial degloving incisionss.

(2) Septal Reconstruction

Reduction of a septal fracture depends on the site of the fracture. If the fracture occurs at a location other than the L-strut, the displaced cartilage may be resected. However, maintaining the cartilage by reattaching it rather than removing it is recommended. At least 10-15 mm of the caudal and dorsal parts of the L-strut should be maintained. If the fracture includes the L-strut, a "figure of eight" suture or batten graft reinforcement is necessary. If the bony septum is fractured and positioned off-center, a severe greenstick fracture may have occurred and the deviated bone can be corrected by osteotomy. Finally, the frame can be reinforced using a septal splint or quilting sutures.

(3) Osteotomy and Humpectomy

As asymmetry in the size or shape of the nasal bone is common, achieving the proper shape and position by paramedian or double lateral osteotomy is helpful in severely displaced nasal bones. An osteotomy may be necessary to correct old nasal bone fractures. Moreover, malunion is common in deformed nasal bones after an injury; therefore, precise refracturing of the malunited bones by medial, lateral, and percutaneous osteotomies may be necessary. Hump reduction can be performed after septal reconstruction and should be as conservative as possible.

(4) Dorsal Augmentation

When there is a cartilage fracture, it may require dorsal augmentation because the keystone area may have been injured. septal or conchal cartilage can be used as augmentation material. When insufficient cartilage is available, or in cases of severe dorsal saddling, alloplastic implants such as silicone, Gore-Tex or Medpor may be used if the risk of implant-related complications is not that high.

(5) Splinting

A thermoplastic splint is applied after the surgery. Nasal splinting serves to fix and support the corrected nasal bone and septum. In particular, it encourages skin attachment to the nasal bone and prevents hematoma formation. A silastic splint is used to stablize the septum and prevent intranasal adhesions. Nasal packing should be removed within several days.

(6) Follow-up

After reduction of nasal bone fractures, a nasal deformity can occur as the swelling subsides and soft tissues become fibrotic. Regular follow-up visits for three to four weeks after surgery are recommended. If a deformity appears, manual reduction may be necessary to prevent the development of a permanent deformity.

V. Pediatric Nasal Bone Fractures

The nasal bone in pediatric patients is relatively flat and highly elastic compared to that of adults; thus, the probability of fractures is low. Because of incomplete ossification of the nasal bone, radiography is of little diagnostic value. A CT scan is essential for diagnosis and to prevent missing a septal fracture, as well as to detect a hematoma and inflammation of the septum. If a pediatric nasal bone fracture with a septal fracture is not treated properly, partial necrosis of the nasal septum can cause permanent deformities of the nose. This may result in nasal septal deviation or saddle nose deformity. Closed reduction is recommended whenever possible; rhinoplasty and open reduction should be postponed until after the growth period. Since bone union occurs earlier in pediatric patients, it is well known that surgery should be performed within a week of injury; however, the evidence in the literature is insufficient. A recent study indicated that treating children within ten days as in adults is not associated with increased complications.

References

1. Atighechi S, Karimi G. Serial nasal bone reduction: a new approach to the management of nasal bone fracture. J craniofac Surg 2009; 20: 49-52.
2. Bull TR, Mackay IS. Rhinoplasty. In: AlanGK eds. Scott-Brown's Otolaryngology. 5th ed. London: Butterworths 1987: 248-71.
3. Chen CT, Hu TL, Lai JB, Chen YC, Chen YR. Reconstruction of traumatic nasal deformity in Orientals. J Plast Reconstr Aesthet Surg 2010; 63: 257-64.
4. Cook JA, McRae RD, Irving RM. A randomized comparison of manipulation of the fractured nose under local and general anesthesia. Clin Otolaryngol 1990; 15: 343-6.
5. Fernandes SV. Nasal fractures: the taming of the shrewd. Laryngoscope 2004; 114: 587-92.
6. Han SK, Chun KW, Park DK, Min BD, Kim WK. Corrective osteotomy technique for a posttraumatic deviated nose. J Craniofac surg 2008; 19: 476-81.
7. Higuera S, Lee EI, Cole P, Hollier LH, Stal S. Nasal trauma and the deviated nose. Plast Reconstr Surg 2007; 120: 64S-75S.
8. Illum P. Role of fixation in the treatment of nasal fractures. Clin Otolaryngol 1983; 8: 191-5.
9. Lee DH, Jang YJ. Pediatric nasal bone fractures: Does delayed treatment really lead to adverse outcomes? Int J Pediatr Otorhinolaryngol 2013; 77: 726-31.
10. Mondin V, Rinaldo A, Ferlito A. Management of nasal bone fractures. Am J Otolaryngol 2005; 26: 181-5.
11. Murray JA, Maran AG, Mackenzie IJ, Raab G. Open v closed reduction of the fractured nose. Arch Otolaryngol 1984; 110: 797-802.
12. Murray A, Maran AG. The treatment of nasal injuries by manipulation. J Laryngol Otol 1980; 94: 1405-10.
13. Park CH, Kim DY, Chun JH. The clinical and radiological evaluation of results about closed reduction for children with nasal bone fractures. Korean J Otolaryngol 2005; 48: 34-9.
14. Renner GJ. Management of nasal fractures. Otolaryngol Clin North Am 1991; 24: 195-213.
15. Ridder GJ, Boedecker CC, Fradis M. Technique and timing for closed reduction of isolated nasal fractures: a retrospective study. Ear Nose Throat J 2002; 81: 49-54.
16. Rohrich RJ, Adams Jr WP. Nasal fracture management: minimizing secondary nasal deformities. Plast Reconstr Surg 2000; 106: 266-73.
17. Rubinstein B, Strong EB. Management of nasal fractures. Arch Fam Med 2000; 9: 738-42.
18. Waldron J, Mitchell DB, Ford G. Reduction of fractured nasal bones; local versus geberal anesthesia. Clin Otolaryngol 1989; 14: 357-9.
19. Watson DJ, Parker AJ, Slack RW et al. Local versus general anesthesia in the management of the fractured nose. Clin Otolaryngol 1988; 13: 491-4.

Case 1 Operated by Prof Jang

A male patient visited for a nasal bone fracture with a septal fracture 11 days ago.

Analysis Frontal: S-shaped deformed dorsum
Basal: Tip tilt to the left and asymmetric nostrils
Lateral and Oblique: Slight saddle deformity

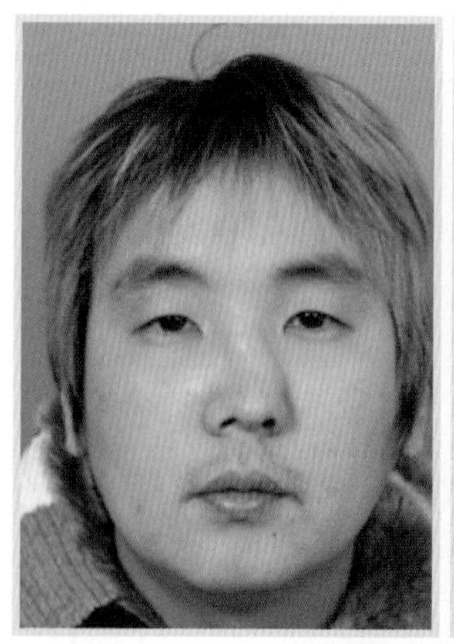
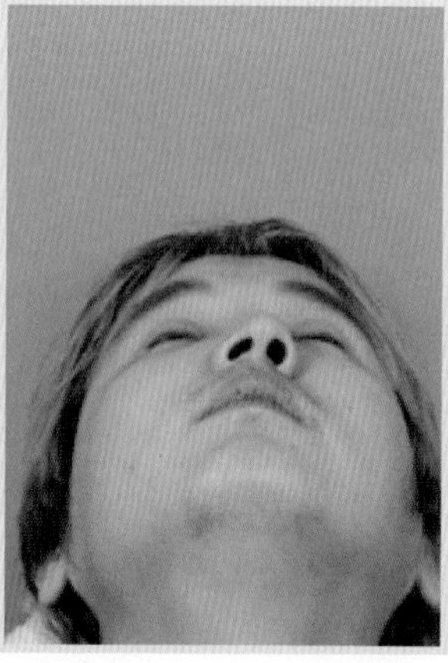
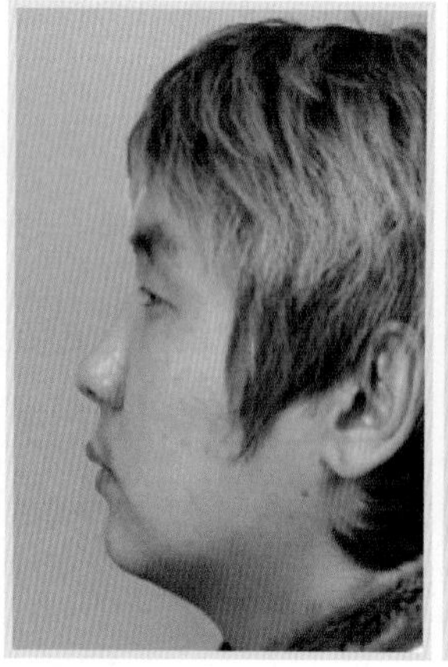
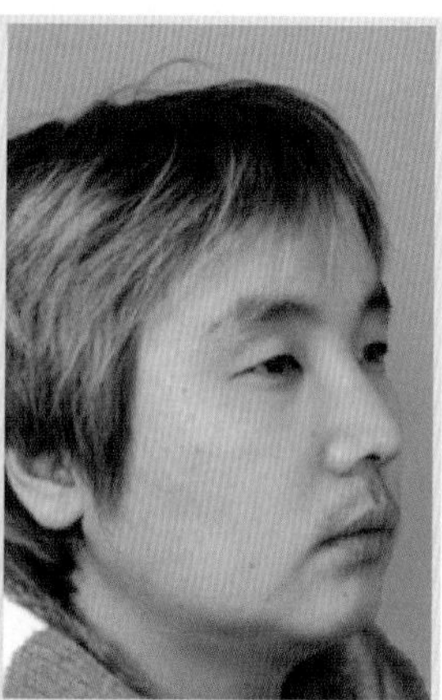

CT Severe nasoseptal fracture

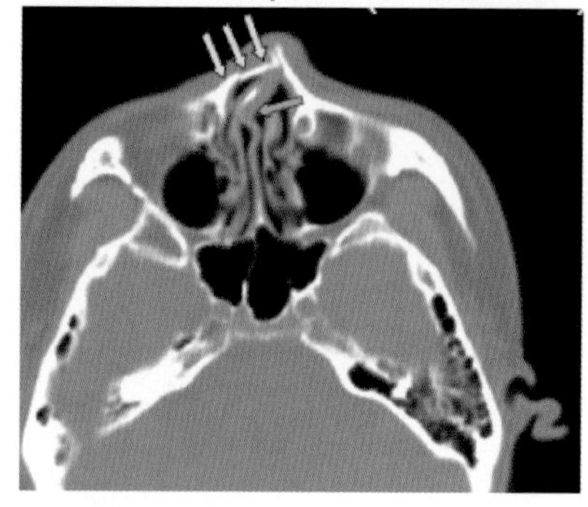

Operative Procedures

Open rhinoplasty approach
Extracorporeal septoplasty
Nasal bone reduction
Unilateral osteotomy (left)
Columellar strut application
Multilayer tip grafting
Tip onlay grafting with fascia lata
Dorsal augmentation using processed fascia lata and crushed cartilage

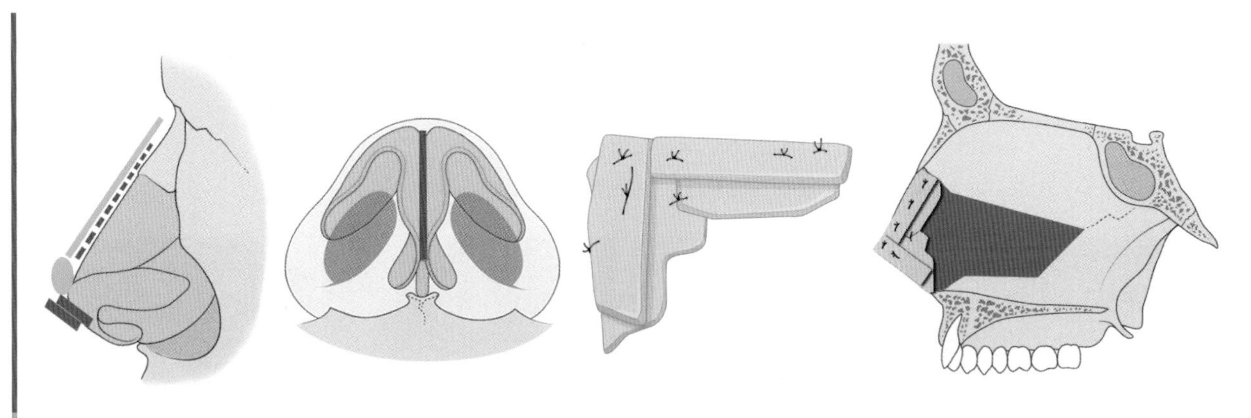

Postoperative Changes

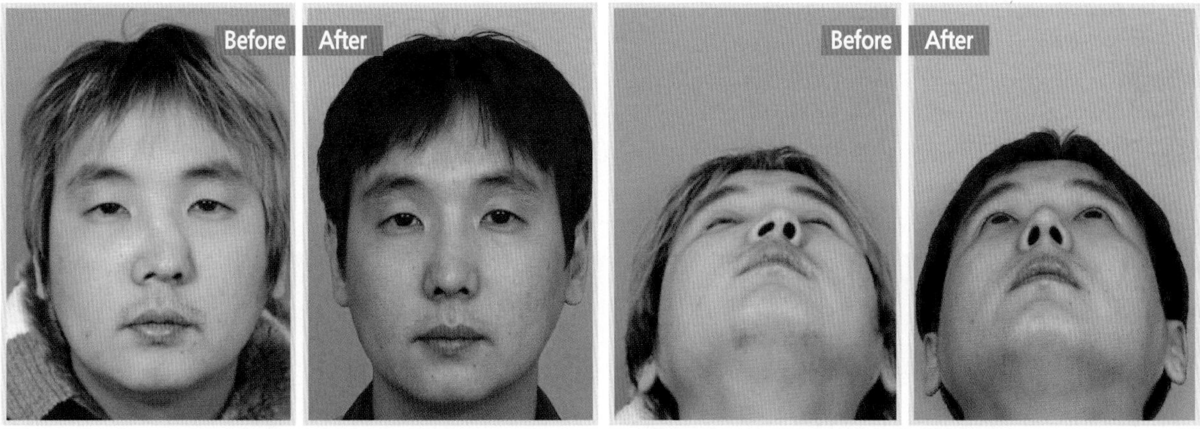

Frontal: Severely deviated nose was corrected.

Basal: Left-tilting tip was improved. Appropriate tip projection was achieved.

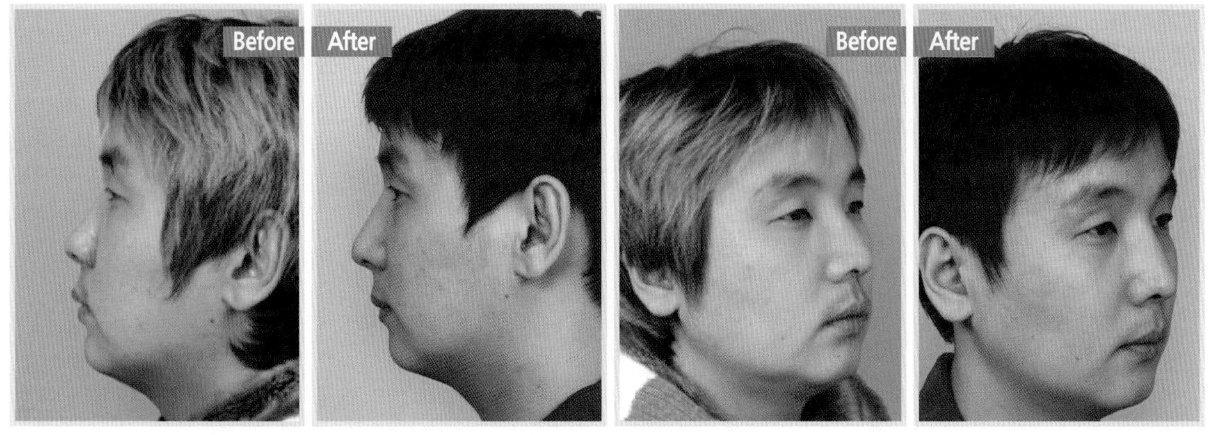

Lateral and Oblique: Dorsal height was augmented.

A 17-year-old male visited for a flat nose deformity resulting from severe nasal trauma.

Analysis Frontal: Flat nose, wide dorsum
Basal: Thick skin, poor tip projection
Lateral and Oblique: Low dorsal height

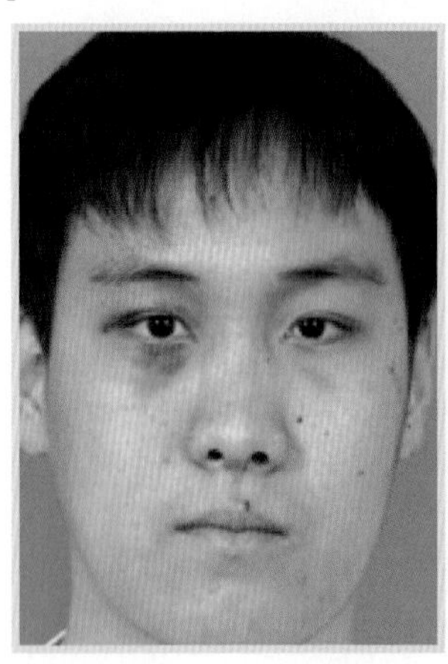
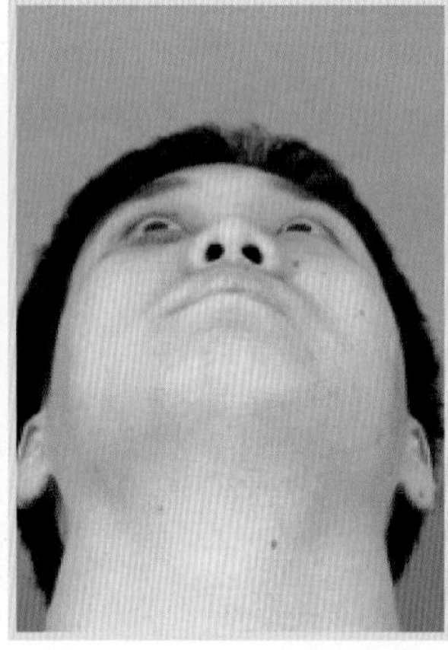
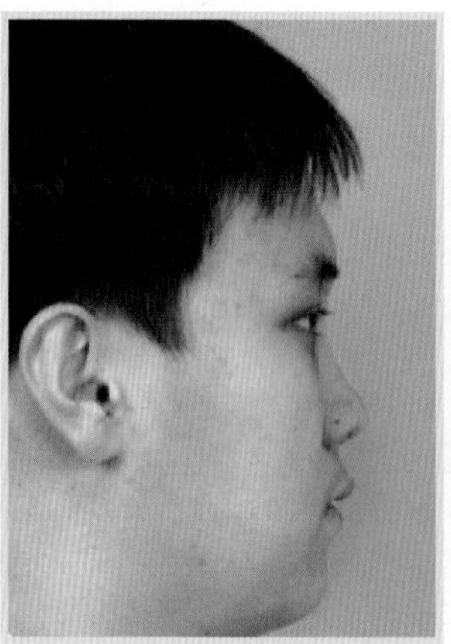
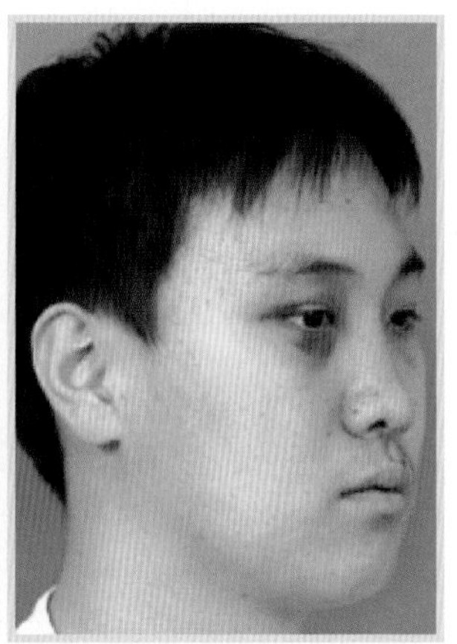

CT and Endoscopy Severe nasoseptal fracture

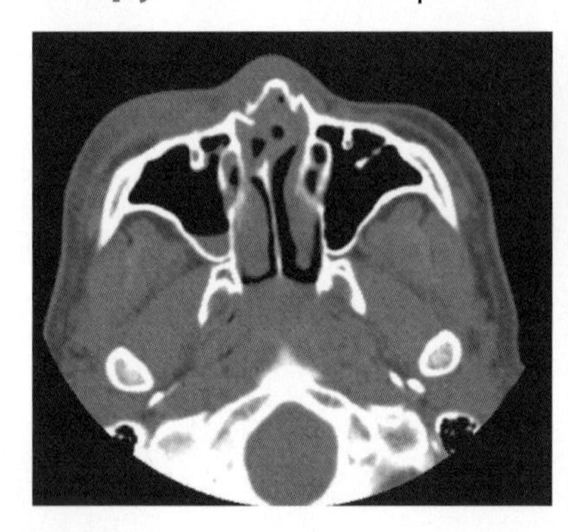
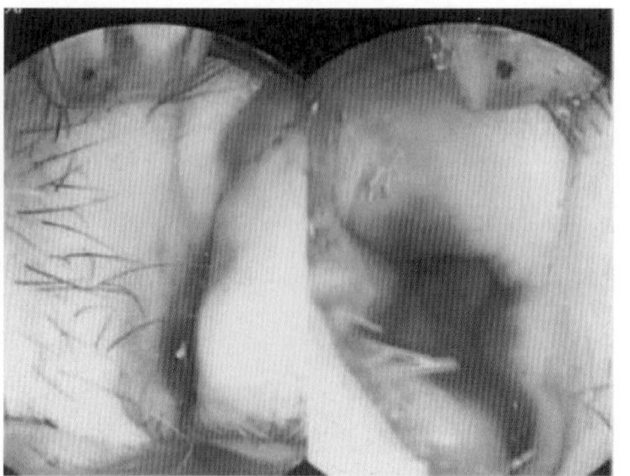

Operative Procedures

Endoscopic reduction (medial blowout fracture of orbit)
Open rhinoplasty approach
Total septal reconstruction (one caudal septal extension graft was sandwiched between two extended spreader grafts)
Lateral osteotomy (bilateral)
Columellar strut application
Dorsal augmentation using processed fascia lata and conchal cartilage

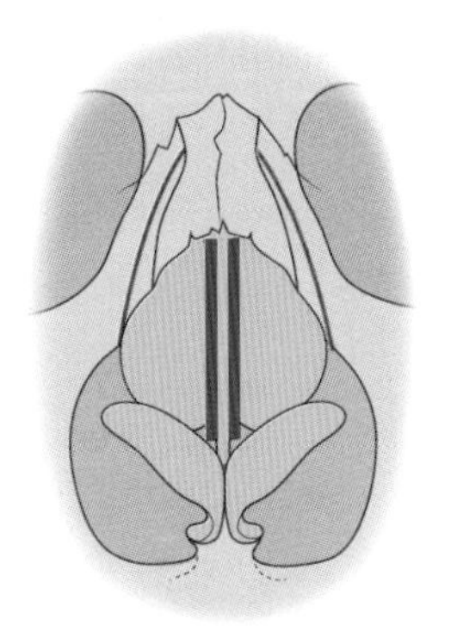
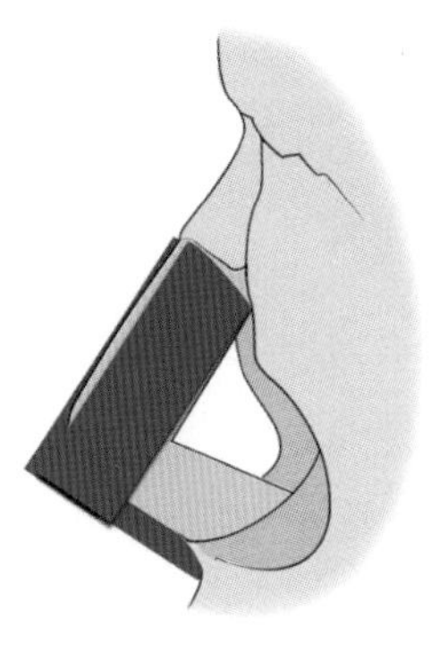
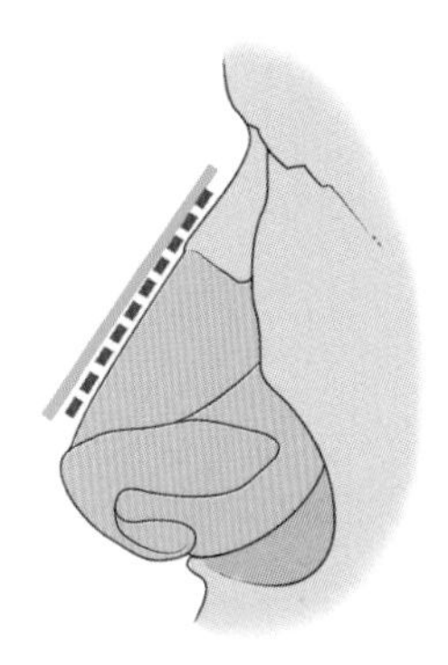
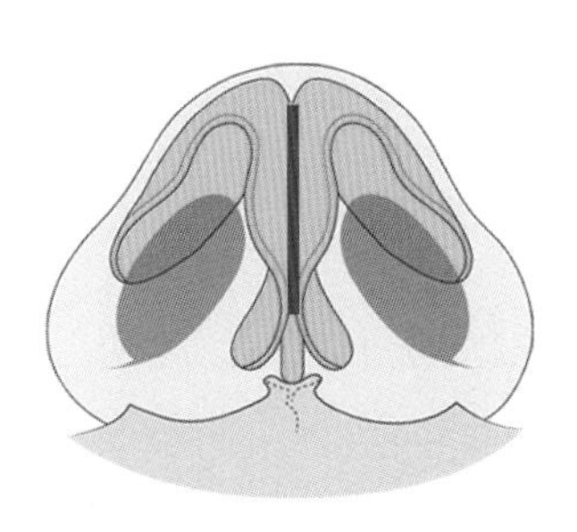

Postoperative Changes

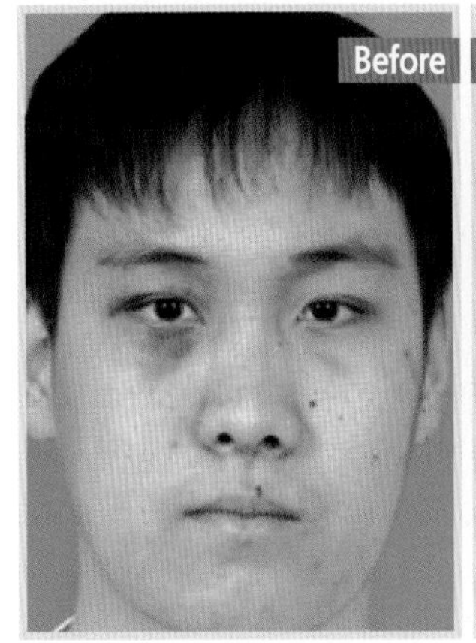

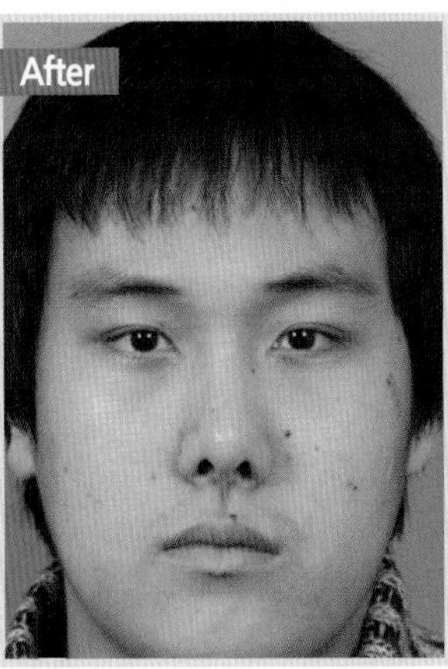

Frontal: Dorsal aesthetic lines were improved. Wide dorsum was narrowed.

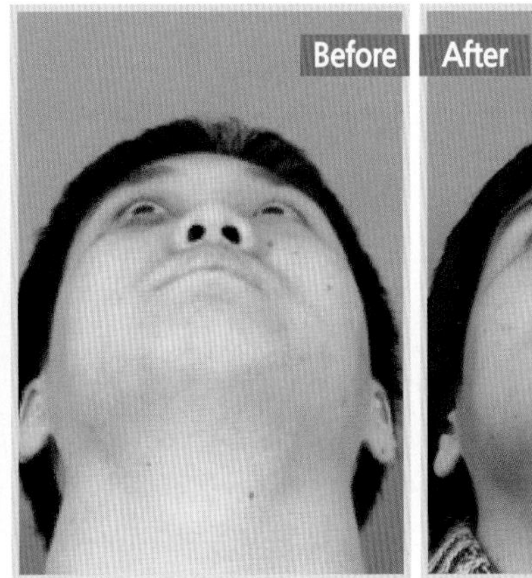

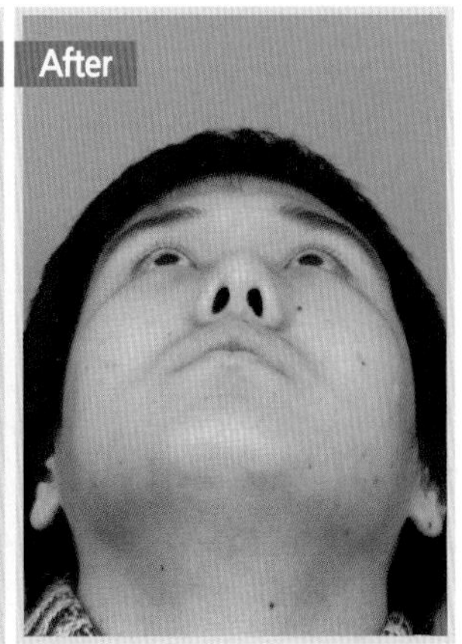

Basal: Tip projection was improved. Ideal nostril shapes were formed.

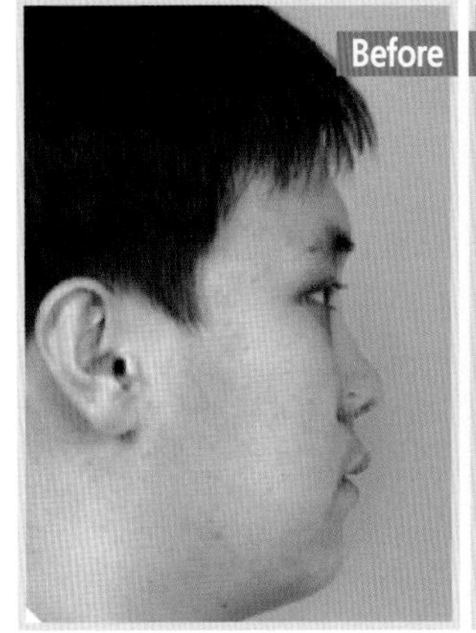

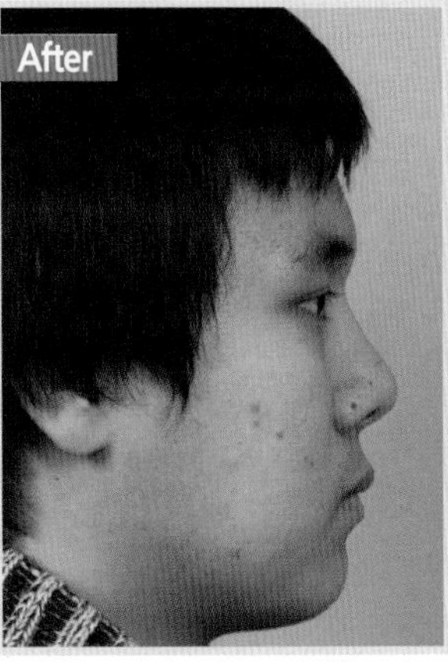

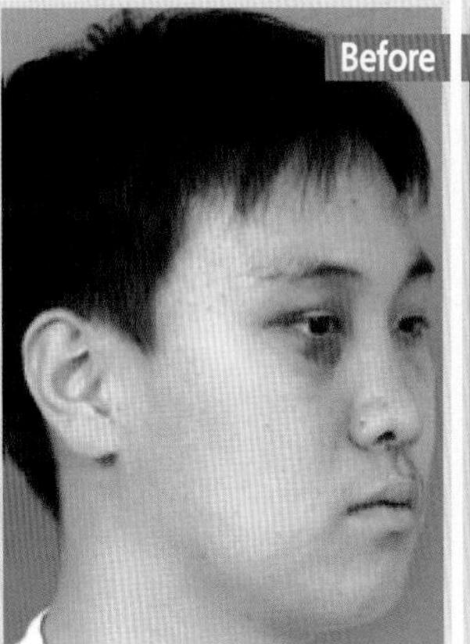

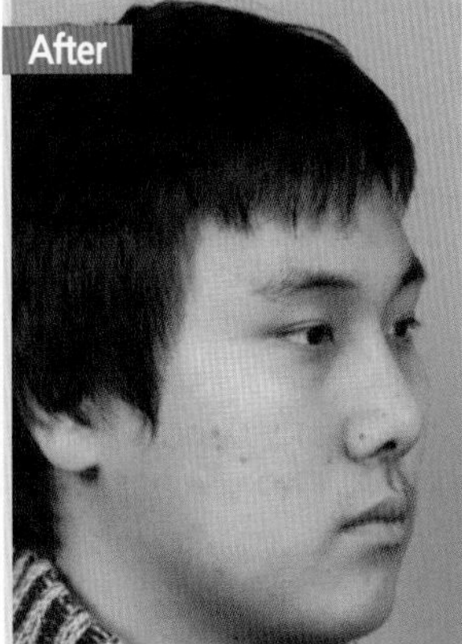

Lateral and Oblique: Dorsal height and tip projection was increased.

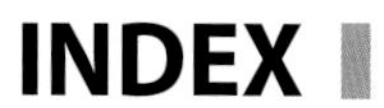

A

B

C

D

E

F

I

J

K

L

M

N

O

P

Q

R

S

T

U

V

W

X

Z

Rhinoplasty and Septoplasty

By Yong Ju Jang, MD, PhD

1st Print : 2014-03-20
1st Publication : 2014-04-07

Publisher : Jooyeon Jang
Editor : Taekyeong Kim
Text Designer : Hyeonjeong Shim
Illustrator : Hyeok Lee
Cover Designer : Suna Jun
Cover Images : By Illustrator

Permissions may be sought at Koonja's rights depatment:
Tel: (82)-2-762-9193
Fax: (82)-2-764-0209
nufunlife@koonja.co.kr
www.koonja.co.kr

Printed in South Korea
First Edition, © 2014 Koonja publishing
ISBN 978-89-6278-876-1